Procedural Coding and Reimbursement for Physician Services
Applying Current Procedural Terminology and HCPCS

2016

Lynn Kuehn, MS, RHIA, CCS-P, FAHIMA

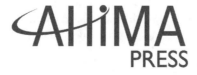
AHIMA PRESS

ISBN: 978-1-58426-456-9
AHIMA Product No.: AC201316

AHIMA Staff:
Caitlin Wilson, Assistant Editor
Jason O. Malley, Vice President, Business and Innovation
Pamela Woolf, Director of Publications, AHIMA Press

American Health Information Management Association
233 North Michigan Avenue, 21st Floor
Chicago, Illinois 60601-5809
ahima.org

Contents

About the Author xxi

Preface.. xxiii

Acknowledgments.. xxv

Chapter 1   Introduction to Coding Basics 1

Chapter 2   Evaluation and Management Coding 39

Chapter 3   Anesthesia.. 85

Chapter 4   Surgery 101

                Coding Used in the Surgery Section 102

                Integumentary System 109

                Musculoskeletal System...................................... 124

                Respiratory System... 136

                Cardiovascular, Hemic, and Lymphatic Systems.................. 144

                Digestive System 160

                Urinary System.. 175

                Male Genital System 183

                Female Genital System and Maternity Care and Delivery 186

                Nervous System 194

                Eye and Ocular Adnexa Systems............................... 205

                Auditory System... 209

Chapter 5   Radiology. 219

Chapter 6   Pathology and Laboratory 239

Chapter 7   Medicine. 259

Chapter 8   HCPCS Level II Coding 293

Chapter 9   Modifiers 301

Chapter 10   Reimbursement Process. 319

Chapter 11   Coding and Reimbursement Reports and Databases. 347

Chapter 12   Evaluation of Coding Quality 371

Appendix A   References and Bibliography. 393

Appendix B   Review Exercises. 397

                 Multiple Choice 398

                 Office Visit/Operative Report Exercises 412

                 Crossword Puzzles. 424

                 Surgical Case Audit Exercise 430

                 Evaluation and Management Audit Exercise 442

Appendix C   Acronyms and Abbreviations 449

Appendix D   Glossary 455

Appendix E   Answers to Odd-Numbered Chapter Review Exercises 467

Index 471

Online Appendices

Appendix F.1   1995 Documentation Guidelines for Evaluation
                 and Management Services

Appendix F.2   1997 Documentation Guidelines for Evaluation
                 and Management Services

Appendix G   Instructions for Completing the CMS-1500 Claim Form

Appendix H   AHIMA's Code of Ethics

Appendix I   AHIMA Position Statement on Quality Healthcare Data and Information

Appendices F.1 through I are located on the companion website to this book. The files are in PDF format and are available to download in zip file posted to www.ahimapress.org /kuehn4569/. Use password AH4569IMA to access the appendices.

Detailed Table of Contents

About the Author xxi

Preface. xxiii

Acknowledgments. xxv

Chapter 1 Introduction to Coding Basics 1

      The Health Record 2

      Organizations That Direct Health Record Content 3

      Standard Formats of the Health Record. 4

        Source-Oriented Health Record 4

        Integrated Health Record 4

        Problem-Oriented Medical Record 4

        Mixed Formats 5

      Basic Information in the Health Record. 5

        Administrative Data 6

        Clinical Data 8

      Basic Elements of Health Record Documentation. 11

      Resources Used to Assign Diagnostic and Procedure Codes 12

        Diagnostic Codes 13

        HCPCS Level I (CPT). 13

        HCPCS Level II 14

        Modifiers. 14

CPT Structure and Conventions. 14

    CPT Code Format. 16

    The Semicolon and Code Structure 17

    Unlisted Procedure Codes 19

    Coding Notes and Instructions 19

    Appendices 19

    Index 20

    Code Organization 21

Sources of Documentation That Generate Physician
Codes and Charges. 22

    Place of Service 22

    Data Collection. 24

General CPT Coding Instructions 26

Identification of Codable Procedural Statements. 27

Identification of Codable Diagnostic Statements. 29

    Signs and Symptoms 30

    Ambulatory Coding Guidelines for ICD-10-CM 30

    External Causes of Injury. 33

Identification of Codable Statements in Physician
Office Documentation 34

Coding Credentials. 35

Chapter 2   Evaluation and Management Coding. 39

Documentation Guidelines. 40

Evaluation and Management Services 41

Terms Commonly Used in Reporting E/M Services 41

    New or Established Patient 41

    Concurrent Care. 42

Levels of E/M Services 42

    Components in Selecting the Level of E/M Service 43

Modifiers. 52

    Modifiers Available for Use with E/M Services Codes. 52

    HCPCS Level II Modifiers 53

Evaluation and Management Categories 54

    Office or Other Outpatient Services 54

    Hospital Observation Services 56

    Hospital Inpatient Services 57

    Consultations 60

    Emergency Department and Other Emergency Services 62

    Critical Care Services 63

    Nursing Facility Services 64

    Domiciliary, Rest Home, or Custodial Care Services 65

    Domiciliary, Rest Home, or Home Care Oversight Services 66

    Home Services 66

    Prolonged Services 66

    Case Management Services 67

    Care Plan Oversight Services 68

    Preventive Medicine Services 68

    Non-Face-to-Face Services 70

    Special Evaluation and Management Services 71

    Newborn Care 71

    Care Management Services 75

    Advanced Care Planning 76

    Other Evaluation and Management Services 76

HCPCS Codes Used in Evaluation and Management Coding 76

Chapter 3   Anesthesia 85

Format and Arrangement of Codes in the Anesthesia Section 86

The Anesthesia Package 86

Modifiers Commonly Used in Reporting Anesthesia Services 87

    Physical Status Modifiers 88

    CPT Modifiers Used in Anesthesia Coding 88

    HCPCS Level II Modifiers Used in Anesthesia Coding 89

    Modifiers Specific to CRNA Coding 89

Codes Used in Reporting Qualifying Circumstances. 90

Steps in Coding Anesthesia Services 90

Calculating Fees for Anesthesia Services 91

Medical Direction. 92

Concurrency 93

Monitored Anesthesia Care 94

    Medicare Modifiers Specific to MAC Anesthesia Coding. 94

Pain Management Services. 95

Chapter 4   Surgery 101

Coding Used in the Surgery Section 102

    Subsections 102

    The Surgical Package 102

    Follow-up Care for Diagnostic and Therapeutic
        Surgical Procedures 104

    Separate Procedures. 104

    Codes for the Laparoscopic Surgical Approach 105

    Modifiers for Reporting More Than One
        Procedure or Service 105

    Add-on Codes 105

Modifiers Used in Surgery Coding 106

    Anatomical Modifiers 107

Integumentary System 109

    Incision and Drainage 109

    Excision-Debridement 110

    Lesions 110

    Nails 111

    Repairs 112

    Adjacent Tissue Transfer or Rearrangement 113

    Skin Replacement Surgery and Skin Substitutes. 114

    Flaps 116

Other Procedures 116

Pressure Ulcers (Decubitus Ulcers) 117

Burns, Local Treatment 117

Destruction of Lesions 117

Breast Procedures 118

HCPCS Codes Used in Integumentary System Coding 119

Musculoskeletal System 124

Wound Exploration 124

Excision, Including Biopsies 125

Introduction and Removal 125

Bone Grafts 126

Fracture and/or Dislocation Treatment Codes 126

Repair, Revision, and/or Reconstruction Codes 127

Spine (Vertebral Column) 127

Bunion Repairs 128

Casts and Strapping 130

Endoscopy/Arthroscopy 130

HCPCS Codes Used in Musculoskeletal System Coding 131

Respiratory System 136

Nose 136

Accessory Sinuses 138

Larynx 138

Trachea and Bronchi 139

Lungs and Pleura 140

HCPCS Codes Used in Respiratory System Coding 141

Cardiovascular, Hemic, and Lymphatic Systems 144

Pacemaker or Implantable Defibrillator 144

Electrophysiologic Procedures 147

Cardiac Valves 148

Coronary Artery Bypass Grafting 148

Heart/Lung Transplantation. 150

Extracorporeal Membrane Oxygenation (ECMO) or
Extracorporeal Life Support (ECLS) Services 150

Arteries and Veins. 150

Vascular Embolization and Occlusion 155

Hemic and Lymphatic Systems 155

Mediastinum and Diaphragm. 155

Miscellaneous Guidelines. 155

HCPCS Codes Used in Cardiovascular System Coding 156

Digestive System 160

Laparoscopies. 162

Endoscopy. 162

Lips 165

Tongue and Floor of Mouth 165

Dentoalveolar Structures 165

Pharynx, Adenoids, and Tonsils 166

Esophagus. 166

Stomach. 166

Intestines, Appendix, and Rectum. 167

Anus 168

Biliary Tract 168

Abdomen, Peritoneum, and Omentum 168

Hernia Repair. 169

HCPCS Codes Used in Digestive System Coding 171

Urinary System. 175

Miscellaneous Guidelines. 176

Laparoscopic Codes 177

Kidney. 177

Ureter 178

Bladder 178

Urethra 180

HCPCS Codes Used in Urinary System Coding. 180

Male Genital System 183

Penis 184

Testis 185

Vas Deferens 185

Spermatic Cord 185

Prostate 185

Reproductive System Procedures 185

Intersex Surgery 185

Female Genital System and Maternity Care and Delivery 186

Vulva, Perineum, and Introitus 187

Vagina 187

Cervix Uteri 187

Corpus Uteri 187

Oviduct 189

Ovary 190

Maternity Care and Delivery 190

HCPCS Codes Used in the Female Genital System 192

Nervous System 194

Skull, Meninges, and Brain 195

Spine and Spinal Cord 198

*Extracranial Nerves, Peripheral Nerves, and Autonomic
Nervous System* 201

HCPCS Codes Used in the Nervous System 202

Eye and Ocular Adnexa Systems 205

Eyeball 206

Anterior Segment 206

Posterior Segment 208

Ocular Adnexa 208

Auditory System 209

HCPCS Codes Used in the Eye and Auditory Systems 211

Operating Microscope 211

Chapter 5   Radiology 219

Radiology Section Format and Arrangement 220

Diagnostic Radiology 220

Diagnostic Ultrasound 221

Interventional Radiology 222

Radiation Oncology 224

Nuclear Medicine 227

Modifiers Used in Radiology Coding 228

Anatomical Modifiers 229

Administration of Contrast Materials 229

HCPCS Codes for Diagnostic Radiology 230

HCPCS Codes for Diagnostic Ultrasound 230

Other HCPCS Codes for Radiology Services 230

Chapter 6   Pathology and Laboratory 239

Pathology and Laboratory Section Structure and Content 240

Alphabetic Index 240

On-Site Testing versus Reference Lab Testing 240

Blood Draws 240

Clinical Laboratory Improvement Amendments
of 1988 (CLIA) 241

Quantitative and Qualitative Studies 242

Guidelines Pertaining to Pathology and
Laboratory Subsections 242

Organ or Disease-Oriented Panels 242

Drug Procedures 242

Evocative/Suppression Testing 243

Consultations in Clinical Pathology 243

Chemistry 243

Hematology and Coagulation. 244

Immunology 244

Microbiology. 244

Anatomic Pathology 245

Cytopathology. 245

Cytogenetic Studies. 247

Surgical Pathology 247

In Vivo (eg, Transcutaneous Laboratory Procedures). 248

Modifiers Used in Pathology and Laboratory Coding. 248

HCPCS Codes Used in Pathology and Laboratory Coding. 249

Chapter 7   Medicine. 259

Medicine Section Content and Structure 260

Immunization Against Disease 260

Psychiatry. 262

Biofeedback. 264

Dialysis 264

Gastroenterology 265

Ophthalmology 265

Special Otorhinolaryngologic Services 267

Cardiovascular. 267

Noninvasive Vascular Diagnostic Studies 272

Pulmonary. 273

Allergy and Clinical Immunology. 273

Endocrinology. 274

Neurology and Neuromuscular Procedures. 275

Central Nervous System Assessments/Tests 276

Health and Behavior Assessment/Intervention. 276

Hydration, Therapeutic, Prophylactic, Diagnostic Injections and Infusions, and Chemotherapy and Other Highly Complex Drug or Highly Complex Biologic Agent Administration 276

Photodynamic Therapy. 279

Special Dermatological Procedures. 279

Physical Medicine and Rehabilitation 279

Medical Nutrition Therapy. 280

Acupuncture 280

Osteopathic and Chiropractic Manipulative Treatment. 280

Education and Training for Patient Self-Management 281

Non-Face-to-Face Nonphysician Services. 281

Special Services, Procedures, and Reports 282

Qualifying Circumstances for Anesthesia 282

Moderate (Conscious) Sedation 282

Other Services and Procedures 282

Home Health Procedures/Services and
Home Infusion Procedures/Services. 283

Medication Therapy Management Services 283

Modifiers Used in Coding Medicine Services. 283

Anatomical Modifiers 284

HCPCS Codes Used in Coding Medicine Services. 284

Immunization Services 284

Vision Services 285

Neurology and Neuromuscular Procedures. 285

Cardiac Procedures 285

Pulmonary Services 286

Special Services, Procedures, and Reports 286

Chapter 8   HCPCS Level II Coding. 293

Code Assignment Hierarchy. 294

Steps in HCPCS Code Assignment. 294

The Effect of HIPAA on HCPCS. 295

HCPCS Level II Codes Inappropriate for Professional Billing. 295

HCPCS C Codes. 295

HCPCS D Codes. 295

Temporary Codes 295

Durable Medical Equipment Carriers. 296

Drugs Administered Other Than Oral Method 296

Chapter 9   Modifiers. 301

How to Use Modifiers 302

Types of Modifiers 302

CPT Modifier Descriptions and Examples 302

CPT Anesthesia Physical Status Modifiers. 309

HCPCS Level II Modifier Descriptions and Examples. 309

Anatomical Modifiers 310

Chapter 10   Reimbursement Process 319

Reimbursement Mechanisms 320

Standard Charges 320

Discounted Charges 320

Usual and Customary Fee Profile 320

Fee Schedule, Negotiated 321

Capitation 321

RBRVS Medicare Fee Schedule 321

Participating Provider Agreements 324

Fee Schedule Management. 324

Sources of Coding and Reimbursement Guidelines. 326

Payer-Specific Guidelines 326

Medical Necessity and Medicare Coverage Policies 326

Diagnoses Linked to Procedures 330

Specific CPT or HCPCS Code Requirement 330

Component Billing (Modifiers –26 and –TC). 331

Medicare's National Correct Coding Initiative (NCCI) Edits 331

Claims Submittal 333

National Provider Identifier 333

HIPAA Transaction and Code Sets. 333

Electronic Claims. 334

Other Claims-Generation Guidelines. 335

Data Elements of a Computerized Internal Fee Schedule 336

The Claims Process 337

Patient Visit through Final Payment 337

Accounts Receivable Management. 338

Chapter 11   Coding and Reimbursement Reports and Databases 347

Data Evaluation 348

Qualitative Analysis 348

Quantitative Analysis 351

Custom Reports. 355

Common Coding Errors Identified through Reports 357

Computerized Internal Fee Schedule Reports 360

Payer Remittance Report 361

Codes and Code Edits. 362

Coder and Biller as a Team 363

Chapter 12   Evaluation of Coding Quality. 371

Tools for Evaluating Quality 372

Collecting Information 372

Correcting Information. 372

Analyzing Information 373

Steps in Performing an Internal Audit 378

Identifying the Need for an Audit 378

Preparing for the Audit. 378

Conducting the Audit 379

Steps in the Audit Process. 379

Audit Follow-up 380

Ongoing Monitoring for Improvement. 381

Common CPT Coding Errors. 381

Compliance Regulations. 383

    Health Insurance Portability and Accountability Act 383

    Office of the Inspector General. 385

    National Correct Coding Initiative. 386

Appendix A   References and Bibliography 393

Appendix B   Review Exercises 397

    Multiple Choice 398

    Office Visit/Operative Report Exercises 412

        Case 1—Office Note 412

        Case 2—Operative Report 412

        Case 3—Operative Report 413

        Case 4—Office Note 413

        Case 5—Office Note 414

        Case 6—Pathology Report 414

        Case 7—Office Note 415

        Case 8—Operative Report 415

        Case 9—Office Note 416

        Case 10—Office Note 417

        Case 11—Office Note 418

        Case 12—Operative Report 419

        Case 13—Hospital Note 419

        Case 14—Day Surgery 420

        Case 15—Operative Report 420

        Case 16—Day Surgery 421

        Case 17—Operative Report 421

        Case 18—Operative Report 422

        Case 19—Operative Report 422

        Case 20—Operative Report 423

    Crossword Puzzles 424

        Reimbursement Puzzle 424

Coding Puzzle 426

Cross-Code Puzzle 428

Surgical Case Audit Exercise 430

Case 1—Day Surgery 432

Case 2—Operative Report 434

Case 3—Operative Report 436

Case 4—Operative Report 438

Case 5—Operative Report 440

Evaluation and Management Audit Exercise 442

Audit Case #1—Visit Note 443

Audit Case #2—Visit Note 444

Audit Case #3—Visit Note 445

Audit Case #4—Visit Note 446

Audit Case #5—Visit Note 447

Appendix C   Acronyms and Abbreviations 449

Appendix D   Glossary 455

Appendix E   Answers to Odd-Numbered Chapter Review Exercises 467

Exercise 1.1. Introduction to Coding Basics 467

Exercise 2.1. Evaluation and Management Coding 467

Exercise 3.1. Anesthesia 467

Exercise 4.1. Surgery Section 467

Exercise 4.2. Integumentary System 467

Exercise 4.3. Musculoskeletal System 468

Exercise 4.4. Respiratory System 468

Exercise 4.5. Cardiovascular, Hemic, and Lymphatic Systems 468

Exercise 4.6. Digestive System 468

Exercise 4.7. Urinary System 468

Exercise 4.8. Male and Female Genital Systems 468

Exercise 4.9. Nervous System 468

Exercise 4.10. Eye and Ocular Adnexa, and Auditory Systems 468

Exercise 5.1. Radiology 468

Exercise 6.1. Pathology and Laboratory 469

Exercise 7.1. Medicine 469

Exercise 8.1. HCPCS Level II Coding 469

Exercise 9.1. Modifiers 469

Exercise 10.1. Reimbursement Process 469

*Exercise 11.1. Coding and Reimbursement Reports
and Databases* 469

Exercise 12.1. Evaluation of Coding Quality 470

Index 471

Online Appendices

Appendix F.1   1995 Documentation Guidelines for Evaluation
                      and Management Services

Appendix F.2   1997 Documentation Guidelines for Evaluation
                      and Management Services

Appendix G   Instructions for Completing the CMS-1500
                      Claim Form

Appendix H   AHIMA's Code of Ethics

Appendix I   AHIMA Position Statement on Quality Healthcare
                      Data and Information

Appendices F.1 through I are located on the companion website to this book. The files are in PDF format and are available to download in zip file posted to www.ahimapress.org /kuehn4569/. Use password AH4569IMA to access the appendices.

About the Author

Lynn Kuehn, MS, RHIA, CCS-P, FAHIMA, is president of Kuehn Consulting in Waukesha, Wisconsin. Previously, she has served in health information management and coordination positions in a variety of healthcare settings. In her volunteer role, Ms. Kuehn has served as secretary and chair of the Ambulatory Care Section of AHIMA and the chair of several national committees. She was a member of the AHIMA Board of Directors from 2005–2007 and served as the chair of the AHIMA Foundation Board of Directors in 2011–2012. She has been active as a presenter at numerous meetings and seminars in the field of physician office management, coding, and reimbursement. Previous AHIMA publications include *CCS-P Exam Preparation*, which she wrote with Anita Hazelwood and Carol Venable, *Effective Management of Coding Services*, which she edited with Lou Ann Schraffenberger, *Documentation and Reimbursement for Physician Offices*, which she coauthored with LaVonne Wieland, and *The Learning Guide for Ambulatory Care*. Her newest AHIMA publication is *ICD-10-PCS: An Applied Approach*, 2016 Edition, which she authored with Teri Jorwic. Ms. Kuehn has been the recipient of the AHIMA Educator-Practitioner Award, the AHIMA Literary Legacy Award, and the Wisconsin Health Information Management Association Distinguished Member Award and Educator Award. She holds an MS in health services administration and a BS in medical record administration, is a certified coding specialist–physician based, and is a Fellow of the American Health Information Management Association.

Preface

The coding process requires a range of skills that combines knowledge and practice. *Procedural Coding and Reimbursement for Physician Services: Applying Current Procedural Terminology and HCPCS* was designed to provide a comprehensive text for students of physician-based procedural coding, as well as practitioners who want to strengthen their knowledge.

This publication introduces the basic principles and conventions of CPT coding, illustrates the application of these principles with examples and exercises based on actual case documentation, and teaches the student how to analyze clinical data for the purposes of coding and reimbursement.

Chapter 1, Introduction to Coding Basics, discusses the content of the health record, sources of documentation that generate physician charges, resources used to assign diagnostic and procedure codes, and basic CPT/HCPCS coding conventions.

Chapter 2, Evaluation and Management Coding, provides detailed instruction in E/M coding and takes the student through each step of the process, using case examples to illustrate how the physician assigns level of service codes. This chapter reflects the Evaluation and Management Documentation Guidelines developed jointly in 1995 and 1997 by the AMA and the Centers for Medicare and Medicaid Services (CMS). For additional information on these guidelines or to check for additional revisions, visit the CMS website (www.cms.gov).

Chapters 3 through 7 cover the clinical areas of anesthesia, surgery, radiology, pathology and laboratory, and medicine. These chapters closely follow the structure of the CPT codebook and provide coding basics, advanced applications, modifier usage, and HCPCS Level II codes for each of the major categories and subcategories of CPT.

Chapter 8, HCPCS Level II Coding, discusses the CMS-developed codes that describe supplies, medications and services not included in the CPT codebook.

Chapter 9, Modifiers, presents both CPT and HCPCS Level II modifiers that help the coder fully describe the physician services by providing extra detail about location, extent of service, or other specific information.

Chapter 10, Reimbursement Process, explores payment methodologies and claims management.

Chapter 11, Coding and Reimbursement Reports and Databases, discusses the purpose and use of a variety of reports and data management techniques that are particularly relevant to physician services.

Chapter 12, Evaluation of Coding Quality, presents tools for evaluating quality, guidelines for preparing an internal audit, critical information on fraud and abuse, and a discussion of compliance.

As in previous editions, review exercises are included in each chapter and in appendix B. The 2016 edition of *Procedural Coding and Reimbursement for Physician Services: Applying Current Procedural Terminology and HCPCS* includes an appendix with keys to these chapter review exercises for student reference. Also included is a chapter test at the conclusion of each chapter. Keys to the chapter tests and appendix B exercises and operative reports are available in the supplementary materials for educators. See Note to Educators.

The index and appendixes make information easily accessible and provide additional resources for the physician-based coder.

This book must be used with the current edition of *Current Procedural Terminology (CPT 2016)* (code changes effective January 1, 2016), published by the American Medical Association.

Appendices F.1 through I are located on the companion website to this book. The files are in PDF format and are available to download in zip file posted to www.ahimapress.org /kuehn4569/. Use password AH4569IMA to access the appendices.

Note to Educators:
The HCPCS Level II codes included in this publication are current as of October 1, 2015. A file containing the most current versions of the HCPCS Level II codes can be found at the following CMS website page: http://www.cms.gov/Regulations-and-Guidance/HIPAA -Administrative-Simplification/TransactionCodeSetsStands/index.html.

AHIMA provides supplementary materials for educators who use this book in their classes. Materials for this book include lesson plans, PowerPoint slides, answer keys, and other useful resources. Visit http://www.ahima.org/education/press for further instruction for accessing the materials. If you have any questions regarding the instructor materials, please contact AHIMA Customer Relations at (800) 335-5535 or submit a customer support request at https://secure .ahima.org/contact/contact.aspx.

Please note: The instructor materials are available *only* to verified instructors.

Acknowledgments

This book was originally published with the coauthorship of LaVonne Wieland, RHIA, CHP. AHIMA and the author wish to acknowledge the tremendous contribution Wieland made to the 1999 to 2005 editions. Without her partnership, this work would not be the comprehensive text it is today.

This book combines instructional material formerly published by AHIMA under the following titles:

CPT/HCPCS for Physician Office Coding,
by Therese M. Jorwic, MPH, RHIA, CCS, CCS-P

CPT: Beyond the Basics, by Gail I. Smith, MA, RHIA, CCS-P

Intermediate CPT/HCPCS for Physician Office Coding,
by Donna M. Didier, MEd, RHIA, CCS

Documentation and Reimbursement for Physician Offices,
by Lynn Kuehn, MS, RHIA, CCS-P, FAHIMA, and LaVonne Wieland, RHIA, CHP

AHIMA wishes to acknowledge all of the preceding authors for their contributions to this work.

AHIMA Press would like to thank Rachael Gagner D'Andrea, MS, RHIA, CHTS-TR, CPHQ, for her work as technical reviewer of this edition.

Chapter 1

Introduction to Coding Basics

Objectives

Upon completion of this chapter, the student should be able to do the following:

- Define the health record

- Identify organizations that direct the content of the physician office health record and indicate which ones are voluntary and which ones are mandatory

- Describe the content, purpose, and various arrangement patterns of the basic components of health records

- Describe documentation guidelines appropriate for use in the physician office health record

- Describe the basic concepts and resources used to assign diagnostic and procedure codes in physician office health record documentation

- Describe the two levels of HCPCS and the types of codes contained in both levels

- Discuss the basic structure, organization, conventions, and symbols used in CPT coding

- List the methods used to locate terms and codes in the CPT Index

- Identify sources of documentation that generate physician charges

- Interpret health record documentation to identify codable diagnostic and procedure statements resulting from a physician service

This chapter introduces the basic tools and concepts necessary for the coding and reimbursement process. In addition to knowing the various coding systems, books, and other resources used in the practice of coding, the coding professional must learn where the information that substantiates the codes to be assigned is located. The primary source of that information is the patient's health record.

The Health Record

The health record is the source of information on all aspects of an individual's healthcare. It is vital to patient care because it documents demographic data, reasons for visits, results of examinations and tests, treatments ordered, and plans for follow-up. In short, the health record explains the who, what, when, where, why, and how of patient care.

In addition to providing information about healthcare, the health record serves several other purposes. It is:

- The document that ensures optimal reimbursement

- A potent defense against malpractice and general liability suits

- The database for evaluation activities (Joseph, Tucker, and Fox 1986)

This chapter discusses how to ensure appropriate and optimal reimbursement through full documentation to substantiate all charges. Submitting unsubstantiated charges can open the physician practice to a possible lawsuit for billing fraud. Chapter 12 describes how to perform coding audits that assess the accuracy of submitted claims versus the corresponding health record documentation, using the health record as the database of information.

To be an effective tool in the provision of healthcare, the health record must be valuable as a key source of information in determining the reimbursement of care. The primary functions of the health record are to:

- Facilitate the ongoing care and treatment of individual patients

- Support clinical decision making and communication among clinicians

- Document the services provided to patients in support of reimbursement

- Provide information for the evaluation of the quality and efficacy of the care provided

- Provide information in support of medical research and education

- Help facilitate the operational management of the facility

- Provide information as required by local and national laws and regulations (LaTour et al. 2013, 241)

Figure 1.1 shows the uses of the health record and the value of record documentation in the healthcare field.

Figure 1.1. The uses and value of the health record

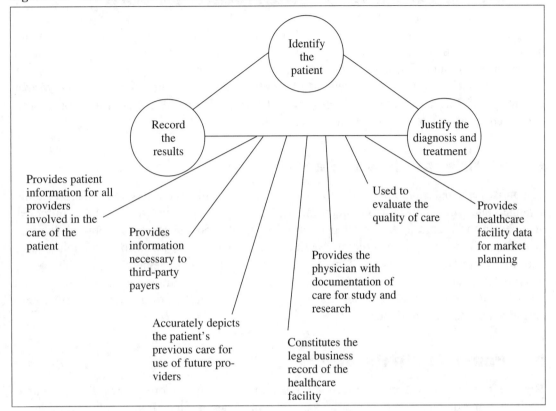

Organizations That Direct Health Record Content

The content of the health record is directed by several organizations and agencies whose standards are voluntary. Accreditation organizations such as the Joint Commission, the Accreditation Association for Ambulatory Health Care (AAAHC), and the National Committee for Quality Assurance (NCQA) publish accreditation standards that list basic record content requirements. Accreditation by any of these organizations, and therefore compliance with their standards, is voluntary. The Joint Commission's standards are published in the *Comprehensive Accreditation Manual for Ambulatory Care.* The manual's chapter on Information Management requires standardized data collection throughout the organization and dissemination of data and information in useful formats. Section 6, Clinical Records, of AAAHC's *Accreditation Handbook for Ambulatory Health Care* contains that association's documentation requirements. NCQA accreditation may be required by some managed care organizations for participation in their plans because NCQA is their accreditation association of choice. The NCQA standards for record content are minimal.

When a physician office or clinic wishes to become accredited voluntarily, it must apply for a survey by an accreditation organization. If the office is found to be in substantial compliance with the organization's published standards, it will receive accreditation. Thus, in preparing for the survey process, the health information professional should evaluate whether the facility's records are indeed in compliance with the organization's accreditation standards.

Standard Formats of the Health Record

The health record is a collection of all the information available on the patient and should be organized so that the information is easy to locate and use. The information in the health record is of no value if it is disorganized and difficult to reference. Three standard formats are available for use in the arrangement of health information: the source-oriented format, the integrated format, and the problem-oriented format. Sometimes these three formats are combined to produce a hybrid format.

Source-Oriented Health Record

The most typical arrangement of information in the health record is the source-oriented arrangement. Information from departments, physician specialties, or other sources is grouped in the record and then filed in chronological order within that grouping. Thus, it provides each department or specialty with easy access to its own information about examinations, treatments, and results. One disadvantage to this arrangement is that the source, or type of document, must be known before the information can be correctly filed into the record or located for use. Another disadvantage is the inability to determine the patient's entire health status at a glance.

Integrated Health Record

The integrated format organizes information in strict chronological order, regardless of source. The forms and documentation from the various sources are grouped by date of creation, making the patient's full health status easier to determine at any given time. However, determining the status of a particular problem is more difficult. The creation date of the form or documentation is the only criterion needed to file the information correctly. One disadvantage to this arrangement is the inability to locate a particular piece of information when the date of service or receipt is unknown.

Problem-Oriented Medical Record

The problem-oriented medical record format, more commonly called the POMR, was developed in the 1960s by Lawrence L. Weed to address the problems associated with the source-oriented record format. The POMR format of documenting information supports a logical, organized approach by the physician to patient diagnosis and treatment. It involves the use of four basic record documentation parts: the database, the problem list, the initial plan, and the progress notes.

"The database is formatted much like the source-oriented health record and contains the following information: chief complaint, present illness(es), social history, medical history, physical examination, and diagnostic test results" (Sayles 2014, 126).

The problem list is an ongoing list of all of the patient's problems, both past and present, identified by a unique number that serves as an index to the record.

The initial plan is the list of steps that will be taken to evaluate and learn about the patient's condition, with each plan referenced back to the associated problem number.

Progress notes are made each time follow-up is done with patients or on their behalf and also are referenced back to the associated problem number.

Progress notes have a specific format in the POMR system. They are documented using four major categories of information, commonly referred to as the acronym SOAP:

- **S**ubjective: The symptoms and history as stated by the patient

- **O**bjective: The measurable and observable findings that the physician determines about the problem

- **A**ssessment: The diagnostic statement made by the physician

- **P**lan: The specific actions to be taken for this patient about this problem

A new format of progress notes incorporates all of the SOAP elements and adds three additional elements. The new elements are the nature of the presenting problem (**N**), counseling and/or coordination of care (**C**), and medical decision making (**M**). Together with the SOAP elements, these compose the new SNOCAMP acronym. Documentation using the SNOCAMP format helps coders more readily determine what information is necessary to confirm the evaluation and management (E/M) code assignment, such as the medical decision-making element, which is difficult to determine in the SOAP note (Larimore and Jordan 1995).

Following is an example of a simple SNOCAMP note:

S: Patient returns for suture removal 10 days after laceration repair in the emergency department; no complaints

N: Minor

O: Wound healed well; sutures removed without difficulty

C: Discussed with patient and her mother expected course of healing, wound protection, and sun protection

A: Arm laceration, healed

M: Low complexity

P: Follow-up PRN

Mixed Formats

Hybrids of the three basic formats discussed above incorporate the best attributes of each. Many records use the problem list concept from the POMR, with the chronological order format for urgent care records and source-oriented divisions for ongoing primary care. Others may divide a source-oriented record by episode of care or use other creative options.

Regardless of the format chosen or developed, consistency is the main requirement. All providers and staff must use a common record order for record maintenance to make the record usable. The record order should be written and widely distributed to help all staff members understand how the record should be organized.

Basic Information in the Health Record

A patient's health record contains a vast amount of information. This information falls into two basic categories: administrative data and clinical data.

Administrative Data

Two health record forms are necessary for the administrative functioning of the practice rather than for the provision of healthcare: the registration record and the release/assignment of benefits form.

Registration Record

The basic demographic data collected before or during the initial patient visit is documented in the registration record. This information is maintained and updated, as needed, on subsequent visits. The registration record should collect all the information necessary to enter the patient into the computer system, create the health record, and complete all data submission requirements for claims payment. The registration record also is commonly referred to as the face sheet of the record. Following are examples of the information to be collected:

- Patient surname, first name, middle name, or initial
- Unique identifying number
- Residence address/telephone
- Date of birth
- Gender
- Marital status
- Race or ethnic origin
- Social security number
- Primary insurance company name and address (insurance identification and group numbers, subscriber of insurance policy, and patient's relationship to subscriber)
- Secondary (or subsequent) insurance company name and address (insurance identification and group numbers, subscriber of insurance policy, and patient's relationship to subscriber)
- Guarantor for the patient's account
- Patient's employer name, address, and telephone number
- Guarantor's employer name, address, and telephone number
- Parent information, if a pediatric/minor patient
- Occupation
- Business address and/or telephone
- Name, address, and telephone number of nearest relative or emergency contact
- Any other emergency contact
- Primary care physician, if different from physician being seen
- Referring physician name, address, and telephone number, if applicable

Figure 1.2 is an example of a registration record used for collecting administrative data.

Figure 1.2. Registration record

Patient Information

Account _____ Medical Record #_____ Date seen_____

Last name _____ First name _____ Middle _____

Street address _____ Apt # _____

City _____ State _____ Zip _____

Home phone ( ) _____ Work phone ( ) _____ S.S. # _____

Sex _____ Marital Status _____ Race _____

Date of birth _____ Age _____

Maiden or other previous name(s)_____

Employer _____

Address _____ City _____ State _____

Occupation_____

Spouse's name _____ Spouse's employer _____

Address _____ Phone # ( ) _____

Contact name (not living with you) _____ Phone # ( ) _____

Relationship_____

Referred by _____ Referring physician _____

Personal physician _____ Phone # ( ) _____

Patient Insurance Information

Primary insurance company name _____

Address _____ Effective date _____

Subscriber # _____ Policy # _____ Group # _____

Secondary ins co. _____ Subscriber # _____ Group # _____

Name of insured policy holder (as it appears on card)_____

Date of birth of subscriber _____ Sex of subscriber _____

Patient's relationship to subscriber _____

Responsible Party Information Complete if someone other than patient is responsible for the bill

Name _____ Address _____

City _____ State _____ Zip _____

Home phone ( ) _____ Relationship to patient _____

Employer _____ Employer's address _____

City _____ State _____ Zip _____

Employer phone ( ) _____

Payment is required at time of service unless prior arrangements have been made. I authorize the payment of medical benefits directly to the physician on my behalf.

Your signature here indicates your consent for treatment and responsibility for paying the associated charges, regardless of insurance status. Thank you.

Signature _____ Date_____

Assignment of Benefits Form

The assignment of benefits form authorizes the physician practice to release information to an insurance company and authorizes the insurance company to pay the practice directly for billable services. Completion of this form also may indicate that the patient assumes responsibility for charges not covered by the insurance company.

Physicians serving Medicare patients ask them to sign an assignment of benefits form specific to Medicare, called a Medicare signature on file. (See figure 1.3.) This form serves the same purpose of authorizing Medicare payments directly to the provider and also more fully describes the patient's payment responsibilities when covered by Medicare.

Clinical Data

Information documented during the care process is clinical data. The forms frequently used to record clinical data include the problem list, the medication list, the medical history, the physical examination, physician orders, progress notes, laboratory reports, and x-ray/diagnostic test reports. Many other names for forms containing the same information are found within physician practices.

Problem List

The Joint Commission requires that a problem list be maintained for all patients who receive continuing ambulatory services. Maintaining a problem list on a patient helps both caregivers

Figure 1.3.   Medicare signature on file

I authorize payment of Medicare benefits on my behalf to the provider listed below. I authorize medical information about me to be released to the Centers for Medicare and Medicaid Services (CMS) if needed to determine benefits payable for the services provided.

If "other health insurance" is indicated in Item 9 of the CMS-1500 form or electronically submitted claim, my signature authorizes release of the information to the insurer shown. If the provider accepts Medicare assignment, it agrees to accept the amount approved by the Medicare program as the full charge, and I am responsible only for the deductible, coinsurance, and charges for noncovered services. Coinsurance and the deductible are based upon the amount approved by the Medicare program.

Provider Name: _____

Provider Address: _____

Patient Name (please print): _____

Patient Signature: _____

Date Signed: _____

Account Number: _____

Medical Record Number: _____

and coders know the patient's diagnoses and problems at a glance. In addition to the diagnosis or problem title, the problem list should contain the date of the problem's onset, whether the problem is currently active or inactive, and its date of resolution.

Medication List

The Joint Commission requires that the use of medications be indicated in the record. This listing contains the names of all medications prescribed, the dosage and amount dispensed, dispensing instructions, the prescription date and discontinued date, and the problem number for which it was prescribed, if using numbered problem lists. It also should contain the list of known allergies to medications. The medication list helps physicians know which medications are being used currently so that drug interactions and duplications of therapy can be avoided.

Medical History

A complete medical history establishes the foundation for comprehensive care by documenting current complaints and symptoms in addition to past medical, personal, and family history. It also should include pertinent aspects of basic physiological systems. The major categories of information to be included in a medical history are:

- Chief complaint
- History of present illness
- Review of systems
- Past medical history
- Family medical history
- Social (or personal) history

Physical Examination

The medical history contains information obtained from the patient; the physical examination is a record of the physician's assessment of the patient. The physical examination is organized into two sections: body areas and organ systems. The body areas to be documented, as appropriate to the case, are:

- Head, including the face
- Neck
- Chest, including breasts and axillae
- Abdomen
- Genitalia, groin, buttocks
- Back, including spine
- Each extremity

The organ systems to be documented, as appropriate to the case, are:

- Constitutional
- Eyes

- Ears, nose, mouth, and throat
- Cardiovascular
- Respiratory
- Gastrointestinal
- Genitourinary
- Musculoskeletal
- Skin
- Neurological
- Psychiatric
- Hematologic/lymphatic/immunologic

The final element of the physical examination is the diagnostic impression or diagnosis statement assigned by the physician after completing the medical history and reviewing the body areas and organ systems.

Physician Orders

The physician orders represent the treatment plan developed by the physician. These orders indicate the diagnostic tests to be performed, the treatments/medications to be given in the office, and the medications the patient is to obtain and use at home. Medication orders must include the medication name, dose, quantity, and route (oral, topical, or self-injectable); dispensing instructions; number of refills; and signature, including name and title. Physician orders also may take the form of standing orders such as "measles-mumps-rubella injection for any unimmunized child at or near 18 months of age." In the physician's office, these orders are frequently found within the progress notes.

Progress Notes

As discussed previously, progress notes provide a chronological record of ongoing patient follow-up and changes in condition. They can be done in the SOAP format as described earlier or they can be completely narrative, describing the patient's symptoms and the physician's examination and response. Regardless of format, all progress notes must contain:

- Date of encounter
- Department, if practice is departmentalized
- Provider name and professional title
- Chief symptom or purpose of visit
- Clinical findings
- Diagnosis or medical impression
- Studies ordered, such as laboratory or x-ray
- Therapies administered
- Disposition, recommendations, and instructions given to the patient
- Signature or initials of practitioner

Laboratory Reports

All laboratory test results must be reported to the physician in a timely manner and must include the date, time, and results of the test, including reference values for the test's normal range. When performing a test manually, the technician should initial or sign the test result slip.

X-ray/Diagnostic Test Reports

X-ray reports, also called radiology reports or medical imaging reports, describe the findings of diagnostic services. Diagnostic procedures include plain film radiography, ultrasonography, computed tomography, and magnetic resonance imaging. A radiologist interprets the films from these examinations and provides a signed interpretation report for inclusion in the record.

Other forms and information may be found in a physician office record. Most health records contain only the information generated by the facility. The physician office or clinic record can be quite different, however. The physician is the overall care manager for the patient and, as such, receives copies of the documentation generated in other care settings. This can allow the physician office or clinic health record to be the source of a wealth of information for both physician and coder.

Basic Elements of Health Record Documentation

Accrediting agencies such as the Joint Commission, the NCQA, and the AAAHC have set standards that describe the basic elements of health records. The basic elements of health record documentation listed here apply to all types of medical and surgical services in all settings:

- *Separate records:* All patients should have their own records. Multiple family members' information should not be contained in one record.

- *Patient information:* Entries into the patient record should identify the patient's name, unique identifier, date and time of service, department/physician seeing the patient, and signature of person documenting the information.

- *Black ink:* Handwritten entries in the health record should be made in ink, preferably black. Black ink produces clear, dark writing on photocopies and facsimiles. The use of pencil may arouse suspicion of alteration during litigation involving health records.

- *Legible handwriting:* Handwriting must be legible to the physician, other health care professionals, and anyone else who may need to read the patient's record. Submitting legible documentation to private payers will make correct and timely reimbursement easier. When poor handwriting is a problem, dictation of the information is recommended. Many physicians are switching from handwritten notes to dictated notes or automated recording systems because they are able to record more information in less time. In this case, a summary of events during the patient visit should be documented in the health record to provide continuity of care in the event of a lag time in transcribing the dictation, physician review and signature of the dictated information, and timely filing into the patient's health record.

- *Prompt entries:* Information should be entered into the patient's record at the time of service, or immediately following, while it is still fresh in the mind of the person making the entry. The more time that elapses before information is recorded, the more details will be lost.

- *Date and time on all entries:* This may seem more than obvious, but this critical piece of information is often missed. Recording the date of service is critical because the patient's record is a legal document and thus is invalid without dates. Including the time of service is important to allow a patient's medical treatment to be reconstructed at a later time. Including time of contact with the patient in any documentation, especially if the patient was seen more than once on any given date, assists in determining the sequence of events. This also may assist in determining the appropriate CPT service when time is the element that determines the code used to report that service. An example is time spent providing prolonged or critical care services to a patient.

- *Blank spaces:* Information in the patient's record should always be listed chronologically. Any spaces left blank between entries should be crossed out to prevent entries from mistakenly being placed out of order or alterations of the record.

- *Signatures:* The service performed during a patient encounter should be signed and dated at the time of service. The physician should sign/initial all diagnostic test results and correspondence to indicate review of the information or case.

- *Changes to the health record:* The best way to show that inaccurate information has been discovered is to draw a single, fine line through it. This enables the information to still be read and avoids giving the impression that it is being concealed. The person making the change should then date and sign the alteration. The best way to enter information that has been omitted is to include it in an addendum. The addendum should be dated, signed, and attached chronologically. However, the original notes should not be replaced. Rather, a reference to the addendum should be included in the original notes (Seare 1996).

Resources Used to Assign Diagnostic and Procedure Codes

The processing of claims for medical services is an impersonal, highly computerized industry. Third-party payers use codes for three reasons:

- Computers can sort and match codes more quickly than they can words.

- Codes are more specific than words; they represent a standard means of reporting diagnoses and injuries as well as the services and procedures used to treat them.

- Because not all third-party payers cover the same or similar services in the same way, codes allow payers to match the service provided by the provider with payment guidelines and the patient's policy to determine the extent of coverage.

A physician's assessment of a condition is a diagnostic statement. The ICD-10-CM diagnostic coding system is used to assign a code that describes the written diagnostic statement.

Services provided are assigned an appropriate code from the CPT and/or HCPCS code books. The code assigned will accurately describe the service performed.

Diagnostic Codes

Codes are assigned to diagnostic statements to classify the statements for billing and collection of research statistics. There are many different classification systems available for use but the only systems used in the United States are based on the International Classification of Diseases.

ICD-10-CM Diagnostic Codes

The system currently in use in the United States is the *International Classification of Diseases, Tenth Revision, Clinical Modification (ICD-10-CM)*. The ICD-10-CM book contains two sections: the Index and the Tabular sections. The Index is an alphabetic listing, and the Tabular section is an alphanumerical listing. An ICD-10-CM code consists of three to seven alphanumeric characters, always starting with an alphabetic character. The code should always be assigned to its highest specificity. Examples of ICD-10-CM codes are:

R54   Age-related physical debility
N02.0   Recurrent and persistent hematuria with minor glomerular abnormality
C40.01   Malignant neoplasm of scapula and long bones of right upper limb
Q76.426   Congenital lordosis, lumbar region
T48.1x1A   Poisoning by skeletal muscle relaxants [neuromuscular blocking agents], accidental (unintentional), initial encounter

The ICD-10-CM code book is updated annually in October, and errata may be published throughout the year. The ICD-10-PCS code set is never used by physicians. The ICD-10-PCS code set is only used by hospitals to report inpatient services. The American Hospital Association's Central Office serves as the official US source for coding advice on diagnostic code assignment using the ICD-10-CM system through their publication, *AHA Coding Clinic for ICD-10-CM/PCS. Coding Clinic* is available for purchase from the AHA website (AHA 2015).

The ICD-10-CM files and the associated guidelines are available for download from the Centers for Disease Control (CDC 2015). AHIMA provides many helpful resources on the ICD-10 website, such as introductory webinars and a free monthly ICD-TEN e-newsletter (AHIMA 2015).

HCPCS Level I (CPT)

Physicians assign codes for services provided using the *Current Procedural Terminology, Fourth Edition (CPT)* (referred to in this volume as the "CPT code book"), first developed by the American Medical Association (AMA) in 1966 and updated annually in recent years. The Centers for Medicare and Medicaid Services (CMS) has included the CPT code book as the first level of codes in the *Healthcare Common Procedure Coding System* (HCPCS) (AMA 2015a). The CPT code book is a listing of more than 9,000 codes and descriptions used for reporting medical services and procedures performed by physicians and other medical professionals. "The purpose of the coding system is to provide a uniform language that accurately describes medical, surgical, and diagnostic services, and provides an effective means for reliable nationwide communication among physicians, patients, and insurance carriers" (Practice Management Information Corporation 2001).

There are three categories of *CPT* codes: Category I, Category II, and Category III. A Category I CPT code is a five-digit number grouped by type of service or body system. Examples of CPT codes include:

51550   Cystectomy, partial; simple

85002   Bleeding time

Category II and Category III CPT codes are five-digit alphanumeric codes consisting of four numeric characters followed by one alphabetic character.

The AMA revises and publishes *CPT* each year. Revisions to the code book may include the addition of new codes, new terminology, and new cross-references, and the deletion of codes. The revisions are prepared by the AMA's CPT Editorial Panel, with the assistance of physicians representing all specialties of medicine. Physician offices should always use the most current publication to ensure accurate code submission and payment. The AMA also publishes the *CPT Assistant* newsletter, the official source of coding guidance for CPT code assignment for physician services (AMA 2015b).

Due to rapid advances in the field of medicine, the AMA recently started issuing new codes and modifiers throughout the year for new procedures or services. These new codes and modifiers are listed on the AMA website (AMA 2015c), but the AMA issues the complete CPT code book just once a year.

HCPCS Level II

The HCPCS Level II codes, also known as the National Codes, are created and updated quarterly by the CMS. This coding system is used to bill supplies, materials, and injectable medications. It also is used to bill for certain procedures and services, such as ambulance or dental, that are not defined by the CPT code book.

HCPCS Level II are five-digit alphanumeric codes, beginning with the letters A through V, and are divided into 23 sections. (See chapter 8 for a detailed discussion of HCPCS Level II coding.)

Modifiers

Modifiers consist of two digits and may be alphabetic, numeric, or alphanumeric. These modifiers are appended at the end of the CPT or HCPCS code to indicate that a service or procedure that has been performed has been altered by some specific circumstance but has not changed in its definition or code. Modifiers may communicate an increase or a decrease in level of service, indicate bilateral or multiple procedures, or provide other information valuable in determining payment for a service. Both the CPT and the HCPCS coding systems contain modifiers.

Additional information on the modifiers appropriate to each section of the CPT code book is provided in each corresponding chapter of this book. Also, chapter 9 of this text contains a detailed discussion of modifiers.

CPT Structure and Conventions

The CPT code book is a single volume that includes an introduction, a numerical list of codes and descriptions, 14 appendices, and an Index. Within the numerical list are the six sections of Category I CPT codes: evaluation and management, anesthesia, surgery, radiology, pathology and laboratory, and medicine.

In addition, Category II codes describe services and/or tests that are agreed upon as contributing to positive health outcomes and high-quality patient care. They are supplemental tracking codes that can be used for performance improvement but are never to be used to replace a Category I code for reimbursement. These codes are five-digit codes beginning with four numeric digits and ending with an alphabetic character, and their use is optional. This section is organized into nine groups:

0001F–0015F	Composite Codes
0500F–0584F	Patient Management
1000F–1505F	Patient History
2000F–2060F	Physical Examination
3006F–3776F	Diagnostic/Screening Processes or Results
4000F–4563F	Therapeutic, Preventive or Other Interventions
5005F–5250F	Follow–up or Other Outcomes
6005F–6150F	Patient Safety
7010F–7025F	Structural Measures
9001F–9007F	Nonmeasure Code Listing

In addition, there are four modifiers (1P, 2P, 3P, and 8P) that are to be used to describe exclusions to the performance measures on a particular patient, such as for medical reasons and due to patient choice.

The AMA updates Category II three times per year in January, April, and July. The version released for January of the current year can be found in the CPT code book following the medicine section. CMS's quarterly changes can be found at https://www.cms.gov/Medicare /Coding/HCPCSReleaseCodeSets/HCPCS-Quarterly-Update.html.

Category III codes are codes for new and emerging technologies. These codes are updated twice per year. The codes are released semiannually via electronic distribution on the AMA CPT website and then published in the next edition of the CPT code book following the medicine section. Some examples include:

0308T	Insertion of ocular telescope prosthesis including removal of crystalline lens or intraocular lens prosthesis
0345T	Transcatheter mitral valve repair, percutaneous approach, via the coronary sinus

Category II codes are accessed through the regular CPT Index and reported using the same methods as other CPT codes. Category III codes must be used when they describe the specific service performed and are required in place of unlisted codes in that section. Refer to the notes at the beginning of the Category III code section of CPT for more information. Additional information about both Category II and Category III codes can be found at ama-assn .org/go/CPT.

The introduction to the CPT code book includes several explanations and general instructions. A review of the introduction shows that the listing of procedures or services and their codes by section does not restrict use of these codes to certain specialty groups. For example, a surgeon may use any of the codes in the book and is not limited to just the surgery section.

For a procedure to be included in the CPT code book, it must meet two criteria: first, many physicians throughout the country must commonly perform it; and, second, it must be consistent with contemporary medical practice. However, inclusion of a procedure in the code book does not imply endorsement by the AMA nor does it mean that the procedure will be covered and paid for by a given third-party payer.

The AMA publishes several formats of the CPT code book each year. Although each format contains the same basic information, some formats are enhanced with helpful information. A beginning coder should consider purchasing the professional edition format of CPT, which includes extra definitions, illustrations, and coding tips that explain procedures in greater detail. Coding tips provide helpful hints and draw the coder's attention to areas of known difficulty with coding. This information can be valuable for all coding professionals, especially beginners, and is only found in the *CPT Professional Edition*.

CPT Code Format

The CPT code book uses code formats that include symbols, modifiers, notes, unique code ranges, sequencing, and other formatting conventions to convey different kinds of information. A good understanding of the format of CPT codes, Index, and appendices is essential to accurate coding.

Symbols

The CPT code book uses several symbols to indicate special circumstances about a code.

The filled-in dot (•) appearing to the left of a CPT code designates a new code in the current edition of the code book.

> • 39401   Mediastinoscopy; includes biopsy(ies) of mediastinal mass (eg, lymphoma), when performed

Code 39401 is a new code in *CPT 2016* and is preceded by a filled-in dot. If this code is still in use in the year 2017, it will not be shown with a filled-in dot in that year's edition of the code book because it no longer will be new.

The pyramid, or triangle, symbol (▲) is used to indicate that a code's terminology has been revised. The code existed before, but the wording has been altered. Such changes in terminology may affect the use of a code; therefore, the new and old versions of the CPT code book should be compared to be sure that the correct code is assigned.

> ▲ 77057   Screening mammography, bilateral (2-view study of each breast)

In *CPT 2015*, the text for this code read:

> 77057   Screening mammography, bilateral (2-view film study of each breast)

Facing triangle symbols (►◄) are used to indicate new and revised text in coding notes. As with the filled-in dot and the triangle, these symbols will not appear in the next version of CPT for a code that has not changed in any way.

> ►Time spent performing separately reportable services other than the E/M or psychotherapy service is not counted toward the prolonged services time.◄

This new message is found in the Evaluation and Management guidelines to help clarify the method used for calculating prolonged services time. Because this note is new in the current edition, it is surrounded by the facing triangle (▶◀) symbols.

The + symbol indicates that the code following the symbol is an add-on code. A full list of add-on codes is found in appendix D of the CPT code book.

+22632   Each additional interspace (List separately in addition to code for
          primary procedure.)

Because code 22632 is an add-on code, it would never be reported alone. Add-on code guidelines are discussed in greater detail in chapter 4 of this book.

The null zero symbol (⊘), or universal no code, indicates that the code is exempt from use of the −51 modifier but is not an add-on code. A comprehensive list of such codes is found in appendix E of the CPT code book.

⊘20974   Electrical stimulation to aid bone healing; noninvasive (nonoperative)

The symbol ⊘ indicates that the −51 modifier cannot be used with code 20974.

The symbol ⊙ indicates that a code includes conscious sedation. A complete listing of the codes associated with this symbol is found in appendix G of the CPT code book.

The symbol ∥ indicates that the approval for the immunization associated with the code is pending FDA approval. A listing of these codes is found in appendix K of the CPT code book.

The symbol # is used to indicate that the code does not appear in numerical sequence. For example, code 21552 describes a concept that should follow code 21555 in sequence but code 21556 was already assigned. Code 21552 was chosen because of the proximity to code 21555 and the fact that it is out of sequence is indicated with a # symbol. In addition, a cross-reference is located in the position where code 21552 should be found, stating that the code number is out of sequence and where it can be found. Code 21552 is an indented code, which is discussed in the next section.

21555   Excision, tumor, soft tissue of neck or anterior thorax, subcutaneous;
         less than 3 cm
#21552   3 cm or greater

The Semicolon and Code Structure

The format of the CPT code book is designed to provide descriptions of procedures that can stand alone without additional explanation. To conserve space, many descriptions refer to a common portion of the procedure listed in a preceding entry rather than repeat the description in its entirety. When this occurs, the incomplete description or descriptions are indented under the main entry. The common portion of the main entry is followed by a semicolon (;). Each indented portion can be substituted as the ending of the coding description of the main code above, replacing the original ending that followed the semicolon. Following are examples of a semicolon application:

1. The indented information may provide diagnostic data.

49520	Repair recurrent inguinal hernia, any age; reducible
49521	incarcerated or strangulated

    The common portion of the description for code 49520 (the part before the semicolon) should be considered part of code 49521. Therefore, the full description of code 49521 reads: Repair recurrent inguinal hernia, any age; incarcerated or strangulated.

2. The indented information may provide alternate anatomical sites.

27705	Osteotomy; tibia
27707	fibula
27709	tibia and fibula
27712	multiple, with realignment on intramedullary rod (for example, Sofield type procedure)

    The full description of code 27707 reads: Osteotomy; fibula.

3. The indented information may describe specific procedures.

44155	Colectomy, total, abdominal, with proctectomy; with ileostomy
44156	with continent ileostomy
44157	with ileoanal anastomosis, includes loop ileostomy, and rectal mucosectomy, when performed
44158	with ileoanal anastomosis, creation of ileal reservoir (S or J), includes loop ileostomy, and rectal mucosectomy, when performed

    The full description of code 44158 reads: Colectomy, total, abdominal, with proctectomy; with ileoanal anastomosis, creation of ileal reservoir (S or J), includes loop ileostomy, and rectal mucosectomy, when performed

4. The indented information also may describe extensive procedures requiring assignment of two codes. The CPT system often designates more extensive procedures by using both the code for a stand-alone procedure and the code for an indented procedure to fully describe the extent of the surgery. When both codes are appropriate, the indented description contains the words "each" or "each additional."

15200	Full-thickness graft, free, including direct closure of donor site, trunk; 20 sq cm or less
15201	each additional 20 sq cm or part thereof (List separately in addition to code for primary procedure.)

When a 40 sq cm graft is performed on a patient, both numbers are assigned. The performance of a 60 sq cm graft requires the following codes to be reported: 15200, 15201, and 15201.

Unlisted Procedure Codes

The CPT system provides codes for unlisted services or procedures for circumstances in which a more specific code does not exist. This might occur when a procedure is new or unusual and a specific code has not been assigned in the CPT code book. However, the unlisted codes should not be used indiscriminately. In cases where the documentation is unclear or the system's nomenclature is difficult to translate, the physician should be consulted for more information or clarification. Unlisted codes are to be used only when there is actually no code for the procedure, not when the coder does not understand the procedure or the documentation.

If an unlisted code is used, additional information must be submitted with the claim. This describes the procedure, the time and effort necessary to perform the procedure, and other variables such as type of equipment required, medical reason for the procedure, and other pertinent information.

A list of all unlisted codes for a given section is included at the front of the section in the guidelines. The codes relate to a specific portion of that subsection. For example, 59899 is the unlisted code for maternity care and delivery.

Coding Notes and Instructions

Many notes and instructions are provided throughout the body of the CPT code book. It is important to read each note and determine whether it applies to the assigned code. A note may be preceded by the word "Note," may be enclosed in parentheses, or may appear within the text.

One function of a note is to define terms. For example, the note before the code series 11400–11471, Excision—Benign Lesions, includes definitions and descriptions of the term *excision* as it relates to this type of lesion.

A note also is used to direct coders to another section of the code book. For example, the last sentence of the first paragraph under Excision—Benign Lesions tells the coder to see the 11300 series for shave removal and 17000 series for electrosurgical or other methods of removal.

Finally, a note may advise coders that a particular code has been deleted and direct them to the new code or coding instruction. For example, a note following code 49062 directs the coder by stating "49080, 49081 have been deleted. To report, see 49082–49084."

Appendices

The CPT code book includes 15 appendices directly before the Index. Appendix A includes a comprehensive list and description of the modifiers. Although some HCPCS modifiers are listed, coders must refer to the HCPCS code book for a complete listing.

Appendix B includes a comprehensive listing of new codes, revised terminology, and deleted codes.

Appendix C includes clinical examples for evaluation and management (E/M) codes. These are examples only and not a complete list of potential E/M coding situations.

Appendix D is a comprehensive list of CPT add-on codes, indicated throughout the book by the + symbol.

Appendix E is a comprehensive list of CPT codes exempt from use of the –51 modifier, but not designated as add-on codes. These codes are preceded by the ⊘ symbol.

Appendix F is a listing of codes that are exempt from modifier –63, indicating that the procedure was performed on an infant weighing less than 4 kg. The codes in this list describe procedures that are normally performed on newborns of this weight.

Appendix G is a comprehensive listing of codes that include moderate (conscious) sedation as part of the procedure.

Appendix I indicates that the modifiers to be used with the genetic testing codes have been removed from CPT and where to locate information on molecular pathology.

Appendix J includes a list of each sensory, motor, and mixed nerve with its appropriate nerve conduction study code to enhance accurate reporting codes 95907-95913.

Appendix K lists the codes associated with products that are pending FDA approval.

Appendix L lists the vascular families and specifies their first, second, third and beyond the third order branches for use in coding vascular access procedures.

Appendix M is the crosswalk to all previously deleted and renumbered CPT codes for continuity of information.

Appendix N is the summary of the CPT codes that are out of numerical sequence.

Appendix O is the listing of multianalyte assays with algorithmic analyses.

Index

The CPT code book includes a comprehensive Index. The Index has been expanded and revised extensively in recent years.

Main terms appear in boldface type and can have modifying subterms. The primary classes of main entries are procedure or service (**Capsulorrhaphy**); organ or site (**Carotid body**); condition (**Carbuncle**); or synonym (**Craniotomy**), eponym (**Campbell procedure**), or abbreviation (**CT scan**).

The codes that follow the main terms and/or subterms may be a code range, a group of codes, or a single code. For example, under the main term **Cholecystectomy**, the subterm for Any Method, with Cholangiography contains three codes separated by commas; the subterm for Any Method (without cholangiography) contains a code range; and the main term **Choledochoscopy** contains only one code.

Often following main entries, subterms provide additional information that must be reviewed before selecting a code, such as:

Hand
Amputation
    at Metacarpal 25927, 26910
    at Wrist. 25920
        Revision. 25922
    Ray amputation 26910
    Revision 25924, 25929, 25931

The Alphabetic Index offers at least one code for review under each entry, although in some cases more than one code or a range of codes is provided. However, whatever the circumstance, each code with its description must be reviewed carefully to ensure accurate assignment and appropriate payment. To illustrate:

Mastectomy
Gynecomastia 19300
Modified Radical 19307
Partial 19301–19302
Radical 19303–19306
Simple, Complete 19303
Subcutaneous 19304
with axillary lymphadenectomy 19302

When reporting a partial mastectomy, the coder should review the descriptions of the codes in the 19301–19302 range before assigning a final code.

The code or codes listed must be checked in the main body of the CPT code book. Even if only one code is listed, this step should not be omitted. Important notes or other instructions may impact code assignment. Also, the Index contains only a portion of the terminology of the code and more careful review may lead the coder away from this code assignment. Coders should never code directly from the Index.

A cross-reference term, *See*, is used in the CPT Index. The *See* cross-reference directs the coder to another possible term in the Index. This is often applicable for synonyms, eponyms, and abbreviations. If the procedure is not listed under the first entry, more information is found under the cross-reference.

For example:

Finney Operation
See Gastroduodenostomy

Code Organization

As stated earlier, the CPT code book consists of six sections: evaluation and management, anesthesia, surgery, radiology, pathology and laboratory, and medicine. Each of these sections is discussed in detail in subsequent chapters.

Moreover, each section is subdivided. For example, the surgery section has 19 subsections, most representing body systems. The first subsection is general and the second is the integumentary system.

The next level is the heading. The headings can be for anatomical sites. For example, in the integumentary system, the first heading is skin, subcutaneous and accessory structures.

Sometimes subheadings are included to provide greater specificity. For example, the first subheading under the skin, subcutaneous and accessory structures heading is incision and drainage.

Understanding how the CPT codes are organized will ensure correct code assignment.

Sources of Documentation That Generate Physician Codes and Charges

Physicians, physician assistants, midwives, nurse practitioners, nursing staff, and ancillary staff all may generate charges during a patient encounter. Insurers/payers have specific guidelines about how to submit claims for nonphysician charges. Some insurance payers may credential nonphysicians to allow charges to be submitted under their own provider number. Other insurers/payers may prefer to bill nonphysician services under the physician's provider number.

Place of Service

Charges may be generated when services are provided in the clinic/office setting, inpatient hospital, same-day surgery center, nursing home, home visit, outpatient hospital, emergency department, and urgent care center. Typically, copies of the history and physical examination, operative notes, and emergency/urgent care visits not originating in clinic/office settings are sent to the clinic for inclusion in the patient's health record. This information can be used for reference while coding.

Clinic/Office Setting

Both physicians and nonphysicians will generate charges. These charges will consist of the following:

- Office visits, consultation visits, and/or procedures performed within the office

- Diagnostic services, such as laboratory, x-ray, EKGs, and spirometry

- Injections

- Immunizations

- Supplies

The documentation to support these charges is found in the progress notes, laboratory reports, x-ray reports, and diagnostic services reports.

Inpatient Hospital

Attending physicians, surgeons, and consultants generate charges in the inpatient hospital setting. These charges consist of the following:

- Initial hospital care, documented in the history and physical examination

- Daily visits, billed as subsequent hospital care, documented in the daily progress notes

- Consultations, documented in the consultation report, that are provided by specialist physicians (Physicians who provide consultations may bill for their services as inpatient consultations to patients not covered by Medicare.)

- Surgical services, documented in operative notes

Observation Area

Physicians attending patients in the observation area of the hospital may bill for these services. The source of documentation will be initial observation care (similar to a history and physical examination) and progress notes for subsequent observation care. If a patient is admitted from the observation area, charges are billed using inpatient visit services rather than observation care services.

Same-Day Surgery Center

Surgical service charges are generated by the surgeon or person performing the procedure, and the operative/procedure note is the source of documentation.

Nursing Facility

Nursing facility, or nursing home, charges are generated by physicians and, in some areas of the nation, nurse practitioners and physician assistants. These charges may occur as follows:

- Initial nursing home care is charged as initial nursing facility services, and the documentation is in the form of a history and physical examination.

- Periodic visits to the nursing home patient by the physician or the nurse practitioner may be charged as subsequent nursing facility visits. Progress notes are the source of documentation for these charges.

- Health insurance coverage determines the frequency with which subsequent nursing home visits can be submitted for payment.

Home Visit

When patients are homebound, services provided by physicians and/or home health agency personnel may be charged. Progress notes are the source of documentation to support physician charges. Typically, the health records for these services are located in the home health agency. When a physician provides home visit services to an established patient from the clinic, the documentation needs to be in the clinic/office health record.

Outpatient Hospital

In the outpatient hospital, charges are generated by a physician; a midlevel practitioner, such as a physician assistant or nurse practitioner; and/or a consultant. Documentation may be a dictated procedure note and/or a progress note indicating the services provided.

Emergency Department

Physicians and midlevel practitioners may generate charges in an emergency department. Their charges may be documented as follows:

- Services provided in the emergency department may be documented on a form, a dictated note, or a consultation note.

- Procedures done during an emergency department visit may be documented in the emergency department form and/or dictated.

Urgent Care Visits

Urgent care visits may generate physician office charges, procedures, and ancillary and diagnostic services. The physician visit and/or procedure is documented in an urgent care form or as a dictated note. Physicians and midlevel practitioners generate the charges.

Data Collection

To ensure that all charges are collected and billed, a data collection form should be used for each place of service. Clinic appointment lists should be verified against the day's completed charges to confirm that all charges are submitted. Many computer systems that have automated scheduling and billing perform this verification after charges have been entered. A report from the computer system may list the patient names and dates of service that have not been entered. This report should be reconciled in a timely manner to ensure the timely filing of charges.

A number of tools can be used to collect information about services requiring coding. The tool most commonly used is a document that captures the services performed. For the purposes of this chapter, the term charge ticket is used for this document (although it also is known as the superbill, fee ticket, encounter form, charge slip, route tag, route slip, fee slip, billing slip, and so on). There may be one charge ticket for the clinic or many different charge tickets for specialties or physicians. The charge ticket may include the following:

- Patient name

- Insurance information

- Date of service

- Physician/provider name

- CPT and/or unique identifier codes specific to the services provided at the clinic or by a specific physician

- Diagnosis codes or narratives

- Area to write additional services or diagnoses

- Area for modifiers

- Area for fees

The charge ticket should be revised at least annually to incorporate any CPT and ICD-10-CM changes or changes in the practice that may have an impact on the information on the charge ticket. It is beneficial to have the most commonly used services on the charge ticket by CPT or unique identifier, rather than having them handwritten each time, which requires individual coding. The revenue production report discussed in chapter 11 of this book can be used to verify that most frequently used codes are included on the charge ticket. Figure 1.4 is an example of a charge ticket for office services.

For ease of completion, many practices use a combined data collection tool for all off-site services. Figure 1.5 is a service record for a physician who performs a variety of different services in a hospital.

Figure 1.4. Clinic charge ticket

INTERNAL MEDICINE SERVICES	D.O.S. _____

☐ CASH	☐ CHECK #	☐ CO-PAY	☐ RECEIPT #	AMT

Control #

SIGNED IN _____
APPT TIME _____
TIME IN _____

☐ WALK-IN   ☐ CONSULT   ☐ APPOINTMENT

PATIENT NAME (Last, First, MI)	SEX	SSN	DOB	Physician 1
				Physician 2
				Physician 3
ADDRESS	CITY	STATE	ZIP	Physician 4

PRIMARY INS: ☐ MEDICARE ☐ EDS ☐ COMM   ☐ SELF-PAY ☐ PCP:
SECONDARY INS: ☐ MEDICARE ☐ EDS ☐ COMM   ☐ SELF-PAY ☐ PCP:

ELIGIBLITY:	APPROVED BY:

DX 1:_____   DX 2:_____   DX 3:_____   DX 4:_____

DESCRIPTION	CODE	CODE	DX	DESCRIPTION	CODE	DX	DESCRIPTION	CODE	DX
HEALTH CHECK SERVICES				**INJECTIONS/MEDICATIONS**		DX	**IMMUNIZATIONS**		DX
	NEW PATIENT	ESTAB PATIENT	DX	Albuterol per 1 mg	☐ J7611		Hepatitis A	☐ 90632	
				Allergy Injection Single	☐ 95115		Hepatitis B Adult	☐ 90746	
☐ Infant 0-11 Months	☐ 99381	☐ 99391		Allergy Injection 2 or >	☐ 95117		Medicare Administration	☐ G0010	
☐ 1 - 4 Years	☐ 99382	☐ 99392		B-12 1000 mcg	☐ J3420		Influenza Vaccine	☐ 90658	
☐ 5 - 11 Years	☐ 99383	☐ 99393		Bicillin 100K units	☐ J0558		Medicare Administration	☐ G0008	
☐ 12 -17 Years	☐ 99384	☐ 99394		D5W 1000cc	☐ J7070		MMR	☐ 90707	
☐ 18 - 39 Years	☐ 99385	☐ 99395		Imitrex	☐ J3030		Pneumovax Vaccine	☐ 90732	
☐ 40 - 64 Years	☐ 99386	☐ 99396		Insulin 5 units	☐ J1815		Medicare Administration	☐ G0009	
☐ 65 Years and Older	☐ 99387	☐ 99397		Kenalog 10 mg	☐ J3301		Td Adult	☐ 90714	
				Rocephin 250 mg	☐ J0696		Varicella	☐ 90716	
NEW PATIENTS			DX	Toradol 15 mg	☐ J1885		Vac Admin < 18 yrs of age	☐ 90460	
☐ Level I - PF, PF, SF	10 min	☐ 99201		Vancomycin 500 mg	☐ J3370		with counseling, 1st		
☐ Level II - EPF, EPF, SF	20 min	☐ 99202		Zithromax	☐ J0456		Vac Admin < 18 yrs of age	☐ 90461+	
☐ Level III - DET, DET, LOW	30 min	☐ 99203		Injection, SubQ/IM	☐ 96372		with counseling, each additional		
☐ Level IV - C, C, MOD	45 min	☐ 99204		IV, drip - 1st hr	☐ 96365		Vac Administration 1st	☐ 90471	
☐ Level V - C, C, HIGH	60 min	☐ 99205		IV, drip each additional hr	☐ 96366		Vac Administration		
ESTABLISHED PATIENTS			DX	IV, push	☐ 96374		each additional vaccine	☐ 90472+	
☐ Level I - MD not required	5 min	☐ 99211							
☐ Level II - PF, PF, SF	10 min	☐ 99212							
☐ Level III - EPF, EPF, LOW	15 min	☐ 99213							
☐ Level IV - DET, DET, MOD	25 min	☐ 99214					**PROCEDURES**		DX
☐ Level V - C, C, HIGH	40 min	☐ 99215		**LABORATORY**		DX	Lumbar puncture	☐ 62270	
NON–MEDICARE OFFICE CONSULTATIONS			DX	Hemoglobin	☐ 85018		MDI Teaching	☐ 94664	
☐ Level I - PF, PF, SF	15 min	☐ 99241		Hematocrit	☐ 85014		Nebulizer Treatment	☐ 94640	
☐ Level II - EPF, EPF, SF	30 min	☐ 99242		Occult Blood	☐ 82270		Pack anterior nasal hem.	☐ 30901	
☐ Level III - DET, DET, LOW	40 min	☐ 99243		One Touch Blood Glucose	☐ 82962		Pack posterior nasal hem.	☐ 30905	
☐ Level IV - C, C, MOD	60 min	☐ 99244		Pap smear collection	☐ Q0091		Simple Repair face, ears		
☐ Level V - C, C, HIGH	80 min	☐ 99245		PPD Test	☐ 86580		Less than 2.5 cm	☐ 12011	
PROCEDURES			DX	Pregnancy Test, Urine	☐ 81025		2.6 cm to 5.0 cm	☐ 12013	
Cerumen removal, irrigation/lavage		☐ 69209		Pulse Oximetry	☐ 94760		Simple Repair trunk, extremities		
Cerumen removal, instruments		☐ 69210		Rapid Strep Test	☐ 87880		Less than 2.5 cm	☐ 12001	
Change burn dressing		☐ 16020		Urinalysis	☐ 81002		2.6 cm to 7.5 cm	☐ 12002	
Chemical cautery		☐ 17250		Wet Prep	☐ 87210		Strapping, ankle	☐ 29540	
I & D Abscess		☐ 10060		Lab Handling	☐ 99000		Strapping, elbow or wrist	☐ 29260	
I & D Hematoma		☐ 10140		Venipuncture	☐ 36415		Strapping, hand	☐ 29280	
I & D Post Op Infection		☐ 10180					Strapping, knee	☐ 29530	
Inject Tendon Sheath/Ligament		☐ 20550					Surgical Tray	☐ A4550	
Inject Tendon Origin/Insertion		☐ 20551							
Inject Trigger Points (1-2)		☐ 20552							
Inject Trigger Points (3 or more)		☐ 20553					**WRITE IN SERVICES HERE:**		DX
Removal of Foreign Body	Ear	☐ 69200							
	Nose	☐ 30300		**EKG**		DX			
	Eye	☐ 65205		EKG, 12 lead total	☐ 93000				
	Skin	☐ 10120		EKG, tracing	☐ 93005				
Removal of Skin Tags (up to 15)		☐ 11200		EKG, intrepretation	☐ 93010				
Removal of Skin Tags (additional 10)		☐ 11201+							
Wart Removal (1st wart)		☐ 17000		**AFTER HOURS/SPECIAL CARE**		DX			
Wart Removal (2-14 additional)		☐ 17003+		After posted hours	☐ 99050+				
				Other than office - special	☐ 99056+				
				Emergency care in office	☐ 99058+				

Figure 1.5. Service record

Patient Name:					Location:	Inpt	SDS/OP		
Date of Birth:					Hospital A [ ] [ ]				
					Hospital B [ ] [ ]				
Med Rec #					Hospital C [ ] [ ]				
Acct #					Diagnoses 1) _____ 2) _____				
					3) _____ 4) _____				

Initial Inpatient Care (Admit)	Date	Prov	Code	DX #	Inpatient Consult	Date	Prov	Code	Dx #
Det Comp Hx & Exam - SF/Low Complex			99221		Requesting Physician				
Comp Hx & Exam - Mod Complex			99222		Name:				
Comp Hx & Exam - High Complex			99223		Initial	Date	Prov	Cpde	Dx #
Subsequent Inpatient Care (Per Day)					PF Hx & Exam - SF			99251	
Level 1 - Problem Focused Hx & Exam/ Straight-forward - Low Complexity (Patient is usually stable, recovering or improving)					EPF Hx & Exam - Sf			99252	
					D Hx & Exam - Low			99253	

Date	Prov	Code	Dx #	Date	Prov	Code	Dx #	Comp Hx & Exam - Mod			99254	
		99231				99231		Comp Hx & Exam - High			99255	
		99231				99231						
		99231				99231						
		99231				99231						

Level 2 - Exp Problem Focused Hx & Exam - Moderate Complex (Patient is responding inadequately or has developed minor complication)								Newborn Care	Date	Prov	Code	Dx #

Date	Prov	Code	Dx #	Date	Prov	Code	Dx #	Initial Normal Newborn			99460	
		99232				99232		Subsequent Routine			99462	
		99232				99232		Subsequent Routine			99462	
		99232				99232		Subsequent Routine			99462	
		99232				99232		Subsequent Routine			99462	

Level 3 - Detailed Hx & Exam - High Complexity (Patient is unstable or had developed a significant complication or new problem)								Subsequent Routine			99462	
								Discharge Mgmt 30 /less			99238	

Date	Prov	Code	Dx #	Date	Prov	Code	Dx #	Discharge Mgmt over 30			99239	
		99233				99233		Same Day admit/disch			99463	
		99233				99233		Attendance at delivery			99464	
		99233				99233		Circumcision			54150	
		99233				99233		Obstetrical Care	Date	Prov	Code	Dx #

Discharge Management	Date	Prov	Code	Dx #	Delivery [ ] Vag [ ] C-Section				
Discharge Mgmt, 30 min or less			99238		[ ] VBAC				
Discharge Mgmt, over 30 minutes			99239		Post partum daily care				
Same Day Admit/Discharge	Date	Prov	Code	DX #	Post partum daily care				
(Observation Area or Inpatient)					Post Partum daily care				
Det-Compr Hx & Exam - SF-low Complex			99234		PP tubal , abd/vaginal			58605	
Comp Hx & Exam - Mod Complex			99235		PP tubal w/C-Section			58611	
Comp Hx & Exam - High Complex			99236		PP curettage (SP)			59160	
Observation Area Care (Per Day)	Date	Prov	Code	Dx #	Delivery ot placenta (SP)			59414	
Det-Compr Y\Hx & Exam - SF - Low Comp			99218		Amniocentesis			59000	
Comp Hx & Exam - Mod Complex			99219		External version			59412	
Comp Hx & Exam - High Complex			99220		Fetal non-stress test			59025-26	
Discharge Mgmt - Not on same day			99217		Insertion of dilator (SP)			59200	
Prolonged Care	Date	Prov	Code	Dx #	Prenatal care only 4-6			59425	
Beyond Primary Service, to 1 hour			99356		Prenatal care only 7 +			59426	
Each addl 30 min _____ units			99357		Post partum care only			59430	
Critical Care (ICU, SCU, CCU)	Date	Prov	Code	Dx #	Other Proc/Service	Date	Prov	Code	Dx #
See CPT Guidelines for specifics									
Critical Care, First 30–74 minutes			99291						
Each addl 30 min _____ units			99292						

General CPT Coding Instructions

The instructions listed will assist coders in selecting the correct code(s). As with any process that is repeated, the steps will soon become automatic. In the meantime, however, students should follow each step carefully.

1. Identify the procedures and services to be coded by carefully reviewing the health record documentation.

2. Consult the Index under the main term for the procedure performed and consult any subterms under the main term.

3. If the term is not located under the procedure performed, check the organ or site, condition, or eponym, synonym, or abbreviation.

4. Note the code number(s) found opposite the selected main term or subterm.

5. Check the code, codes, or code range in the body of the CPT code book:

   • When a single code number is provided, locate the code in the body of the CPT code book.

   • When two or more codes separated by a comma are shown, locate each code in the body of the CPT code book.

   • When a range of codes is shown, locate the range in the body of the CPT code book.

6. Read and be guided by any coding notes under the code, at the subheading, heading, subsection, or section level.

7. Never code directly from the Index.

8. Assign the appropriate modifier(s), when necessary, to complete the code description.

9. Assign the appropriate code.

10. Continue coding all components of the procedure/service using the above steps.

In many cases, following these general guidelines is not an easy task. The CPT system sometimes assumes that the coding professional or clinician has a wide knowledge of medical terminology and anatomy, as well as pathophysiology. Even when the coder has this extensive background, it is advisable to have medical dictionaries and other medical texts available for reference. An additional challenge may be the lack of complete medical reports, for example, laboratory, radiology, or pathology results. Because many CPT codes are very specific, it may be necessary to delay coding until the most complete and accurate information is available. The documentation in the health record must fully support the codes reported.

Identification of Codable Procedural Statements

Procedural statements are assigned codes using the CPT and/or the HCPCS system. The procedure and/or service completed during a visit for physician services must be documented in the patient's health record.

> **Example:** We anesthetized a large lesion, 3.5 cm in size, at the junction just anterior and lateral to the left tonsil with 1% local anesthetic, and then with a sharp scissors and a forceps, we dissected out the lesion. This will be sent to the laboratory for microscopic examination.

The procedure in the above example would be coded as excision of a lesion of the mouth.

However, assigning a procedure code to the level of the office visit is not as easy. Complete instructions for coding E/M services are provided in chapter 2 of this book, and the documentation guidelines are included in appendix F. The physician's documentation must meet the documentation guidelines for history, examination, and medical decision making to determine the appropriate CPT office visit code. In most physicians' offices, physicians select the level of service they want to report and/or charge. As the student learns CPT coding and applies the documentation guidelines, levels of service will be identified more easily.

Coding from an operative report requires a few extra steps. The following operative report illustrates the additional steps required:

Example:

Operative Report

Preoperative Diagnosis: History of colon cancer

Postoperative Diagnosis: Rectosigmoid polyp

Procedure Performed: Colonoscopy and polypectomy

Indications: The patient has had three previous resections of three different primary carcinomas of the colon. His last resection of carcinoma was in 1998. He has been doing well in general.

Premedications: Demerol 50 mg IV and Versed 2.5 mg IV

Description of Procedure: The CF100-L video colonoscope was passed without difficulty from the anus up through the anastomosis, which appears to be in the distal transverse colon. The instrument was advanced into the distal small bowel and then slowly withdrawn with good view obtained throughout. A small, 3-mm polyp was found near the rectosigmoid junction, removed with hot biopsy forceps, and retrieved. Otherwise, the patient has a satisfactory postoperative appearance of the colon. It is shortened due to previous resections, but there is no other evidence of neoplasm. The instrument was withdrawn completely without other findings.

The coding process includes the following steps:

1. Scan the documentation and indicate the procedure performed. (Colonoscopy and polypectomy)

2. Search the Index for Colonoscopy, Removal, Polyp, and record the coding selection. (45384–45385)

3. Review the coding descriptions to determine what additional documentation is needed before a code can be selected accurately. (How was the polyp removed? Hot biopsy, forceps, snare, and so forth.)

4. Read the operative report again to determine the method of removal utilized. ("and this polyp was removed with hot biopsy forceps and retrieved")

5. Choose the code that reflects the documentation. (45384)

In the following operative report, the coder also must reference the pathological diagnosis to assist with code assignment. The steps in the coding process include a review of the additional documentation to clarify the diagnosis and assist in selection of the correct code.

Example:

Operative Report

Preoperative Diagnosis: Subepidermal nodular lesion of the forearm

Operation: Excision of lesion of the forearm

Procedure: Under local anesthesia, the lesion is opened with a linear-elliptical incision. The 2.6-cm lesion and 0.2-cm margins are excised and submitted to pathology. Bleeding is controlled with electrocautery, and the wound is closed with five vertical mattress sutures of 5-0 nylon. Polysporin and dressing are applied to the wound.

Pathological Diagnosis: Well-organized basal cell carcinoma

The coding process includes the following steps:

1. Scan the documentation and record the main procedure to be located in the alphabetic Index. (Excision)

2. Search the Index for the main terms/subterms and record the code selections. (Can be located under Excision, lesion, skin; or Lesion, skin, excision. Selections: Benign, 11400–11471, or Malignant, 11600–11646)

3. Review the code descriptions to determine what additional documentation is needed before a code can be selected accurately. (Pathological diagnosis indicates that the lesion was malignant, 11600–11646.)

4. Read the operative report and the pathological diagnosis again to determine the additional documentation to clarify the selection. (Documentation to code: Malignant lesion, size [2.6 cm], margins [0.2 cm + 0.2 cm], and site [arm])

5. Choose the code that reflects the documentation of 3.0-cm total excised diameter. (11603)

Identification of Codable Diagnostic Statements

Diagnostic statements obtained from the physician's notes are assigned a code number from the ICD-10-CM coding system. Coders must learn the rules of ICD-10-CM coding to understand which diagnostic statements need to be coded. Although this is a CPT/HCPCS instructional text, the concept of coding diagnostic statements is also vitally important. Some concepts that affect reimbursement are covered here, and coders are encouraged to seek a full instructional text on ICD-10-CM coding.

Diagnostic statements or diagnoses can be found in many places within the health record, most commonly in the physician's notes in the assessment or diagnosis portion of the note. Examples of a codable diagnostic statement are

Assessment: Upper respiratory infection (URI)
Diagnosis (Dx):   Right wrist fracture

When a patient presents for a laboratory-only or a radiology-only appointment, the diagnosis may be found:

- On the order requisition for the test

- In a previous note where the test was ordered

- In a phone message, if the patient called and was requested to come in for tests

- On the problem list, if it is a chronic condition requiring ongoing monitoring

Signs and Symptoms

When a definitive diagnosis or assessment statement is unavailable, the chief complaint should be used for coding. The chief complaint is often a sign or symptom of disease and is reported by the patient when first checking in for the appointment.

As an example, the patient's chief complaint is blood in the stool. Although the physician may suspect a colon tumor, coding a colon tumor without diagnostic evidence is inappropriate. Instead, the physician should use blood in the stool as the reason for ordering diagnostic testing, such as a barium enema. If the results from a barium enema show a questionable mass, "abnormal radiology examination" should be used as the reason for an additional test, such as a colonoscopy, rather than the questionable mass.

Coding questionable diagnoses as fact will label the patient's insurance history with unconfirmed and potentially incorrect findings. Additional important items to remember about diagnosis coding are covered below.

Ambulatory Coding Guidelines for ICD-10-CM

ICD-10-CM Official Guidelines for Coding and Reporting are presented jointly by the CMS and the National Center for Health Statistics (NCHS). These official guidelines are approved by four organizations that make up the Cooperating Parties for the ICD-10-CM: the American Hospital Association (AHA), AHIMA, CMS, and NCHS. These guidelines, effective 10/1/2015, can be accessed and downloaded from http://www.cdc.gov/nchs/data /icd/10cmguidelines_2016_Final.pdf.

Section I of the guidelines is applicable to all settings. Section IV is specific to ambulatory services and is reprinted here. This version of the guidelines was in effect when this publication went to press.

Section IV. Diagnostic Coding and Reporting Guidelines for Outpatient Services

These coding guidelines for outpatient diagnoses have been approved for use by hospitals/providers in coding and reporting hospital-based outpatient services and provider-based office visits.

Information about the use of certain abbreviations, punctuation, symbols, and other conventions used in the ICD-10-CM Tabular List (code numbers and titles), can be found in Section IA of these guidelines, under "Conventions Used in the Tabular List." Section I.B. contains general guidelines that apply to the entire classification. Section I.C. contains chapter-specific guidelines that correspond to the chapters as they are arranged in the classification. Information about the correct sequence to use in finding a code is also described in Section I.

The terms encounter and visit are often used interchangeably in describing outpatient service contacts and, therefore, appear together in these guidelines without distinguishing one from the other.

Though the conventions and general guidelines apply to all settings, coding guidelines for outpatient and provider reporting of diagnoses will vary in a number of instances from those for inpatient diagnoses, recognizing that:

- The Uniform Hospital Discharge Data Set (UHDDS) definition of principal diagnosis applies only to inpatients in acute, short-term, long-term care and psychiatric hospitals.

- Coding guidelines for inconclusive diagnoses (probable, suspected, rule out, etc.) were developed for inpatient reporting and do not apply to outpatients.

A. Selection of first-listed condition

In the outpatient setting, the term first-listed diagnosis is used in lieu of principal diagnosis.

In determining the first-listed diagnosis the coding conventions of ICD-10-CM, as well as the general and disease specific guidelines take precedence over the outpatient guidelines.

Diagnoses often are not established at the time of the initial encounter/visit. It may take two or more visits before the diagnosis is confirmed.

The most critical rule involves beginning the search for the correct code assignment through the Alphabetic Index. Never begin searching initially in the Tabular List as this will lead to coding errors.

1. Outpatient Surgery

   When a patient presents for outpatient surgery (same day surgery), code the reason for the surgery as the first-listed diagnosis (reason for the encounter), even if the surgery is not performed due to a contraindication.

2. Observation Stay

   When a patient is admitted for observation for a medical condition, assign a code for the medical condition as the first-listed diagnosis.

   When a patient presents for outpatient surgery and develops complications requiring admission to observation, code the reason for the surgery as the first reported diagnosis (reason for the encounter), followed by codes for the complications as secondary diagnoses.

B. Codes from A00.0 through T88.9, Z00-Z99

The appropriate code(s) from A00.0 through T88.9, Z00-Z99 must be used to identify diagnoses, symptoms, conditions, problems, complaints, or other reason(s) for the encounter/visit.

C. Accurate reporting of ICD-10-CM diagnosis codes

For accurate reporting of ICD-10-CM diagnosis codes, the documentation should describe the patient's condition, using terminology which includes specific diagnoses as well as symptoms, problems, or reasons for the encounter. There are ICD-10-CM codes to describe all of these.

D. Codes that describe symptoms and signs

Codes that describe symptoms and signs, as opposed to diagnoses, are acceptable for reporting purposes when a diagnosis has not been established (confirmed) by the provider. Chapter 18 of ICD-10-CM, Symptoms, Signs, and Abnormal Clinical and Laboratory Findings Not Elsewhere Classified (codes R00-R99) contain many, but not all codes for symptoms.

E. Encounters for circumstances other than a disease or injury

ICD-10-CM provides codes to deal with encounters for circumstances other than a disease or injury. The Factors Influencing Health Status and Contact with Health Services codes (Z00-Z99) are provided to deal with occasions when circumstances other than a disease or injury are recorded as diagnosis or problems.

See Section I.C.21. Factors influencing health status and contact with health services.

F. Level of Detail in Coding

1. ICD-10-CM codes with 3, 4, 5, 6 or 7 characters

   ICD-10-CM is composed of codes with 3, 4, 5, 6 or 7 characters. Codes with three characters are included in ICD-10-CM as the heading of a category of codes that may be further subdivided by the use of fourth, fifth, sixth or seventh characters to provide greater specificity.

2. Use of full number of *characters* required for a code

   A three-character code is to be used only if it is not further subdivided. A code is invalid if it has not been coded to the full number of characters required for that code, including the 7th character, if applicable.

G. ICD-10-CM code for the diagnosis, condition, problem, or other reason for encounter/visit

List first the ICD-10-CM code for the diagnosis, condition, problem, or other reason for encounter/visit shown in the medical record to be chiefly responsible for the services provided. List additional codes that describe any coexisting conditions. In some cases the first-listed diagnosis may be a symptom when a diagnosis has not been established (confirmed) by the physician.

H. Uncertain diagnosis

Do not code diagnoses documented as "probable", "suspected," "questionable," "rule out," or "working diagnosis" or other similar terms indicating uncertainty. Rather, code the condition(s) to the highest degree of certainty for that encounter/visit, such as symptoms, signs, abnormal test results, or other reason for the visit.

Please note: This differs from the coding practices used by short-term, acute care, long-term care and psychiatric hospitals.

I. Chronic diseases

Chronic diseases treated on an ongoing basis may be coded and reported as many times as the patient receives treatment and care for the condition(s)

J. Code all documented conditions that coexist

Code all documented conditions that coexist at the time of the encounter/visit, and require or affect patient care treatment or management. Do not code conditions that were previously treated and no longer exist. However, history codes (categories Z80-Z87) may be used as secondary codes if the historical condition or family history has an impact on current care or influences treatment.

K. Patients receiving diagnostic services only

For patients receiving diagnostic services only during an encounter/visit, sequence first the diagnosis, condition, problem, or other reason for encounter/visit shown in the medical record to be chiefly responsible for the outpatient services provided during the encounter/visit. Codes for other diagnoses (e.g., chronic conditions) may be sequenced as additional diagnoses.

For encounters for routine laboratory/radiology testing in the absence of any signs, symptoms, or associated diagnosis, assign Z01.89, Encounter for other specified special examinations. If routine testing is performed during the same encounter as a test to evaluate a sign, symptom, or diagnosis, it is appropriate to assign both the Z code and the code describing the reason for the non-routine test.

For outpatient encounters for diagnostic tests that have been interpreted by a physician, and the final report is available at the time of coding, code any confirmed or definitive diagnosis(es) documented in the interpretation. Do not code related signs and symptoms as additional diagnoses.

Please note: This differs from the coding practice in the hospital inpatient setting regarding abnormal findings on test results.

L. Patients receiving therapeutic services only

For patients receiving therapeutic services only during an encounter/visit, sequence first the diagnosis, condition, problem, or other reason for encounter/visit shown in the medical record to be chiefly responsible for the outpatient services provided during the encounter/visit. Codes for other diagnoses (e.g., chronic conditions) may be sequenced as additional diagnoses.

The only exception to this rule is that when the primary reason for the admission/encounter is chemotherapy or radiation therapy, the appropriate Z code for the service is listed first, and the diagnosis or problem for which the service is being performed listed second.

M. Patients receiving preoperative evaluations only

For patients receiving preoperative evaluations only, sequence first a code from subcategory Z01.81, Encounter for pre-procedural examinations, to describe the pre-op consultations. Assign a code for the condition to describe the reason for the surgery as an additional diagnosis. Code also any findings related to the pre-op evaluation.

N. Ambulatory surgery

For ambulatory surgery, code the diagnosis for which the surgery was performed. If the postoperative diagnosis is known to be different from the preoperative diagnosis at the time the diagnosis is confirmed, select the postoperative diagnosis for coding, since it is the most definitive.

O. Routine outpatient prenatal visits

See Section I.C.15. Routine outpatient prenatal visits.

P. Encounters for general medical examinations with abnormal findings

The subcategories for encounters for general medical examinations, Z00.0-, provide codes for with and without abnormal findings. Should a general medical examination result in an abnormal finding, the code for general medical examination with abnormal finding should be assigned as the first-listed diagnosis. A secondary code for the abnormal finding should also be coded.

Q. Encounters for routine health screenings

See Section I.C.21. Factors influencing health status and contact with health services, Screening

External Causes of Injury

In addition to diagnostic statements, the ICD-10-CM system can be used to code the reason for an accident or injury as a supplemental code. The codes starting with V, W, X, and Y in the ICD-10-CM code book are used for this purpose. A separate Index, the Index to External Causes, following the main ICD-10-CM Index, is used to assign these codes. External cause codes are never assigned alone. They must follow the code that describes the injury.

By placing the date of the accident or injury in box 14 of the CMS-1500 claim form (see appendix G for the form and directions to the online instructions) and listing one or more external cause codes as secondary diagnoses, the physician can fully explain why the care was given. Although External cause codes are not required for use by physicians, using them with ICD-10-CM diagnosis codes when applicable, such as with the injury and poisoning categories (S and T categories), can reduce the number of inquiries from insurance companies about whether they are the primary payer on a claim.

For example, the physician sees a small child who fell out of bed at home and has a fractured radius and ulna. By submitting these codes, the insurance company would clearly know that the accident happened at home and that no other personal injury or motor vehicle carrier is primary:

S52.541A   Smith's fracture of right radius, initial encounter for closed fracture
W06.XXXA   Fall from bed, initial encounter

Y92.032	Bedroom in apartment as the place of occurrence of the external cause
Y93.E9	Activity, other interior property and clothing maintenance
Y99.8	Other external cause status

As another example, the physician sees a patient who injured a hand at work. By submitting these codes to the workers' compensation carrier, the coder tells the insurance company that the accident happened at work and gives basic information about how it happened:

S67.22XA	Crushing injury of left hand, initial encounter
W23.0XXA	Caught, crushed, jammed, or pinched between moving objects, initial encounter
Y92.59	Other trade areas as the place of occurrence of the external cause
Y93.E2	Activity, laundry
Y99.0	Civilian activity done for income or pay

Identification of Codable Statements in Physician Office Documentation

One of the important skills that a coder must learn is to assess the health record for key statements that require code assignment. The physician visit documented below contains a number of statements that need to be coded:

S: Patient is having a follow-up for an abrasion of his right arm following a fall at home. He has fallen again and now has abrasions on his left arm. The most recent fall occurred while he was doing some gardening. His other complaints include a skin tag on his neck that continues to be irritated from shirt collars. In addition, he is due for a vitamin B_{12} injection. Because it is flu season, he also is requesting a flu shot. Finally, he reports a slow heartbeat. The patient is on Toprol 100 mg daily.

ROS: Patient denies any contact with other sick people. He last had a vitamin B_{12} injection 4 weeks ago. He denies any fevers or night sweats. Other ROS unremarkable.

PFSH: Patient has a history of cardiac arrhythmia diagnosed in 1979. He has been vitamin B_{12} deficient for the past 2 years due to pernicious anemia. Patient is happily married; his wife is in good health. He has three adult children and six grandchildren who keep him very busy. All are in good health.

O: The patient has marked bradycardia and normal blood pressure. He has some mild PVCs with irregularity in the rhythm; however, this appears to be sinus rhythm. The lungs are clear. There is no peripheral edema. He is generally unsteady in his gait. His right arm abrasion is healing well; the left arm abrasion is fresh and appears to be healthy and appropriately dressed at this time. The skin tag on his neck is irritated and loose. The area was anesthetized with 1% lidocaine, and the skin tag was excised. The skin was cauterized and a bandage applied.

A: Multiple forearm abrasions due to instability and falling.
Bradycardia.

Skin tag on neck.
Vitamin B$_{12}$ deficiency due to pernicious anemia.
Requests flu shot.

P: Vitamin B$_{12}$ injection given. Flu shot given. Decrease Toprol to 50 mg daily. Keep neck area clean and dry for 48 hours. Return as needed.

Procedure statements to be coded:

1. E/M service (CPT)

2. Skin tag removal (CPT)

3. Vitamin B$_{12}$ injection (CPT—HCPCS Level II)

4. Flu vaccination (CPT—HCPCS Level II)

Diagnostic statements to be coded:

1. Bradycardia (ICD-10-CM)

2. Arm abrasion due to fall (ICD-10-CM)

3. Pernicious anemia (ICD-10-CM)

4. Prophylactic flu vaccination (ICD-10-CM)

5. Skin tag, neck (ICD-10-CM)

Coding Credentials

In addition to the American Health Information Management Association (AHIMA) credentials of Registered Health Information Administrator (RHIA) and Registered Health Information Technician (RHIT), several credentials specific to the coding field are available to coding professionals.

Certified Coding Associate (CCA): An AHIMA credential awarded to individuals who have demonstrated entry-level coding expertise in a variety of settings, by passing a certification examination.

Certified Coding Specialist (CCS): An AHIMA credential awarded to individuals who have demonstrated skill in classifying medical data from patient records, generally in the hospital setting, by passing a certification examination.

Certified Coding Specialist—Physician-based (CCS–P): An AHIMA credential awarded to individuals who have demonstrated coding expertise in physician-based settings, such as group practices, by passing a certification examination.

Certified Professional Coder (CPC): An American Academy of Professional Coders (AAPC) credential awarded to individuals who have demonstrated coding proficiency by passing a certification examination.

Exercise 1.1. Introduction to Coding Basics

Choose the best answer for each of the following questions.

1. Which code set is used to describe new and emerging technologies?
   a. Category I codes
   b. Category II codes
   c. Category III codes
   d. HCPCS Level II codes

2. Which system is used to code medications, supplies, and durable medical equipment provided in a physician office?
   a. CPT
   b. HCPCS Level II
   c. ICD-10-CM, Volumes 1 and 2
   d. ICD-10-PCS

3. Which form contains information that substantiates treatment given in the physician office on today's visit?
   a. Problem list
   b. Medical history
   c. Physical examination
   d. Progress notes

4. Code 3120F represents which type of code?
   a. HCPCS Level II
   b. CPT Category I
   c. CPT Category II
   d. CPT Category III

Identify the section of the CPT code book in which the following codes are located.

5. 21310 _____

6. 70486 _____

7. 99232 _____

8. 00840 _____

9. 96401 _____

Fill in the blanks.

10. The ● symbol, or filled-in dot, means that this code _____ _____.

11. The (▲) symbol, or pyramid/triangle, means that the _____ has been _____.

12. The ⊘ symbol indicates that the _____ modifier does not apply.

Exercise 1.1. (Continued)

13. The (▶◀) symbol signifies _____ or _____ coding notes.

14. The + symbol indicates that this is a(n) _____-___ code.

Fill in the blanks.

Refer to the notes immediately preceding code 45300 and the code series 45300–45398.

15. True or false? Surgical endoscopy always includes a diagnostic endoscopy. _____

16. Which type of examination may include the terminal ileum? _____

17. What code would be used for a sigmoidoscopy with removal of a polyp by the snare technique? _____

18. What code would be used for a diagnostic proctosigmoidoscopy with brushings?
_____

19. What action should the coder take when an entry such as the following is seen in the Index: 42810–42815?
    a. Assign both codes listed in the Index.
    b. Assign the first code listed in the Index.
    c. Review the codes in the Tabular to find the best code.
    d. Query the physician regarding which code to assign.

20. What is the complete description of code 27333?
    _____

Chapter 1 Test

Choose the best answer for each of the following questions.

1. The physician orders a throat culture to rule out strep throat because the patient has a fever, sore throat, and lymphadenopathy. What diagnosis(es) would be submitted with the claim for the throat culture?
   a. Fever, sore throat, and lymphadenopathy
   b. Fever and sore throat
   c. Fever and strep throat
   d. Strep throat

2. The correct description of CPT code 44370 is:
   a. Small intestinal endoscopy, enteroscopy beyond second portion of duodenum, not including ileum; with transendoscopic stent placement (includes predilation)
   b. Small intestinal endoscopy, enteroscopy beyond second portion of duodenum, not including ileum; diagnostic, with or without collection of specimen(s) by brushing or washing (separate procedure)
   c. Small intestinal endoscopy, enteroscopy beyond second portion of duodenum, not including ileum; diagnostic, with or without collection of specimen(s) by brushing or washing, with transendoscopic stent placement (includes predilation)
   d. With transendoscopic stent placement (includes predilation)

(Continued on next page)

Chapter 1 Test (Continued)

3. When completing a yearly code update on data collection forms, what source(s) could best help this process?
   a. Appendix B of CPT
   b. Appendix B and the Tabular of CPT
   c. Appendix L
   d. Appendix L and the Tabular of CPT

4. Vital signs assessed by the physician are part of which type of data in the health record?
   a. Administrative data
   b. Assessment data
   c. Objective/examination data
   d. Subjective/history data

5. The physician develops a new technique for performing a procedure that is not currently described in the CPT or HCPCS book. How should the coder code this case?
   a. Ask the physician to select the code that most closely describes the procedure.
   b. Select the code number designated in that section for unlisted procedures.
   c. Select code 99199 to describe the procedure.
   d. Send a letter to the insurance carrier asking for advice on how to code the procedure.

6. Which coding system would be used to code the following statement: "Penicillin G potassium, up to 600,000 units"?
   a. CPT
   b. ICD-10-CM
   c. HCPCS
   d. Place of Service

7. What type of code is 0387T, Transcatheter insertion or replacement of permanent leadless pacemaker, ventricular?
   a. HCPCS code Level I code
   b. CPT Category I code
   c. CPT Category II code
   d. CPT Category III code

8. What type of action would the coder take when an entry such as the following is seen in the Index: 27310, 27330, 27403?
   a. Assign all of the codes listed in the Index.
   b. Review the codes in the Tabular to find the best code.
   c. Assign the first code listed in the Index.
   d. Consult the physician to determine which code to assign.

9. In which section of CPT is code 99605 found?
   a. Radiology
   b. Pathology and Laboratory
   c. Medicine
   d. Evaluation and Management

10. The lightning bolt symbol (⚡) represents what information in the CPT book?
    a. A new code has been added for the current year.
    b. The code includes moderate sedation.
    c. The code is exempt from modifier –51 usage.
    d. The code is for a vaccine that is pending FDA approval.

Chapter 2

Evaluation and Management Coding

Objectives

Upon completion of this chapter, the student should be able to do the following:

- Understand the definitions pertaining to evaluation and management (E/M) services

- Apply knowledge of E/M services guidelines to locate the correct code for the level of service provided during the encounter or visit

- Understand and apply modifiers to codes for E/M services

This chapter discusses the evaluation and management (E/M) section of the CPT code book. The E/M section requires a thorough understanding of CPT guidelines and the ability to interpret and understand the documentation provided by physicians and other qualified healthcare professionals. In addition, it requires that coders be aware of any payer-specific guidelines that may affect coding. For the purposes of this text, the word "physician" should be interpreted to mean "physician or other qualified healthcare professional."

The various levels of the E/M codes describe the wide variations in skill, effort, time, responsibility, and medical knowledge required for the prevention, diagnosis, and treatment of illness or injury, and the promotion of optimal health.

The basic format of E/M service codes consists of five elements:

1. Are listed by unique code numbers beginning with 99

2. Generally identify the place or type of service (for example, office or other outpatient service, initial or subsequent hospital care)

3. Define the content, extent, or level of the service (for example, detailed history or detailed examination)

4. Describe the nature of the presenting problem (for example, moderate severity)

5. Identify the time typically required to provide a service

Documentation Guidelines

Documentation is the basis for all coding, including E/M services. In 1995, the American Medical Association (AMA) and the Centers for Medicare and Medicaid Services (CMS) implemented documentation guidelines to clarify E/M code assignment for both physicians and claims reviewers. These basic guidelines provided a framework for physician documentation that supported the codes chosen for billing. Although they described the necessary elements in greater detail than the profession had seen previously, they still left far too much to interpretation. Physicians and claims reviewers often differ widely on the extent of documentation needed to fully support a chosen code.

In 1997, CMS (formerly known as the Health Care Financing Administration [HCFA]) and the AMA collaborated on a revised edition of the documentation guidelines that delineated specific elements to be performed and documented for general multisystem and selected single-specialty examinations. However, these guidelines were not implemented as expected in 1998. CMS and the AMA continue to work on a mutually accepted set of guidelines that meets both payer and provider requirements for professional service coding levels.

The purpose and content of these guidelines will become clear in the course of this chapter. The 1995 and 1997 documentation guidelines are presented in online appendix F. The 1995 guidelines are used as the basis for the majority of instruction and examples in this text, although some pertinent comparisons are provided.

Both the 1995 and 1997 guidelines are acceptable for use in determining an E/M code. There is no need to standardize the usage of one method over the other. In fact, when coding, physicians are encouraged to use the set of guidelines that is most advantageous for that particular visit. For example, the 1997 guidelines can be more beneficial to physicians in specialties that have a specific exam identified, such as ophthalmology, orthopedics, dermatology, or psychiatry. Physicians in these specialties typically have a much more difficult time using the generalized examination criteria of the 1995 guidelines to achieve a code that appropriately compensates them for their work. However, physicians in primary care specialties completing generalized exams frequently find the simplicity of the 1995 guidelines much easier to understand and to memorize.

When submitting insurance claims for payment, physicians use E/M codes to report professional services rendered to patients. Their documentation must support the charges (CPT) and diagnoses (ICD-10-CM) submitted. Each CPT code or service has a unique dollar amount assigned. Periodically, payers conduct audits to verify that the charges submitted are accurate. In addition, an ICD-10-CM code must be assigned to its highest level of specificity. Many payers have edit systems that deny or reject claims if the highest level of specificity of a diagnosis code is not submitted. Submitting a code that is not supported in the health record may constitute fraud and abuse. Fraud and abuse cases carry stiff penalties, including fines and imprisonment.

Careful understanding of the rules and guidelines is essential to correct E/M code assignment or validation. Moreover, physicians and coders must work together to ensure that clinical documentation substantiates the level of service code assigned. Physicians who understand these guidelines and perform quality and validation reviews will help prevent allegations of fraud or billing abuse during health plan audits.

Chapter 12 of this book continues the discussion of fraud and abuse and describes how to complete documentation reviews to improve physician documentation and charge submission accuracy.

Evaluation and Management Services

Although E/M codes begin with the number 99201, which places them at the end of the CPT numbering sequence, they are found at the front of the CPT code book. Coders should review and become familiar with the E/M services guidelines in *CPT*. These guidelines are the backbone of the E/M section and should be applied to all of its subsections.

E/M codes are divided into broad categories based on the type of service or the type of location in which the E/M service was performed.

Terms Commonly Used in Reporting E/M Services

The E/M services guidelines contain definitions of certain key terms in order to reduce the potential for differing interpretations and to increase consistency in reporting E/M codes by physicians in different specialties. Three of these terms—new patient, established patient, and concurrent care—are discussed here.

New or Established Patient

The definitions of new patient and established patient have been modified over time. In these definitions, professional services are those face-to-face services rendered by physicians and other qualified healthcare professionals who may report evaluation and management services reported by a specific CPT code(s).

- A new patient is one who *has not* received any face-to-face professional services from the physician or qualified healthcare professional, or another physician or qualified healthcare professional of the exact same specialty and subspecialty who belongs to the same group practice, within the past three years.

- An established patient is one who *has* received professional services from the physician or qualified healthcare professional, or another physician or qualified healthcare professional of the exact same specialty and subspecialty who belongs to the same group practice, within the past three years.

When the physician is on call or covering for another physician, the patient's encounter is classified in the same manner as if the physician had been available. When a physician sees a patient in the hospital (for example, a newborn) and the patient then presents to the clinic, the patient is considered an established patient upon his or her first encounter with the physician at the clinic.

Coders should note that the following E/M services are the only categories that provide separate code ranges to identify new and established patients: Office or Other Outpatient Services; Domiciliary, Rest Home, or Custodial Services; Home Services; and Preventive Medicine Services.

Concurrent Care

When two or more physicians provide similar services (for example, hospital visits or consultations) to the same patient on the same day, the CPT code book defines this as concurrent care. Health plans often limit reimbursement to one physician per day unless the physicians have different specialties and the services of more than one physician are medically necessary. Correct assignment of ICD-10-CM codes plays an important role in billing and receiving payment for concurrent care services. The physicians involved in the concurrent care episode must identify the appropriate ICD-10-CM code for each service provided.

> **Example:** Patient is admitted to the hospital complaining of unstable angina and uncontrolled type 2 diabetes mellitus. Dr. Smith treats the patient's angina, and Dr. Reynolds follows the patient's diabetes. The following codes should be reported:
>
> Dr. Smith: I20.0, Intermediate coronary syndrome, and the appropriate E/M level of service code from the hospital inpatient services category
>
> Dr. Reynolds: E11.65, Diabetes mellitus, type II, with hyperglycemia and the appropriate E/M level of service from the hospital inpatient services category

Levels of E/M Services

Each of the E/M categories and subcategories have been assessed and broken down into several levels of service to be used for reporting purposes. These levels are based on the extent and type of treatment provided in various settings, and they correspond with the physician resources (skill, effort, knowledge, time, responsibility, and so forth) expended in providing the service. Before an E/M service code can be assigned, three questions must be considered:

- What type of service is the patient receiving? Initial or subsequent care? Consultation? Critical care?

- What is the place of service? Physician's office or clinic? Hospital inpatient or outpatient department? Emergency department? Nursing facility or rehabilitation unit?

- Is the patient new or established?

Components in Selecting the Level of E/M Service

Seven components, applicable to the entire spectrum of E/M services, must be considered before selecting a code and should be available in the associated documentation:

History Examination Medical decision making	Key Components
Counseling Coordination of care Nature of presenting problem Time	Contributing Components

History, examination, and medical decision making are the key components, or essential factors, that must be considered first when selecting an E/M service code. The key components represent services that are provided at one level or another at every patient encounter. When applicable, the remaining four components are factored in. Documentation in the health record must support code-level selection by describing the key components and the pertinent contributing factors. Physician selection of E/M codes is recommended to ensure clinical validity for service levels. Coders may verify code selection with documentation and assist physicians in meeting the current guidelines for code selection.

Appendix C of the CPT code book includes a supplement of clinical examples illustrating the appropriate selection of E/M service codes for specific medical specialties. However, these examples are only guidelines and the documentation in the health record remains the final source when reporting a particular level of service code.

The CPT code book defines each level of E/M service by basing it on a unique combination of the three key components. The combination of the key components that defines an E/M service for Office or Other Outpatient Services, Established Patient, is reflected in the following table.

Code	History	Examination	Medical Decision Making
99211	Minimal service (not requiring the presence of a physician)		
99212	Problem focused	Problem focused	Straightforward
99213	Expanded problem focused	Expanded problem focused	Low complexity
99214	Detailed	Detailed	Moderate complexity
99215	Comprehensive	Comprehensive	High complexity

Five codes can be used to report services provided to an established patient in the office or other outpatient setting. Each of these codes represents a different level of service, based on the extent or type of history, examination, and medical decision making provided to the patient in this particular setting.

A physician who consistently reports the same level of service for all patient encounters may look suspicious to claims auditors. With the exception of certain specialists, physicians treat all types of patients in their offices, and office treatment requires use of most of the levels of E/M. The level selected depends on the work done and the resources expended in providing the services. This concept is discussed further in chapter 12.

Each category of E/M service may require that a different number of the key components be considered when determining the level of service. Some categories require the history, examination, and medical decision making for a given encounter to meet or exceed a given level to bill for that level of service. Others require that only two of the three key components meet or exceed the stated requirements to qualify for a particular level of service. As this chapter presents each E/M category, the text indicates whether two of the three key components or all three key components must meet or exceed the requirements stated in the code descriptor to qualify for a specific level of service.

A detailed discussion of each of the key components and how they are used in determining a level of service follows. The levels of service may be thought of as building blocks, as the documentation required for each level builds from the previous level.

History

The history component consists of documentation of some or all of the following:

- Chief complaint

- History of the present illness

- Review of systems

- Past medical, family, and social history

Chief Complaint

The CPT code book defines the chief complaint as a "concise statement describing the symptom, problem, condition, diagnosis, or other factor that is the reason for the encounter, usually stated in the patient's words" (AMA 2015).

History of the Present Illness

The level of the history of the present illness (HPI) is distinguished by the amount of detail that is documented. The HPI is defined as brief or extended based on how many of the eight elements, as defined in table 2.1, are documented. A brief HPI will have one to three elements documented; an extended HPI will have four or more elements documented.

Review of Systems

The review of systems (ROS) is an inventory of body systems obtained through a series of questions asked of patients that may identify signs and symptoms they may be experiencing or have experienced in the past. The recognized body systems are listed in the front of the CPT code book in the E/M service guidelines section. Items of ROS can also be found under the heading of history and counted as part of the ROS. However, the same item may not be counted in both sections.

Three levels of review are considered when determining the level of ROS documented:

- Problem-pertinent ROS, which entails review of one body system that is related directly to the presenting problem

- Extended ROS, which involves review of the body systems that are related directly to the presenting problem as well as additional body systems, for a total of two to nine body systems

- Complete ROS, which includes review of 10 or more body systems

Table 2.1.   Elements of the history of the present illness

HPI Element	Definition	Example
Location	Where on the body the symptom is occurring	Leg, head, arm, abdomen
Quality	Characteristics, grade	Burning, gnawing, stabbing, fullness, nagging
Severity	How hard it is to endure; rank from 1 to 10	Severe, slightly worse, worst I've ever had, mild, intense
Duration	How long; length of time	2 days, past month, over the past few hours
Timing	When it occurs	At night, after meals, after or during exercise, intermittent, frequent
Context	Situation associated with the symptom	Big meal, since beginning a walking program, after sitting
Modifying factors	Things that make symptoms worse or better	Took Tylenol and pain was less, lay down and slept for awhile
Associated signs and symptoms	What else happens when this symptom is present	Chest pain leads to shortness of breath, feeling of chills

The physician may document those systems that have findings and state "All others reviewed and are negative" if the patient denies any other issues. This qualifies the visit for a complete review of systems. Check with your Medicare contractor to see if this statement is allowed.

Past Medical, Family, and Social History

Two levels of documentation are considered when determining the level of past medical, family, and social history:

- Pertinent, which includes at least one item from one of the areas of past history

- Complete, which entails at least two specifics from at least two history areas documented for an established or emergency patient or discussion of all three areas of the past history for a new patient

Bringing all of these individual parts of the history together is demonstrated in the grid in table 2.2. The E/M service levels recognize four types of history (problem focused, expanded problem focused, detailed, or comprehensive). The history component is equal to the lowest type of history documented in the health record.

Table 2.2. Breakdown of history component

History Component (equal to lowest category documented)	Problem Focused	Exp. Problem Focused	Detailed	Comprehensive
Chief Complaint _____ HPI—History of Present Illness __ Location __ Duration __ Severity __ Quality __ Context __ Timing __ Modifying factors __ Associated signs and symptoms	Brief 1–3 HPI elements documented	Brief 1–3 HPI elements documented	Extended ≥ 4 HPI elements documented	Extended ≥ 4 HPI elements documented
ROS—Review of System(s) __ Constitutional (wt loss, etc.) __ Integumentary __ Eyes __ GI __ Endocrine __ ENT, Mouth __ GU __ Hem/lymph __ Respiratory __ MS __ Allergy/Immun __ Cardiovasc __ Neuro __ Psychiatric __ All others negative	None	Problem Specific (1 system)	Extended (2–9 systems)	Complete (Greater than 10 systems or some with all others negative)
PFSH (past medical, family, and social histories) __ Previous medical (past experience with illness, injury, surgery, medical treatments, etc.) __ Family medical history (diseases which may be hereditary or with increased risk of occurrence) __ Social (relationships, diet, exercise, occupation, etc.)	None	None	Pertinent At least 1 item from at least 1 history	Complete Specifics of at least 2 history areas documented Initial = all 3

Examination

The examination component is the second of the three key components used to determine a level of E/M service. The level of examination is determined by the number of body areas or organ systems documented. It should be noted that any body area or organ system can be documented for the visit to qualify for a detailed examination. A comprehensive examination requires an exam of eight body systems (body areas do not qualify for a comprehensive exam). The examination component is also equal to the lowest type of examination (problem focused, expanded problem focused, detailed, or comprehensive) documented in the patient's health record. Table 2.3 shows a breakdown of this component when using the 1995 guidelines. Table 2.4 shows a comparison of the Examination Component in the 1995 and 1997 guidelines.

Table 2.3. Breakdown of examination component

Exam Component	Problem Focused	Exp. Problem Focused	Detailed	Comprehensive

Body Areas   Organ Systems
 __ Head, Face   __ Const.
 __ Neck   (Vitals, Gen. appear)
 __ Chest,   __ Eyes   __ GU
 Breasts   __ ENT,   __ Integ
 __ Abdomen   mouth   (skin)
 __ Genit   __ Respirat   __ MS
 Groin   __ Cardio   __ Neuro
 __ Back, Spine   __ Gastro   __ Psych
 __ Each Extrem   __ Lymph/
   Hem/
   Immun
	1 body area or system	2–4 body systems incl. affected area or 2–7 basic body areas and/or organ systems	5–7 detailed systems incl. affected area or 2–7 body areas and/or organ systems with one in detail	8 or more systems

Table 2.4. Comparison of examination key component in 1995 and 1997 guidelines

Level of Examination	1995 Guidelines	1997 General Multisystem Examination	1997 Single Organ System (except Eye and Psych) Examinations	1997 Eye and Psychiatric Examinations
Problem Focused	At least 1 Body Area or Organ System	1 to 5 Elements	1 to 5 Elements	1 to 5 Elements
Expanded Problem Focused	2–4 OR 2–7 Basic Body Areas and/or Organ Systems	At least 6 Elements	At least 6 Elements	At least 6 Elements
Detailed	5–7 OR 2–7 Body Areas and/or Organ System with One in Detail	At least 2 Elements from each of 6 Areas/Systems or at least 12 Elements in 2 or more Areas/Systems	At least 12 Elements	At least 9 Elements
Comprehensive	8 out of 12 Organ Systems	At least 2 Elements from Each of 9 Areas/Systems	All Bulleted Elements in shaded boxes plus 1 Element in each unshaded box	All Bulleted Elements in shaded boxes plus 1 Element in each unshaded box

Not all Medicare contractors interpret the requirements for Expanded Problem Focused and Detailed exams in the same way. Table 2.3 displays both methods currently in use in the industry. Check with your Medicare contractor to determine their requirements.

Medical Decision Making

Medical decision making is the third key component used in determining a level of service. Medical decision making can be a subjective area, which makes it one of the most difficult components to determine. There are four types of medical decision making: straightforward, low complexity, moderate complexity, or high complexity. The type of medical decision making is determined by the following:

- The number of possible diagnoses and/or the number of management options that must be considered

- The amount and/or complexity of medical records, diagnostic tests, and/or other information that must be obtained, reviewed, and analyzed

- The risk of significant complications, morbidity, and/or mortality, as well as comorbidities associated with the patient's presenting problem(s), the diagnostic procedure(s), and/or the possible management options

Table 2.5 illustrates the factors that comprise the medical decision-making process. Results from the three tables are combined to calculate the medical decision making element.

Box A describes the number of diagnoses or treatment options. The number of problems that the patient presents with will determine the score on this table. Self-limited or minor problems, such as sunburn or a minor rash, provide one point. Points are allowed for a maximum of two self-limited or minor problems. Problems that are established to the examiner and are stable or improved provide one point each. If the established problem is worsening, then two points are assigned for each. New problems to the examiner that don't require any workup

Table 2.5. Factors in the medical decision-making process

A. Number of Diagnoses or Tx Options		
Categories of Problem	**# × Points = Subtotal**	
Self-limited or minor; stable, improved, or worsening	1	(max = 2)
Established problem (to examiner); stable, improved	1	
Established problem (to examiner); worsening	2	
New problem (to examiner); no additional workup planned	3	
New problem (to examiner); additional workup planned	4	
	Total	

B. Amount/Complexity of Data Reviewed	
Categories of Data Reviewed	
Order and/or review clinical lab tests	1
Order and/or review tests from radiology section	1
Order and/or review tests from medicine section (i.e., EKG, EMG, allergy tests, audiometry)	1
Discussion of test results with performing provider	1
Decision to obtain old records/Obtain history from other than patient/Discuss case with other provider	2
Independent visualization of image, tracing, or report	2
Total	

C. Complication Risk Factor(s) (select highest assigned to any category)			
Level of Risk	**Presenting Problem**	**Dx Procedures Ordered**	**Management Options Selected**
Minimal	• One self-limited or minor problem	• Lab tests, x-rays, EKG, EEG	• Rest, superficial dressings, none required
Low	• Multiple self-limited or minor problems • One stable chronic illness • Acute, uncomplicated illness or injury	• Physiologic tests w/o stress • Imaging studies w/contrast • Superficial needle biopsy • Skin biopsy • Arterial blood draw	• Over-the-counter remedy • Minor surgery w/o risk factor • Physical, occupational therapy • IV fluids w/o additive
Moderate	• One or more chronic illness with exacerbation, progression, or treatment side effects • Two or more chronic stable illnesses • Undiagnosed new problem with uncertain prognosis • Acute complicated injury • Acute illness with systemic symptoms	• Stress tests • Endoscopies w/o risk factors • Cardiovascular imaging study w/o identified risk factor • Deep needle or incisional biopsy • Centesis of body cavity fluid	• Minor surgery with identified risk factors • Elective major surgery without identified risk factors • Prescription drug management • Therapeutic radiology • IV fluids with additives • Closed treatment of skeletal injury
High	• One or more chronic illnesses with severe exacerbation, progression, or treatment side effects • Acute or chronic illness or injury that may pose a threat to life or bodily functions • An abrupt change to mental status	• Cardiovascular imaging studies with identified risk factors • Cardiac electrophysiological tests • Endoscopy with identified risk factors	• Elective major surgery with identified risk factors • Emergency major surgery • Parenteral-controlled substance • Drug therapy requiring intensive monitoring • DNR status

D. Medical Decision Making (MDM) (Highest 2 out of 3)		**Straightforward**	**Low Complexity**	**Moderate Complexity**	**High Complexity**
A	Diagnoses/Management Options	Minimal (≤1)	Limited (2)	Multiple (3)	Extensive (≥4)
B	Amount/Complexity of Data	Min/Low (≤1)	Limited (2)	Moderate (3)	Extensive (≥4)
C	Highest Risk (highest from any category)	Minimal	Low	Moderate	High

(treatment may be provided but there is no planned testing or further investigation) provide three points each. A new problem that requires additional workup provides four points.

Box B describes the amount and/or complexity of data that need to be ordered or reviewed at the visit. One point is assigned for any amount of orders or data reviewed in the categories of clinical lab tests, radiology section tests (plain films, CT, MRI, and ultrasound) and medicine section tests (EKG, EMG, allergy, audiometry, and pulmonary). One point is also provided for discussing test results with the performing provider such as Pathology or Radiology. Two points are provided for the decision to obtain old records, obtaining history from someone other the patient, and independent visualization of an image or tracing.

Box C is also referred to as the Table of Risk. To determine the level of risk with the table, the physician or coder should select the one statement from any column that best describes the clinical picture of the patient on that visit. Frequently used statements are "Prescription drug management" from the Management Options column (moderate risk) or "One stable chronic illness with severe exacerbation, progression or treatment side effects" from the Presenting Problem column (high risk), but any statement that describes the patient can be assigned, if it applies. The statement with the highest value determines the result for Table C.

Box D shows the determination of the medical decision making component. When the results of two out of the three tables (criteria) meet or exceed a level, that level is assigned.

Example 1: Box A = 3 points (or multiple problems)
Box B = 1 point (or minimal/low)
Box C = moderate

The result is moderate complexity decision making because two criteria meet the requirements in the column for moderate.

Example 2: Box A = 2 points (or limited)
Box B = 2 points (or limited)
Box C = moderate

The result is low complexity decision making because two criteria meet or exceed the requirements in the column for low.

By combining all of the information from these three key components (history, examination and medical decision making), the physician and the coding professional are able to determine the level of E/M service provided. Table 2.6 shows the E/M levels for the office or other outpatient services category. The three key components are used to determine the level of service for any type of E/M service. The case example in figure 2.1 illustrates how the correct level of E/M service is derived from

Table 2.6.   E/M levels for office and other outpatient services

Selection of E/M Level Based on Above Components												
Established Patient (requires 2 of 3 elements)						New Patient or Consultation (requires 3 of 3 elements)						
			E/M—Office/OP						E/M Office/OP		E/M OP Consult	
History	Exam	MDM	Min	Level		History	Exam	MDM	Min	Level	Min	Level
Min service, may not require MD			5	99211		PF	PF	SF	10	99201	15	99241
PF	PF	SF	10	99212		EPF	EPF	SF	20	99202	30	99242
EPF	EPF	Low	15	99213		Det	Det	Low	30	99203	40	99243
Det	Det	Mod	25	99214		Comp	Comp	Mod	45	99204	60	99244
Comp	Comp	High	40	99215		Comp	Comp	High	60	99205	80	99245

Figure 2.1.   Case example

Dr. Williams documents the following information after seeing an established patient, Fred Fuller, in the office.

S: Fred presents today complaining of headaches. Review of his chart reveals that he has had intermittent complaints of headaches for some time. Some of these have been thought to be related to overexertion in the sun and some possibly consistent with migraine or caffeine withdrawal. Patient states he has decreased his cola consumption considerably. He has most recently been working on the weekends and not sleeping late. Has onset now of headache for the past 2 days, which is associated with phonophobia, photophobia, and nausea. Has been taking Tylenol, Ibuprofen 600 mg per dose, and Excedrin Migraine, without significant improvement. He was seen by his chiropractor on Tuesday with some adjustments made on the day of onset of headache. Seen again yesterday, and chiropractor was unable to find any muscle alignment to explain his complaints and suggested he may need further workup. Patient is anxious about the headaches because he had a friend whose wife was recently diagnosed with leukemia whose presenting complaint had been headaches. Review of the patient's food intake reveals he had pizza with pepperoni on Sunday and then Monday and Tuesday had beef jerky and M&Ms. Patient has not previously distinguished types of headaches but on review probably has two types of headaches. One is associated with discomfort in the neck and the other is more distinguished by the phonophobia and photophobia. Has not noted any particular food intake to be associated with headaches.

O: Vitals: Ht 5'11"; Wt 173 lbs; BP 104-88; T 98.3; P 64
HEENT: TMs within normal limits. Pupils are equal, round and reactive to light. Fundi are within normal limits. Cup to disc ratio is normal. Throat within normal limits.
Neck: Without lymphadenopathy
Neuro: Finger to nose is within normal limits. Heel to shin reflexes are 2+ and bilaterally symmetrical.

A: Cephalgia. Patient has two types of headaches and the current one seems more characteristic for migraine headache. May have been precipitated by intake of pizza/pepperoni/chocolate.

P: Midrin two tablets p.o. with onset of migraine headache and then on q 1 hour, maximum of 5 per 12 hours; for tension headache, 1–2 tablets q 4–6 hours, maximum 8 per day, #30 with no refills. Had a long discussion about possible dietary contributions to the headache as well as scheduling issues, sleep cycles, etc. Follow-up PRN not improving. Would consider MRI and/or referral to neurology PRN.

Selection of E/M Level of Service

History Component

1. Chief complaint: Recurring headaches

2. History of Present Illness: Extended HPI (four or more elements are documented)

>   Timing: Intermittent for some period of time
>   Duration: Last 2 days
>   Context: Related to overexertion in the sun
>   Associated signs and symptoms: Phonophobia, photophobia, and nausea

3. Review of Systems: Extended ROS (a total of three body systems were evaluated)

>   Constitutional: Fred has not noted any particular food intake associated with his headaches.
>   Musculoskeletal: Two types of headaches are present, one is associated with neck discomfort.
>   Neurological: The other type of headache is distinguished by phonophobia and photophobia.

4. Past Medical, Family, and Social History: Comprehensive PFSH (at least two history areas are documented)

>   Medical: Headaches. Fred sees a chiropractor. Current meds are Excedrin Migraine. Allergies: NKDA
>   (The current meds and allergies are documented in the nursing assessment.)
>   Social: Fred works weekends. His friend's wife recently was diagnosed with leukemia with presenting complaint of headache.

Dr. Williams has documented an extended HPI, an extended ROS, and a comprehensive PFSH. According to table 2.2, Breakdown of history component, this documentation constitutes a detailed history component.

Examination Component

A review of the documentation reveals that Dr. Williams examined four body areas or organ systems (HEENT, eyes, neck, neurological). According to table 2.3, Breakdown of examination component, this documentation supports a detailed examination component.

Figure 2.1.   (Continued)

Medical Decision-Making Component

1. Number of diagnoses or treatment options: Fred's headaches were an established problem to Dr. Williams, although he found them worsening. According to table 2.5, A, the diagnoses/management options are limited (2) or of low complexity.

2. Amount/complexity of data to be reviewed: None were reviewed. Therefore, according to table 2.5, B, this factor would be considered minimal/low or straightforward.

3. Level of risk: Dr. Williams documented that Fred was experiencing two types of headache of a chronic nature, with exacerbation, progression, or treatment side effects. No diagnostic procedures were ordered. The management option selected was the prescription of Midrin. Therefore, according to table 2.5, C, the level of risk factor would be rated as of moderate complexity.

According to table 2.5, D, when the three elements of medical decision making are each assigned a different level (straightforward, low complexity, and moderate complexity), the middle level is assigned. Therefore, the documentation in Fred Fuller's case supports medical decision making of low complexity.

Selection of E/M Level of Service

According to table 2.6, E/M levels for office and other outpatient services, documentation supports a detailed level of service, code 99214, as indicated below in bold type. With an established patient, only two of the three key components need to be met at a specific level.

CPT Code	History	Examination	Medical Decision Making
99211	Minimal service		
99212	Problem focused	Problem focused	Straightforward
99213	Expanded problem focused	Expanded problem focused	**Low complexity**
99214	**Detailed**	**Detailed**	Moderate complexity
99215	Comprehensive	Comprehensive	High complexity

---

the clinical data in a patient's health record. Some Medicare contractors utilize a different point scale. Check with your Medicare contractor to determine the point scale requirements currently in use.

Time as a Factor in Selecting the Level of E/M Service

To determine whether time is the key, or controlling, factor that qualifies a particular level of E/M service, the coder should carefully review the final section of E/M guidelines in the CPT code book, titled "Select the Appropriate Level of E/M Services Based on the Following." A common coding error occurs when time is used as the only factor in selecting an E/M code.

Although physicians may feel most comfortable with the component of time, coding by time alone is inaccurate unless counseling or coordination of care dominates the visit (that is, it takes up more than 50 percent of the visit). Documentation guidelines require that documentation in the patient record clearly specify the amount of time spent on counseling and coordination of care in order for this component to be supported and used as the determining factor in selecting the E/M level of service.

When coding based on time, the physician should report both the time spent counseling and the total time of the visit. The E/M level should be chosen based on the total time of the visit. Table 2.6 on page 49 shows the minutes associated with each level of new and established office visit for reference in choosing the level based on time.

Modifiers

As discussed in both chapter 1 and in greater detail in chapter 9, modifiers are two-digit additions to the CPT code that enable physicians to describe special circumstances that may affect a service or procedure. Appending a modifier to an E/M service does not guarantee reimbursement. Reimbursement is determined by multiple factors and, ultimately, is at the discretion of the insurance payer.

Modifiers Available for Use with E/M Services Codes

Following are some of the most frequently used modifiers for E/M services. It is important to note that HCPCS Level II modifiers also may need to be applied. (Examples of modifiers that apply to different E/M categories are provided in the next section.)

–24 **Unrelated Evaluation and Management Service by the Same Physician or Other Qualified Health Care Professional during a Postoperative Period:** Modifier –24 can be reported with an E/M service provided during the postoperative period by the same physician who performed the original procedure. However, the E/M service must be unrelated to the condition for which the original procedure was performed.

> **Example:** An office visit is provided to a patient who is in the postoperative period for a cholecystectomy performed three weeks earlier. The patient's current complaint is a possible infection of a finger that was lacerated four days earlier. The physician may report the appropriate office visit code and attach modifier –24 to identify this activity as an unrelated service provided during the postoperative period of the cholecystectomy.

–25 **Significant, Separately Identifiable Evaluation and Management Service by the Same Physician or Other Qualified Health Care Professional on the Day of a Procedure or Other Service:** Modifier –25 may be reported to indicate that the patient's condition required a separate E/M service on the day a procedure or other service was performed because the care provided went beyond the usual procedures associated with the activity. The E/M service may be prompted by the symptom or condition for which the procedure and/or service was provided. As such, different diagnoses are not required for reporting of the E/M services on the same date. Modifier –25 is appropriate with procedures that Medicare designates as "minor," which are generally those with a ten-day global fee period or zero-day global fee. Chapter 4 discusses the global surgical concept in detail.

> **Example:** An office visit is provided to a patient for evaluation of diabetes and associated chronic renal failure, as well as a mole on the arm that has increased

in size. Suspecting that the mole is malignant, the physician excises it. The pathology report confirms a 1.1-cm malignant lesion. The physician can bill for the malignant lesion removal and use the office visit code accompanied by modifier –25 to identify that a separate condition—in this example, the diabetes and the renal failure—was addressed during the visit. Generally, two diagnosis codes are required to explain the reporting of two separate services during the same encounter, although CPT guidelines do not require it.

–32   **Mandated Services:** Modifier –32 is reported when someone, such as a third-party payer, quality improvement organization, or governmental, legislative or regulatory requirement mandates a service. This modifier is reported most often when a patient is sent for a consultation.

–55   **Postoperative Management Only:** When one physician or other qualified health care professional performs the postoperative management and another physician has performed the surgical procedure.

–56   **Preoperative Management Only:** Modifier –56 should be reported when one physician or other qualified health care professional performs the preoperative care, such as surgical clearance, and another physician performs the surgical procedure.

–57   **Decision for Surgery:** Modifier –57 is reported along with the appropriate E/M services code when an E/M service results in the initial decision to perform surgery on a patient. It is appropriate to use this modifier with procedures that Medicare designates as "major," which are generally those with a 90-day global period assigned. Generally, it is not required when the decision for surgery occurs at a time earlier than the day of or before surgery. Some insurance plans include consultation and/or visit codes when the decision is made in the global period for surgery and do not provide separate payment.

      Example: An office visit is provided to a Medicare patient with complaints of acute right upper-quadrant pain and tenderness to the right scapula, nausea and vomiting, and anorexia. A low-grade fever and an elevated white blood count are noted. An ultrasound confirms the diagnosis of acute cholecystitis with cholelithiasis (gallbladder disease). The physician recommends that surgery be performed later that day. The physician can report the appropriate visit code along with modifier –57 to identify that, during this visit, it was decided to perform a cholecystectomy (removal of the gallbladder).

HCPCS Level II Modifiers

HCPCS Level II modifiers are not reported as frequently as CPT modifiers are, but they are important to consider when identifying the service provided. HCPCS Level II modifiers include:

–FP   Service provided as part of a family planning program

–GC   Service performed in part by a resident under the direction of a teaching physician

–GE   Service performed by a resident without the presence of a teaching physician under the primary care exception

–GT   Via interactive audio and video telecommunication systems (Modifier –GT is reported with an E/M service to indicate that the physician performed the service via interactive audio and video telecommunication systems, such as telemedicine.)

–Q5   Service furnished by a substitute physician under a reciprocal billing arrangement

–Q6   Service furnished by a locum tenens physician (A locum tenens physician is a physician who is filling a temporary position or a vacancy and/or who is filling in for a physician on vacation.)

Evaluation and Management Categories

Health record documentation is the source for substantiating the correct E/M category (such as office visit or consultation) and level of visit. To ensure that the appropriate E/M category is used, the guidelines in each subcategory should be reviewed. The following sections discuss each of these categories in varying detail.

Office or Other Outpatient Services

The office or other outpatient services category covers E/M services provided in either the physician's office or an outpatient facility or other ambulatory facility. When a physician provides a service in an urgent care area, he or she reports that service from this category of codes.

Codes 99201–99215 are based on the definitions for new and established patients mentioned earlier. The extent of services documented for all three key components (history, examination, and medical decision making) must meet or exceed the specified requirements to determine the level of new patient visit, whereas the extent of services documented for only two of the three key components must meet or exceed the stated requirements to determine the level of service for an established patient. Table 2.6 shows the documentation requirements for each level of service in this category.

It is important to note that the verbiage in the CPT code book describing the levels of service for new and established patients does not correlate exactly between the two subcategories.

Reporting an office visit code is inappropriate if, during the course of events within a specific encounter, the physician admits the patient into the hospital as an inpatient or an observation patient or into a nursing care facility. Only the resulting admission service should be reported in this situation, and the code selected should incorporate the level of care provided in the office. Only one E/M service code can be submitted per day, per physician. There may be a rare circumstance when the patient receives office services early in the day and then returns later and must be admitted to the hospital from the office. Such a situation would merit the use of modifier –25 to show that the services were separately identifiable.

Coders also should understand when to use CPT code 99211. This is the only E/M office visit code in which the descriptor states "may not require the presence of a physician." Many physician practices report code 99211 incorrectly and lose reimbursement as a result. This code should be used to report those occasions when either the physician or a nurse or technician sees a patient for a minimal service—for example, to perform a medically necessary blood pressure check, weight check, or wound check. Generally, this code is not used when the physician sees the patient.

New Patient

For new patients seen in the office, all three key components of history, exam, and medical decision making must meet or exceed stated requirements to qualify for a given E/M service code.

Example: Martha Peters is visiting friends in a neighboring town and needs to have a prescription filled because she forgot her hay fever medication. Dr. Jones, who is seeing her for the first time, prescribes her medication.

Code 99201 is assigned in this case. Dr. Jones performed a problem-focused history and examination, with straightforward medical decision making (addressing only the hay fever).

Example: The following documentation was charged as a high-level office visit, code 99204:

New patient. Arm pain. Sling applied. Return as needed.

The documentation in the second example does not support a high-level office visit for many reasons, including the following:

- To report a new patient office visit, the documentation must include all three key components (history, examination, and medical decision making) of an E/M service. No exam is documented.

- The history needs to include, at a minimum, the chief complaint and a brief history of the present illness. This example indicates only arm pain as a chief complaint.

- Medical decision making would be implied as straightforward, the lowest level of medical decision making.

Established Patient

For established patients, the requirements differ depending on the level of service. The first level (99211) does not require a history, an exam, or medical decision making. Moreover, it may not require the presence of a physician. However, higher levels of service (99212–99215) specify that at least two of the three key components (history, examination, and medical decision making) meet or exceed the stated requirements to qualify for a given E/M service code.

Example: A 55-year-old male visits his physician, Dr. Smith, complaining of a cough and productive sputum. The physician obtains a history, performs a physical examination, and orders a chest x-ray and laboratory tests. The results reveal a diagnosis of pneumonia in an otherwise healthy patient.

Dr. Smith's history focused on the chief complaint and included a brief history of the problem as well as pertinent system review of the problem. The problem-focused examination involved only the affected organ system. The medical decision making was of low complexity because it included a minimal number of diagnoses and management options, low risk of complications and/or morbidity and mortality, and a limited amount and/or complexity of data to be reviewed. Code 99213 is assigned in this case. At least two of the three key components were met: an expanded problem-focused history, a physical examination, and a medical decision of low complexity.

Modifiers Commonly Used in Reporting Office or Other Outpatient E/M Visit Codes

Several modifiers are commonly used in reporting office or other outpatient E/M visit codes.

Modifier –24 is used to indicate that an E/M service was performed during a postoperative period for a reason unrelated to the original procedure.

Example: When a patient is seen for evaluation of a twisted ankle during his post-operative recovery period for a humeral shaft fracture, modifier –24 is appended to the appropriate established patient E/M office visit code. It is important to keep in mind, however, that the diagnosis code should link to the current problem, which in this case is the twisted ankle.

Modifier –25 is used to indicate that on the day a procedure or service with a separate CPT code was performed, the patient's condition required a significant, separately identifiable E/M service either above and beyond the other service provided or beyond the usual pre- and postoperative care associated with the procedure. The modifier is appended to the appropriate level of service.

Example: A physician performs the history, examination, and medical decision making for a patient suffering from a sinus infection and an infected leg wound. The physician determines that antibiotics are needed for the sinus infection and that a full-thickness skin debridement should be performed immediately to minimize the leg wound infection. In this case, the appropriate E/M service should be coded with modifier –25 and the debridement should be reported with a surgical CPT code. It should be noted that a different diagnosis code is not required for the use of modifier –25.

Modifier –57 is used when the E/M service resulted in the initial decision to perform a surgery.

Example: A patient is seen for evaluation of a bulging, painful abdomen, with a history of previous hernia repairs. Upon examination, the physician identifies another hernia and determines that additional hernia repair surgery is needed. In this case, modifier –57 is appended to the appropriate-level E/M service code. Some Medicare carriers suggest the use of modifier –25 for surgical decisions with a zero- to 10-day global period and reserve modifier –57 for major (90-day) procedures. The coder should check the appropriate third-party payer manual to determine what modifier to use under the circumstance.

Hospital Observation Services

The codes in the hospital observation services category are used to report services provided to a patient designated as an observation patient in a hospital. The patient does not need to be located in an observation area for these codes to be used. The coder should review the guidelines for initial observation care and observation care discharge services. The code descriptor states "per day," which means that all services performed within the day should be accumulated to determine the appropriate level of code to report.

It should be noted that CPT codes 99218–99220 are used for initial observation care, which includes services for the first day of care. Code 99217, Observation care discharge, is used for services on the final day of observation care (as long as it is not the same date as initial care).

When the patient is admitted to observation status during the course of an encounter at another service site (such as a hospital emergency department, a physician's office, or a nursing facility), all E/M services that are performed by the supervising physician on that day and that relate to initiating observation status are considered part of the initial observation care. The level of service reported should reflect all of the E/M services provided at sites other than the hospital.

The codes in this category are not to be used for postoperative recovery if the procedure is considered a global surgical procedure. To qualify for a particular level of service, all three key components must meet or exceed stated requirements as defined within each level.

Code	History	Examination	Medical Decision Making
99218	Detailed or comprehensive	Detailed or comprehensive	Straightforward or low complexity
99219	Comprehensive	Comprehensive	Moderate complexity
99220	Comprehensive	Comprehensive	High complexity

When subsequent observation care is provided on any days other than the initial or discharge observation day (usually the middle day of an observation stay spanning three calendar days), codes 99224–99226 are assigned for this service. Documentation should include changes in the patient's history, physical condition, response to treatment since the physician's last assessment of the patient, and the results of any tests performed since the last assessment.

All the levels of service for subsequent observation care require two of the three key components, as defined within each level, to qualify for the selection of a particular level of service. In addition, both initial and subsequent observation care codes have typical times listed in the code descriptions and, therefore, these visits are eligible to be coded using time as the key component, previously described.

Code	History	Examination	Medical Decision Making
99224	Problem focused interval history	Problem focused	Straightforward or low complexity
99225	Expanded problem focused interval history	Expanded problem focused	Moderate complexity
99226	Detailed interval history	Detailed	High complexity

Hospital Inpatient Services

The hospital inpatient services category is divided into four parts: initial hospital care, subsequent hospital care, observation or inpatient care services, and hospital discharge services. Services provided to patients in a so-called partial hospital setting are included in this category.

Partial hospitalization is used for crisis stabilization, intensive short-term daily treatment, or intermediate-term treatment of psychiatric disorders. There is no distinction between new and established patients in this category. It should be noted that initial and subsequent hospital care codes are reported per day; therefore, services for the physician should be accumulated for the entire day before the coder can choose the appropriate level of visit for that day.

When counseling and coordination of care dominate the visit (comprising more than 50 percent of the visit), time is the key factor in determining the code. For hospital care E/M codes, time is based on unit/floor time.

Initial Hospital Care

The codes in the initial hospital care subcategory are used to report the first hospital inpatient encounter with the patient by the admitting physician (admitting physician is equivalent to attending physician). For Medicare, the admitting physician must append modifier –AI to the code for the initial hospital care to indicate that they were the principal physician of record. This change was initiated to differentiate the admitting physician from any specialists who may see the patient during the stay, due to Medicare change in payment for consultations. See the section on Consultations (99241–99255) later in this chapter.

A physician whose patient is admitted to the hospital while being seen at another site (for example, a hospital emergency department, observation status at a hospital, a nursing facility, or a physician's office) can assign only the service code describing the initial hospital care. The physician may not assign separate E/M codes for services provided at the other sites because these services are considered part of the initial hospital care when performed on the same date as the admission by the same physician.

In this subcategory, all three key components must meet or exceed stated requirements for a given level of service.

Code	History	Examination	Medical Decision Making
99221	Detailed or comprehensive	Detailed or comprehensive	Straightforward or low complexity
99222	Comprehensive	Comprehensive	Moderate complexity
99223	Comprehensive	Comprehensive	High complexity

Subsequent Hospital Care

All levels of subsequent hospital care include a review of the entire health record. Documentation should include changes in the patient's history, physical condition, and response to treatment, as well as the results of diagnostic studies since the physician's last assessment of the patient.

All the levels of service for subsequent hospital care require two of the three key components, as defined within each level, prior to code selection.

Code	History	Examination	Medical Decision Making
99231	Problem focused interval history	Problem focused	Straightforward or low complexity
99232	Expanded problem focused interval history	Expanded problem focused	Moderate complexity
99233	Detailed interval history	Detailed	High complexity

Observation or Inpatient Care Services (Including Admission and Discharge Services)

The codes in the observation or inpatient care services subcategory are used to report observation or inpatient care services provided to patients admitted and discharged on the same date. When the patient is admitted to the hospital from observation status on the same date, the physician should report only the initial hospital care code. The initial hospital care code should include the services related to the observation status services provided to the patient on the same date of his or her admission to the hospital.

When the patient is admitted to observation status during the course of an encounter at another service site (such as a hospital emergency department, a physician's office, or a nursing facility), all the E/M services performed by the supervising physician on the same date that relate to the admission to observation status are considered part of the initial observation care. The level of service reported should reflect all of the E/M services provided at sites other than the hospital as well as in the observation setting when provided by the same physician.

For patients admitted to observation or inpatient care and discharged on a different date, the coder should refer to codes 99217, 99218–99220, or 99221–99223, 99224–99226, and 99238–99239.

All the codes for observation or inpatient care services specify that two of the three key components must meet or exceed stated requirements, as defined within each level, to qualify for selection at a particular level of service.

Code	History	Examination	Medical Decision Making
99234	Detailed or comprehensive	Detailed or comprehensive	Straightforward or low complexity
99235	Comprehensive	Comprehensive	Moderate complexity
99236	Comprehensive	Comprehensive	High complexity

Hospital Discharge Services

The codes in the hospital discharge services subcategory are used to report the total duration of time spent by the physician in managing the patient's discharge. Code 99238 is assigned for 30 minutes or less; code 99239 is assigned for more than 30 minutes. These codes include final examination of the patient, discussion of the hospital stay, instructions for continuing care, and preparation of discharge records.

A hospital discharge service code should *not* be used when the patient is admitted and discharged on the same date. When this occurs, the coder should refer to codes 99234–99236.

Modifiers Commonly Used in Reporting Hospital Inpatient Services

Modifiers commonly used in reporting hospital inpatient services include –24, –25, and –57.

Modifier –24, Unrelated E/M Service by the Same Physician during a Postoperative Period, is appended to the appropriate E/M hospital visit code.

> **Example:** When a patient is admitted for evaluation (by the same physician) because of multiple lacerations after an auto accident during the postoperative recovery period for a cholecystectomy (gallbladder removal).

Modifier –25 is appended to the appropriate level of service code to indicate that on the day a procedure or service (with a separate CPT code) was performed, the patient's condition required a significant, separately identifiable E/M service above and beyond the usual pre- and postoperative care associated with the procedure that was performed.

Modifier –57, Decision for Surgery, is appended to the appropriate level of E/M hospital inpatient service code.

> **Example:** When a surgeon sees an inpatient and during the course of the examination determines the patient must have surgery.

Consultations

It should be noted that CMS has eliminated payment for the consultation codes, both Office and Other Outpatient Consultations and Inpatient Consultations. CMS instructs physicians who perform consultations to code the outpatient services using the New or Established Office or Other Outpatient Services codes, following the current definition of New versus Established patients. Inpatient services should be coded using Initial Hospital Care codes if the service was the first service provided to that patient during the admission or Subsequent Hospital Care codes for additional services provided during that admission. It is unclear whether other third-party payers will adopt this change in payment policy in the future. Check with the payer for current policies.

According to the CPT code book, a consultation is a type of service provided by the physician whose opinion or advice regarding the evaluation and management of a specific problem is requested by another physician or other appropriate source.

Specific guidelines apply to using consultation codes. These include the following:

- The consulting physician may initiate diagnostic and/or therapeutic services during the same or a subsequent visit.

- The written or verbal request for a consult may be made by a physician or other appropriate source and documented in the patient's health record.

- Documentation in the health record of the consultant's opinion and of any services ordered or performed is required (and should be referenced in the record).

- Communication between the attending physician or other appropriate source and the consulting physician is required.

- Specific, identifiable procedures performed on or after the date of the initial consultation should be reported separately.

The consulting physician may initiate diagnostic and/or therapeutic services during the same encounter of the consultation services. If responsibility is assumed for this condition, subsequent services are reported with the appropriate E/M services setting code. Also, consultation codes should not be reported by the physician who has agreed to accept the transfer of care before an initial evaluation but are appropriate to report if the decision to accept the transfer of care cannot be made until after the initial consultation evaluation, regardless of site of service. Also, if the physician explicitly agrees to accept responsibility for the patient from a physician who was managing some or all of the patient's problems, this is not a consultation. Documentation in the health record to support a consultation is essential and should include the request and need for a consultation, the opinion of the consultant, and any services ordered and/or performed. All of this information should be documented in the health record and communicated by written report to the requesting physician or other appropriate source.

When a consultation is requested by the patient or his or her family, but not by another physician, the consulting physician should report the service using the office or other outpatient codes. Reporting a consultation code would be inappropriate in this case because the consultation was not performed at the request of another physician.

Office or Other Outpatient Consultations

The office or other outpatient consultations subcategory designates the locations where such services may be provided: in the consultant physician's office; in an outpatient or ambulatory facility; or through a hospital observation service, home services, a domiciliary, a rest home, custodial care, or the emergency services department. When the consultant initiates additional follow-up visits, they are reported using the appropriate level of established patient office visit codes (99211–99215).

All three of the key components, as defined within each level, must meet or exceed stated requirements to qualify for a particular level of E/M service or selection of the consultation code.

Code	History	Examination	Medical Decision Making
99241	Problem focused	Problem focused	Straightforward
99242	Expanded problem focused	Expanded problem focused	Straightforward
99243	Detailed	Detailed	Low complexity
99244	Comprehensive	Comprehensive	Moderate complexity
99245	Comprehensive	Comprehensive	High complexity

Inpatient Consultations

The codes in the inpatient consultation subcategory are used for physician consultations provided to hospital inpatients, residents of nursing facilities, or patients in a partial hospital setting (for example, psychiatric) without distinction as to new and established patients. The consultant should report only one consultation per admission. When the consulting physician begins treatment at the consultation and later participates in the management of the patient, the codes for subsequent hospital care are reported for the later management services.

All three key components must meet or exceed the stated requirements to qualify for a given level of service for inpatient consultations.

Code	History	Examination	Medical Decision Making
99251	Problem focused	Problem focused	Straightforward
99252	Expanded problem focused	Expanded problem focused	Straightforward
99253	Detailed	Detailed	Low complexity
99254	Comprehensive	Comprehensive	Moderate complexity
99255	Comprehensive	Comprehensive	High complexity

Modifiers Commonly Used in Reporting Consultations

Modifier –25, Significant, Separately Identifiable E/M Service by the Same Physician on the Same Day of the Procedure or Other Service, may be used with the consultation codes.

Modifier –32, Mandated Service, may be assigned to a confirmatory consultation that is required or mandated, such as by a third-party payer.

Modifier –57, Decision for Surgery, may be reported with consultation codes.

> **Example:** When an attending physician asks a cardiac surgeon to render an opinion on the cardiac status of a patient and the cardiac surgeon recommends insertion of a pacemaker, modifier –57 is appended to the appropriate consultation code.

Emergency Department and Other Emergency Services

The codes in the emergency department services category are used to report E/M services provided in the emergency department. New patient and established patient definitions do not apply to emergency department codes. The CPT code book defines the emergency department as an organized, hospital-based facility for the provision of unscheduled episodic services to patients who present for immediate medical attention. In addition, the facility must be available 24 hours a day. Any physician performing E/M services in the emergency department may use these codes.

Coders should review the definition of emergency services carefully. A common coding error occurs when a coder reports emergency services codes for urgent care or minor medical facilities. The codes in this category should *not* be used for E/M services performed at an urgent or immediate care center. The coder should use office and outpatient E/M codes (99201–99215) for these services.

Special attention should be given to the description of code 99285, "which requires these three key components within the constraints imposed by the urgency of the patient's clinical condition and mental status. . . ." This description allows the code to be assigned, even if all the documentation does not meet the criteria as stated.

Coders are directed to codes 99291 and 99292 when critical care services are provided in the emergency department and exceed 30 minutes in length. An emergency department service E/M code is not assigned in addition to critical care codes. Physicians who see their patients in the observation area of the hospital are referred to code ranges 99217–99220 or 99234–99236.

All three of the key components must meet or exceed the services stated within a given level of the emergency department services codes to qualify for code selection at that level. It should be noted that the difference between codes 99282 and 99283 is in the complexity of medical decision making required, whereas the difference between codes 99283 and 99284 is in the type of history and examination required.

Code	History	Examination	Medical Decision Making
99281	Problem focused	Problem focused	Straightforward
99282	Expanded problem focused	Expanded problem focused	Low complexity
99283	Expanded problem focused	Expanded problem focused	Moderate complexity
99284	Detailed	Detailed	Moderate complexity
99285	Comprehensive	Comprehensive	High complexity

Modifier Commonly Used in Reporting Emergency Department Services

Modifier –25 should be appended to the appropriate level of emergency services visit.

> **Example:** An emergency services physician evaluates a patient with possible head injury during a bicycle accident. The physician repairs several wounds

on the patient's extremities in addition to the E/M service. Codes for the wound repairs may be reported in addition to the appropriate E/M emergency services visit code appended with modifier –25.

Critical Care Services

The codes in the critical care services category are used to report the total duration of time spent by the physician in providing direct critical care services for a critically ill/injured patient on a given date, even if the time spent by the physician on that date is not continuous. According to the guideline, the physician's full attention must be devoted to the patient during the time reported as providing critical care services; he or she cannot provide services to any other patient during the same period of time. Types of medical emergencies that may require critical care services include cardiac arrest, shock, overwhelming infection, respiratory failure, postoperative complications, or trauma cases.

Critical care is usually, but not always, given in a critical care area, such as the intensive care unit (ICU), coronary care unit (CCU), pediatric intensive care unit, respiratory care unit, or emergency facility.

Codes 99291 and 99292 are used to report critical care services provided to patients in any care setting. Code 99291 is used once per date to show the first 30 to 74 minutes spent in critical care services with the patient. Add-on code 99292 is used as often as necessary for each additional 30-minute period. Critical care services of less than 30 minutes on a given date should not be reported with 99291; instead, the appropriate E/M service code should be used. CPT provides specific codes for reporting inpatient critical care to neonates (28 days of age or younger), infants or young children from age 29 days through 24 months and children age two through five years. See CPT code range 99468–99476. The time spent with a critically ill or injured pediatric (24 months of age or less) patient during transport should be reported with the appropriate transport codes (99466–99467).

Time spent with the individual patient should be recorded in his or her health record. The time that can be reported as critical care is the time spent engaged in work directly related to the individual patient's care whether the time was spent at the immediate bedside or elsewhere on the floor or on the unit.

Services included, but not billed separately, in the critical care code(s) are the following:

- Interpretation of cardiac output measurements (93561, 93562)

- Chest x-rays (71010, 71015, 71020)

- Pulse oximetry (94760, 94761, 94762)

- Blood gases and information data stored in computers (for example, EKGs, blood pressures, hematologic data) (99090)

- Gastric intubation (43752, 43753)

- Temporary transcutaneous pacing (92953)

- Ventilator management (94002–94004, 94660, 94662)

- Vascular access procedures (36000, 36410, 36415, 36591, 36600)

Any services not listed above should be reported separately when supported by documentation. Services provided for patients who are not critically ill in a CCU should be reported using the subsequent hospital care codes (99231–99233) or hospital consultation codes (99251–99255), as appropriate.

Nursing Facility Services

The codes in the nursing facility services category are divided into four subcategories: initial nursing facility care, subsequent nursing facility care, annual nursing facility assessment, and nursing facility discharge services. There is no differentiation between new and established patients when assigning these service codes, and the codes in this category are used "per day," meaning that all services provided in a 24-hour period are to be included in one code. These codes are used to report E/M services provided to patients in nursing facilities (also known as skilled nursing facilities [SNFs], intermediate care facilities [ICFs], long-term care facilities [LTCFs]), or psychiatric residential treatment centers.

Assessing the functional capacity of each patient via the resident assessment instrument (RAI) is a requirement of these nursing facilities. All RAIs include the Minimum Data Set (MDS), resident assessment protocols (RAPs), and utilization guidelines. It should be noted that the typical times listed in each code description include time at the bedside and on the patient's facility floor or unit.

Initial Nursing Facility Care

When a patient has an encounter in another site of service (for example, emergency services facility or physician's office) and is admitted to the nursing facility, all E/M services provided by that physician in conjunction with that admission are considered part of the initial nursing facility care when performed on the same date as the admission or readmission.

All three of the key components must be met in these cases before code selection.

Code	History	Examination	Medical Decision Making
99304	Detailed or comprehensive	Detailed or comprehensive	Straightforward or low complexity
99305	Comprehensive	Comprehensive	Moderate complexity
99306	Comprehensive	Comprehensive	High complexity

Subsequent Nursing Facility Care

The codes in the subsequent nursing facility care subcategory are used to report E/M services provided to residents who are not newly admitted to the facility. All levels require that the physician review the health record, note changes in the resident's status since the last visit, and review and sign orders.

Subsequent nursing facility care codes require that only two of the three key components meet or exceed stated requirements at any given level before assigning a specific level of service code.

Code	History	Examination	Medical Decision Making
99307	Problem focused interval history	Problem focused	Straightforward
99308	Expanded problem focused interval history	Expanded problem focused	Low complexity
99309	Detailed interval history	Detailed	Moderate complexity
99310	Comprehensive interval history	Comprehensive	High complexity

Nursing Facility Discharge Services

The codes in the nursing facility discharge services subcategory are used to report the total time spent by a physician on the final discharge of a patient from a nursing facility. The services include final examination of the patient and discussion of the nursing facility stay, even if the time spent on that date is not continuous. Instructions are given for continuing care to all relevant caregivers and for preparation of discharge records, prescriptions, and referral forms.

Applicable codes are 99315 for services of 30 minutes or less and 99316 for services of more than 30 minutes. According to *CPT Assistant* (May 2002), it is appropriate to report 99315 or 99316 in the case of a patient's death, if all of the above services are provided, including a face-to-face examination of the patient.

Other Nursing Facility Services

CPT provides one code to describe the process of completing an annual nursing facility assessment, requiring that all three key components be met or exceeded.

Code	History	Examination	Medical Decision Making
99318	Detailed interval history	Comprehensive	Low to moderate complexity

Domiciliary, Rest Home, or Custodial Care Services

Physician visits to patients being provided room, board, and other personal assistance services, usually on a long-term basis, are reported using codes 99324–99337. A medical component is not part of the facility's services. Such facilities may include group homes, correctional facilities, and assisted living facilities.

This category has two sections—new and established patients. All three key components, as defined in the levels of service, must be met before code assignment in the new patient subcategory (99324–99328).

Code	History	Examination	Medical Decision Making
99324	Problem focused	Problem focused	Straightforward complexity
99325	Expanded problem focused	Expanded problem focused	Low complexity
99326	Detailed	Detailed	Moderate complexity
99327	Comprehensive	Comprehensive	Moderate complexity
99328	Comprehensive	Comprehensive	High complexity

Only two of the three key components must meet or exceed established service levels to qualify for any given code in the established patient subcategory (99334–99337).

Code	History	Examination	Medical Decision Making
99334	Problem focused interval history	Problem focused	Straightforward
99335	Expanded problem focused interval history	Expanded problem focused	Low complexity
99336	Detailed interval history	Detailed	Moderate complexity
99337	Comprehensive interval history	Comprehensive	Moderate to high complexity

Domiciliary, Rest Home, or Home Care Oversight Services

The two codes in this section are similar to the care plan oversight codes, 99374–99380, and the coding notes found in that section apply to all of these codes. These services involve the regular development and/or revision of care plans, review of ancillary studies, and telephone calls. When 15 to 29 minutes are spent per calendar month, code 99339 is reported. When 30 minutes or more are spent per calendar month, code 99340 is reported.

Home Services

The codes in the home services category are used to report E/M services provided in a private residence. This category is subdivided to distinguish between a new patient and an established patient.

All three key components must meet or exceed stated requirements as defined within the levels of service to qualify for any given code in the new patient subcategory.

Code	History	Examination	Medical Decision Making
99341	Problem focused	Problem focused	Straightforward
99342	Expanded problem focused	Expanded problem focused	Low complexity
99343	Detailed	Detailed	Moderate complexity
99344	Comprehensive	Comprehensive	Moderate complexity
99345	Comprehensive	Comprehensive	High Complexity

However, the established patient subcategory requires that only two of the three key components meet or exceed the stated service-level requirements.

Code	History	Examination	Medical Decision Making
99347	Problem focused interval history	Problem focused	Straightforward
99348	Expanded problem focused interval history	Expanded problem focused	Low complexity
99349	Detailed interval history	Detailed	Moderate complexity
99350	Comprehensive interval history	Comprehensive	High complexity

Prolonged Services

The codes in the prolonged services category are used when a physician provides prolonged services or when the time spent is beyond the usual service in either the inpatient or outpatient setting. These codes are reported in addition to other physician services, including E/M services at any level or 90837 Psychotherapy, 60 minutes with patient and/or family member. This category has four subcategories: prolonged physician service with direct patient contact (99354–99357); prolonged physician service without direct patient contact (99358–99359); prolonged clinical staff services with physician or other qualified health care professional supervision (99415–99416); and physician standby services (99360).

Codes are selected based on the total time spent, which does not need to be continuous, on a given date. In three of the subcategories, the time spent must total at least 30 minutes or more to assign codes from this category (such as 99354 or 99356, based on place of service). Each additional 30 minutes of time spent beyond the first Prolonged Services hour is coded with the appropriate add-on code, based on place of service. Coders should note that prolonged service of less than 30 minutes should not be reported separately for physician or other qualified health care professional prolonged services. The CPT book coding notes within this section provides a chart to assist in code assignment. For the prolonged clinical staff services with physician or other qualified health care professional supervision subcategory, prolonged services of less than 45 minutes total duration on a given date is not separately reportable. The times used to calculate prolonged care in this subcategory are slightly different and have a separate table in CPT to determine the code assignment.

Codes 99354–99357 are used when a physician provides prolonged services involving direct contact with the patient that is beyond the usual service. Codes 99354 and 99355 indicate prolonged services provided in the office or other outpatient setting (physician office, emergency department). Codes 99356 and 99357 are to be used when services are provided in the inpatient setting.

Codes 99358–99359 describe prolonged physician services without direct contact with the patient that is beyond the usual service. This type of service can involve prolonged communication with other healthcare professionals or prolonged review of extensive health record and diagnostic tests. These codes may be reported along with other services, including E/M services at any level and can be reported on a different day than the primary service to which it is related. They are also used to report services related to other non–face-to-face services codes that have a published maximum time, such as telephone services.

According to *CPT Assistant* June 2008, the lack of typical times as published in the CPT book for most services makes it impossible to determine when services have been prolonged, and thus, these add-on codes cannot be used for services beyond E/M. In most cases other than E/M, significantly prolonged time is associated with additional work, and modifier –22 is the appropriate reporting mechanism.

Code 99360 is used to report physician standby services requested by another physician, which involves prolonged physician attendance without face-to-face contact with the patient. The standby physician may not provide care or services to other patients during this time. Code 99360 should not be used if the standby period ends with the performance of a procedure subject to a surgical package by the physician on standby. Standby service of less than 30 minutes' total duration on a given date is not reported separately. For example, when a neonatologist is on standby for one hour during a high-risk delivery and his or her services are not needed, the neonatologist should report code 99360 twice (once for each 30-minute interval). (Note that code 99360 may not be reported in conjunction with 99464.)

Case Management Services

Case management services include services in which a physician is responsible for the direct care of a patient, as well as for coordinating and controlling access to, or initiating and/or supervising other healthcare services for, the patient. This category includes two subcategories: team conferences and telephone calls.

Anticoagulant Management

Codes 99363–99364 describe the process of managing patients on warfarin (commonly known as Coumadin) and their frequent dosage changes. Code 99363 is assigned for the management of the initial 90 days of treatment and 99364 is assigned for the management of each subsequent 90-day period of treatment.

Team Conferences

Code 99366 describes participation by a nonphysician qualified healthcare professional as part of an interdisciplinary team with direct face-to-face contact with the patient and/or family. If the physician is involved in an interdisciplinary team conference where there is direct face-to-face contact, the E/M service codes should be used.

Codes 99367–99368 describe medical team conferences that do not involve direct face-to-face contact. Code 99367 is for use by a physician, and code 99368 is for use by a nonphysician qualified healthcare professional.

All codes in this series describe participation for 30 minutes or longer and are used to code coordination of care with other physicians, other healthcare professionals, or agencies without a patient encounter on that day.

Care Plan Oversight Services

Care plan oversight services are reported separately from other E/M services and refer to physician supervision of patients under the care of home health agencies, hospices, or nursing facilities requiring complex or multidisciplinary care modalities. These services involve regular physician development and/or revision of care plans, review of patient status, review of studies or laboratory results, and coordination with other healthcare professionals. The codes in this category are based on time spent within a 30-day period. The services provided are reported when the time spent is 15 minutes or more during a 30-day period. Documentation must substantiate the codes billed.

Only one physician may report this type of service within a 30-day period. Work involved in providing very low-intensity services or infrequent supervision is included in the pre- and postencounter work for the home, office/outpatient, and nursing facility or domiciliary visit codes and should not be reported with care plan oversight codes.

Preventive Medicine Services

The codes in the preventive medicine services category are used to report the preventive medicine E/M of infants, children, adolescents, and adults. They are assigned based on the patient's age and whether the patient is new or established. The comprehensive history and examination of the preventive medicine services are not synonymous with the comprehensive requirements in E/M codes 99201–99350. The extent and focus of the services depend largely on the patient's age and gender. Counseling, risk factor reduction, and anticipatory guidance appropriate for the age of the patient are included in the preventive medicine code.

Immunizations and ancillary studies involving laboratory, radiology, or other procedures, or screening tests identified with a specific CPT code, are reported separately when supported by documentation.

According to the AMA, when less than the preventive medicine code description is provided, office visit codes (99201–99215) should be reported rather than preventive care codes. Any insignificant conditions/abnormalities discovered during the preventive medicine services that do not require additional workup should not be reported separately.

A common coding oversight is to code only the preventive medicine service when additional services are performed; however, some health plans allow only one code per visit.

> **Example:** An annual preventive medicine exam of a 2-year-old patient revealed a tightened chest and some breathing difficulty, which prompted the physician to order a chest x-ray, obtain additional medical information,

and prescribe antibiotics for possible pneumonia. In this case, the preventive medicine service and the appropriate level of office and other outpatient service should be coded. Modifier –25 should be appended to the office or other outpatient service code (99201–99215) to indicate that the same physician provided a significant, separately identifiable E/M service on the same day as the preventive medicine service.

Initial Preventive Physical Examination and Annual Wellness Visits for Medicare Patients

From the inception of the Medicare program, preventive medicine services have been considered a noncovered benefit. The Medicare Prescription Drug, Improvement, and Modernization Act of 2003 (MMA) directed the Medicare program to provide a covered preventive medicine service to new beneficiaries for the first time, beginning on January 1, 2005.

This benefit is called the Initial Preventive Physical Examination, also known as an IPPE or "Welcome to Medicare Physical," because it is only available to new Medicare Part B enrollees and must be delivered within the first 12 months of Medicare Part B entitlement. The IPPE service is coded as G0402 and has specific performance and documentation requirements that differ from any of the other published documentation requirements for E/M codes:

1. Review of the individual's medical and social history

2. Review of the individual's potential risk factors for depression, using various screening methods

3. Review of the individual's functional ability and level of safety based on the use of appropriate screening questions or a screening questionnaire

4. An examination to include measurement of the individual's height, weight, blood pressure, a visual acuity screen, measurement of body mass index, and other factors deemed appropriate based on the patient's medical and social history

5. End-of-life planning

6. Education, counseling, and referral based on the above information

7. Education, counseling, and referral for appropriate screening examinations

A screening EKG is payable as one of the appropriate screening examinations when performed as a part of an IPPE, but is not a mandatory component. G0403 is used for the performance of the complete EKG (tracing, interpretation, and report), code G0404 is used for the tracing only, and code G0405 is used for only the interpretation and report of the EKG performed elsewhere. Codes from the 93000 series cannot be used to describe the EKG done as part of the IPPE. (See chapter 10 for a thorough discussion of component billing.) Note that CPT Level I codes cannot be used to report the IPPE and the associated services. Payment is provided only for the HCPCS codes.

"For dates of service on or after January 1, 2011, Medicare will cover an Annual Wellness Visit (AWV), providing Personalized Prevention Plan Services (PPPS) at no cost to the beneficiary, so beneficiaries can work with their physicians to develop and update a personalized prevention plan. This new benefit will provide an ongoing focus on prevention that can be adapted as a beneficiary's health needs change over time.

The first AWV (G0438) is a one-time Medicare benefit that includes the following elements:

- Establishment of the beneficiary's medical/family history, including the following:
  - Past medical and surgical history
  - Use or exposure to medications and supplements
  - Medical events in the beneficiary's parents, siblings, and children
- Measurement of beneficiary's height, weight and body mass index (BMI), blood pressure, and other vital signs
- Establishment of a list of current providers and suppliers regularly used
- Detection of any cognitive impairment
- Review of beneficiary's functional ability and level of safety, including the following:
  - Hearing impairment
  - Ability to perform activities of daily living
  - Fall risk
  - Home safety
- Establishment of a written screening schedule
- Establishment of a list of risk factors
- Provision of personalized health advice and appropriate referrals" (CMS 2014).

Subsequent AWVs (G0439) will begin on or after January, 1, 2012 and include updates to the above collected information. A subsequent AWV can only take place if at least 12 months have passed since the last AWV.

Counseling Risk Factor Reduction and Behavior Change Intervention

The codes in the counseling and/or risk factor reduction intervention subcategory are used to report services provided to healthy individuals, at a separate encounter, for the purpose of promoting health and preventing illness or injury. Counseling and/or risk factor reduction intervention varies with age and should address issues such as family problems, diet and exercise, substance abuse, sexual practices, injury prevention, dental health, and diagnostic and laboratory test results available at the time of visit. These codes are not to be used in counseling a patient with symptoms or an established illness.

Codes 99401–99429 apply to both new and established patients. The following subcategories are recognized: preventive medicine, individual counseling (99401–99404); behavior change interventions (99406–99409); preventive medicine, group counseling (99411–99412); and other preventive medicine services (99420 and 99429).

Codes 99401–99412 are assigned based on the amount of time spent counseling the patient.

Non-Face-to-Face Services

This section describes codes for telephone services and online medical evaluation services provided by physicians.

Telephone Services

Coders should carefully read the guidelines for this section. Physicians may report CPT codes 99441–99443 for telephone calls initiated by patients or guardians if the call is not related to another E/M service within the past seven days. If the telephone call results in a decision to see the patient within 24 hours or the next available urgent visit appointment, the codes cannot be reported, as the call is considered preservice work.

Online Medical Evaluation

Physicians may report an E/M service that was provided using Internet resources in response to a patient's inquiry using CPT code 99444. This code cannot be used to report an online service related to another E/M service that was provided in the last seven days or as part of a postoperative period of a completed procedure.

Special Evaluation and Management Services

The codes in the special E/M services category were developed to report services that can be performed in the office setting or other setting to establish baseline information before life or disability insurance certificates are issued. Coders should note that no active management of the patient's problem is performed during this visit. If other E/M services and/or procedures are performed on the same date, the appropriate E/M services codes also should be reported, with modifier –25.

Newborn Care

The codes in the newborn care category are used to report the services provided to normal or high-risk newborns in different settings. Code 99460 is reported for history and examination of the *normal* newborn, initiation of diagnostic and treatment programs, and preparation of hospital records. This code is appropriate for birthing room deliveries. Code 99462 is reported to indicate subsequent hospital care for the E/M of a normal newborn on a per day basis. Code 99463 should be reported for discharge services provided to the newborn admitted and discharged on the same date. Code 99464 is used to report attendance at a delivery, at the request of the delivering physician, for initial stabilization of the newborn. According to *CPT Assistant* (April 2004), a history and physical performed on a newborn that is not "normal" should be reported using initial hospital care codes (99221–99223) or neonatal intensive and critical care services (99466–99469, 99477–99480).

Delivery/Birthing Room Attendance and Resuscitation Services

Attendance at delivery (when requested by the delivering physician) and initial stabilization of the newborn is reported with code 99464. The request should be clearly documented in the medical record.

Newborn resuscitative services are reported with code 99465, which includes the provision of positive-pressure ventilation and/or chest compressions in the presence of acute inadequate ventilation and/or cardiac output. Code 99465 cannot be reported with code 99464. When other procedures are performed in addition to the resuscitative services, additional codes should be reported. It should be noted that the parenthetical statement under code 99465 supports that 99465 may be reported in conjunction with 99460, 99468, and 99477.

Pediatric Critical Care Patient Transport

The codes in the pediatric patient transport category are used to report the time a physician is in attendance of a critically ill or injured pediatric patient (24 months of age or younger) during the transport to or from a facility or hospital, for example, the time spent with the patient in the ambulance or a helicopter. Only the actual face-to-face time is reported.

Code 99466 is reported for the first 30 to 74 minutes of direct face-to-face time during transport and should be reported only once on a given date. Code 99467 is reported for each additional 30 minutes on a given date.

Inpatient Neonatal and Pediatric Critical Care

The codes in the inpatient neonatal critical care category (99468–99469) are used to report services provided by a physician directing the care of a critically ill neonate (28 days of age or less). These codes are applicable as long as the neonate qualifies for critical care services. Inpatient critical care services provided to infants and young children from 29 days through 24 months of age are coded using 99471–99472 and inpatient critical care services provided to young children from 2 through 5 years of age are coded using 99475–99476.

Critical care services performed in an outpatient setting (for example, an emergency services department or a physician's office) on a neonate or pediatric patient should be reported with codes 99291–99292, the hourly critical care codes. When the same physician provides an outpatient critical care service on the same day as an inpatient critical care service on the same patient, report only the appropriate inpatient neonatal or pediatric critical care code (99468–99476).

The inpatient neonatal and pediatric critical care codes are reported only once per day, per patient, not as hourly services. The pediatric and neonatal critical care codes include those procedures listed above for the hourly critical care (99291–99292) and the additional services listed here. All of these codes are bundled into the critical care codes and are not separately reportable. In addition, the following codes are not separately reportable with pediatric and neonatal critical care codes 99468–99472, 99475–99476, and the intensive care services codes 99477–99480:

- Invasive or noninvasive electronic monitoring of vital signs

- Vascular access procedures

    o Peripheral vessel catheterization (36000)

    o Other arterial catheters (36140, 36620)

    o Umbilical venous catheters (36510)

    o Central venous catheterization (36555)

    o Vascular access procedures (36400, 36405, 36406)

    o Vascular punctures (36420, 36600)

    o Umbilical arterial catheters (36660)

- Airway and ventilation management

    o Endotracheal intubation (31500)

    o Ventilatory management (94002–94004)

    o Bedside pulmonary function testing (94375)

- o Surfactant administration (94610)
- o Continuous positive airway pressure (CPAP) (94660)
- Monitoring or interpretation of blood gases or oxygen saturation (94760–94762)
- Car seat evaluation (94780–94781)
- Transfusion of blood components (36430, 36440)
- Oral or nasogastric tube placement (43752)
- Suprapubic bladder aspiration (51100)
- Bladder catheterization (51701, 51702)
- Lumbar puncture (62270)

Any services performed that are not listed above should be reported separately when supported by documentation.

Codes 99360 (standby service), 99464 (present at the delivery and newborn stabilization), or 99465 (newborn resuscitation) are coded in addition to the neonatal intensive care codes. It should be noted that standby services (99360) should not be reported together with attendance at delivery services (99464) but any of the three codes can be used with the neonatal intensive care codes.

Each code description should be read carefully because specific services are delineated for each level of service.

Code	Description of Service
	Inpatient Neonatal Critical Care
99468	Initial inpatient neonatal critical care, per day, for the evaluation and management of a critically ill neonate, 28 days of age or younger
99469	Subsequent inpatient neonatal critical care, per day, for the evaluation and management of a critically ill neonate, 28 days of age or younger
	Inpatient Pediatric Critical Care
99471	Initial inpatient pediatric critical care, 29 days through 24 months of age, per day, for the evaluation and management of a critically ill infant or young child, 29 days through 24 months of age
99472	Subsequent inpatient pediatric critical care, 29 days through 24 months of age, per day, for the evaluation and management of a critically ill infant or young child, 29 days through 24 months of age
99475	Initial inpatient pediatric critical care, per day, for the evaluation and management of a critically ill infant or young child, 2 through 5 years of age
99476	Subsequent inpatient pediatric critical care, per day, for the evaluation and management of a critically ill infant or young child, 2 through 5 years of age

Based on the age and weight of the patient, severity of illness, and what day of hospitalization is being coded, table 2.7 may help to demonstrate how each of the codes is used.

Table 2.7. Coding summary for neonatal and pediatric critical care services

Day(s) of Stay	1st Day	2nd–28th Day	29th Day or More	2nd Day or More
Critical Neonate	99468	99469	99472	— —
Noncritical Neonate	9922X	9923X	9923X	— —
Noncritical Premature Infant	9922X 99477	— —	— —	99478* (<1500 g) 99479* (1501–2500 g) 99480* (2501–5000 g) 99231–99233* (>5000 g)
Critical infant, 29 days to 24 months	99471	— —	— —	99472
Critical child, 2 to 5 years of age	99475	— —	— —	99476

*Based on present body weight of the infant
Source: Adapted from Crow 2002.

When the critically ill neonate or pediatric patient is transferred to a lower level of care, the codes in this series are not reported by the transferring physician. Instead, the transferring physician should report a subsequent hospital care code (99231–99233) or critical care code (99291–99292), based on the condition of the patient. The receiving physician should report a subsequent intensive care code (99478–99480) or a subsequent hospital care code (99231–99233) based on the condition of the patient.

Initial and Continuing Intensive Care Services

Initial hospital care provided to a neonate of 28 days or age or younger who is not critically ill but requires intensive observation, frequent interventions, and other intensive care services can be reported with code 99477. This code is reported only once per day.

Infants born at a low birth weight (LBW) have a body weight of less than 2,500 g. Very low birth weight (VLBW) infants have a body weight of less than 1,500 g. When these infants require ongoing management after they are no longer critically ill, their subsequent care should be reported with 99478 for VLBW and 99479 for LBW infants.

Code	Description of Service
	Initial and Continuing Intensive Care Services
99477	Initial hospital care, per day, for the evaluation and management of the neonate, 28 days of age or younger, who requires intensive observation, frequent interventions, and other intensive care services
99478	Subsequent intensive care, per day, for the evaluation and management of the recovering very low birth weight infant (present body weight less than 1,500 g)
99479	Subsequent intensive care, per day, for the evaluation and management of the recovering low birth weight infant (present body weight of 1,500–2,500 g)

99480   Subsequent intensive care, per day, for the evaluation and management of the recovering infant (present body weight of 2,501–5,000 g)

As with Neonatal and Pediatric Critical Care codes, the codes in this section should not be reported by the transferring individual when a patient is transferred to a lower level of care. Subsequent hospital care codes (99231–99233) should be used on the day of transfer. The receiving individual should use a code that describes the appropriate level of care as provided.

Care Management Services

Care Management is patient-centered management and support services. It is provided by physicians, qualified healthcare professionals, and clinical staff. Patients reside at home, in a domiciliary, rest home or assisted living facility, and patients have two or more chronic conditions that are expected to last 12 months or until the death of the patient, or the conditions place the patient at a significant risk of death, acute exacerbation, decompensation or functional decline. The goal of this care is coordination of care by multiple disciplines and agencies.

Chronic Care Management Services

Code 99490 requires that a care plan be established and the clinical staff directed by a physician or other qualified healthcare professional provide at least 20 minutes per calendar month of chronic care management services.

Complex Chronic Care Management Services

Complex chronic care management involves meeting the definition of chronic care management plus the inability to adhere to a treatment plan, the presence of psychiatric or other medical comorbidities that complicate their care, and social support requirements or difficulty with access to care. Code 99487 describes the first 60 minutes of clinical staff time per calendar month. Code 99489 describes each additional 30 minutes of clinical staff time per calendar month.

Transitional Care Management Services

Transitional care management services assist patients in the transition to the community setting following inpatient care. These include the day of discharge and the next 29 days following discharge from inpatient care. The patient must be discharged to his or her home, domiciliary, rest home, or assisted living facility. These services require an interactive contact within two business days following discharge and a face-to-face visit for problems that require moderate to high complexity medical decision making with medication reconciliation completed no later than the face-to-face visit. Documentation requirements are noted in the coding notes at this section of CPT 2016. Transitional care services begin on the day of discharge and are reportable on the 30th day.

Two codes are available for transitional care services. Code 99496 is used when the medical decision making is high and a visit takes place within seven days. Code 99495 is used when the medical decision making is moderate and the visit takes place within 14 days or when the decision making is high but the visit takes place between day 8 and day 14. Refer to the chart in the coding notes at this section of CPT 2016.

Advanced Care Planning

Advance care planning relates to discussion of advance directives between a healthcare provider and the patient, family, or surrogate to appoint an agent or record future wishes. Code 99497 describes the first 30 minutes of face-to-face service and 99498 describes each additional 30 minutes of service.

Other Evaluation and Management Services

CPT code 99499 is the sole code in the E/M services category that is used to report an E/M service that does not fit into the previous categories.

HCPCS Codes Used in Evaluation and Management Coding

The following HCPCS Level II codes are used for evaluation and management services involving:

G0402　　Initial preventive physical examination; face-to-face visit, services limited to new beneficiary during the first 12 months of Medicare enrollment

G0403　　Electrocardiogram, routine ECG with 12 leads; performed as a screening for the initial preventive physical examination with interpretation and report

G0404　　Electrocardiogram, routine ECG with 12 leads; tracing only, without interpretation and report, performed as a screening for the initial preventive physical examination

G0405　　Electrocardiogram, routine ECG with 12 leads; interpretation and report only, performed as a screening for the initial preventive physical examination

G0438　　Annual wellness visit; includes a personalized prevention plan of service (PPS), initial visit

G0439　　Annual wellness visit, includes a personalized prevention plan of service (PPS), subsequent visit

Exercise 2.1. Evaluation and Management Coding

Choose the best answer for each of the following questions.

1. A patient is seen in the office. His last visit was four years ago, although documentation in his record reveals that the physician has ordered prescription medicine several times in the past three years. The physician performed an expanded problem focused history; an expanded problem focused examination; and straightforward medical decision making. Which CPT code should be reported for the E/M services?

   a. 99202
   b. 99203
   c. 99212
   d. 99213

2. Which CPT service is *not* considered part of critical care and can be reported separately?

   a. Chest x-rays
   b. Cardiopulmonary resuscitation
   c. Vascular access procedures
   d. Ventilator management

3. Which code group is used to report E/M services provided to patients in a psychiatric residential treatment center?

   a. Hospital inpatient services
   b. Nursing facility services
   c. Office or other outpatient services
   d. Psychiatric services

4. The middle day of an observation stay that spans three calendar days should be coded with which sequence of codes?

   a. 99211–99215
   b. 99218–99220
   c. 99224–99226
   d. 99231–99233

5. Which CPT codes should be reported for critical care services for an adult requiring constant physician attendance for 110 minutes?

   a. 99291
   b. 99291, 99292
   c. 99291, 99291
   d. 99291, 99292, 99292

Assign the appropriate E/M codes to the following scenarios. Do not assign procedure codes. Assign modifiers if necessary.

6. A patient is seen in his home due to deteriorating health by a physician who has been treating him for years in the office. A detailed history, comprehensive exam, and high medical decision making are documented.

   _____

7. A middle-aged patient visited his physician complaining of chest pain. This was the patient's first visit to this physician, so a comprehensive history and a physical examination were performed. An electrocardiogram (EKG) was performed immediately and revealed some evidence of coronary insufficiency. An automated complete blood count also was ordered and performed.

   _____

(Continued on next page)

Exercise 2.1. (Continued)

8. A 4-year-old boy sees his physician for an annual physical. During the examination, the physician locates a significant lymph node mass. An extended problem focused history and examination are done, and a CT scan is ordered for further evaluation.

   _____

9. A physician sees a neonate that weighs 2,440 g who requires management and continual monitoring of breathing and temperature control issues but overall is progressing well.

   _____

10. The physician saw a child for suspicion of child abuse. At the conclusion of the physician services, Child Protective Services was contacted to provide protective placement and a clinical staff member monitored the child apart from the parent for 95 additional minutes to prepare the patient and accomplish the transfer. In addition to the E/M code for the visit, which E/M code(s) would be assigned?

    _____

11. Dr. Jones asks Dr. Matthews to confirm his diagnosis and treatment plan for a 5-day-old inpatient with a congenital heart defect of tetralogy of Fallot. The patient's insurance company requires this service before authorizing payment for an operation. Dr. Matthews obtains a comprehensive history and reviews the medical records, including diagnostic test results from Dr. Jones. He performs a comprehensive examination, including a complete organ system evaluation. He provides medical decision making of high complexity by evaluating all treatment options and considering the high risk of mortality with this type of defect.

    _____

12. The patient is seen by the physician in the office for chest pain and is directly admitted to the telemetry unit as an inpatient for monitoring. The physician also sees the patient later that day in the telemetry unit to reassess their condition. A detailed history, comprehensive exam and high level medical decision making is documented.

    _____

13. The patient is sent to an OB/GYN physician by her primary care physician, who arranged the appointment. After a detailed history and a comprehensive examination, the physician suggested an endometrial biopsy, which was completed on that day. Medication was prescribed and the findings communicated to the primary care physician.

    _____

14. A 55-year-old patient with rectal bleeding was seen by a gastroenterologist in the physician's office at the recommendation of the patient's internist. The consultant conducted a comprehensive history, noting the patient's dietary habits, current medications, and bowel habits, as well as a family history of colon cancer. A comprehensive physical examination was performed, including a digital rectal examination. A barium enema and a complete blood count were ordered and performed. A report goes back to the internist.

    _____

15. A pediatrician directs the care of a critically ill neonate immediately after delivery.

    _____

Exercise 2.1. (Continued)

16. An endocrinologist is asked to provide an opinion regarding a 26-year-old patient who is covered by commercial insurance and is being evaluated in the emergency department. The endocrinologist documents a comprehensive history, detailed exam, and high complexity decision making after seeing the patient.

17. The patient sees a new ophthalmologist on an urgent basis for conjunctivitis. A detailed history and comprehensive eye examination are done. The physician suspects an allergy to contact lens solution and prescribes oral and ophthalmic medication.

18. An 8-year-old boy is seen by a new physician for evaluation of ADHD. The physician documents a comprehensive history, an expanded-problem focused exam, and moderate medical decision making, stating, "I spent 45 minutes of a 60-minute visit counseling the patient and family about my findings and the nature of the disease."

19. Assign the appropriate E/M code(s) to the following emergency department report.

Emergency Department Report

Patient: Peter Poe   **Health Record #** 28-28-02

Presenting Complaint: Motorcycle accident with laceration, left leg

T 37   P 72   R 18

History: Patient was involved in a motorcycle accident 1 hour prior to admission, falling on his left leg and sustaining a laceration to the pretibial area. He experienced no loss of consciousness or head trauma. This was the patient's first time on a motorcycle, and he was unsure of how to manipulate it.

Physical Examination:
HEENT: Normal
Neck: No adenopathy, supple
Lungs: Clear
Abdomen: Soft
Cardio: Normal sinus rhythm

Extremities reveal a well-demarcated pinpoint 5-cm laceration over the mid-pretibial area. The wound is well marginated and discrete with a small amount of grassy debris inside. The depth is penetrating down to the periosteum of the tibia. There is no arterial bleeding, but there is small venous capillary bleeding.

Vascular Exam: Bilateral venous pulses in the posterior tibial and dorsalis pedis. Capillary refill time is normal.

Neurologic Exam: Normal. Motor and sensory examination is normal, without any paresthesia to the left leg or numbness.

Treatment: Irrigated wound copiously with normal saline. Wound infiltrated with 1% Xylocaine. Patient prepared/draped in a sterile fashion. Skin and deeper tissues closed in layers. Skin edges reapproximated with 12 3-0 prolene sutures and alternating vertical mattress interrupted. Skin reapproximated with slight difficulty. Sterile dressing. Bacitracin ointment. Compression dressing.

Diagnosis: Acute laceration to the left pretibia, with extension down to the periosteum

Disposition and Condition of the Patient at Discharge: Patient instructed in wound care precautions. To return tomorrow between 1:00 p.m. and 11:00 p.m. for recheck. Patient given prescriptions for Tylenol #3, 1 to 2 tablets prn every 4 to 6 hours for pain; Keflex 250 mg, 1 per mouth, 4 times daily.

20. Assign the appropriate E/M code(s) to the following office visit note.

(Continued on next page)

Exercise 2.1. (Continued)

Office Visit Note—Established Patient

Patient: Mary Raab   **Health Record #** 16-86-59

Presenting Complaint: Head congestion

T 38   P 68   R 22   BP 110/72

History: This 33-year-old female comes in with congestion, sinus discomfort, and headache. Her ears have been popping. The throat is somewhat sore but she has not been coughing. She is currently on no medication.

Physical Examination: She is alert and in no acute distress.
HEENT: Ears are clear. TMs pearly bilaterally. Maxillary sinuses are tender with palpation. Nose: Positive rhinorrhea. Pharynx: Positive postnasal discharge. Slight erythema.
Neck: Supple and shotty lymphadenopathy
Lungs: Clear to auscultation.
Abdomen: Soft, nontender with good bowel sounds
Cardio: Regular rate and rhythm

Assessment: Acute sinusitis

Disposition: Amoxicillin 500 mg one po t.i.d × 7 days. Increase fluids and follow up with me in 7 to 10 days if symptoms are not resolved.

Chapter 2 Test

Choose the best answer for each of the following questions.

1. The physician performs a second consultation for the same diagnosis during the patient's hospital stay. What series of E/M codes would the physician use to report this service?
    a. Initial Hospital Care
    b. Initial Inpatient Consultations
    c. Subsequent Hospital Care
    d. Office and Other Outpatient Consultations

2. Assign an E/M code to the following service, based on the contents of the office note and information that follows:

    CC: URI

    S: This 69-year-old patient has URI-type symptoms, dry tickling cough of five days' duration. He is due to see Dr. B next week to follow up on his prostate CA.

    O: His blood pressure is 124/82, left arm sitting, right arm supine 122/76, sitting 124/76, standing 120/78. Oropharynx is benign. Nose is not particularly congested. Lungs sound clear.

    A: URI, hypertension, and prostate CA.

    P: Symptomatic care. Continue present medications for hypertension. Run PSA next week in preparation for visit to Dr. B. See back in three months.

    HISTORY: EXPANDED PROBLEM FOCUSED
    EXAMINATION: EXPANDED PROBLEM FOCUSED
    MEDICAL DECISION MAKING: MODERATE

    a. 99202
    b. 99203
    c. 99212
    d. 99213

3. The patient was discharged from a skilled nursing facility on June 10th. The provider's RN has an interactive contact with the patient to do medication reconciliation and check

Chapter 2 Test (Continued)

progress on June 12th. The patient is seen by the provider on June 21st in their assisted living apartment for two chronic problems which are reasonably stable. Prescription drug management is performed. Which of the following correctly describes how this care should be reported?

a. Code 99495 on June 12
b. Code 99496 on June 21
c. Code 99495 on July 10
d. Code 99496 on July 12

4. Assign an E/M code to the following service, based on the contents of the office note and information that follows:

CC: Hip pain. 2 months status post right knee arthroscopy for medial meniscectomy and debridement of ACL tear.

S: The patient has become symptom-free with regard to the knee I repaired, except for a feeling that his knee might want to give way when he goes up and down stairs. He has had no locking, catching, buckling, or giving way. There is no swelling and there is really no pain.

The patient is being sent as a new consult from Dr. A for his left hip, which is painful with walking and with turning certain ways. It will catch and lock and the pain is primarily in the groin. There is no pain in the right hip. He has not been taking anything for the hip other than Tylenol for the pain, which provides little relief. No other musculoskeletal issues. General health otherwise is good except for hypertension, on HCTZ daily. Lives with his wife in a bilevel home.

O: Examination of the left hip: The patient has marked loss of motion. He can flex to about 45 degrees. Internal rotation is 0 degrees, external rotation is 20 degrees. Extension, however, is full. Abduction is about 20 to 25 degrees. Adduction is 15 degrees. With regard to the right hip, his flexion is about 100 degrees, internal rotation is 10 degrees, external rotation is 30 degrees, and abduction is 45 degrees. Adduction is 30 degrees. Examination of the knees reveals well-healed surgical wound about the right knee. He has excellent range of motion. There is good stability, except for a slight hint of anterior drawer sign.

Diagnostic tests: Tests are reviewed. The x-rays of the hips done last week by his primary physician reveal he has a rather significant osteoarthritis of the left hip, and somewhat lesser osteoarthritis of the right hip.

A: Osteoarthritis of the hips, bilaterally, left worse than right.

Status post right knee arthroscopy for debridement of torn medial meniscus and debridement of stump of ACL tear.

P: I have given him an order for an ACL brace and prescription for Ibuprofen 600 mg 1, p.o. t.i.d., with two refills for the hip. I would like to see him back in a month for reevaluation. If there is no improvement, will discuss the possibility of a joint injection to the hip.

cc: Dr. A
HISTORY: DETAILED
EXAMINATION: EXPANDED PROBLEM FOCUSED
MEDICAL DECISION MAKING: LOW

a. 99242
b. 99242–24
c. 99243
d. 99243–24

5. Assign an E/M code to the following service, based on the contents of the hospital note and information that follows:

HPI: The patient is an 11-year-old child who was admitted for abdominal pain. He was sent over from his primary care physician's office because of this pain. Mom states that the pain started today at about 2:00 pm when it just suddenly hit him. He started to bend over and writhe in pain. It seems to be somewhat constant with worsening periods at times. He states that it is somewhere in the suprapubic area. It is not associated with meals or with urination. Mom also states that he has never had these troubles before. He has not had any associated constipation, vomiting, or diarrhea and has not had any fever at all with this episode. While in the PCP's office, he did have a UA that did show blood microscopically. There is no gross hematuria. He does have ADHD for which he takes Adderall and he takes clonidine for sleep at night. He had been treated in the past 2 weeks for URI with

(Continued on next page)

Chapter 2 Test (Continued)

Zithromax, of which he has 2 days left. He also was given prednisone, 3 days left and is also doing albuterol nebulizations at home. All other systems are reviewed and are negative.

Medications:	As above.
Allergies:	None.
Surgeries:	None.
Immunizations:	Up to date.
Family History:	Not significant for any type of renal problems or renal stones. There is a history of alcoholism on both sides of the family and no history of CA.
Social History:	He lives at home with parents and four other siblings. Attends St. Joseph School in the 5th grade.

Examination: General: He is alert and active. He is obviously in pain and writhing on the bed.

HEENT: Head is normocephalic, atraumatic. His pupils are equal, round and reactive to light. His oropharynx seems to be somewhat dry. TMs are clear. He does have poor dentition. Neck: Supple without adenopathy. Lungs: To my examination are clear. I do not hear any wheezing. His air entry is good and he does not have a prolonged expiratory phase. Cardiovascular: Regular rate and rhythm without any murmur. Abdomen: Soft. Seems to be tender in the suprapubic area only. He has no other point tenderness. The right quadrant does not have any point tenderness. He has no rebound. He does not appear to be distended. He does have bowel sounds in all four quadrants. Extremities: He moves all four. Pulses are 2+ in all extremities. Neurologic: DTRs are 2+. There appear to be no motor or sensory deficits. Skin: Well perfused. Capillary refill is less than 2 seconds. He does not have any rashes.

Assessment and Plan: Suprapubic abdominal pain.

1. Will admit him and do an ultrasound of the kidneys and urinary collecting system to image for any possible kidney stones. In addition, we will also do an abdominal series to investigate for any intra-abdominal pathology.

   We will strain his urine for any stones while he is here and will get a basic metabolic panel, UA with micro, spot urine for calcium and creatinine, calcium/creatinine ratio, and CBC to rule out v infectious cause.

2. We gave him a bolus of fluid due to some mild dehydration and placed him on IV fluids at maintenance after that. We will place him on morphine overnight every 3 hours as needed for his pain control. He can have a diet as tolerated if he is able and wants to eat.

3. Will keep him on his normal psych meds of clonidine and Adderall.

4. Will continue his Zithromax to completion and will make albuterol nebs prn for sats below 98%. My suspicion is that his lungs have cleared and he won't need these any longer.

5. Discharge tomorrow if pain is resolved.

   HISTORY: COMPREHENSIVE
   EXAMINATION: COMPREHENSIVE
   MEDICAL DECISION MAKING: HIGH

   a. 99223
   b. 99236
   c. 99245
   d. 99255

6. The physician office note states: "Counseling visit, 15 minutes counseling in follow-up with a patient newly diagnosed with diabetes." If the physician codes a 99214 visit, which vital piece of documentation is missing to substantiate this code?

   a. Chief complaint
   b. History component
   c. Exam component
   d. Total length of visit

7. A patient is admitted and discharged from the hospital on the same date. Which category(ies) of E/M services should the physician use to code these services?

   a. Initial Hospital Care and Hospital Discharge Services
   b. Initial Observation Care and Observation Care Discharge Services
   c. Observation or Inpatient Care Services (Including Admission and Discharge Services)
   d. Initial Inpatient Consultations

Chapter 2 Test (Continued)

8. Assign an E/M code to the following service, based on the contents of the hospital note and information that follows:

ADMITTING DIAGNOSIS: Suicide attempt.

HPI: The patient is a 17-year-old girl with salicylate overdose as a suicide attempt. She has a 3-year history of depression, suicide attempts, and self-mutilating behavior. She had a determined suicide attempt last night at about 7 pm by an overdose of aspirin. She has been depressed chronically and has had over 10 suicide attempts, the most recently being 3 weeks ago when she cut her left wrist, the most serious to date. She did write a suicide note stating that she loved and missed her friends in Maryland. She took approximately 30 aspirin over a several-hour period because she had a headache. She went to bed and then awoke not able to hear and with her ears ringing. She states she explained this to her mother at that point because as long as she was still alive, she did not want to have that awful ringing in her ears, which is why she sought help.

She complains of a chronic, depressed mood, low energy, early morning awakening, low level of interest and concentration. She reports having felt this way since about the 4th grade. She has chronic suicidal ideations but does not have a plan to hurt herself while here at the hospital. She states she will ask for help if she is feeling this way while here. The separation from her friends in Maryland appears to have tipped her over the edge last night.

PAST PSYCHIATRIC HISTORY: She had had three previous inpatient hospitalizations on psychiatric wards for about 1 month each, most recently being 1 year ago. She has been diagnosed with depression but has had no improvement on any medications. Some of her medications have included Celexa, Wellbutrin, Prozac, and Effexor, and she has been on no meds in the past year.

She has not seen a psychiatrist since moving back 3 months ago. She did have a psychiatrist that she got along with quite well near the end of her stay in Maryland.

SUBSTANCE ABUSE HISTORY: She drinks alcohol about four times a month and drinks at parties. She smokes marijuana frequently, and she usually does this by herself. She has used cocaine, heroin, and speed, all in the past but nothing at this time. She smokes half a pack of cigarettes a day, drinks 2+ cups of coffee a day, and also takes caffeine tablets.
ALLERGIES: No known drug allergies. Her immunizations are reportedly up-to-date.

PAST MEDICAL HISTORY: History of headaches behind the right eye since about the 4th grade. These headaches are associated with nausea, resolve with sleep, and come about once a week. Usual trigger is stress. She had an appendectomy at 12 years of age. She reports no other significant past medical history.

SOCIAL HISTORY: She is the second of four daughters in the family. She complains of frequent moves by the family so she feels very disconnected from friends she has made in multiple places. Most recently feels alone without her father. She reports that she has no respect for her mother who is a "fake." Dad visits sometimes on weekends but is still trying to find a job here.

EMERGENCY ROOM COURSE: Upon arrival to the emergency department, she was given a gastric lavage with charcoal, of which she drank 50 g without a problem. She had numerous labs done of which her salicylate level was 47.3, about 12 hours out from the ingestion. Her urine tox screen was otherwise negative. Pregnancy test is negative. Other labs in records. The patient was started on IV fluids with two amps of bicarbonate and 20 mEq of KCL at 250 cc per hour.

PHYSICAL EXAMINATION: Patient was afebrile with normal vital signs. Generally, she was alert and oriented x3. She was a well-developed and well-appearing female looking her stated age. She is very pleasant and cooperative through the examination. She was very articulate with a depressed mode though animated when talking. Her speech was appropriate in rate, volume, and tone. Her attention and concentration were quite good. HEENT: Pupils are equal, round, reactive to light. Extraocular movements are intact. TMs clear bilaterally. Oropharynx clear with moist mucous membranes. NECK: Supple with shoddy adenopathy. LUNGS: Clear to auscultation with equal breath sounds bilaterally. HEART: Normal S1 and S2, no murmur or gallop. ABDOMEN: Positive bowel sounds, soft, nontender, nondistended, no masses or hepatosplenomegaly. EXTREMITIES: No cyanosis, clubbing, or edema. SKIN: Both arms and legs have numerous old scars from self-mutilation. Her right forearm has a more recent abrasion from when she fell down some stairs. There is a more recent cut on the left wrist from the recent suicide attempt 3 weeks ago.

ASSESSMENT: This is a 17-year-old with salicylate overdose as a suicide attempt. She is in the toxic range for salicylate overdose.

(Continued on next page)

Chapter 2 Test (Continued)

After discussion with toxicology, because her mental status is normal and she is afebrile and appropriate, we decided to admit her to the medicine unit, monitoring her salicylate level, electrolytes, and venous pH every 4 hours, alkalizing her urine to a pH greater than 8. We will use D5 .45 normal saline with 3 amps of bicarb at 20 mEq of KCL at a rate of 200 cc per hour as I discussed with Poison Control. We will continue to do checks on her every hour and obtain a psychiatric consult for recommendations on further plans for discharge. We will plan that after 24 hours if her salicylate level is falling and is less than toxic level times 2 greater than 4 hours apart and her electrolytes are stable, we will discharge per the recommendation of the psychiatrist. Suicide precautions while in house.

HISTORY: DETAILED
EXAMINATION: COMPREHENSIVE
MEDICAL DECISION MAKING: HIGH

   a.   99221
   b.   99222
   c.   99223
   d.   99236

9. Critical care delivered to a 10-year-old patient for 85 minutes is coded as:

   a.   99291 × 3
   b.   99291, 99292
   c.   99291, 99292 × 2
   d.   99291, 99292 × 3

10. A patient is seen in the emergency room, admitted to an inpatient bed and discharged on the same calendar date. To code these services, the coder would choose the CPT code(s) from which of the following categories:

   a.   Emergency Department Services, Initial Hospital Care and Hospital Discharge Services
   b.   Emergency Department Services and Hospital Discharge Services
   c.   Observation or Inpatient Care Services (Including Admission and Discharge Services)
   d.   Initial Hospital Care

Chapter 3

Anesthesia

Objectives

Upon completion of this lesson, the student should be able to do the following:

- Describe the anesthesia section and its codes

- List the services included in the anesthesia code package and describe services that may be included in addition to the anesthesia services

- Define modifiers and their use with anesthesia codes

- Describe the anesthesia code format and the arrangement of the section

- Assign anesthesia codes to given cases

- Calculate fees for anesthesia services

- Assign appropriate codes for analgesia services provided by the anesthetist

This chapter discusses the codes used to report anesthesia services usually provided by anesthesiologists, certified registered nurse anesthetists (CRNAs), or anesthesiologist assistants (AAs). It is important to distinguish the anesthesia codes from the surgery codes, which are assigned for the performance of the actual surgery. At one time, anesthesia providers were required by most third-party payers to bill for their services by using the same surgical CPT code that would be submitted by the surgeon. The anesthesia provider would indicate that the charge was for anesthesia by submitting a type of service code 07, Anesthesia, in box 24C of the CMS 1500 insurance claim form. With the passage of HIPAA, third-party payers are required to accept all CPT codes, including the anesthesia section of codes, when submitted by physicians for payment. However, some third-party payers are still in the process of updating their software and are not yet capable of accepting and processing anesthesia codes. Medicare and Medicaid require anesthesia codes. Most large third-party payers will also accept them. Because workman's compensation payers are exempt from these HIPAA statues and many of them still require the use of either surgical CPT codes or carrier-created codes when billing for anesthesia services, coders should verify the requirements of each of the different payers prior to submitting claims.

Format and Arrangement of Codes in the Anesthesia Section

The anesthesia codes (00100–01999) are arranged first by body site, beginning with the head, and then by specific surgical procedure performed. They may be found in the Index of the CPT code book by referencing either of the main terms Anesthesia or Analgesia.

Within the subsections, codes may be very specific or very general. For example, consider the differences between codes 00560 and 00580. Code 00560 is very broad in scope, including any heart, pericardium, and great vessel procedure, whereas code 00580 is for only two types of transplant procedures.

00560	Anesthesia for procedures on heart, pericardial sac, and great vessels of chest; without pump oxygenator

00580	Anesthesia for heart transplant or heart/lung transplant

The Anesthesia Package

Basic types of anesthesia services include general, block, regional, epidural, and monitored anesthesia care (MAC) and are provided by or under the responsible supervision of an anesthesiologist. The anesthesia "package" includes the following services:

- Routine preoperative and postoperative visits to evaluate the patient for the appropriate anesthesia and to monitor the patient's post surgical recovery from anesthesia

- Anesthesia care during the procedure, including induction and emergence

- Administration of fluids and/or blood, and blood products

- Usual monitoring services such as EKG, temperature, blood pressure, oximetry (measurement of oxygen saturation of blood) capnography (measurement of carbon dioxide in the blood) and mass spectrometry (analyzing a substance via electrical particles in a magnetic field)

Invasive forms of monitoring are not included in the standard anesthesia package and should be reported separately. These monitoring devices include intra-arterial catheters (also known as arterial lines or A-Lines), central venous lines (also known as CVPs), and Swan-Ganz (pulmonary artery) catheters. Because CPT states that these items are not a part of the standard anesthesia package, a –59 modifier is not normally required when billing these devices. However, please note that, when placing a Swan-Ganz catheter, a central venous line is normally placed first to serve as an introducer, and the Swan-Ganz is then threaded through the CVP. Because the CVP has been placed only for the purpose of introducing the Swan-Ganz, it would not be billed separately; only the charge for the Swan-Ganz would be billed. In certain circumstances it may be necessary for patient care to insert both a Swan-Ganz (via a CVP placed solely as an introducer) and an additional central venous line, using a different insertion site for each device. In this case, it would be appropriate to bill for both the Swan-Ganz and the second CVP, including modifier –59 on the CVP charge to indicate that the second CVP is a separate procedure from the Swan-Ganz.

Only one code from the anesthesia section is reported per anesthesia session (that is, continuous time period during which the patient is anesthetized). Anesthesia codes are chosen based upon the anatomical site of the procedure and the type of procedure performed, not the type of anesthesia used. If multiple surgical procedures are performed during a single anesthesia session, the anesthesia code that describes the most complicated and resource-intensive procedure is reported. The time should be the combined total of all procedures in the anesthesia session. Anesthesia add-on codes are the exception to this and are reported in addition to the primary anesthesia code.

Example: Neuraxial epidural anesthesia is provided to a patient for a planned vaginal delivery: continued fetal monitoring shows distress necessitating a Cesarean delivery. The add-on codes reported for these services would be 01967 for the epidural anesthesia for the planned vaginal delivery and 01968 for the anesthesia for the Cesarean delivery following the neuraxial labor analgesia.

Per Medicare guidelines, only anesthesiologists, certified registered nurse anesthetists (CRNAs), or anesthesiology assistants (AAs) performing solely anesthesia services should bill using anesthesia codes. A surgeon who also administers sedation should not bill a separate anesthesia charge using an anesthesia code. Some private/commercial insurance carriers will reimburse a surgeon for conscious sedation during a surgical procedure, provided a trained observer is present to monitor the patient's vital signs. (See Moderate (Conscious) Sedation codes 99143–99150). However, Medicare regards any type of anesthesia provided by the surgeon a component of the surgical package and will generally not provide separate payment for these services.

Modifiers Commonly Used in Reporting Anesthesia Services

Modifiers commonly used with anesthesia codes include physical status modifiers to report the physical condition of the patient. The guidelines at the beginning of the anesthesia section of the

CPT code book also address other modifiers that may be used in reporting anesthesia codes. CPT modifiers are two-digit modifiers attached to the basic code and are used to report circumstances such as unusual or distinct procedures or services, mandated services, multiple procedures, and discontinued procedures. HCPCS modifiers provide additional information on how the anesthesia was administered. (See chapter 9 for additional information on modifiers.)

Physical Status Modifiers

Physical status modifiers are used to indicate the patient's condition and thus the complexity of the anesthesia service. They are consistent with the ranking system used by the American Society of Anesthesiologists (ASA). Physical status modifiers are assigned by a member of the anesthesia staff prior to surgery, usually during a "preanesthetic interview" with the patient. These modifiers indicate the complexity of the proposed anesthesia, and allow the anesthesia staff to be prepared for possible problems that might arise during the course of the anesthesia due to any chronic conditions or diseases from which the patient might suffer.

The physical status modifiers and their definitions are as follows:

–P1   A normal healthy patient

–P2   A patient with mild systemic disease

–P3   A patient with severe systemic disease

–P4   A patient with severe systemic disease that is a constant threat to life

–P5   A moribund patient who is not expected to survive without the operation

–P6   A declared brain-dead patient whose organs are being removed for donor purposes

Some third-party payers recognize the physical status modifiers and allow additional reimbursement in recognition of the increased difficulty in administering anesthesia to such a patient. When used, the modifier is appended to the basic anesthesia code. Many anesthesia practices do not assign modifier –P1, A normal healthy patient; modifier –P2, A patient with mild systemic disease; or modifier –P6, A declared brain-dead patient, to their billing charges. Because these modifiers represent patients whose physical condition should have little or no clinical impact on their anesthesia, the ASA ranks these modifiers as having no impact on reimbursement. Therefore, many anesthesia providers choose to use only the –P3, –P4, and –P5 modifiers, which represent patients who are inherently more at risk due to their physical condition. Because not all carriers recognize these modifiers, it is important to adhere to individual third-party payer rules and regulations when billing for anesthesia services. Neither Medicare nor Medicaid recognizes physical status modifiers. Some practices use these modifiers to analyze patient outcomes so it is advisable to check first before omitting these modifiers.

CPT Modifiers Used in Anesthesia Coding

The following CPT modifiers are commonly used in the anesthesia section. As mentioned in the above discussion of physical status modifiers, it is important to follow third-party payer guidelines when assigning CPT modifiers in coding anesthesia services.

–22   **Increased Procedural Services:** Modifier –22 may be reported when the work required to provide the service is substantially greater than typically required. Supportive documentation may need to be submitted to the third-party payer to justify use of this modifier (that is, increased intensity, time, technical difficulty of procedure, severity of patient's condition, or physical and mental effort required).

–23 **Unusual Anesthesia:** Modifier –23 may be reported when general anesthesia is administered for a procedure that usually requires local anesthesia or none at all. This modifier would be attached to the appropriate code describing the anesthesia service.

–51 **Multiple Procedures:** Modifier –51 may be reported to identify that multiple services were provided during the same operative episode. This modifier would not be used with an anesthesia code, but it might be necessary to report if, for example, multiple intra-arterial catheters (A-Lines) were placed via separate insertion sites during the same operative session. The first procedure listed should identify the major service provided or the most resource-intensive service provided. Subsequent or secondary services should be appended with modifier –51.

–53 **Discontinued Procedure:** Modifier –53 is appropriate for circumstances when the physician elects to terminate or discontinue a procedure, usually because of risk to the patient's well-being. However, this modifier is not meant to report the elective cancellation of a procedure before the patient's surgical preparation or induction of anesthesia. Also, the appropriate ICD-10-CM code should be assigned to identify the reason for the procedure's termination or discontinuation.

–59 **Distinct Procedural Service:** Modifier –59 may be used to identify that a procedure/service was distinct or independent from other services provided on the same day.

HCPCS Level II Modifiers Used in Anesthesia Coding

A number of HCPCS Level II modifiers may be required when coding anesthesia services. These include

–AA   Anesthesia services performed personally by anesthesiologist

–AD   Medical supervision by a physician: more than four concurrent anesthesia procedures

–G8   Monitored anesthesia care (MAC) for deep complex, complicated, or markedly invasive surgical procedure

–G9   Monitored anesthesia care for patient who has history of severe cardiopulmonary condition

–QK   Medical direction of two, three, or four concurrent anesthesia procedures involving qualified individuals

–QS   Monitored anesthesia care (MAC) service

–QY   Medical direction of one certified registered nurse anesthetist (CRNA) by an anesthesiologist

Modifiers Specific to CRNA Coding

Two modifiers are specific to CRNA coding. These are

–QX   CRNA service with medical direction by a physician

–QZ   CRNA service without medical direction by a physician

Codes Used in Reporting Qualifying Circumstances

Four codes have been provided to report unusually difficult circumstances for anesthesia administration. Such circumstances refer to patient conditions, operative conditions, and/or unusual risk factors.

The qualifying circumstance codes are actually from the medicine section of the CPT code book but also are listed in the guidelines at the beginning of the anesthesia section. These codes are not used alone; rather, they are used in conjunction with an anesthesia code/physical status modifier. If more than one qualifying circumstance applies, more than one code may be assigned. The qualifying circumstance codes are

99100   Anesthesia for patient of extreme age, under 1 year and over 70 (List separately in addition to code for primary anesthesia procedure)

99116   Anesthesia complicated by utilization of total body hypothermia (List separately in addition to code for primary anesthesia procedure)

99135   Anesthesia complicated by utilization of controlled hypotension (List separately in addition to code for primary anesthesia procedure)

99140   Anesthesia complicated by emergency conditions (specify) (List separately in addition to code for primary anesthesia procedure)

An emergency, as applicable to code 99140, is defined as existing when delay in treatment of the patient would lead to a significant increase in the threat to life or body part.

Some third-party payers recognize the codes for qualifying circumstances and allow additional reimbursement in recognition of the increased difficulty in administering anesthesia to such a patient; Medicare does not. Therefore, it is important to review all third-party payer rules and regulations when reporting anesthesia services.

Steps in Coding Anesthesia Services

To correctly code for anesthesia services, the coder must first determine if it is necessary to assign an anesthesia code or a surgical CPT code to the service. Again, this will be determined by which third-party payer will be processing the claim. When an anesthesia code is required, follow these steps to determine the correct code:

1. Refer to the main term, Anesthesia, in the Index.

2. Search for a subterm to indicate the anatomic site of the procedure and/or the actual procedure performed.

3. Reference the code or codes noted in the Index within the tabular portion of the CPT code book.

4. Read and apply any notes or cross-references that may appear in the Tabular section.

5. Choose the anesthesia code associated with the procedure or, if multiple procedures were performed, the anesthesia code for the most complicated or resource-intensive procedure.

6. Review anesthesia record for any techniques that would change the code selection (that is, one-lung ventilation, positioning-field avoidance, with pump oxygenator).

7. Assign the applicable physical status modifier (if recognized by the patient's insurance carrier).

8. Assign codes for any qualifying circumstances (if recognized by the patient's insurance carrier).

If it is necessary to assign a surgical CPT code rather than an anesthesia code, follow the process outlined in chapter 4, Surgery, to determine the primary surgical code for the procedure. Once the coder has determined the correct code, assign the applicable physical status modifier and/or code for qualifying circumstance as appropriate.

Calculating Fees for Anesthesia Services

Unlike a surgeon's office, which submits a flat fee for a surgical package, anesthesia charges can vary from case to case. Instead of billing a flat fee, the anesthesia charge is determined by the complexity of the procedure and the amount of time that the anesthesia personnel are required to spend with the patient. Every anesthesia code is assigned a weighted value that reflects the complexity of the case. The American Society of Anesthesiologists (ASA) publishes the *Relative Value Guide* each year to provide a resource for establishing basic values for anesthesia used in most surgical procedures, as well as base values for both the physical status modifiers and the codes for qualifying circumstances. The base units for a procedure include the usual preoperative interview and evaluation, intraoperative care including induction/administration of the anesthetic, administration of IV fluids and/or blood products, interpretation of non-invasive monitoring, care during emergence from the anesthesia and postoperative visits by the anesthesiologist. The base units and time units are added to the modifying units for physical status to establish the charge for anesthesia services. It should be noted that the ASA guide is a relative value study and not a fee schedule, but it is widely accepted as a method of establishing fees for anesthesia services. When multiple surgical procedures are performed during a single anesthetic session, the anesthesia code for the most complex (highest base value) should be assigned as the appropriate anesthesia code for the case.

In addition to the anesthesia code, time must be reported separately when anesthesia services are billed. To determine the amount of anesthesia time, time begins with the preparation of the patient by the anesthesiologist, CRNA, and/or AA for induction of the anesthesia (usually in the OR) and ends when the patient is safely placed under the care of a non-anesthesia provider for postoperative supervision. This is the point where the anesthesiologist is no longer in attendance. It should be noted that when multiple surgical procedures are performed during a single anesthetic administration, only the anesthesia code representing the most complex procedure is reported but the time reported is the combined total for all procedures. Also, the time reported should only reflect time involved in the actual anesthesia. For procedures performed by the anesthesia staff that will be billed separately, such as placement of central lines or injections for postoperative pain control, the time spent performing these procedures should not be included within the total anesthesia time. However, if a block such as an epidural is placed preoperatively to be used as the primary anesthetic, the block will not be billed separately and time spent in placement should be included within the total anesthesia time.

Anesthesia time is calculated in units. For Medicare billing, a 15-minute block of time is equal to one time unit. Other third-party payers may use a different measure of minutes to determine time unit increments. It is important to maintain an accurate profile for each third-party payer to ensure accurate and compliant claim submission and to receive full and timely reimbursement for all anesthesia services provided.

The charge for anesthesia services is based on the following formula:

$$\text{Base unit} + \text{time unit} + \text{modifying factors} \times \text{conversion factor} = \$\$\$$$

The conversion factor is the dollar amount that the anesthesia provider elects to bill per anesthesia unit.

Example: (5 base units + 8 time units + 1 modifying factor) × $50
5 + 8 + 1 = 14 × 50.00 = $700

Medical Direction

To bill Medicare and Medicaid for anesthesia services, anesthesia providers must also provide information regarding who provided the anesthesia service itself. Anesthesia can be provided by an anesthesiologist working alone, a certified registered nurse anesthetist (CRNA) working alone, or by a care team approach involving both an anesthesiologist and a CRNA or an anesthesiologist assistant (AA) working in concert. Anesthesiologist assistants cannot provide anesthesia or surgical services unless they are working under the direct supervision of an anesthesiologist; therefore, an AA will never submit a claim for solo service.

When either an anesthesiologist or a CRNA working alone provides the anesthesia services for a Medicare or Medicaid patient, the provider receives 100 percent of the allowed payment amount. When an anesthesiologist and an anesthetist provide anesthesia under the team approach, the fee is divided and billed out in each provider's name and the allowed Medicare and Medicaid payment is divided between both providers.

When anesthesia is provided under the team approach, the anesthesiologist is responsible for managing as well as participating in the overall anesthesia plan for the patient while the anesthetist is responsible for the administration of the anesthesia itself and the continuous monitoring of the patient during the procedure. The anesthesiologist might be responsible for anesthesia plans for multiple patients in multiple rooms at the same time. This is referred to as either medical direction or medical supervision. Medical direction occurs when the physician is directing two, three, or four concurrent cases; medical supervision occurs when the physician is directing more than four concurrent cases. For a case to qualify as medically directed, the anesthesiologist must also document certain items within the medical record, in addition to ensuring that the concurrency rate is no greater than four cases being performed simultaneously. Per Medicare guidelines, the physician must do the following:

1. Perform a preanesthetic examination and evaluation of the patient

2. Prescribe the anesthesia plan for the case

3. Personally participate in the most demanding aspects of the anesthesia plan, including induction and emergence, if applicable

4. Ensure that any procedures not personally performed by the physician are performed by a qualified anesthetist

5. Monitor the course of the anesthesia at frequent intervals

6. Remain physically present and available for immediate diagnosis and treatment of emergencies

7. Provide indicated postanesthesia care

Other services allowed during medical direction include the following:

- Addressing an emergency of short duration in the immediate area
- Administering an epidural or caudal anesthetic to a laboring patient
- Performing periodic, rather than continuous, monitoring of an OB patient
- Receiving patients entering suite for the next surgery
- Checking on or discharging patients in the PACU
- Coordinating scheduling matters

Cases that are billed to Medicare or Medicaid as medically supervised receive a reduced rate of reimbursement. Therefore, both Medicare and Medicaid track the concurrency rate (how many cases an anesthesiologist is concurrently managing) for all anesthesia charges submitted by the anesthesiologist. Increasingly, many other third-party payers are also beginning to require this information on claims.

Concurrency

It is the responsibility of the coding and billing staff to determine the concurrency rate of all anesthesia services billed to Medicare or Medicaid (or any other payers that may require this information). Many anesthesia computerized billing programs offer an automatic concurrency calculator within their software. If such a program is not available, the concurrency must be manually calculated. To manually calculate the concurrency rate, the coder must compare all anesthesia cases performed by the physician on the date in question to determine if cases overlap. Every case must be included, not just the cases for Medicare or Medicaid patients.

Example: Dr. Smith is managing CRNA Wilson in room one from 8:00 to 10:00, CRNA Peterson in room two from 9:30 to 10:00, and CRNA Howard in room three from 9:45 to 10:15. From 9:45 to 10:00, all three cases are concurrent—that is, they are all being performed at the same time. This is the point of maximum concurrency—when the most cases are being performed simultaneously. The concurrency for each of these cases would be 3 to 1.

To indicate the concurrency of a case when billing the charge, the coder should attach one of the previously listed HCPCS Level II modifiers to the anesthesia code. In the preceding example, if CRNA Wilson's case was for a patient covered by Medicare, the physician portion of the fee would be billed with the appropriate anesthesia code plus modifier –QK (for medical direction of two, three, or four concurrent anesthesia providers), and the CRNA portion of the fee would be billed with the appropriate anesthesia code plus modifier –QX (CRNA service with medical direction by a physician). An anesthesiologist acting as the only anesthesia provider for a Medicare patient would submit a claim for the full fee in the anesthesiologist's name and modifier –AA (anesthesia services personally performed by anesthesiologist) would be attached to the anesthesia code. A CRNA acting as the only anesthesia provider for a Medicare patient would submit a claim for the full anesthesia fee in the CRNA's name and modifier –QZ (CRNA service without medical direction by a physician) should be attached to the anesthesia code.

Beginning in 2010, Medicare will reimburse at 100 percent for cases involving residents when the supervision by the teaching physician is no greater than 2 to 1. For these cases, the coder should attach the modifiers –AA and –GC to the appropriate anesthesia code. If the teaching physician is directing two to four residents, the appropriate modifiers would be –QK and –GC.

Monitored Anesthesia Care

Monitored anesthesia care (MAC) is a controversial reimbursement issue among many third-party payers. The term is used to describe situations where the patient remains able to protect his or her airway for the majority of the procedure, usually a diagnostic or therapeutic procedure such as a breast biopsy or colonoscopy. Monitored anesthesia care includes the following:

- All services routinely provided during any anesthesia encounter, including a preoperative and postoperative visit as well as intraprocedural care including monitoring vital signs and maintaining the patient's airway

- Diagnosing and treating clinical problems during the procedure

- Administering medications, as necessary

- Providing other medical services, as needed, to complete the procedure safely

Some insurance carriers, including Medicare and Medicaid, require that any anesthesia cases performed under MAC be identified by the addition of a specific modifier to the charge when billing. HCPCS Level II modifier –QS, Monitored anesthesia care (MAC) service, should be attached to the anesthesia code to indicate that the anesthesia service was provider under MAC.

Carriers also may require that medical necessity be documented to support the need for MAC. To demonstrate medical necessity, anesthesia billers may be required to attach an additional diagnosis code to the charge line indicating that the patient suffers from a condition or chronic disease that might possibly have a negative impact on the patient's outcome, which would warrant the use of continuous monitoring during the case.

If, during the course of a procedure, a patient loses consciousness and the ability to respond purposefully, the anesthesia care then becomes a general anesthesia whether or not instrumentation is required to maintain the airway. If this occurs and the case is being medically directed, the anesthesiologist *must* be present for induction. If this is a possibility, the anesthesiologist may want to participate on the induction of MAC cases just as they would for general anesthesia cases.

Medicare Modifiers Specific to MAC Anesthesia Coding

Two modifiers specific to MAC Anesthesia coding are

- –G8   MAC for deep, complex, complicated, or markedly invasive surgical procedures
- –G9   MAC for patient who has history of severe cardiopulmonary condition

Medicare will allow certain anesthesia codes that would normally require proof of medical necessity when performed under MAC to pass through the system if certain conditions are met. For example, if a patient has a history of a severe cardiopulmonary condition, the coder may communicate that information to Medicare by attaching HCPCS Level II modifier –G9, Monitored anesthesia care for a patient who has history of severe cardiopulmonary condition, to the anesthesia code instead of modifier –QS.

Billing policies for MAC anesthesia may vary widely from carrier to carrier. Some carriers require a modifier and others do not. Carriers may develop individual lists as to what (if anything) must be documented to demonstrate the medical necessity of MAC anesthesia, and information that supports the use of MAC for one payer will not be recognized by another payer. Coders must verify what each third-party payer requires regarding MAC anesthesia before submitting any claims for payment.

Pain Management Services

In addition to providing anesthesia services, many anesthesiologists also perform procedures that are related to analgesia, the control of pain. These services may be provided within the hospital, in conjunction with anesthesia services, or as a completely separate function in a freestanding pain management practice. Pain management services are usually provided by an anesthesiologist as opposed to a CRNA. When billing for pain management services, it is important to remember that the anesthesiologist is actually performing the procedure itself and that the charges should be submitted as surgery codes rather than anesthesia codes.

Probably the best-known type of analgesia routinely provided by an anesthesiologist is an epidural for labor and delivery. This procedure is intended to minimize the pain and discomfort that can occur during labor without reducing the patient's awareness or ability to respond and without affecting the unborn child. Billing policies for labor epidurals vary greatly from one third-party payer to another. Some payers prefer that claims be submitted with the surgical CPT code for a continuous lumbar epidural infusion (see CPT code 62319); others require submission of anesthesia CPT code 01967 for neuraxial labor analgesia/anesthesia. Some payers require that the claim be submitted with the total time that the catheter is infusing attached to the charge; other payers do not recognize a time factor for the code. Once again, it is vital that the coder verify billing requirements with the third-party payers prior to the submission of claims.

Pain management services may also be provided in conjunction with anesthesia services. The anesthesiologist may perform injections or pain blocks, which, like a labor epidural, provide the patient with adequate postoperative pain control while allowing the patient to remain alert and responsive without experiencing some of the side effects present in some other forms of pain medications. These injections may be performed either immediately prior to or immediately following surgery and can be placed in many areas of the body depending upon the operative site. For example, for certain extremely invasive abdominal surgeries, the anesthesiologist might place a continuous epidural infusion catheter in the patient's back immediately prior to surgery. While an epidural can be used as an anesthetic, in this case the epidural is placed solely for the purpose of providing postoperative pain relief to the patient. General anesthesia is provided for the surgery itself and is billed with the appropriate anesthesia code. A separate charge line is billed for the continuous epidural, using CPT code 62318 if the epidural is placed within the cervical or thoracic areas of the spine or CPT 62319 if it is placed with the lumbar or sacral areas of the spine.

Unlike an intra-arterial catheter (A-line) or central venous line (CVP), an epidural catheter is not inherently separate from the anesthetic itself—an epidural can also be used as an adjunct anesthetic. Therefore, if a block is ordered by the surgeon for postoperative pain management only, it is necessary to convey to the third-party payer that this is an entirely separate procedure. CPT modifier –59, Distinct Procedural Service, or appropriate HCPCS modifier such as –XU for a patient covered by Medicare, should be attached to the code for the epidural or other block. Conversely, if the epidural is placed and used for *both* the anesthetic and postoperative pain, the provider may not bill separately for the epidural placement. In this case, it is included within the anesthesia charge itself. These policies should be followed regardless of the type of block performed.

Postoperatively, the epidural catheter is attached to an infusion pump that delivers a measured dose of medication to the patient at a regular interval. This infusion can be left in place for several hours or several days, depending upon the needs of the patient. Normally, if the catheter is left in place for several days, the anesthesiologist will check the patient daily to verify that the catheter is functioning correctly and that the patient is not experiencing any complications. This daily management of the catheter can be billed using CPT anesthesia code 01996, Daily management of epidural or subarachnoid continuous drug administration. This charge is billed as a single fee per day; no time is attached. Some third-party payers do not recognize and separately pay for epidural management; others recognize the code but only pay for a set number of days. Billers need to verify individual billing policy with third-party payers prior to submitting claims.

Anesthesiologists may also be called upon to perform a pain injection for a patient who is not having surgery. For example, a patient is admitted with multiple rib fractures. The patient will not be undergoing any kind of surgical repair in the operating room. However, the patient is experiencing severe chest wall pain from the fractures. The anesthesiologist may be asked to perform multiple injections into the patient's intercostal nerves to reduce the pain of the fractures. To bill for these injections, the coder would submit CPT code 64420, Injection, anesthetic agent; intercostal nerves, multiple, regional block. Because this is the only procedure performed, CPT modifier –59, Distinct Procedural Service, is not required.

Codes for the various types of injections may be found under Injection in the CPT Index and following the appropriate subheading for either Epidural or Nerve—Anesthetic. Injection charges are submitted as surgical fees; no anesthesia time is required. Because these are not anesthetic services, no concurrency modifiers are required. Physical status modifiers and qualifying circumstances codes would not be attached to these injection codes because the injections are considered surgical procedures instead of anesthesia.

Exercise 3.1. Anesthesia

Choose the best answer for each of the following questions.

1. A patient is brought to the emergency department with a ruptured aortic aneurysm and is taken immediately into surgery for operative repair. Which qualifying circumstance code is assigned to indicate that anesthesia for the surgery will be affected by the emergency status of this patient?

   a. 99140
   b. 99100
   c. 99116
   d. 99135

2. Which modifier is used to indicate that a pain injection performed by the anesthesiologist prior to surgery is a separate procedure from the anesthesia service?

   a. –22
   b. –32
   c. –AA
   d. –XU

3. Which modifier would be added to the anesthesia code for the physician's services to indicate that the physician was medically directing two cases at the same time?

   a. –QK
   b. –P6
   c. –QZ
   d. –AA

Exercise 3.1 (Continued)

Assign anesthesia code(s), including physical status modifiers and any other applicable modifiers and codes, to the following scenarios for Medicare claims.

4. Patient has anesthesia for radical mastectomy with internal mammary node dissection. The anesthesia was administered by a CRNA working without medical direction.

   _____

5. Patient has anesthesia for triple coronary balloon angioplasty. The procedure was aborted when the patient went into atrial fibrillation. The anesthesiologist personally administered the anesthesia.

   _____

6. Patient had general anesthesia administered for extensive debridement of the shoulder joint by arthroscopy. Team care anesthesia was provided by an anesthesiologist medically directing two CRNAs. The anesthesiologist performed a brachial plexus injection for post-operative pain control.

   _____

7. Patient has MAC anesthesia for excision of a basal cell carcinoma on the lower leg. Team care anesthesia was provided by an anesthesiologist medically directing one CRNA.

   _____

Assign the appropriate codes and physical status modifiers to describe anesthesia services for the following scenarios for non-Medicare claims. Assume that all payers require that charges be submitted using anesthesia codes.

8. Anesthesia services for tympanostomy with insertion of ventilating tubes for recurrent otitis media. The patient is 9 months old.

   _____

9. Anesthesia services for triple coronary artery bypass graft. The grafting was performed with the use of a pump oxygenator. Preoperatively, the anesthesiologist placed a Swan-Ganz catheter and an arterial line. The patient had suffered a massive myocardial infarction and was assigned a –P4 physical status.

   _____

10. Anesthesia services for laparoscopic cholecystectomy with cholangiography for acute chole-cystitis. The patient has well-controlled diabetes mellitus and was assigned a –P3 physical status rating by the anesthesiologist preoperatively.

   _____

Chapter 3 Test

Choose the best answer for each of the following questions.

1. Assuming the following parameters are correct, choose the appropriate anesthesia code(s) from the following list and calculate the charge(s).

   A 55-year-old patient is brought urgently to the operating room for an appendectomy for ruptured appendix. The patient has severe chronic obstructive pulmonary disease, and the anesthesiologist has assigned a physical status of four. The total anesthesia time for the procedure is 50 minutes. The anesthesiologist's conversion factor is $25.

   00790—Anesthesia for intraperitoneal procedures in upper abdomen including laparoscopy; not otherwise specified (Base unit value of 7)

   00840—Anesthesia for intraperitoneal procedures in lower abdomen including laparoscopy; not otherwise specified (Base unit value of 6)

   00860—Anesthesia for extraperitoneal procedures in lower abdomen, including urinary tract; not otherwise specified (Base unit value of 6)

   99135—Anesthesia complicated by utilization of controlled hypotension (Base unit value of 5)

   99140—Anesthesia complicated by emergency conditions (Base unit value of 2)

   P2—A patient with mild systemic disease (Base unit value of 0)

   P3—A patient with severe systemic disease (Base unit value of 1)

   P4—A patient with severe systemic disease that is a constant threat to life (Base unit value of 2)

   a. 00840–P4 for $300
   b. 00790–P4 for $325
   c. 00840–P4 for $300; 99140 for $50
   d. 00860–P4 for $350; 99140 for $50

2. Anesthesia services for an endovascular repair of an abdominal aortic aneurysm using a modular bifurcated prosthesis in a 70-year-old Medicare patient, performed on an emergent basis. The patient also has peripheral vascular disease and uncontrolled diabetes. How are the anesthesia services coded?

   a. 00770, 99140
   b. 00770, 99100
   c. 34803, 99100
   d. 34803, 99140

3. Which of the following is true about coding for the services of an anesthesiologist?

   a. They can only use the anesthesia and surgery codes.
   b. They can use any CPT/HCPCS codes that describe the work they do.
   c. HIPAA requires that anesthesiologists use only anesthesia codes.
   d. The use of modifiers is always optional in anesthesia coding.

4. For a 45-year-old patient with renal cell carcinoma, mild coronary artery disease, and hypertension who is not on Medicare, anesthesia services for laparoscopic partial nephrectomy would be coded as:

   a. 00862–P4
   b. 00868–P4
   c. 50543–P2
   d. 50543–P3

Chapter 3 Test (Continued)

5. Anesthesia services for a CABG surgery of five vessels with pump oxygenator are provided. The patient is covered by commercial insurance, has severe coronary artery disease, as well as hypertensive end-stage renal disease and is undergoing hemodialysis. How are the anesthesia services coded?

   a. 00560–P3
   b. 00562–P4
   c. 33518–P2
   d. 33518–P4

6. The anesthesiologist must reduce and maintain a decreased body temperature for a patient with severe systemic disease who is undergoing surgery. How is this additional service reported to the insurance carrier?

   a. By adding modifier –P3
   b. By adding modifier –23
   c. By adding CPT code 99116
   d. By adding CPT code 99149

7. Anesthesia services for left lobectomy due to lung carcinoma in a 65-year-old Medicare patient. The patient also has severe chronic obstructive pulmonary disease and emphysema treated with bronchodilators. How are the anesthesia services coded?

   a. 00541
   b. 00540
   c. 32480
   d. 32440

8. When a patient has a history of a severe cardiopulmonary condition and cannot have general anesthesia, what modifier should be assigned when monitored anesthesia care is provided?

   a. –AA
   b. –QS
   c. –G8
   d. –G9

9. Assuming the following parameters are correct, choose the appropriate anesthesia code(s) from the attached list and calculate the charge(s).

   A 69-year-old Medicare patient is admitted to the hospital for treatment of pneumonia. The patient has a history of a previous prostatectomy for prostate cancer. In addition to the pneumonia, the patient complains of severe groin pain at the site of his previous surgery. Upon the request of the patient's attending physician, the anesthesiologist evaluates the patient and elects to perform a pain injection at the site of the previous surgery. The anesthesiologist's conversion factor is $30.

   00800—Anesthesia for procedures on lower anterior abdominal wall; not otherwise specified (Base unit value of 4)

   64420—Injection, anesthetic agent; intercostal nerve, single (Base unit value of 5)

   64425—Injection, anesthetic agent, ilioinguinal, iliohypogastric nerves (Base unit value of 5)

   a. 64420 for $150
   b. 64425 for $150
   c. 00800 for $120
   d. 00800 for $120; 64420 for $150

(Continued on next page)

Chapter 3 Test (Continued)

10. Anesthesia services for a radical abdominal hysterectomy in a 55-year-old woman with commercial insurance. She is otherwise in good health. How are the anesthesia services coded?

    a. 00846–P1
    b. 00846–P2
    c. 58210–P1
    d. 58210–P2

Chapter 4

Surgery

Objectives

Upon completion of this chapter, the student should be able to do the following:

- Describe the format and basic contents of the surgery section of the CPT code book and its subsections

- Define the surgical package and the services included in it

- Describe the significance of add-on codes and separate procedures in the surgery section

- Describe the coding conventions specific to each subsection of the surgery section

- Understand and apply the definitions pertaining to the surgery section

- Assign CPT codes to given procedures within the surgery section

- Determine when a procedure is a component of a larger procedure

- Apply modifiers to codes within the surgery section based on documentation provided

- Determine when HCPCS Level II codes are required in the surgery section

This chapter discusses the codes listed in the largest section of the CPT code book—surgery. Included in this section are codes and descriptions for services that range from minor procedures to major surgeries.

Coding Used in the Surgery Section

CPT is a nomenclature, or listing, of preferred terms. For this reason, the code descriptions are very detailed and distinctions among codes may be very discrete. Choosing the correct code in a detailed subsection of the surgery section can be difficult. Careful review of the source document, usually the operative report or progress note, is necessary. The body system involved, the approach, the procedure itself, and methods of closure all can affect code assignment. Physician and coder must work together to ensure that the documentation in the health record supports the code(s) selected.

The coder should review the guidelines located at the beginning of the surgery section and many of the subsections of the CPT code book. These guidelines provide the information necessary to ensure proper code assignment. The notes that usually appear in parentheses after individual codes also provide valuable information. Together, they help the coder understand the intended use of the codes, alert the coder to special circumstances regarding code assignment, and direct the coder to alternate codes that may be more appropriate.

Subsections

There are 19 major subsections in the surgery section, most representing body systems. Within each subsection, codes are broken down by anatomical site for that system. This breakdown follows the universal anatomical position, from the top of the body proceeding down. For example, in the respiratory system subsection, the first anatomical position is the nose; in the digestive system, it is the mouth; and so on.

Within each anatomical site, there is a somewhat predictable order of procedures: incision, excision, endoscopy, repair, grafts, and other/miscellaneous. Not every type of procedure exists for every site, and additional procedures may be listed depending on body system and site. The predictability of this arrangement can be helpful in locating codes. For example, all the potential endoscopy codes for the nose are located together in codes 31231–31297.

The Surgical Package

In the CPT code book, the surgical procedures performed include certain services that are considered part of the procedure, are designated as the surgical or global package, and are covered by a single fee. These include the following:

- The operation itself

- Any local infiltration, metacarpal/metatarsal/digital block, or topical anesthesia

- Subsequent to the decision for surgery, one related E/M encounter on the date immediately prior to or on the date of procedure (including history and physical)

- Immediate postoperative care, including dictating operative notes, talking with the family and other physicians

- Associated activities such as writing orders

- Evaluation of the patient in the postanesthesia recovery area

- Typical postoperative follow-up care

Postoperative care includes the care given within the payer's designated follow-up period. For administrative purposes, postoperative visits may be reported with code 99024, Postoperative follow-up visit, included in global service. No charge should be associated with such visits. Chapter 10 discusses how to determine the number of days in the Medicare global surgical package using the Fee Schedule file. The Medical global surgical package for a procedure performed in the operating room is typically 90 days, although some minor procedures may have a 10-day global period.

The surgical package does not include encounters for a complication or a new condition within the follow-up period. Also, preoperative visits or consultations other than the routine presurgical history and physical are not included in the surgical package but can be billed separately. As always, the documentation in the patient's health record must support the code assigned. For example, if a patient develops a complication that requires additional care, this should be documented thoroughly in the health record. The diagnosis code for the complication also should be included and linked appropriately to the CPT code for the additional services provided.

> **Example:** A new patient is seen for abdominal pain:
>
> Office visit #1   A comprehensive history and physical examination and high medical decision making lead to the conclusion that an appendectomy is necessary immediately.
>
> Code Assigned: 99205
>
> Surgery   An appendectomy is performed.
>
> Code Assigned: 44950
>
> Office Visit #2   One week later, the patient returns to the physician's office for a check of the operative wound.
>
> Code Assigned: 99024 (no charge)
>
> Office Visit #3   Four days later, the patient returns for suture removal.
>
> Code Assigned: 99024 (no charge)

The definition of the Medicare surgical package that appears in Chapter 12, Section 40.1 of the Medicare Claims Processing Manual is slightly different from the preceding definition in the CPT code book. The Medicare global surgical includes

- Preoperative visits—Preoperative visits after the decision is made to operate beginning with the day before the day of surgery for major procedures and the day of surgery for minor procedures;

- Intra-operative services—Intraoperative services that are normally a usual and necessary part of a surgical procedure;

- Complications following surgery—All additional medical or surgical services required for the surgeon during the postoperative period of the surgery because of complications that do not require additional trips to the operating room;

- Postoperative visits—Follow-up visits during the postoperative period of the surgery that are related to recovery from the surgery;

- Postsurgical pain management—By the surgeon;

- Supplies—Except for those identified as exclusions; and

- Miscellaneous services—Items such as dressing changes; local incisional care; removal of operative pack; removal of cutaneous sutures and staples, lines, wires, tubes, drains, casts, and splints; insertion, irrigation and removal of urinary catheters, routine peripheral intravenous lines, nasogastric and rectal tubes; and changes and removal of tracheostomy tubes.

In all the surgery subsections, incision and repair (closure) are considered part of the procedure and are not coded separately. The only exception is in the integumentary system, when intermediate and complex repairs may be coded in addition to the primary procedure.

Follow-up Care for Diagnostic and Therapeutic Surgical Procedures

Codes for diagnostic procedures, such as endoscopies, arthroscopies, and injection procedures for radiological studies, include follow-up care only for the specific diagnostic procedure. Any additional follow-up care to initiate or continue treatment for the condition for which the diagnostic test was performed, or for other diseases and conditions that exist, is not included and may be coded separately.

For example, a physician performs a biopsy that shows evidence of a tumor, and the tumor is later excised. The biopsy and the tumor excision would each be coded separately because the excision is not normal routine follow-up for the biopsy. It is a separately definable service.

Therapeutic surgical procedures include follow-up care only for those services that are usually part of the surgical procedure. Any complications, exacerbations, recurrence, or other diseases, conditions, or injuries that require additional services should be reported with separate codes, as appropriate.

For example, if a patient had surgery to repair a compound fracture of the ankle and is readmitted one week later for repair of a fractured hip due to a fall from the crutches, the two procedures are coded separately. The second procedure would require the addition of modifier −79, Unrelated Procedure or Service by the Same Physician during the Postoperative Period. A new follow-up period is started for the second procedure.

Separate Procedures

The designation of separate procedure applies to procedures that are commonly carried out as an integral part of a total service but now are performed independently.

56605	Biopsy of vulva or perineum (separate procedure); one lesion

In the preceding example, code 56605 would be reported only if the biopsy were performed on its own. If the biopsy were an integral part of a larger procedure, for example, a simple vulvectomy, code 56605 would not be used. In general, it is fraudulent to report the codes separately and to charge separate fees for each procedure. This practice is called unbundling.

Codes for the Laparoscopic Surgical Approach

Procedure codes for the laparoscopic surgical approach are available in many of the surgery subsections. When a laparoscopic (or hysteroscopic) approach is documented, a laparoscopic procedure code must be selected. When a laparoscopic code is not available for the particular procedure and anatomic site, the unlisted laparoscopy procedure code for the most precise anatomic site should be used. Moreover, coders should be aware of other operative approaches (for example, percutaneous, endoscopic, arthroscopic, and open surgery) because updated CPT code descriptions increasingly reflect the methods of approach. Coders should not use a laparoscopic approach code for procedures accomplished by other means, such as open surgery, other endoscopy, or percutaneous route.

Modifiers for Reporting More Than One Procedure or Service

When a physician performs more than one procedure or service on the same date, during the same session, or during the global postoperative period, a CPT modifier may apply.

In some instances, more than one procedure or service (other than E/M services) is performed on the same day by the same physician. These circumstances can be reported by coding the most significant procedure first and then all the other procedures performed, with modifier –51 appended to each additional code. For example, if a patient has a 4-cm layer closure repair of the face and a simple suturing of a 5-cm laceration of the neck, the codes would be 12052, 12002–51.

Modifier –58 is used for staged or related procedures or services, that is, a prospectively planned procedure having two or more stages.

Modifier –59 is used for procedure(s) or service(s) not ordinarily performed or encountered on the same day by the same physician, but appropriate under certain circumstances (for example, separate excisions or lesions). Note that for patients covered by Medicare, one of four other modifiers must be used to more clearly define a distinct procedure, instead of modifier –59. The modifiers are:

–XE: Separate encounter
–XP: Separate practitioner
–XS: Separate structure (or organ)
–XU: Unusual non-overlapping service

Modifiers –76 and –77 are used for repeat procedures by the same and another physician, respectively. Modifier –78 is used when a procedure related to the initial procedure requires a return to the operating room, and modifier –79 is used for an unrelated procedure or service by the same physician during the postoperative period.

Add-on Codes

Certain procedures are commonly carried out in addition to the primary procedure performed. The terminology for these codes includes phrases such as "each additional," "each," or "list separately in addition to primary procedure." Because these procedure codes are never reported alone, it is not appropriate to use modifier –51 with add-on codes.

These additional procedures are designated as add-on codes by the + symbol. The add-on concept applies only to procedures performed by the same physician.

+44015   Tube or needle catheter jejunostomy for enteral alimentation, intraoperative, any method (List separately in addition to primary procedure.)

+67335   Placement of adjustable suture(s) during strabismus surgery, including postoperative adjustment(s) of suture(s) (List separately in addition to code for specific strabismus surgery.)

Modifiers Used in Surgery Coding

Modifiers provide additional information relating to the main code. They do not alter the basic definition of the code but, rather, help describe special circumstances or conditions surrounding the procedures.

The following modifiers are available for use with the surgery codes. (For detailed descriptions and examples, see chapter 9 on modifiers.)

- −22   Increased Procedural Services
- −23   Unusual Anesthesia
- −26   Professional Component
- −47   Anesthesia by Surgeon
- −50   Bilateral Procedure
- −51   Multiple Procedures
- −52   Reduced Services
- −53   Discontinued Procedure
- −54   Surgical Care Only
- −55   Postoperative Management Only
- −56   Preoperative Management Only
- −57   Decision for Surgery
- −58   Staged or Related Procedure or Service by the Same Physician during the Postoperative Period
- −59   Distinct Procedural Service
  For patients covered by Medicare, use −XE, −XP, −XS or −XU in place of −59
- −62   Two Surgeons
- −63   Procedure Performed on Infants Less Than 4 kg
- −66   Surgical Team
- −76   Repeat Procedure or Service by Same Physician
- −77   Repeat Procedure by Another Physician
- −78   Unplanned Return to the Operating/Procedure Room by the Same Physician Following Initial Procedure for a Related Procedure during the Postoperative Period
- −79   Unrelated Procedure or Service by the Same Physician during the Postoperative Period
- −80   Assistant Surgeon
- −81   Minimum Assistant Surgeon
- −82   Assistant Surgeon (when qualified resident surgeon not available)

Anatomical Modifiers

Anatomical modifiers help describe exactly which digit or body area is receiving treatment. The anatomical modifiers include:

–LT   Used to identify procedures performed on the left side of the body. This modifier is required on surgical procedures performed on the eye when reported to Medicare.

–RT   Used to identify procedures performed on the right side of the body. This modifier is required on surgical procedures performed on the eye when reported to Medicare.

The anatomical modifiers assigned to each digit are summarized below:

Left Hand	Left Foot	Right Hand	Right Foot
–FA (Thumb)	–TA (Great toe)	–F5 (Thumb)	–T5 (Great toe)
–F1 (2nd Digit)	–T1 (2nd Digit)	–F6 (2nd Digit)	–T6 (2nd Digit)
–F2 (3rd Digit)	–T2 (3rd Digit)	–F7 (3rd Digit)	–T7 (3rd Digit)
–F3 (4th Digit)	–T3 (4th Digit)	–F8 (4th Digit)	–T8 (4th Digit)
–F4 (5th Digit)	–T4 (5th Digit)	–F9 (5th Digit)	–T9 (5th Digit)

Other anatomical modifiers help describe the exact location for procedures on the eyelids:

Left Eyelid	Right Eyelid
–E1 (Upper)	–E3 (Upper)
–E2 (Lower)	–E4 (Lower)

Exercise 4.1. Surgery Section

Choose the best answer for each of the following questions.

1. Which modifier should the coder apply when an unrelated procedure is performed during the global period?

    a. –24
    b. –25
    c. –77
    d. –79

2. How many days are typically included in the global surgical period?
    a. 120
    b. 90
    c. 60
    d. 0

3. Based on CPT guidelines, which service may be coded separately when a surgical procedure is performed?

    a. Provision of local anesthesia
    b. Physician-administered digital block
    c. Care for wound infections
    d. Incision closure services

(Continued on next page)

Exercise 4.1. (Continued)

4. True or false? A patient underwent surgery 5 days ago and now presents to the office with dehiscence. The surgeon codes an E/M code for the evaluation of the wound. The surgeon coded this case correctly.

   _____

5. Code 99024 is associated with which of the following concepts?

   a. Surgical package
   b. Unlisted procedures
   c. Unbundling
   d. Separate procedures

6. Which modifier should a coding professional apply to a procedure performed on the left upper eyelid?

   a. –51
   b. –LT
   c. –E1
   d. No modifier

7. Which modifier would be associated with a procedure that requires two surgeons for the completion of the procedure?

   a. –51
   b. –62
   c. –66
   d. –77

8. When a procedure is normally carried out as an integral part of a total service but is performed independently on a particular day, it is acceptable to use codes that include the phrase _____ in the descriptor.

   _____

9. When the same surgical procedure is performed on two different organs at the same operative session, which modifier is applied to the second procedure code when submitting to Medicare?

   a. –XE
   b. –XS
   c. –XU
   d. –59

10. Which of the following codes are never reported alone and thus are exempt from modifier –51?

    a. Evaluation and management codes
    b. Separate procedure codes
    c. Unlisted procedure codes
    d. Add-on procedure codes

Integumentary System

The codes in the integumentary system subsection of surgery are used to report procedures performed on the skin, the subcutaneous and areolar tissues, the nails, and the breasts. This subsection is arranged by type of procedure and body area.

Procedures included in the integumentary system subsection are incision and drainage, excision of malignant and benign lesions, treatment of burns, wound repair, grafts and flaps, and Mohs' micrographic surgery. Incision, excision, repair, and reconstruction of the breast also are contained in this subsection.

The skin consists of two layers. The epidermis is the outer layer, and the dermis is the inner layer. The dermis provides a thicker covering to the body structures beneath it. Below the dermis lies the subcutaneous tissue. The other areas also included in the integumentary system are hair follicles, nails, and glands. Figure 4.1 shows a cross section of the skin and its components to assist in visualizing the structures.

Coders should be aware that procedures involving skin of some sites, for example, the eyelids and genitalia, could be assigned to other sections of the CPT code book.

Incision and Drainage

Incision and drainage of skin is coded to 10040–10180. When the documentation supports incision and drainage beyond the skin, the coder should reference the CPT Index under the main head of Incision and Drainage and should identify the structure. In this case, the coder should not assign codes from the integumentary system subsection.

For incision and drainage of skin, several codes are identified as simple or complicated. To report a complicated code, the coder should make sure the documentation clearly supports the complication. Examples of complications include extent of the disease, presence of infection, delayed treatment, patient anatomy, and patient condition. Any query should be directed to the physician, requesting that the documentation be clarified in the record.

Figure 4.1.   Depth of split-thickness and full-thickness grafts

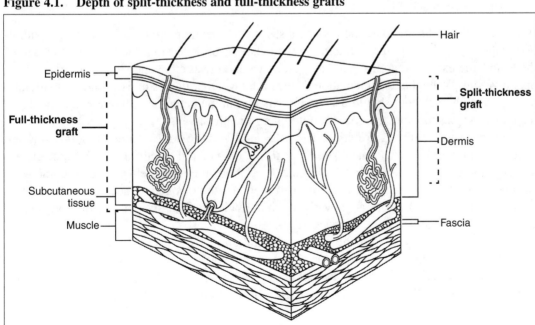

Excision-Debridement

Excision-debridement codes should be used for the debridement of skin, subcutaneous tissue, muscle fascia, muscle, and bone. Codes 11042–11047 should not be used for debridement of nails or burns. This is a common coding error. Codes 11720–11721 are the correct codes to use to report nail debridement. Burn debridement is coded in the 16000 series based on the size of the burn and whether anesthesia was used.

Each debridement is coded to the deepest level and coded based on the size documented in the record. Each successive code includes the layers described in the previous code. For example, debridement of muscle and/or fascia in 11043 includes debridement of subcutaneous, dermis, and epidermis in 11042 at the same location. Code 11042 would not be assigned with 11043 unless debridement was provided at two separate locations. When multiple wounds are debrided, add together the surface areas of those wounds of the same depth, but do not add together the surface areas of wounds of different depths.

Lesions

The size and number of lesions are important factors in code assignment in this subsection. Different codes are assigned for excision of malignant or benign lesions, or any type of lesion removed by destruction.

Certain site measurements are identified by metric measurements rather than inches within the lesion and repair portions of this subsection. The coder must convert the sizes documented in inches to centimeters or square centimeters. For square centimeters, a 4 × 3-cm wound equals 12 sq cm (4 × 3 = 12).

> 1 mm = 0.1 cm
> 10 mm = 1.0 cm
> 0.3937 in = 1.0 cm
> 1 in = 2.54 cm (approximately)
> 1 cm = 0.4 in
> 0.16 sq in = 1 sq cm
> 1 sq in = 6.452 sq cm

Because of these distinctions, the coder must review documentation included in the pathology and/or operative reports to determine the behavior of the lesion, the location and size of the lesion, the excised margins, and any special wound closure beyond simple suturing of the operative site. When the documentation determining whether the lesion is benign or malignant does not match, the coder should use the information in the pathology report. When the documentation is questionable, the coder should query the physician.

Benign lesion removals are coded from the 11400–11446 series. Codes 11400–11446 are differentiated based on anatomical site and excised diameter. To determine the diameter, use the largest area of the lesion plus the margins. If possible, the measurement should come from the operative report or progress notes instead of the pathology report because the specimen shrinks after removal. Lesions are always coded individually. The sizes of two or more lesions are never added together. Each is coded separately.

Even though skin tags are benign tumors found on many areas of the skin, benign lesion removal codes should not be used for skin tag removal. This series of codes specifically excludes skin tags. Skin tag removal should be coded using code 11200 for the first 15 lesions and add-on code 11201 for each additional 10 lesions removed.

Coding the excision of a lesion is based on the total excised diameter of the lesion, including both the lesion size and the size of both margins. To be sure that the correct code is chosen for the work performed, the coder should educate the physician on the importance of documenting the total excised diameter, including both the lesion and the margins.

It is important to note that the lesion excision includes simple repair or closure of the excision site. If an intermediate repair involving layer closure of one or more deeper layers of subcutaneous tissue and superficial fascia also is performed, the repair code would be used in addition to the excision code. Also note that the surgeon makes a defect larger than the actual lesion and skin margins when removing the lesion. This larger defect is made as an ellipse, pictured in the professional edition of *CPT 2016*. This ellipse is created so that the skin can be closed with a straight-line repair. If the defect needs to be closed with intermediate or complex repair, and therefore needs to be coded separately, the length of the repair is the length from one tip of the ellipse to the other tip. Therefore, the size of the lesion, including margins, may be smaller than the size of the defect that is repaired.

The coder is directed to codes 17000–17250 for electrosurgical or other methods of lesion destruction. The codes in this series are intended for benign or premalignant lesions and include destruction by any method including electrocautery, electrodesiccation, chemical treatment, cryosurgery, and laser removal. Code assignment then depends on the type and number of lesions destroyed.

Excision of malignant lesions is coded from the 11600–11646 series. As with benign lesions, excised diameter and anatomical site determine the codes. Simple closure of the excision site is included; more complicated closures are coded in addition to the excision code. Destruction of malignant lesions is coded from the 17260–17286 series.

An excision of malignant lesion code should *not* be used unless the pathology report or other documentation clearly supports a malignant lesion. Coders unfamiliar with the neoplastic behavior of tumors will find the coding system in *International Classification of Diseases, Tenth Revision, Clinical Modification* (ICD-10-CM) helpful in determining whether a tumor is benign or malignant. The Alphabetic Index of *ICD-10-CM* lists neoplasms by their behavior (for example, adenocarcinoma, osteosarcoma, and leiomyoma). Many coders skip this step and go directly to the ICD-10-CM table of neoplasms, thereby missing helpful instructions and exception notes. The Alphabetic Index indicates the correct behavior type (benign or malignant) for each neoplasm. Knowing the neoplastic behavior (the tendency of the lesion to metastasize) is essential information for coding excisions and repairs involving neoplasms of the skin and subcutaneous tissue, as well as of deeper structures.

When malignant lesions are excised, the pathology report may state that the margins removed were questionable for malignancy. This requires that an additional excision be performed to obtain tissue that is free of malignancy. This subsequent excision, at a different operative session, is coded based on the size of the margin excised, with modifier –58 to indicate the staged procedure within the postoperative period. When the additional excision is performed at the same operative session, *CPT Assistant* (August 2004) directs the coder to report only one code, selected based on the final widest excised diameter.

Nails

Several codes are found in CPT to describe nail procedures, covering both fingernails and toenails. The code series 11719–11721 describes trimming and debridement of nails. Many insurers, including Medicare, have special diagnosis requirements for coverage of these services.

Codes 11730, 11750, and 11765 are often confused during the code assignment process. Code 11730 describes the process of removing some or all of just the nail plate (commonly called the toenail) and no other surrounding tissues. Avulsion means pulling or stripping off. This may be performed after injury to the nail and is not performed for permanent removal. Code 11750 describes the excision of both the nail and the nail matrix (the growth plate for the nail found back from the cuticle), all or in part. This is intended to be done for permanent removal of the nail. Completion of this process may involve electrocautery or excision. Code 11765 is a wedge resection of the skin of the nail fold on the side of the nail. This is removed to free the ingrown nail and the nail plate may be cut to help eliminate the ingrown nail.

Repairs

The CPT code book provides codes 12001–13160 for simple, intermediate, and complex wound repairs.

A *simple* repair is a suturing (stitching) of a superficial wound involving primarily epidermis or dermis, or subcutaneous tissues without significant involvement of deeper structures, and requires one layer closure. It is important to note that methods involving adhesive strips, such as butterfly bandages, are not coded in the surgery section but instead are included in the code for the evaluation and management (E/M) service. Some third-party payers may require the use of HCPCS code G0168 for wound closure utilizing tissue adhesive only, such as Dermabond.

An *intermediate* repair involves layered closure of one or more of the deeper layers of subcutaneous tissue and superficial fascia in addition to the skin closure. Also included in this classification are single-layer closures of heavily contaminated wounds that require extensive cleansing and removal of debris.

A *complex* repair involves services beyond that of intermediate repair. It may include scar revision, debridement, placement of stents, or retention sutures. A wound may require complex repair because of its anatomical location, such as an injury of the face.

To report multiple wound repairs, the repairs in the same classification are added together and reported once. The code descriptions include a description of the anatomic site of the repair. Lengths of wound repairs of the same type within the same anatomic site category are added together.

When more than one classification of wound repair is performed, all codes are reported, with the code for the most complicated procedure listed first. Modifier –59 should be added to the secondary code(s). For patients covered by Medicare, instead of modifier –59, one of four other modifiers must be used to more clearly define a distinct procedure. The modifiers are:

–XE: Separate encounter
–XP: Separate practitioner
–XS: Separate structure (or organ)
–XU: Unusual non-overlapping service

Example: A patient involved in a knife fight had superficial wounds of the scalp, 5 cm; neck, 3.5 cm; and nose, 1.5 cm which required simple repair. He had lacerations that required layered closure on the hands, 5.5 cm; neck, 4 cm; and ears, 1.75 cm. Also, plastic surgery was required to perform a complex repair of a left cheek wound, 2 cm.

1. List the most complicated repair first: Complex repair cheek, 2 cm, 13131.

2. Add wound repairs in the same classification/anatomic site together and report as one code.

Intermediate:	Hands	5.5 cm	
	Neck	4.0 cm	
	Total:	9.5 cm	12044–51

Intermediate:	Ears	1.75 cm	12051–51
Simple:	Scalp	5.0 cm	
	Neck	3.5 cm	
	Total:	8.5 cm	12004–51
	Nose	1.5 cm	12011–51

Codes reported: 13131, 12044–51, 12051–51, 12004–51, 12011–51.

Debridement and decontamination of the wound are included in the wound repair code. These procedures are coded separately only when gross contamination requires longer-than-usual cleansing, when considerable amounts of tissue are removed, or when debridement is done separately with the wound repair performed later.

When a wound is repaired, the simple exploration of surrounding nerves, blood vessels, and tendons is a normal component of the repair. Ligation, or the tying off of blood vessels, also is considered part of the repair. However, if any of these underlying structures requires extensive repair, they are coded under the appropriate subsection. The wound repair then becomes a portion of this more comprehensive procedure unless the repair is complex, in which case the codes for both the repair of the blood vessel, nerve, or tendon and the complex wound repair are used.

Also, if the wound is penetrating (for example, a knife or gunshot wound) and the exploration requires that it be enlarged with other associated services, such as removal of foreign bodies, but without thoracotomy or laparotomy, the wound exploration codes from the musculoskeletal system should be used. The coder should see codes 20100–20103, which are discussed in the Musculoskeletal subsection of this chapter.

Proper coding for wound repair requires a careful review of the documentation to determine exactly which services were provided.

Adjacent Tissue Transfer or Rearrangement

Codes for adjacent tissue transfer or rearrangement include the excision of lesions as well as the local skin graft, such as Z–plasty, W–plasty, V–Y plasty, rotation flap, advancement flap, or double pedicle flap. The codes include information on size of the defect area and anatomical site involved. The size of the defect is determined by adding the size of the primary defect (from the excision) and the secondary defect (created to do the repair) together. The following definitions are used in code assignment:

- **Z–plasty:** A tissue transfer that surgically releases tension in the skin caused by a laceration, a contracted scar, or a wound along the flexion crease of a joint. It is characterized by a Z-shaped incision that is above, through, and below the scar or defect.

- **W–plasty:** A tissue transfer performed to release tension along a straight scar. A W-shaped incision creates a series of triangular flaps of skin. The triangular flaps on both sides of the scar are removed, and the remaining skin triangles are moved together and sutured into place.

- **V–Y plasty:** A tissue transfer that begins with a V-shaped skin incision and with advancement and stretching of the skin and tissue. The defect is covered and forms a Y when sutured together.

- **Rotational flap:** Flaps that are curved or semicircular and include the skin and subcutaneous tissues. A base is left, and the remaining portion of the flap is freed and rotated to cover the defect and then sutured into place.

Skin Replacement Surgery and Skin Substitutes

The coding notes at the beginning of this subsection of the CPT code book are vital for proper code selection. In addition, the following definitions will help the coder understand the terminology being used for these procedures:

Autografts

- An autograft or autologous skin graft is a graft of skin from elsewhere on the patient's body.

- A tissue cultured autograft is created from the patient's own skin cells in the laboratory. The skin cells are cultured to grow into large, thin sheets and then are applied to the recipient site. Because they are the patient's own tissue, they are not rejected. This type of autograft requires harvesting (15040) of the patient's own skin two weeks prior to the grafting, to allow time for the skin to grow in the laboratory.

- A pinch graft is a piece of skin graft about one quarter inch in diameter that is obtained by elevating the skin with a needle and slicing it off with a knife.

- A split-thickness graft consists of only the epidermal (superficial) layers of the skin, epidermis, and dermal tissue.

- A full-thickness skin graft is composed of skin and subcutaneous tissue graft.

Skin Substitutes

"Skin substitute grafts include non-autologous human skin (dermal or epidermal, cellular or acellular) grafts (homografts or allografts), non-human skin substitute grafts (xenograft), and biological products that form a sheet scaffolding for skin growth" (AMA 2016, 84).

- An **allograft** is a graft obtained from a genetically dissimilar individual of the same species; also known as allogenic graft or homograft.

- A **xenograft** is a graft obtained from a species different from the recipient, as in animal to human; also called xenogeneic graft, heterograft, or hetero-transplant. A pigskin graft is an example of a xenograft.

- **Acellular dermal grafts** are made from chemically treated cadaver skin that has been cleansed of all living material. It provides the matrix needed for the patient's own skin to regrow while covering the defect.

Figure 4.1 displays the depths of split-thickness and full-thickness grafts, and Figure 4.2 displays the autologous skin graft process.

Free skin grafts are coded by the size and location of the defect, also called the recipient area, or where the graft tissue will be placed. These codes include procedures in which the skin graft is separated completely from the donor site in a one-step process. The type of graft, anatomic site, and size of the defect determine the code assignment. Simple debridement and removal of granulations or recent avulsion are included in the code.

Figure 4.2. Skin graft

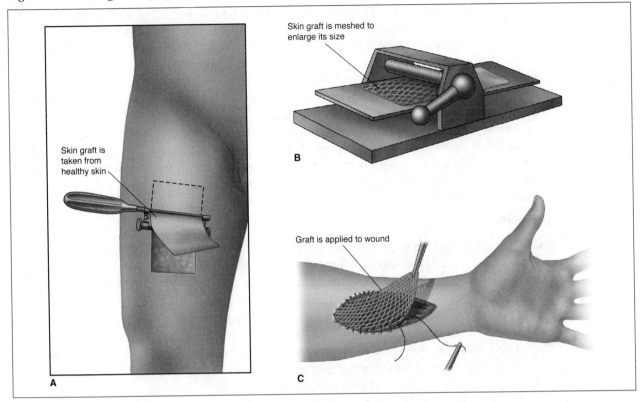

A

Skin graft is taken from healthy skin

B

Skin graft is meshed to enlarge its size

C

Graft is applied to wound

When the primary, or most important, procedure requires a skin graft to complete the operative closure, a skin graft code is reported in addition to the primary procedure. For example, a radical mastectomy may require a skin graft in addition to the breast removal.

In determining body size, the measurement of 100 sq cm is applicable to adults or children age 10 and older, and percentages apply to infants and children under the age of 10.

Generally, the donor site, or where the graft comes from, requires only simple closure. If, however, the donor site requires more extensive skin grafting and/or local flaps, this is coded as a separate procedure.

Surgical preparation of the recipient site is coded with 15002–15005, regardless of the type of graft that will be placed. To code the surgical preparation of the recipient site, the physician must excise an open wound, eschar, or scar, or perform an incisional release of scar tissue.

The use of these codes requires more than just debridement of the wound bed. Surgical preparation is completed to allow healing by primary intention. *Primary intention healing* means that the wound edges heal by directly touching each other, such as when a wound is sutured. This method is used to minimize the growth of granulation tissue, which can distort the skin and cause contracture later. At times, wounds start to heal by secondary intention, or without skin approximation, and this causes granulation tissue to develop. The process of surgically preparing the wound removes nonviable tissue or incisional release of a scar contracture that would interfere with healing by primary intention. Surgical preparation provides a clean and viable wound surface for adjacent tissue transfer, placement of a graft, flap, skin replacement or skin substitute, or the application of negative pressure wound therapy. Do not report 15002–15005 when the wound is left to heal by secondary intention.

Autografts are coded using codes 15050–15261. Within that series, codes 15150–15157 are used when the autograft is tissue cultured skin. Application of skin substitutes such as allografts and xenografts are coded with codes 15271–15278. When a biological implant is used for soft tissue reinforcement, such as the product Alloderm, this is coded as code 15777 in addition to the code for the primary procedure.

When surgical preparation is performed on different body sites, add together the surface area of all wounds from all anatomic sites that are named in the code description. Procedures that involve the wrist are reported with codes that include "arm" in the description and procedures that involve the ankle are reported with codes that include "leg" in the description.

Flaps

Codes for flaps include procedures such as pedicle flaps, muscle, myocutaneous, or fasciocutaneous flaps, and delayed flap transfers. The code ranges listed refer to the recipient site rather than the donor site when the flap is being attached in transfer or to a final site. The donor site is coded from the 15570–15738 code range when a tube is formed for later use or when delay of flap is prior to the transfer. Careful reading of the operative report and the code descriptions is necessary for correct code assignment.

The graft codes do not include extensive immobilization such as plaster casts; these are coded separately. As with other graft codes, an additional code should be listed if the donor site requires any repair beyond simple closure.

Use the following definitions in coding flap grafts:

- A pedicle flap is a flap of detached skin and subcutaneous tissue in which the attached end or base contains an adequate blood supply. This flap is partially transferred to the recipient site with the base still attached to the donor site. After the recipient site has established a good blood supply, the base or pedicle is cut off and the graft is completed.

- A myocutaneous flap involves the transfer of intact muscle, subcutaneous tissue, and skin as a single unit rotated on a relatively narrow blood supply of the muscle.

A variety of other flaps, implants, and grafts are described with codes 15740–15777 including punch grafts for hair transplantation.

Other Procedures

Codes for other procedures include those for removal of sutures and dressing changes performed under anesthesia (15850–15852). Removal of sutures and dressing changes by the physician who performed the initial procedure are considered part of the initial procedure and are not reported separately unless they are performed under anesthesia other than local. For removal of sutures or dressing changes without anesthesia by a physician other than the physician who performed the initial procedure, the coder should report the appropriate level of E/M code and supplies used. Some third-party payers may require the use of HCPCS code S0630 for suture removal done by a physician other than the physician who closed the wound.

Pressure Ulcers (Decubitus Ulcers)

The excision of pressure ulcers is coded based on the location of the ulcer, whether bone is removed and the closure methods used, such as primary closure, skin flap, muscle or myocutaneous flap, or skin graft. These codes describe pressure ulcers of the coccyx, sacrum, ischial tuberosity and greater trochanter areas. The excision of a pressure ulcer of any other area is coded as 15999, Unlisted procedure, excision pressure ulcer.

Muscle or myocutaneous flaps should be coded separately using 15734 and/or 15738 in addition to codes 15936, 15937, 15946, 15956, or 15958. Split skin graft closure should be coded with 15100 and 15101, as appropriate for the size of the graft, in addition to 15936, 15937, 15946, 15956, or 15958. *CPT Assistant* June 2002 tells the coder that reporting an excision of an ischial ulcer in preparation for muscle or myocutaneous flap or skin graft closure but without an osteotomy should be reported as 15946–52, with the –52 modifier indicating that the procedure was not performed in its entirety as described in the code descriptor.

Burns, Local Treatment

Local treatment of burns involves treatment not described with the Skin Replacement Surgery and Skin Substitutes codes. Local treatment may involve debridement and curettement and application or change of dressing to burn wounds. Codes 16020–16030 describe burns in three ways: size (small, medium, and large), a description of the area (whole face, whole extremity, more than one extremity), and percentage of total body surface area (less than 5 percent, 5 percent to 10 percent, and greater than 10 percent). Only one code from 16020–16030 should be reported per treatment session, using the code for the largest body area treated.

Also included in this section is a code for initial treatment of a first-degree burn of any size and two codes for escharotomies, with coding of these based on the number of incisions created.

Destruction of Lesions

Lesion removal requires the coder to differentiate among the various methods. The definition of destruction is provided in the guidelines at the beginning of the 17000 code series in the CPT code book. The premalignant code descriptions are written so that the coder lists a code for the first lesion (17000), and then repeats code 17003 for each additional lesion (two through fourteen). Fifteen or more lesions are identified by listing only code 17004.

> **Example:** Physician destroys three lesions determined to be actinic keratoses. The correct code assignment would be 17000, 17003, and 17003.

For codes 17106–17108, measure the area requiring destruction in square centimeters (sq cm). To determine square centimeters, measure the two longest edges and multiply. Select the code for the appropriate number of square centimeters.

Destruction of malignant lesions is described by size of lesion and anatomic site. Excision of malignant lesions is described in codes 11600–11646.

Breast Procedures

Codes 19000–19499 include procedures performed on both the female and male breast. This series includes codes for incision, excision, introduction, and repair and/or reconstruction.

It should be noted that these codes include only unilateral procedures. When both breasts are involved, the codes for each breast procedure would be reported with the appropriate modifier (–50, –51, –LT, or –RT).

When coding biopsies of the breast, it is necessary to determine the type of biopsy performed. An incisional biopsy is when a small part of a breast lesion or a lump is removed for examination. It is coded as 19101. Excisional biopsies (the entire lump is removed for examination) are coded to 19120. A needle core biopsy, or removal of a core of tissue, is coded to 19100 when performed not using imaging guidance. The coder should note the cross-reference to codes 10021 for fine needle aspiration, the removal of fluid for examination, performed without imaging guidance. Wire localization biopsies are coded to 19125 and 19126. In this procedure, the lesion has been marked by needles placed during a radiological procedure. Code 19125 is used for the first lesion removed, and code 19126 is used for each additional lesion removed. Note that these codes are specific to the breast and should be used instead of code 10035 or 10036 when breast wire localization is performed.

Percutaneous breast biopsies performed using imaging guidance are coded with codes 19081–19086, based on the type of imaging guidance used and whether one or more lesions is biopsied. These codes include the placement of the localization device, the biopsy, and the guidance.

When image-guided placement of a localization device is performed without the actual biopsy, a code from the 19281–19288 series is assigned. These codes include the placement and the imaging. When the lesion is subsequently excised using an open approach, the surgeon assigns code 19125 for the first lesion and 19126 for each additional lesion.

Codes 19300–19307 are used to report various types of mastectomies. The following definitions will assist the coder in determining which procedure was performed:

- A partial mastectomy is the removal of breast tissue from part of the breast and includes specific attention to adequate surgical margins surrounding the breast mass or lesion (*CPT Assistant* 2008, 18:9, 5). Other terms for partial mastectomy are breast lumpectomy and segmental mastectomy.

- A complete mastectomy, simple, is the excision of breast tissue only. The muscles and lymph nodes remain intact.

- A subcutaneous mastectomy is the excision of subcutaneous tissue only. The skin and nipple remain intact.

- A radical mastectomy is the excision of breast tissue, muscle, and lymph nodes. Specific muscles and lymph nodes vary depending on the CPT code.

- A modified radical mastectomy is the excision of breast tissue, including axillary lymph nodes. The pectoralis minor muscle may or may not be removed. The pectoralis major muscle remains intact.

Mastectomies are reported based on what portion of the breast and surrounding tissue is removed. Partial mastectomies are coded to 19301.

CPT Assistant, September 2008 (5–6) states that CPT code 19301 describes a procedure where specific attention to adequate surgical margins of the lesion is given. Therefore, this

Figure 4.3. Modified radical mastectomy

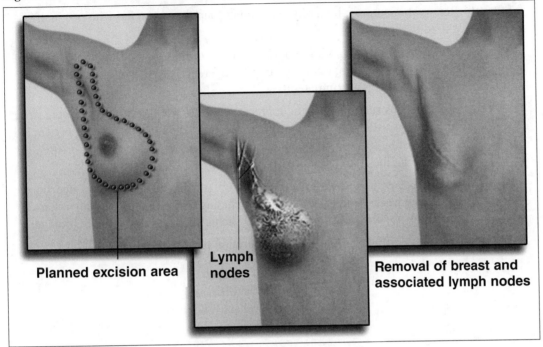

Planned excision area

Lymph nodes

Removal of breast and associated lymph nodes

code is meant to describe the work performed in excising a malignant lesion and whenever attention to surgical margins is required.

If removal of the axillary lymph nodes also is performed during this operative session, code 19302 is used instead of 19301. Lumpectomies with lymph node removals are coded to 19302. Figure 4.3 displays the modified radical mastectomy procedure described in CPT code 19307. For lymph node biopsies or lymphadenectomies performed separately, see CPT codes 38500–38900.

Insertion of a breast prosthesis is coded separately. If done at the same time as the mastectomy, an additional code of 19340 is used. If the prosthesis is inserted at a later time, the code is 19342. The coder is directed to detailed definitions and coding notes found at the beginning of the excision (19100–19499) section.

Breast reconstruction procedures performed using any type of free flap are coded to codes 19364, S2066, or S2068 because the free flap has been completely disconnected from the donor location and moved to the breast location to create the new breast mound. The vascular supply is reattached using the microvascular technique. Individual codes are available for the different tissue flaps used in breast reconstruction. The pedicle tissue flaps are moved to the breast location without being disconnected, similar to the concept of the adjacent tissue transfer procedure.

HCPCS Codes Used in Integumentary System Coding

The following HCPCS Level II codes are used with codes for surgical procedures involving the integumentary system:

A4550   Surgical tray

G0127   Trimming of dystrophic nails, any number

G0168   Wound closure utilizing tissue adhesive(s) only

S0630   Removal of sutures; by a physician other than the physician who originally closed the wound

S2066   Breast reconstruction with gluteal artery perforator (GAP) flap, including harvesting of the flap, microvascular transfer, closure of donor site and shaping the flap into a breast, unilateral

S2067   Breast reconstruction of a single breast with "stacked" deep inferior epigastric perforator (DIEP) flap(s) and/or gluteal artery perforator (GAP) flap(s), including harvesting of the flap(s), microvascular transfer, closure of donor site(s) and shaping the flap into a breast, unilateral

S2068   Breast reconstruction with deep inferior epigastric (DIEP) flap, or superficial inferior epigastric artery (SIEA) flap, including harvesting of the flap, microvascular transfer, closure of donor site and shaping the flap into a breast, unilateral

S9055   Procuren or other growth factor preparation to promote wound healing

Exercise 4.2. Integumentary System

Choose the best answer for each of the following questions.

1. The excision-debridement codes (11000–11047) are used for all of these except _____.

    a. Skin
    b. Nails
    c. Muscle
    d. Bone

2. A wound that is 9 cm × 9 cm measures:

    a. 9 square centimeters
    b. 18 square centimeters
    c. 81 square centimeters
    d. 99 square centimeters

3. Which of the following is a simple repair of a laceration?

    a. Application of adhesive strips
    b. Closure of multiple layers of skin after removing debris
    c. Closure of skin, subcutaneous and fascia layers
    d. Suturing of a single-layer skin wound

4. The surgeon performs a breast reconstruction of the right breast with a free transverse rectus abdominus myocutaneous flap. How is this coded?

    a. 19364
    b. 19367
    c. S2066
    d. S2068

5. The patient has two malignant lesions on the neck, 0.5 cm and 0.8 cm, destroyed by electrosurgery. How is this coded?

    a. 11620, 11621
    b. 17000, 17003
    c. 17270, 17271
    d. 17272

6. Procedure performed: Grafting of right lower leg.

    Indications for procedure: The patient had an extensive partial thickness burn to the lower right leg. He presents for split thickness skin grafting today.

    Description of procedure: After successful induction of general anesthesia and time-out for patient identification, the patient's prior dressings were taken down to the level of the red rubber catheters and his lower leg was prepped and draped in the usual sterile manner. Once this was complete, the remaining dressings were removed and this showed healthy underlying base. A split-thickness graft was then harvested from the lower back and was messed 1:2. The leg defect measured 32 cm x 8 cm. The split-thickness graft was placed and was secured with surgical staples, covered with fine mesh gauze, layers of burn gauze, red rubber catheters, burn gauze, and a Spandex stent. Patient tolerated the procedure well and went without incident back to his room in critical, but stable condition. How is this procedure coded?

    a. 15100, 15101, 15040
    b. 15100, 15101 x 2
    c. 15110, 15111
    d. 15300, 15301 x 2

(Continued on next page)

Exercise 4.2. (Continued)

7. In which of these cases would the coder add the lengths of the defects?
    a. Full- and split-thickness skin grafts
    b. Removal of benign lesions from neck
    c. Simple and intermediate closures of lacerations on arm and face
    d. Simple closure of two lacerations on the trunk

8. A xenograft is:
    a. The same as a full-thickness graft
    b. Used as a permanent skin replacement
    c. Skin taken from a cadaver to be used as a substitute
    d. A temporary wound closure

9. Which of the following is not a method of lesion destruction?
    a. Cryosurgery
    b. Electrosurgery
    c. Excision
    d. Laser removal

10. The skin harvesting code is only used when:
    a. Greater than 100 sq cm is needed.
    b. Skin is sent for tissue culturing.
    c. A split-thickness graft is harvested.
    d. A full-thickness graft is harvested.

11. The physician removes a benign lesion of breast tissue measuring 1.2 cm × 1.8 cm. How is this coded?
    a. 11402
    b. 19101
    c. 19120
    d. 19301

Assign CPT codes for the following scenarios.

12. The surgeon revises a previous breast reconstruction.

    _____

13. Full-thickness graft of the forehead of 15 sq cm is performed. Excisional preparation of the recipient site with excision of extensive scarring also is performed.

    _____

14. A 3-cm laceration of the arm that requires simple closure.

    _____

15. Liquid nitrogen is applied to the face for treatment of acne.

    _____

Exercise 4.2. (Continued)

16. A 75-year-old patient presents to the office with two subungual hematomas, one on the right middle finger and one on the right ring finger. Both are evacuated. No other service is performed.

17. Two punch biopsies are performed on skin lesions. Simple closure is performed.

18. The physician excises a 3 cm × 3 cm benign lesion from the patient's back and uses a rotation flap to repair the skin. The rotational flap is 10 cm × 3.2 cm.

19. Read the following physician office record and determine the appropriate procedure code(s).

Physician Office Record

While chasing his brother, this 13-year-old boy fell through a sliding glass door and sustained three lacerations: one on his left knee, one on his right knee, and one on his left hand.

Left knee: 5.5 cm laceration involving deep subcutaneous tissue and fascia, repaired with layered closure

Right knee: 7.2 cm laceration repaired under local anesthetic, with a single-layer closure

Left hand: 2.5 cm laceration of the dermis, repaired with simple closure under local anesthetic

Assessment: Wounds of both knees and left hand require suture repair using 1% lidocaine for local anesthetic.

Plan: Follow-up in 10 days for suture removal. Call office if there are any problems or complications.

20. Read the following operative report and determine the appropriate surgical procedure code(s).

Operative Report

Preoperative Diagnosis: Pigmented skin lesions: right lateral (1.5 cm excised) and left lateral chest wall (2.0 cm excised). Rule out melanoma.

Postoperative Diagnosis: Seborrheic keratosis, right and left chest wall

Operation: Excision of skin lesions, layered closure

Anesthesia: 2% Xylocaine with .25% Marcaine with epinephrine with sodium bicarbonate

Procedure: After the patient's right lateral chest wall was prepped and draped in the usual manner, and after obtaining satisfactory analgesia with infiltration of local anesthetic, elliptical skin incision was made. The 1.3 cm pigmented skin lesion with a 0.2 cm skin margin was excised, and the specimen was sent for histopathological exam. Subcutaneous tissue was approximated with interrupted 4-0 Dexon, and skin was approximated with subcuticular 4-0. Sterile dressing was applied with Neosporin ointment and OP Site. After having changed the gloves and with a new set of instruments, a 1.8 cm pigmented skin lesion with a 0.2 cm skin margin was excised from the left lateral chest wall. The skin was approximated with subcuticular 4-0 suture. Sterile dressing was applied with Neosporin ointment. Patient tolerated the procedure well.

Musculoskeletal System

The codes in the musculoskeletal subsection of surgery are used to report surgical procedures on the bones, tendons, muscles, and soft tissues. This subsection also includes codes for fracture care and for casting and strapping. The general codes 20005–20999, located at the beginning of the musculoskeletal system subsection, are to be used when a procedure cannot be reported with a more specific site code. Procedures in the rest of the section are listed from head to feet, with subheadings for type of procedure performed. Each anatomical subsection includes subheadings for incision, excision, introduction or removal, repair, fracture and/or dislocation, arthrodesis, and amputation.

Because of the similarity in sections, it is good practice to double-check the subheading to be sure the code selected is from the correct anatomical site. Careful reading of all code descriptions is necessary to ensure correct coding assignment. In addition, the extensive notes and definitions before the first code in this subsection should be reviewed prior to code assignment.

Reporting modifier –50, Bilateral Procedure, can be difficult in the musculoskeletal system subsection. The codes should be read carefully when deciding whether to use this modifier. It should not be used when "bilateral" is stated in the procedure description. However, some procedures are inherently bilateral and their descriptions do not include a reference to being bilateral. As an example, code 21422 is inherently bilateral because it involves open treatment of palatal or maxillary fracture. Because the palate is in the center of the body and the LeFort procedure involves treatment of the palate or maxillary bones, the procedure is considered bilateral. The coder should consult medical references and query the physician for assistance whenever there is a question.

Excision of soft tissue tumors and bone tumors are found throughout the chapter, according to their anatomic site. These codes are assigned by depth and size. The codes for these excisions include either simple or intermediate closure. Complex closure should be coded separately when documented.

Wound Exploration

Codes 20100–20103 for traumatic wound exploration (for example, penetrating gunshot, stab wound) are used to report the trauma services in conjunction with penetrating wound exploration. The codes are subdivided based on the anatomical site of the wound and are found at the beginning of the musculoskeletal system subsection between incisions and excisions in the general heading area.

The codes include surgical exploration and enlargement of the wound and extensive dissection to determine penetration, debridement, and removal of foreign bodies. Also included is ligation or coagulation of minor subcutaneous and/or muscular blood vessels and of the subcutaneous tissue muscle fascia and/or muscle. The codes also include removal of any foreign bodies located during the exploration. These procedures do not include thoracotomy or laparotomy. When more extensive procedures are required to repair major structures or vessels, the codes for these procedures are used instead of the wound exploration codes.

If only simple, intermediate, or complex repair of the wound is performed, and wound enlargement and other exploration are not required, the appropriate codes from the integumentary system subsection should be used instead of the wound exploration codes.

The June 1996 issue of *CPT Assistant* includes several vignettes that are helpful in clarifying these code distinctions.

Excision, Including Biopsies

For biopsy of soft tissue, the coder should choose the code according to the site and should determine whether the biopsy is superficial or deep. For needle or trocar bone biopsies, the coder should choose code 20220 or 20225, depending on the site.

Note: For needle or trocar bone marrow biopsy, code 38221 (from the hemic and lymphatic systems category) should be used.

Introduction and Removal

In the physician's office, codes 20600–20612 are commonly used for either aspiration (removal of fluid) or injection of medication into a joint or ganglion cyst. The codes are specific to the size of the joint involved and are selected based on whether or not ultrasound guidance is used to perform the procedure. Some practices may use codes for injecting tendons and muscles. Specific codes are provided for carpal tunnel (20526), Dupuytren's contracture (20527), other tendons and ligaments (20550–20551), and trigger points (20552–20553).

When a structure is injected, the physician first injects a local anesthetic and then the chosen medication. The medication is coded using the J series of codes from HCPCS. When coding medications with HCPCS, the coder must note the quantity of medication associated with a particular J code. If the physician administers an amount less than or equal to the quantity listed, only one code is used. The code is coded a second time for the second dose or fraction thereof. The same code may be listed multiple times, depending on the dosage given.

An alternative to listing the code multiple times is the use of units on the CMS-1500 form. Units are always expressed as whole numbers when coding the dosage of medication administered. Decimals are never used with units of medication. (See chapter 10 for a complete discussion of and instructions for reporting service units on the CMS-1500 form.)

As noted at the beginning of this chapter, local anesthetic is included in the global surgical package and is not coded separately.

Example: The physician injects the patient's knee with 30 mg of Kenalog 10, without the use of ultrasound guidance. No evaluation and management services were performed on that day. The coder selects code 20610 for the injection of a major joint. When referencing the HCPCS Table of Drugs, the entry for Kenalog 10 refers the coder to Triamcinolone Acetonide, per 10 mg, code J3301.

The correct coding assignment is:

20610, J3301, J3301, J3301

or

20610, J3301 (3 units)

(If the physician had injected 35 mg of Kenalog 10, 4 units of J3301 would have been coded.)

When the physician aspirates a joint or ganglion cyst and then injects the same location, the appropriate code from 20600–20612 is coded only once. *CPT Assistant* (March 2001) directs the coder to use one code because the description indicates "aspiration and/or injection."

Trigger point injection codes are also found in this section. A trigger point is a knot or tight band of muscle that will not relax. These sites can become swollen and tender, and can constrict the blood flow to the remainder of the muscle. Codes 20552 and 20553 are used to describe the process of injecting one or more muscles. Local anesthetic, anti-inflammatory drugs, corticosteroids, and normal saline can all be used to help relieve muscle tension. Codes 20552 or 20553 are reported only once per session. Codes 20550 and 20551 represent similar injections of a tendon sheath, ligament, aponeurosis, or tendon. However, these represent a single injection and are reported once for each injection. Injected materials are coded separately for both types of procedures. Both injection procedures are described in greater detail in the September 2003 issue of *CPT Assistant*. However, it should be noted that the procedure descriptions for codes 20550 and 20551 have changed since this issue was written and the advice is no longer current for codes 20550 and 20551.

Removal of hardware (found in the Index under Removal, implant) is coded in this section. CPT code 20670 is used for removal of superficial hardware, and code 20680 is used for removal requiring a deep approach to the implant, usually below the muscle and/or within the bone. Code 20694 is used for removal of an external fixation system when general anesthesia is required.

Bone Grafts

Codes for obtaining autogenous (from the patient) bone, cartilage, tendon, fascia lata, or other tissue grafts through separate incision (20900–20926) are to be assigned only when obtaining the graft is not already listed as part of the basic procedure. For example, code 21127 includes obtaining autograft; therefore, a second code describing harvesting of the graft is not assigned.

Fracture and/or Dislocation Treatment Codes

The codes found in every subsection under the heading of Fracture and/or Dislocation relate to the type of treatment performed, not to the type of fracture. This is an important distinction because closed fractures may require treatment that is open and/or involves percutaneous fixation.

Fracture treatment can be closed, open, or with percutaneous fixation. Important definitions of terms used in fracture treatment appear at the beginning of the musculoskeletal system subsection. No incision is made in closed fracture treatments, whereas open fracture treatment does involve an incision. Percutaneous fixation is neither open nor closed. Instead, the fracture site has a fixation device placed across the fracture fragments through the skin. Usually, this is accomplished with the assistance of x-ray imaging. For treatment of fractures, it is important to remember that the type of fracture (open, closed) has no coding correlation with the type of treatment provided.

The expression "reduction of a fracture" is commonly used in the medical community, but the CPT classification system uses the term *manipulation*. When the terms *reduce* and *reduction* are found in the health record to describe treatment of a fracture, a code description of manipulation should be used. Manipulation also is used to describe the restoration of a fracture or joint dislocation to its normal anatomical alignment using manual force.

The fracture treatment can include manipulation or manual reduction of the fracture. It also may involve internal or external fixation. *Internal fixation* occurs during open fracture treatment. Pins, rods, nails, or plates are inserted into the bone to stabilize the fracture site. *External fixation* involves the use of pins that extend out through the skin. The pins are attached to a connecting device to hold the bony fragments together. A plaster or fiberglass cast is not an external fixation device.

Traction also may be used and may be of the skeletal or skin variety. Skeletal traction is the application of a force to a limb segment through a wire, pin, screw, or clamp that is attached to bone. Skin traction, on the other hand, is the application of a force to a limb using felt or strapping applied directly to the skin only.

It also should be noted that some code descriptions for fracture treatment of fingers and toes specify the word "each." An example is code 28485, Open treatment of metatarsal fracture, includes internal fixation when performed, each. In these cases, if more than one finger or toe is fractured and treated, a code should be reported for each one. An anatomical multiple modifier also should be used to avoid a denial as a duplicate service if the exact procedure is performed on more than one finger or toe.

The following questions must be answered before coding the treatment of fractures and dislocations:

- What is the site of the fracture or dislocation?
- Is the treatment open or closed?
- Is manipulation part of the treatment?
- Is an internal or external fixation device utilized?

Codes for the treatment of fractures include the application and removal of the initial cast and/or traction device only. However, plaster or fiberglass supplies are coded separately with the appropriate HCPCS Level II code. Reimbursement for these supplies is a payer-specific determination. Codes 29000–29799 are assigned for subsequent replacement of cast and/or traction device. Codes for cast removals should be used only for casts applied by another physician.

Repair, Revision, and/or Reconstruction Codes

Several special definitions apply when coding the repair, revision, and/or reconstruction of tendons:

- A primary repair is the first repair of any structure, such as a tendon.
- A secondary repair is done at some time subsequent to the primary repair.
- "No man's land" is the zone in the palmar or volar surface of the hand between the distal palmar crease (the crease in the palm closest to the finger) and the middle of the middle phalanx (middle finger).

Spine (Vertebral Column)

CPT states that the term "vertebral segment" describes the basic constituent part into which the spine may be divided. It represents a single complete vertebral bone with its associated articular process and laminae. The term "vertebral interspace" is the non-bony compartment between two adjacent vertebral bodies that contains the intervertebral disk and includes the nucleus pulposus, annulus fibrosus, and two cartilaginous endplates (AMA 2015, 122–123).

In coding procedures for the spine (vertebral column), the arthrodesis codes often are used incorrectly. Note that fusion is another word for arthrodesis. The coder should review the guidelines in this subsection, noting that when an arthrodesis is combined with another definitive procedure, both procedures can be reported. Modifier −51, Multiple Procedures, is appropriate with some arthrodesis codes. The symbols + and ⊘ indicate codes that are inappropriate with the use of modifier −51. Spinal instrumentation is reported separately from, and in addition to, the arthrodesis, when performed. Codes 20930–20938 are used to report bone grafts performed after arthrodesis. The bone graft codes are coded in addition to the definitive procedure, such as spinal fusion, and do not require the addition of modifier –51.

Cervical arthrodesis and discectomy are almost always performed together, therefore, a combination code is provided. Arthrodesis of the cervical vertebrae (C2–C7), when performed with a discectomy, is coded with combination code 22551, rather than coding the procedures separately using 22554 and 63075.

A separate code for spinal instrumentation (22840–22848, 22851) is listed in addition to the code for the fracture, dislocation, or arthrodesis of the spine (22325, 22326, 22327, 22548–22812). Codes 22850, 22852, and 22855 are used for removal of instrumentation. The coder is directed to the CPT code notes at the beginning of the arthrodesis section (22548–22830) for additional information.

A common set of spine procedures is described as a posterior lumbar single level interbody arthrodesis at L4-5, allograft bone cage device at L4-5, posterolateral lumbar single level arthrodesis at L4-5, posterior lumbar nonsegmental pedicle screw instrumentation at L4-5 and autograft iliac crest bone graft. Five CPT codes are required to correctly code this common grouping of procedures:

22612	Arthrodesis, posterior or posterolateral technique, single level; lumbar (L4-5)
22630–51	Arthrodesis, posterior interbody technique, including laminectomy and/or discectomy to prepare interspace (other than decompression), single interspace; lumbar (L4-5)
22840	Posterior nonsegmental instrumentation (for example, Harrington rod technique, pedicle fixation across one interspace, atlantoaxial transarticular screw fixation, sublaminar wiring at C1, facet screw fixation (L4-5)
22851	Application of intervertebral biomechanical device(s) (for example, synthetic cage(s), threaded bone dowel(s), methylmethacrylate) to vertebral defect or interspace (L4-5)
20937	Autograft for spine surgery only (includes harvesting the graft); morselized (through separate skin or fascial incision)

Bunion Repairs

Codes for reporting bunion repairs are used to categorize procedures performed to correct a hallux valgus or bunion deformity. These codes are used when the physician removes the medial eminence (bump) from the first metatarsal head of the great toe. Depending on the severity of the deformity, the procedures vary in complexity. Normally, these procedures are done through an incision over the bunion from the proximal phalanx to the metatarsal shaft. Figure 4.4 illustrates the bones of the foot.

Following are brief descriptions of the primary bunionectomy procedures (as mentioned previously, the professional edition of the CPT code book offers diagrams that assist with coding selections):

- Silver procedure (28290) is a simple resection of medial eminence.

- Keller procedure (28292) is the removal of the medial eminence and a resection of the base of the proximal phalanx of the great toe.

- McBride procedure (28292) is the removal of medial eminence, resection of the base of the proximal phalanx of the great toe, plus removal or release of the lateral sesamoid bone.

- Keller-Mayo procedure (28293) includes all elements of Keller procedure, plus a partial resection of the first metatarsal head. Usually, a total double-stem implant is used when this procedure is performed.

- Joplin procedure (28294) is the removal of the medial eminence, plus fusion of the hallux interphalangeal joint of the great toe. The extensor tendon of the great toe is transferred to the head or neck of the first metatarsal.

- Mitchell Chevron (Austin) procedure (28296) refers to the removal of the medial eminence, plus the performance of any type of osteotomy at the first metatarsal neck with repositioning of the metatarsal head.

- Lapidus-type procedure (28297) involves removing the medial eminence of the metatarsal head and cutting a tight tendon that is pulling the toe out of alignment. This may include fusing the first and second metatarsal bases.

- Phalanx osteotomy procedure (28298) is the removal of the medial eminence, plus the performance of an Akin osteotomy.

Figure 4.4. The bones of the foot

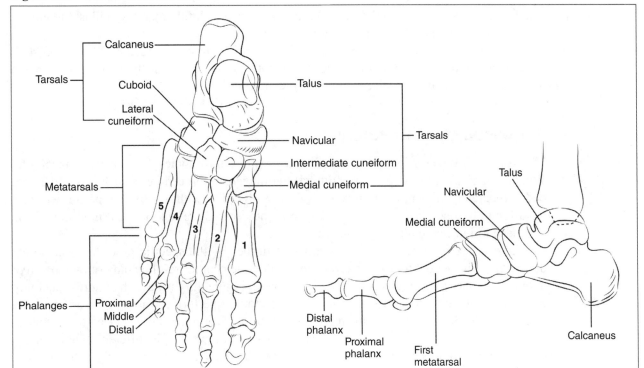

Casts and Strapping

The series of codes describing the application of casts and strapping can be reported in the following scenarios:

- To identify replacement of a cast or strapping during or after the period of normal follow-up care (global postoperative period)

- To identify an initial service performed without any restorative treatment or stabilization of the fracture, injury, or dislocation, and/or to afford pain relief to the patient

- To identify an initial cast or strapping when the same physician does not perform, or is not expected to perform, any other treatment or procedure

- To identify an initial cast or strapping when another physician provided, or will provide, restorative treatment

> **Example:** A patient is seen in the emergency department after being injured in a football game. The emergency department physician determines that the patient's left forearm is fractured. The physician then applies a short arm splint and instructs the patient to follow up with an orthopedic physician to receive the fracture treatment. Code 29125 should be used.
>
> *Note:* When the key components of an E/M service are documented, the appropriate E/M code also is coded. Moreover, plaster or fiberglass supplies are coded in addition to the casts and strapping codes.

The February 1996 issue of *CPT Assistant* includes some helpful vignettes to illustrate how to use these codes in the emergency department.

Applying a multilayer compression system on various limbs is coded as 29581–29584. A multilayer compression system provides therapeutic compression for the treatment of edema associated with venous leg ulcers and related conditions.

Endoscopy/Arthroscopy

The arthroscopy codes include codes for diagnostic arthroscopies in each anatomical site. When a surgical arthroscopy is performed, the diagnostic procedure is included and is not coded separately. When an arthroscopy (viewing the joint with a scope) is performed with an arthrotomy (open inspection of a joint), both procedures are reported and modifier –51 is appended to indicate multiple procedures.

Surgical arthroscopy codes are subdivided further by the specific procedure performed during the arthroscopy, for example, shaving or debridement. Careful reading of the operative note is necessary to ensure correct code assignment. Figure 4.5 displays the internal anatomy of the knee, along with debridement and meniscectomies performed through the arthroscope. The coder should read the documentation carefully to determine the extent of the meniscal work that is performed. Meniscectomy, as displayed in Figure 4.5, is different than meniscal repair, which requires placement of sutures to repair a radial tear that usually extends completely through the sidewall of the meniscal cup.

Figure 4.5. Knee arthroscopy

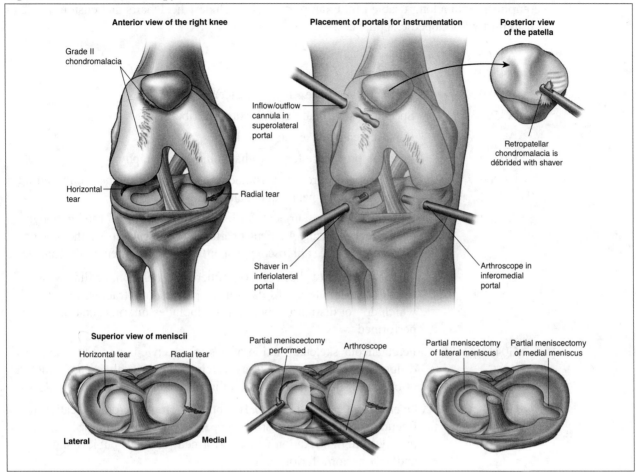

When multiple procedures are performed through the scope, separate codes should be reported for each procedure, when appropriate. Modifier −51, Multiple Procedures, should be used for each subsequent procedure performed through the scope unless they are identified as an add-on code. For example, when an arthroscopy of the knee is performed with a two-compartment synovectomy and medial meniscus repair, codes 29876 and 29882–51 are reported. If an arthroscopic rotator cuff repair is documented with subacromial decompression and distal clavicular resection, three codes are required:

29827	Arthroscopy, shoulder, surgical; with rotator cuff repair
+29826	decompression of subacromial space with partial acromioplasty, with coracoacromial ligament release, when performed
29824–51	Distal claviculectomy including distal articular surface (Mumford procedure)

HCPCS Codes Used in Musculoskeletal System Coding

Many third-party payers reject CPT code 99070 for supplies because they require information on the specific supplies used or provided. A special durable medical equipment (DME) provider number may be required to submit charges for more complex supplies and expensive equipment with a long usable life. Examples would include wheelchairs and custom-made or custom-fitted orthopedic appliances.

A4565	Slings
A4570	Splint
A4580	Cast supplies (for example, plaster)
A4590	Special casting material (for example, fiberglass)
A4635–A4640	Replacement pads and tips for DME
G0259	Injection procedure for sacroiliac joint; arthrography
G0260	Injection procedure for sacroiliac joint; provision of anesthetic, steroid and/or other therapeutic agent and arthrography
G0289	Arthroscopy, knee, surgical, for removal of loose body, foreign body, debridement/shaving of articular cartilage (chondroplasty) at the time of other surgical knee arthroscopy in a different compartment of the same knee
G0412	Open treatment of iliac spine(s), tuberosity avulsion, or iliac wing fracture(s), unilateral of bilateral for pelvic bone fracture patterns which do not disrupt the pelvic ring, includes internal fixation, when performed
G0413	Percutaneous skeletal fixation of posterior pelvic bone fracture and/or dislocation, for fracture patterns which disrupt the pelvic ring, unilateral or bilateral, (includes ilium, sacroiliac joint and/or sacrum)
G0414	Open treatment of anterior pelvic bone fracture and/or dislocation for fracture patterns which disrupt the pelvic ring, unilateral or bilateral, includes internal fixation when performed (includes pubic symphysis and/or superior/inferior rami)
G0415	Open treatment of posterior pelvic bone fracture and/or dislocation, for fracture patterns which disrupt the pelvic ring, unilateral or bilateral, includes internal fixation, when performed (includes ilium, sacroiliac joint and/or sacrum)
Q4001–Q4048 and Q4050	Cast supplies by type of cast and age of patient
Q4049	Finger splint, static
Q4051	Splint supplies
S0395	Impression casting of a foot performed by a practitioner other than the manufacturer of the orthotic
S2112	Arthroscopy, knee, surgical for harvesting of cartilage (chondryoctye cells)
S2115	Osteotomy, periacetabular, with internal fixation
S2117	Arthroereisis, subtalar
S2118	Metal-on-metal total hip resurfacing, including acetabular and femoral components
S2300	Arthroscopy, shoulder, surgical; with thermally induced capsulorrhaphy
S2325	Hip core decompression

S2348	Decompression procedure, percutaneous, of nucleus pulposus of intervertebral disc, using radiofrequency energy, single or multiple levels, lumbar
S2350	Discectomy, anterior, with decompression of spinal cord and/or nerve root(s), including osteophytectomy; lumbar, single interspace
S2351	Discectomy, anterior, with decompression of spinal cord and/or nerve root(s), including osteophytectomy; lumbar, each additional interspace (List separately in addition to code for primary procedure)
S2360	Percutaneous vertebroplasty, one vertebral body, unilateral or bilateral injection; cervical
S2361	Each additional cervical vertebral body (List separately in addition to code for primary procedure)
S8450	Prefabricated digit splint (use digit modifier)
S8451	Prefabricated wrist or ankle splint
S8452	Prefabricated elbow splint

Exercise 4.3. Musculoskeletal System

Choose the best answer for each of the following questions.

1. A physician injects a painful joint at the base of the patient's thumb with 20 mg Depo-Medrol after anesthetizing the joint with 1% lidocaine. Ultrasound guidance is not used. Which codes best describe the services provided?

   a. 20550, J1020
   b. 20550, J2001, J1020
   c. 20600, J1020
   d. 20600, J2001, J1020

2. The term "reduction of a fracture" is most closely related to which term?

   a. Casting of a fracture
   b. Manipulation of a fracture
   c. Internal fixation
   d. Percutaneous fixation

3. A patient suffers a trimalleolar ankle fracture. The physician realigns and casts the fracture in plaster. No E/M services are performed. Which codes best describe the services provided?

   a. 27816, 29405, A4580
   b. 27818, A4580
   c. 27824, A4590
   d. 27818, 29405, A4590

4. Wound exploration does not include which of the following?

   a. Laparotomy
   b. Wound enlargement
   c. Debridement
   d. Foreign body removal

5. A physician uses ultrasound guidance to aspirate fluid from a patient's shoulder joint and then injects 5 mg of dexa-methasone sodium phosphate. Permanent recording and reporting are done. Which codes correctly describe the service provided?

   a. 20605, J7637
   b. 20606, J1100 (5 units)
   c. 20610, 20610–76, J7637 (5 units)
   d. 20611, J1100 (5 units)

6. Read the following operative report and assign the appropriate CPT procedure code(s).

Operative Report

Preoperative Diagnosis: Right intertrochanteric hip fracture

Postoperative Diagnosis: Same

Procedure: Cephalomedullary nailing of right intertrochanteric hip fracture

Implants: A Synthes TFN 360 x 12 mm nail with 85 mm lag screw

Indications: The patient is a 73-year-old female with a fall at the nursing home, resulting in a right hip fracture. She was a direct transfer and is deemed appropriate for surgical fixation of the right hip. Risks and benefits of surgical fixation of the right hip were discussed with the patient in detail. The consent was signed.

Operative Report: The right lower extremity was marked by myself and confirmed by the patient. She was placed under general anesthesia and was placed supine on the Hana fracture table with the right hip in traction, adduction and internal rotation. Fluoroscopic imaging confirmed adequate reduction in AP and lateral views and the right hip was then prepped and draped in normal sterile fashion. Surgical pause was observed confirming the patient and procedure and she received Ancef for prophylaxis. An incision approximately 4 cm above the greater trochanter was then made and a guidewire placed in the tip of the greater

Exercise 4.3. (Continued)

trochanter and on the AP and lateral view advanced down to the level of the lesser trochanter, and the starting reamer was used to gain access to the proximal femur. The guidewire was then placed above the knee. This measured for a 360 mm intramedullary nail and a single pass 13.5 mm reamer was done with minimal chatter. The nail was then placed down and placed in appropriate position for position of the lag screw within center-center in the femoral head, and using the percutaneous guide, an 85 mm lag screw was placed into the center of the femoral head with some gentle compression being made across the fracture site. Then, using a perfect circle technique, two lateral to medial interlocking screws were then placed distally and confirmed in AP and lateral views for correct placement. All wounds were then copiously irrigated. The deep gluteus fascia closed with 0 Vicryl suture, skin closed with 2-0 Vicryl suture and staples. Sterile Xeroform dressing was applied. Anesthesia was reversed and the patient taken to postop recovery in stable condition. All sponge and needle counts correct at the end of the case.

7. Fracture of the right radius and ulna. Long arm splint application by emergency physician on call, will be followed up by orthopedic surgeon tomorrow in the office. How is this coded?

_____

8. Read the following operative report and assign the appropriate CPT procedure code(s).

_____

Operative Report

Preoperative Diagnosis: Painful right elbow hardware

Postoperative Diagnosis: Same

Operation: Removal of elbow hardware

Anesthesia: Local with IV sedation

Procedure: The right elbow was prepared and draped in the usual sterile fashion. A small stab wound was made directly over the prominent screws going up into the humerus both medially and laterally. Dissection was carried down bluntly to the screw head with hemostat, and the screw head was delivered through the incision. Both screws were removed without difficulty. Great care was taken to avoid the ulnar nerve, which was located more lateral and was palpable throughout the procedure well lateral to the incision. The incision was closed with 5-0 nylon interrupted sutures, and the dressing consisted of Owens gauze, 4 × 4; sterile Webril; and a posterior mold.

9. Read the following operative report and assign the appropriate CPT procedure code(s).

_____

Operative Report

Preoperative Diagnosis: Internal derangement medial meniscus tear and degenerative changes

Postoperative Diagnosis: Same

Procedure: Arthroscopic debridement, partial medial meniscectomy

Anesthesia: General

Clinical Note: The patient is a 70-year-old man with a periarthritic/arthritic knee whom we have been following for some time. We have treated him with anti-inflammatory drugs, physical therapy, and injections of cortisone. None of these have helped, and he continues to have significant knee effusion. He comes in for an arthroscopic evaluation.

Procedure: The patient was brought to the OR; and after general anesthetic was obtained and 2 g IV Kefzol given, his knee was prepared and draped in a sterile fashion. The arthroscope was introduced in the lateral portal; after the medial inflow cannula was established, the diagnostic procedure began. The undersurface of the kneecap had a significant plical region that was debrided. The femoral trochlea was much more damaged, with grade III–IV full-thickness loss of cartilage. It was debrided down to stable surfaces, and the lateral joint line was viewed. He had some degenerative fraying of the lateral meniscus, and the lateral

(Continued on next page)

Exercise 4.3. (Continued)

femoral condyle and tibial plateau also had some grade I–II changes, but nothing significant. The medial side had a significant degenerative medial meniscus tear along with the grade II–III changes of the medial femoral condyle and medial tibial plateau. All surfaces were debrided down to stable cartilaginous borders. Partial medial meniscectomy was performed with mechanical and handheld instruments. The knee was irrigated and the wounds closed with nylon. The patient tolerated the procedure well and was transferred to the recovery room in good condition after the knee was injected with Marcaine and epinephrine.

10. Read the following operative report and assign the appropriate CPT procedure code(s).

Operative Report

Preoperative Diagnosis: Bilateral mandible fractures including the open fracture to the right mandible and nondisplaced left angle fracture of mandible

Postoperative Diagnosis: Same

Procedures: 1. Closed reduction with arch bars. 2. Open reduction with internal fixation of right para-symphyseal fractures of the mandible.

Indication for Surgery is the Following: This patient is an 18-year-old female status post assault by kicking to the right face. I recommended the procedure of open reduction with internal fixation of the right parasymphyseal fracture of the mandible along with interdental fixation.

Description of Operation: The patient was taken to the OR and she was placed in supine position and connected to monitor. General anesthesia was induced with propofol general anesthetic medication and the patient was then draped in usual sterile fashion. I inoculated approximately 3 mL of 0.5% Marcaine with 1:100,000 epinephrine to the right parasymphysis area of the gingival mucosa. I placed the arch bar to patient's upper dentition from right first molar to left first molar and was subsequently ligated with 25-gauge wire to each tooth from right first molar to left first molar. Similar approach also applied to the mandibular dentition in the same fashion and the patient was then placed in interdental occlusion. I used #15 blade and made an incision from the right canine extending to the left lateral incisor area. The incision was about a 6 cm long, down to the periosteum and all the way down to the inferior border of the mandible where the fracture can be visualized. I selected a four-hole titanium plate that stayed away from the right mental nerve and was sitting in between the fracture line. Four screws were placed into the Synthes plate. The surgical site was then copiously irrigated with normal saline and subsequently the surgical site then closed with 3-0 chromic gut. At this time, I removed the wire fixation wires and then replaced it with tight rubber bands at the bicuspid and the molar area of both sides. There were no complications during the procedures. The patient was then awakened from general anesthesia and transferred to recovery room for further monitoring.

Respiratory System

Like all the subsections in the CPT code book, the respiratory system subsection is divided by anatomical site, beginning with the nose and including the mouth, pharynx, larynx, trachea, bronchi, and lungs. Codes are provided for many different types of procedures, including endoscopic and open approaches. Figures 4.6 and 4.7 show the respiratory system.

Nose

In coding excision of nasal polyp(s), when the procedure is performed on both sides of the nose, the bilateral modifier −50 must be used. To determine whether the polyps are simple or extensive, the documentation must be reviewed carefully. Simple excision involves polyps that are easy to remove; they are often pedunculated (hanging from a stalk). Extensive polyp

Figure 4.6. The upper respiratory system

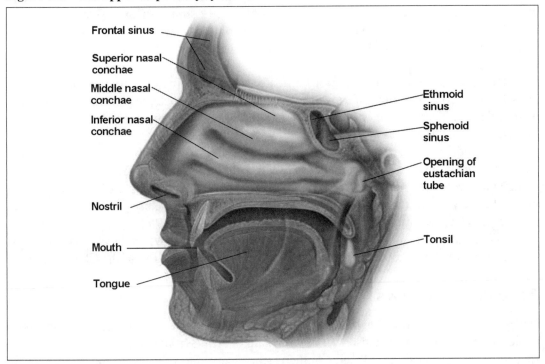

Figure 4.7. The lower respiratory system

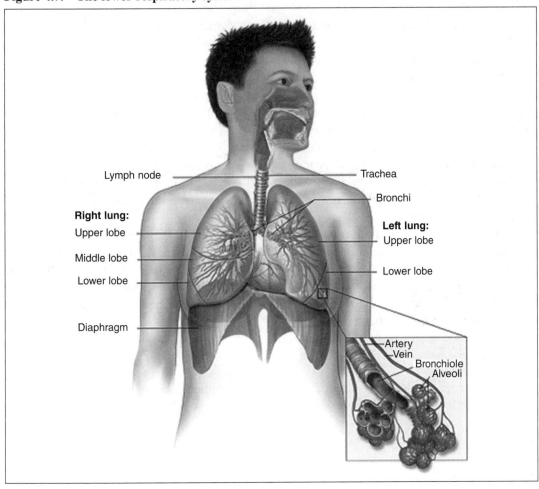

excision usually involves sessile polyps (with a thickened base) whose removal requires more effort and skill. When the documentation does not specify simple or extensive excision, the coder should query the physician. A simple polypectomy (30110) could be completed in an office setting, but an extensive procedure, such as 30115, normally requires the facilities available in a hospital or surgical center.

CPT code 30130, Excision inferior turbinate, partial or complete, any method, and code 30140, Submucous resection inferior turbinate, partial or complete, any method, are considered unilateral. Therefore, modifier −50 should be added when the procedure is performed bilaterally. Nasal turbinates are also referred to as nasal conchae.

When coding secondary rhinoplasties (30430–30450), the following definitions apply: *minor revision* involves a small amount of nasal tip work; *intermediate revision* involves bony work with osteotomies; and *major revision* involves both nasal tip work (cartilage) and osteotomies. The musculoskeletal system codes (20900–20926, 21215) are used for obtaining tissues for some nasal reconstructive procedures.

Codes for the nose subsection often use different approaches. When the approach is external, the coder may be directed to the integumentary system subsection of the CPT code book.

Accessory Sinuses

Codes 31231–31297 describe diagnostic and therapeutic sinus endoscopies. These codes relate to the four paranasal sinuses, all of which are bilateral: frontal, maxillary, ethmoid, and sphenoid. The frontal sinus is located in the forehead area and is accessed for endoscopy via the inner aspect of the eyebrow. The maxillary sinus is located in the cheek area just lateral to each nares. This sinus is accessed through the inferior meatus of the nose. Three small ethmoid sinuses, or cells (anterior, middle, and posterior), are located behind the frontal sinus and the nasal cavity. The sphenoid sinus is located directly behind the posterior ethmoid sinus. The ethmoid and sphenoid sinuses are accessed intranasally.

The surgical sinus endoscopy codes always include a sinusotomy and diagnostic endoscopy. The codes are always unilateral unless otherwise specified and therefore, if the same procedure is performed on bilateral sinuses, a modifier −50 is required. It should be noted that codes 31231–31235 also are used for diagnostic evaluations. They always include an inspection of the interior of the nasal cavity and the middle and superior meatus, the turbinates, and the sphenoethmoid recess. Therefore, a separate code is not required when each area is examined.

The surgical sinus endoscopies are subdivided based on the main procedure performed. When multiple procedures are performed through the nasal endoscope, separate codes should be reported for each procedure, as appropriate.

Modifier −51 should be used for each subsequent procedure performed through the scope. For example, if an anterior ethmoidectomy, polyp removal, frontal sinus exploration, and antrostomy were performed, the codes would be 31254, 31256–51, and 31276–51. It should be noted that polyp removal (removal of tissue from frontal sinus) is included in these codes and thus is not coded separately. Codes 31295–31297 are used to describe the dilation of the various sinus ostium using a balloon.

Larynx

Codes for the larynx describe various procedures performed. Codes 31505–31579 describe procedures performed through an endoscope. There are two types of laryngoscopies—indirect and direct. An indirect laryngoscopy is performed by viewing the larynx with a laryngeal mirror; a direct laryngoscopy is a more complex procedure allowing for direct visualization of the larynx through the endoscope.

Endoscopic procedures on the larynx always include a diagnostic endoscopy with any surgical procedure. Within this grouping, the codes are subdivided based on whether the procedure was indirect, direct, direct operative, or flexible fiberoptic, along with other procedures that are performed during the endoscopy.

Many codes in this section include the use of an operating microscope. However, code 69990 should not be coded when the use of an operating microscope is included in the description of the code itself.

Trachea and Bronchi

Code 31600, Tracheostomy, planned, and code 31601, Tracheostomy, planned; under two years, are considered separate procedures. When a planned tracheostomy is performed as an integral part of another procedure, only the other procedure is coded. Neither code should be reported when the tracheostomy is integral to another procedure.

Codes 31622–31656 describe bronchoscopies, which are procedures performed on the bronchi through an endoscope. The endoscope is passed through the mouth (or nose in some cases), past the vocal cords, through the larynx, and into the trachea and bronchi. Biopsies, tumor excisions, or other procedures may be performed through the scope.

As with other endoscopic codes, a diagnostic bronchoscopy is always included in a surgical endoscopic procedure. The surgical codes then are subdivided based on the additional procedures performed (for example, excision of tumors, biopsy). Diagnostic bronchoscopy codes 31622–31661 include fluoroscopic guidance, when applicable, and are always considered bilateral. Surgical endoscopies where the same procedure is performed on both bronchi or lungs must be reported with a modifier −50, unless a code is provided for an additional location, such as in 31636 and 31637.

It should be noted that a bronchoscopy with brushings and washings is considered a diagnostic bronchoscopy and not a biopsy. Code 31622 is selected to classify cell washings, and code 31623 specifies brushings. Code 31622 is designated as a separate procedure. Code 31624 denotes a bronchoscopy with bronchial alveolar lavage, which should be distinguished from total lung lavage, which is classified as 32997. Code 31643 is for bronchoscopic placement of a catheter for intracavitary radioelement application. Codes 31660 and 31661 describe bronchoscopy for bronchial thermoplasty based on the number of lobes treated.

Bronchoscopy can be performed to place a fiducial marker (31626) within the bronchus or lungs. This marker is placed as a point of reference for later surgery or treatment. In addition, computer-assisted, image-guided navigation (31627) can be used to locate the exact position for diagnostic procedures such as biopsies, for therapeutic procedures such as excision of tumors, or placement of fiducial markers for later surgical procedures or radiation therapy. Code 31627 is an add-on code that can be coded with a variety of bronchoscopy procedure codes.

A bronchial valve is an implantable self-expanding device, delivered by flexible bronchoscopy. The valve that looks like a miniature umbrella acts as a one-way valve to obstruct the airflow into certain areas of the lung, but still allow distal air and mucus flow. It's primary use is to decrease hyperinflation frequently found in emphysema. Code 31647 describes the sizing of the airway and insertion of the valve. Insertion of a valve is coded

Figure 4.8. Bronchial valves

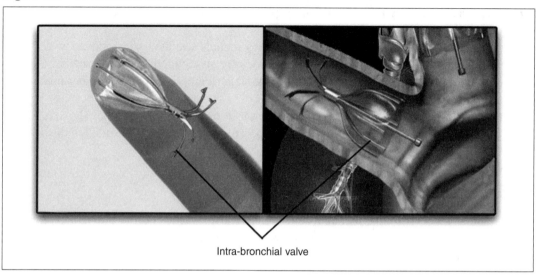

Intra-bronchial valve

separately for each additional lobe using code 31651. There are codes that describe bronchoscopy specifically for the removal of bronchial valves—31648 for the initial lobe and 31649 for each additional lobe where valves are removed. Figure 4.8 shows the size of the valve in comparison to an index finger and the placement of the valve within the bronchial tree after deployment.

Lungs and Pleura

Diagnostic thoracoscopy is always included in surgical thoracoscopy codes. If the code description includes the word "lungs," it is safe to assume that the procedure is bilateral and should be coded only once for bilateral procedures. To code a thoracostomy when a chest tube is inserted, code as 32551.

Codes 32400 and 32405 are for biopsies using a percutaneous needle. The radiological supervision and interpretation is coded separately. If a fine needle aspiration is performed as displayed in Figure 4.9, the coder is directed to code 10021 or 10022.

Lung transplantation codes describe a three-part process of removal of cadaver organs, backbench work to prepare the organ(s) for transplantation, and the actual transplantation of a single- or double-lung allograft. Separate codes are available for each part of the process, specifying a single- or double-lung transplant.

CPT provides codes for various procedures associated with lung excision. Figure 4.10 displays a wedge resection, coded as 32505 when performed through a thoracotomy and 32666 when performed through a thoracoscopy; a lobectomy, coded as 32480 when performed through a thoracotomy and 32669 when performed through a thoracoscopy; and a pneumonectomy, or removal of an entire left or right lung, coded as 32440 when performed through a thoracotomy and 32671 when performed through a thoracoscopy. Both the thoractomy section and the thoracoscopy section include add-on codes for each additional wedge resection performed on the same lung field (the ipsilateral side). If thoracoscopic wedge resections are performed on both lung fields, code 32666 is reported with a −50 modifier. Lobectomy is also referred to as a segmentectomy because a single lung segment is being removed. The extensive coding notes for this section provide valuable information for the coder.

Figure 4.9. Fine needle aspiration of lung

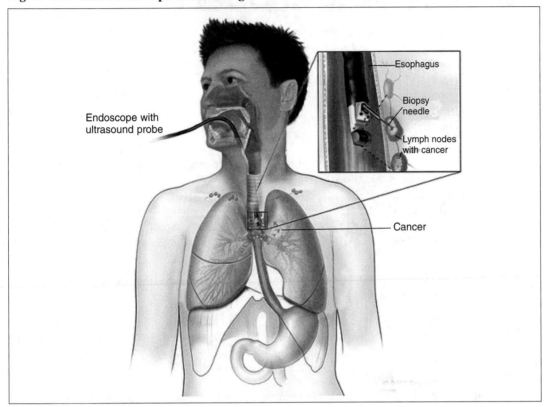

Figure 4.10. Lung excision

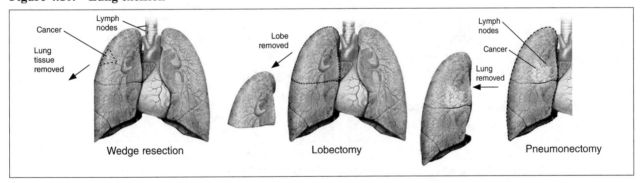

HCPCS Codes Used in Respiratory System Coding

The following HCPCS Level II codes are used with codes for surgical procedures involving the respiratory system:

S2340   Chemodenervation of abductor muscle(s) of vocal cord

S2341   Chemodenervation of adductor muscle(s) of vocal cord

S2342   Nasal endoscopy for postoperative debridement following functional endoscopic sinus surgery, nasal and/or sinus cavity(s), unilateral or bilateral

Exercise 4.4. Respiratory System

Choose the best answer for each of the following questions.

1. Laryngoscopy with operating microscope, direct, with biopsy is coded as _____.
   a. 31536
   b. 31510, 69990
   c. 31530
   d. 31579, 69990

2. The surgeon performs a thoracotomy and performs a biopsy of the pleura and excision of a lung mass. How is this coded?
   a. 32098, 32505
   b. 32096, 32097
   c. 32098, 32097
   d. 32310, 32505

3. After an injury to the chest, the patient requires a thoracentesis with imaging guidance for accumulated air in the pleural cavity. How is this procedure coded?
   a. 32551
   b. 32554
   c. 32555
   d. 32960

4. A patient returns to Dr. X's office after having an epistaxis packed earlier in the day by Dr. X. The anterior nasal passage is again hemorrhaging and requires packing. To properly code this second procedure, which code is required?
   a. 30901
   b. 30901–76
   c. 30905–76
   d. 30906

5. Removal of two lobes of the right lung is coded as _____.
   a. 32440
   b. 32480, 32480–51
   c. 32482–RT
   d. 32484–RT

6. Read the following operative report and assign CPT codes, as appropriate.

Operative Report

Preoperative Diganosis: Right chest pleural effusion

Postoperative Diagnosis: Right chest empyema

Procedure Performed: 1. Right thoracoscopy, surgical. 2. Total pulmonary decortication, including intrapleural pneumolysis.

Findings: There was extensive empyema in the right chest.

Description of Operation: The patient was brought to the operating room and placed in the supine position. All the appropriate monitoring lines were placed by anesthesia. A double-lumen tube was

Exercise 4.4. (Continued)

inserted. The position of the double-lumen tube was confirmed by flexible bronchoscopy. The patient was then repositioned with the right chest up. All the appropriate pressure points were padded. The right chest was then prepped and draped sterilely. I made a small 1-cm incision at the posterior axillary line at the eighth intercostal space. This was the camera port. I made another small 1-inch incision anteriorly at the fourth intercostal space. This was the utility incision. Through these two incisions, the entire operation was performed.

The camera was then inserted. There was extensive empyema. I drained all the empyema fluid which totaled to be about 1 liter. There was extensive fibrinous peel covering the entire right lower lobe and part of the right middle lobe and right upper lobe. I performed extensive total pulmonary decortication by removing all the peel from all the lobes. Afterwards, I irrigated the chest with antibiotic saline solution. I placed a 32-French straight and 32-French angled chest tubes into the pleural space and secured to the skin with Ethibond sutures. Both chest tubes were then connected to suction. The right lung was then allowed to expand under direct visualization. The anterior utility incision was then closed in layers with Vicryl followed by Monocryl for the skin. The needle and sponge counts were correct. There were no complications.

7. Thoracoscopy with three wedge resections of the right lung was performed. How is this coded?

_____

8. Read the following operative report and assign CPT codes, as appropriate.

_____

Operative Report

Preoperative Diagnosis: Left maxillary polyposis

Postoperative Diagnosis: Left maxillary mucous retention cyst

Operation: Removal of contents, left maxillary sinus

Anesthesia: General endotracheal

Procedure: The patient was taken to the OR where general endotracheal intubation was induced.

The head was draped in the usual fashion, allowing visualization of the medial canthus. The posterior insertion of the middle turbinate and lateral wall were injected using 1% lidocaine with 1:100,000 epinephrine after cocaine pledgets had been placed into the nasal cavity containing 4% cocaine. This allowed for vasoconstriction and hemostasis. The 30-degree scope was then used to visualize the contents of the left maxillary sinus, which were photo-documented. The contents were then removed using a combination of microdebrider, micro forceps, and a straight pickup. It appeared mainly to contain mucus with minimal polypoid soft tissue. However, specimens were sent to pathology. Photo documentation was taken at the end of the case. The procedure was then terminated and she was taken to recovery in satisfactory condition.

9. Read the following operative report and assign CPT codes, as appropriate.

_____

Operative Report

Preoperative Diagnosis: Pleural effusion, right side

Postoperative Diagnosis: Metastatic carcinoma of pleura

Operation: Tube thoracostomy—chest tube insertion

Anesthesia: Local

History: This is a 67-year-old woman with a history of squamous cell carcinoma of the cervix. The patient presents with a right pleural effusion that was drained via thoracentesis 3 days ago, and the culture revealed metastatic carcinoma of the pleura. Fluid is reaccumulating, giving the patient symptoms of dyspnea. Chest x-ray reveals a significant pleural effusion up to the midlung region.

Procedure: The patient was taken to the OR at the Surgicenter and was prepared and draped in the usual fashion. She was then anesthetized using 1% lidocaine above the 10th rib. An incision

(Continued on next page)

Exercise 4.4. (Continued)

was made in the skin. The subcutaneous fascia was then opened and the pleura penetrated. There was no unusual hemorrhage, and immediately serosanguineous fluid came forth from the opening. A 36-size chest tube was then inserted after palpation of the diaphragm, which was localized just below the entrance to the pleura. The chest tube was inserted posteriorly extending up to the superior aspects of the left pleural space. The patient tolerated the procedure well. There were no complications. Immediately postop, she was stable. Approximately 400 cc of fluid were drained from the right chest.

10. Read the operative report below and assign CPT codes, as appropriate.

Operative Report

Preoperative Diagnosis: Foreign body in airway

Postoperative Diagnosis: Airway inflammation

Operative Findings: Trachea subglottis inflamed and cobblestoned, tracheal mucosa inflamed and cobblestoned moderate, carina normal and mainstem bronchi cobblestoning, secretions lavaged

Operation: Bronchoscopy

Procedure in Detail: The patient was brought to the operating room and placed on the operating room table in supine position. After successful induction of anesthesia, a shoulder roll was placed. The larynx was uncovered using the intubating laryngoscope and sprayed with 0.5 cc of lidocaine. The patient was then re-mask ventilated. The telescope was then passed between the vocal cords and the tracheobronchial tree was evaluated with the above findings noted. The patient was then intubated without difficulty, using the ventilating bronchoscope after a tooth guard was placed. Secretions were irrigated and lavaged from both main bronchi. Telescope and tooth guard removed. Repeat evaluation with 0 degree telescope negative for FB. The patient was then awakened from anesthesia and brought to the recovery room in satisfactory condition. There were no complications.

Cardiovascular, Hemic, and Lymphatic Systems

The codes in the cardiovascular system subsection are used to report procedures for surgeries performed on the heart and pericardium, valves, veins, and arteries. Also included are codes for insertion of hyperalimentation or hemodialysis catheters and infusion pumps. The codes are categorized first by body part involved and then by procedure performed, such as insertion of pacemaker, coronary artery bypass, embolectomy, and venous and arterial access sites.

Therapeutic and diagnostic cardiovascular system procedures, such as PTCA (percutaneous transluminal coronary angioplasty) and cardiac catheterizations, are coded from the medicine section of the CPT code book (codes 92920–93799). These procedures are discussed in chapter 7. Figure 4.11 shows the arteries of the body and Figure 4.12 shows the veins of the body. Blood flow to and from the heart is shown in Figure 4.13.

Pacemaker or Implantable Defibrillator

The pacemaker or implantable defibrillator subsection addresses the insertion or replacement of a pacemaker or implantable defibrillator system, or part of one of these systems. The guidelines at the beginning of the subsection are specific to what is included in a pacemaker or

Figure 4.11.   Arteries of the body

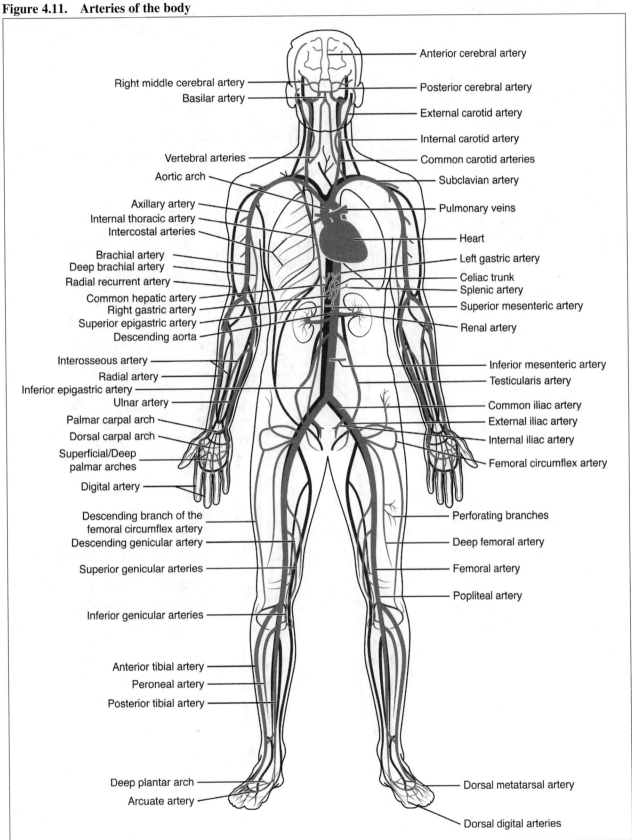

Anterior cerebral artery

Right middle cerebral artery

Basilar artery

Posterior cerebral artery

External carotid artery

Internal carotid artery

Vertebral arteries

Common carotid arteries

Aortic arch

Subclavian artery

Axillary artery

Pulmonary veins

Internal thoracic artery

Intercostal arteries

Heart

Brachial artery

Left gastric artery

Deep brachial artery

Celiac trunk

Radial recurrent artery

Splenic artery

Common hepatic artery

Superior mesenteric artery

Right gastric artery

Superior epigastric artery

Renal artery

Descending aorta

Interosseous artery

Inferior mesenteric artery

Radial artery

Testicularis artery

Inferior epigastric artery

Common iliac artery

Ulnar artery

External iliac artery

Palmar carpal arch

Internal iliac artery

Dorsal carpal arch

Femoral circumflex artery

Superficial/Deep palmar arches

Digital artery

Descending branch of the femoral circumflex artery

Perforating branches

Descending genicular artery

Deep femoral artery

Superior genicular arteries

Femoral artery

Popliteal artery

Inferior genicular arteries

Anterior tibial artery

Peroneal artery

Posterior tibial artery

Deep plantar arch

Dorsal metatarsal artery

Arcuate artery

Dorsal digital arteries

Figure 4.12. **Veins of the body**

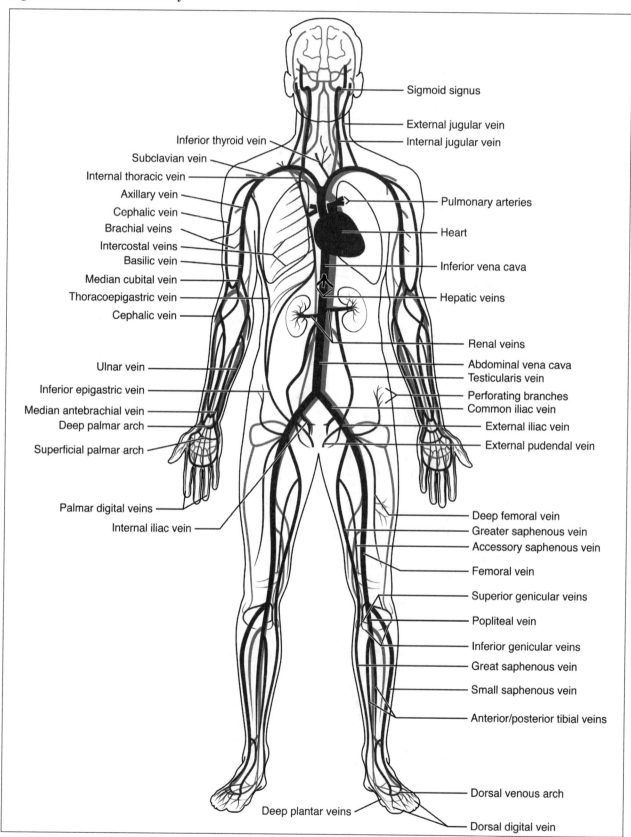

Figure 4.13. Heart blood flow

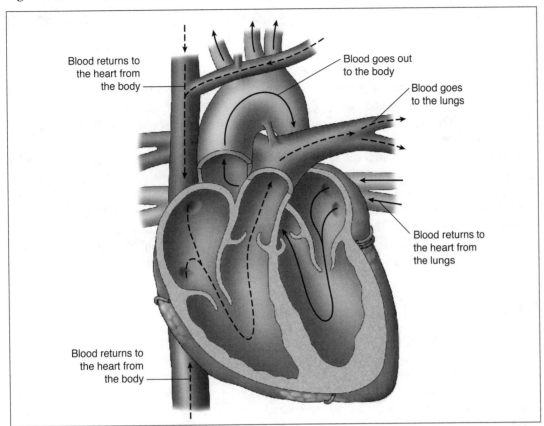

implantable defibrillator system and to how they may be inserted. The CPT code book includes a table in this section that assists the coder in coding the many scenarios of inserting, removing, or replacing pacemakers and implantable defibrillators.

For coding permanent pacemaker and implantable defibrillator procedures, the following documentation is needed:

- Whether the pacemaker or defibrillator is an initial insertion or a replacement

- Whether a component (for example, lead or pulse generator) or the entire system is being placed/replaced

- The specific type of pacemaker/defibrillator system (for example, single- versus dual-chamber or insertion versus removal of a defibrillator system)

- The surgical approach for placement of the electrodes (for example, transvenous versus thoracoscopic or epicardial)

Electrophysiologic Procedures

Electrophysiologic (EP) procedures are operative ablations that render a vessel as nonfunctioning to treat various types of arrhythmias. The use of cardiopulmonary bypass during the procedure determines the appropriate code.

Cardiac Valves

Codes 33361–33366 describe the work of transcatheter aortic valve replacement (TAVR) or transcatheter aortic valve implantation (TAVI). Both of these procedures require two physicians and the codes for all components of the procedure should have modifier –62 applied.

TAVR or TAVI codes describe all components of the procedures, such as percutaneous access when performed, placing the access sheath, balloon aortic valvuloplasty, advancing the valve delivery system into position, repositioning the valve if needed, deploying the valve, temporary pacing, and closure of the arteriotomy (AMA 2012). The coding notes in this section provide guidance on when diagnostic left heart catheterization, supravalvular aortography, and coronary angiography can and cannot be coded with TAVR/TAVI codes. Codes 33418–33419 describe the work of transcatheter mitral valve repair (TMVR), and 33477 describes the work of transcatheter pulmonary valve implantation (TPVI).

One of codes 33367, 33368, or 33369 can be assigned as an add-on code with a TAVR/TAVI, TMVR or TPVI code to describe the specific type of cardiopulmonary bypass support that is provided in association with the primary procedure.

Coronary Artery Bypass Grafting

Codes 33510–33548 describe procedures related to coronary artery bypass grafting (CABG). CABG procedures involve harvesting arteries and/or veins from other body locations and using them to create blood flow bypasses around diseased portions of cardiac vessels. Each bypass is also called a graft because the vessel is "grafted" to the new location. Figure 4.14 contains the anatomy of the coronary arteries and potential blockage points within the arteries. It also shows a cutaway view of diseased cardiac vessels.

The key to using these codes correctly is found in the body of the operative report. The coder must determine the number of coronary grafts performed and whether they were venous, arterial, or combined (vein and artery). The operative report title can be misleading. For example, the report title may list a procedure as a "triple CABG," but a review of the body of the report may reveal that three coronary artery grafts and one vein graft were used. In this case, codes 33535 and 33517 are reported.

Harvesting an upper extremity vein for a lower extremity or coronary artery bypass (35500) or an upper extremity artery (35600) is coded in addition to the primary procedure.

Venous Grafting Only

Codes 33510–33516 describe CABG procedures using venous grafts only. Procurement of the saphenous vein graft is included in these codes.

> **Example:** CABG of two coronary arteries using saphenous vein grafts. The code reported is 33511.

Combined Arterial-Venous Grafts

Arterial-venous grafts must be reported with two codes, an appropriate code from 33533–33536 and an appropriate add-on code from codes 33517–33523. Procurement of the saphenous vein graft is included in the 33517–33523 series and is not coded separately. Procurement of the artery for grafting is included in the 33533–33536 series except when an upper extremity vessel

Figure 4.14. Coronary arteries

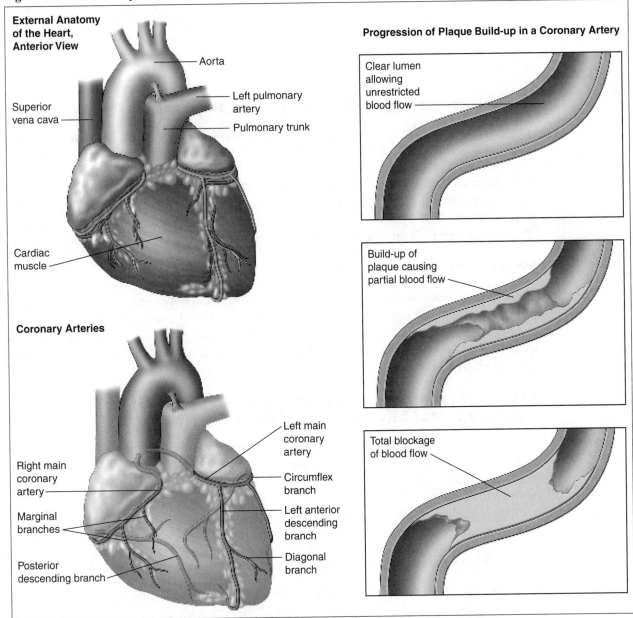

is used. Any of the following types of vessel harvesting are reported separately, in addition to the bypass procedure:

- Artery, upper extremity—report 35600

- Vein, upper extremity—report 35500

- Vein, femoro-popliteal segment—report 35572

The 33517–33523 codes may not be used alone and are exempt from modifier −51, Multiple Procedures.

Arterial Grafting Only

When a bypass procedure uses only the internal mammary arteries or other arteries, a single code from the 33533–33536 series should be reported to indicate the number of arterial grafts used. Codes from this series also are reported when a CABG uses a combination of arterial and venous grafts.

Single Ventricle and Other Complex Cardiac Anomalies

A new hybrid technique for repairing complex congenital heart defects such as hypoplastic left heart syndrome now includes a stage 1 procedure done through a posterolateral thoracotomy. This stage 1 procedure places bands around the right and left pulmonary arteries. A ductal stent is placed to create a patent ductus arteriosus and oxygenate the body. Code 33621 describes the thoracotomy and code 36620 describes the placement of the band. Stage 1 normally takes place within the first week of the patient's life. Stage 2 normally takes place after one year of life, after the child's heart and lungs have matured.

Heart/Lung Transplantation

Similar to lung transplantation, the heart/lung transplantation codes describe a three-part process of removal of cadaver organs, backbench work to prepare the organ(s) for transplantation, and the actual transplantation of the allograft organ(s). Separate codes are available for each part of the process and codes are provided here for a combination heart and lung transplant, or a heart-only transplant.

Extracorporeal Membrane Oxygenation (ECMO) or Extracorporeal Life Support (ECLS) Services

ECMO or ECLS provides cardiac or respiratory support while the organs rest or recover from illness or injury. The process continuously pumps the patient's blood out of the body to an oxygenator where oxygen is added, carbon dioxide is removed, blood is rewarmed and returned to the body.

The guidelines at the beginning of this subsection are specific to which codes may be reported together. To correctly code these services, the following documentation is needed:

- The age of the patient as birth through age 5 years or age 6 years and older

- Whether the service is veno-venous or veno-arterial

- Whether the cannula(e) are inserted peripherally using a percutaneous or open approach or whether the cannula(e) are placed centrally

- Whether the cannula(e) are repositioned or removed

- Whether the service was initiation of care or daily management

Arteries and Veins

The arteries and veins subsection is organized by specific artery or vein involved and approach. The guideline in this subsection states that the primary vascular procedure listing includes establishing both inflow and outflow by whatever procedures necessary. This subsection requires knowledge of the anatomy of arteries and veins.

Codes 34800–34826 describe placement of an endovascular graft for abdominal aortic aneurysm repair under fluoroscopic guidance and include vascular access, all catheter manipulations, balloon angioplasty within the endovascular prosthesis, and closure of the arteriotomy site. The coder should review the note under this heading for additional information on what is included and what radiological procedures may be coded in addition to this series of codes.

The code series 34841–34848 is used to code fenestrated endovascular repair of the visceral aorta, with or without the endovascular repair of the infrarenal aorta at the same session. The portion of the aorta that includes the branching of the celiac, superior mesenteric, and renal arteries is called the visceral aorta because these vessels feed the organs, or viscera. The infrarenal aorta is the area of the abdominal aorta below the level of the renal arteries. A fenestrated endovascular stent used in this procedure has small windows that are situated to allow blood flow to these visceral arteries that branch from the aorta. This fenestrated stent is made specifically for the individual patient based on their anatomy and must be manufactured for them in advance of the surgery. This service is coded as 34839 for the physician planning. Once the fenestrated stent is placed, one or more endoprostheses are placed from the visceral aorta into the branching arteries, such as the renal arteries to maintain lateral blood flow.

Code 34841 describes endovascular repair of the visceral aorta, including placement of one visceral artery endoprosthesis and the associated radiologic supervision and interpretation. When more than one visceral endoprosthesis must be placed into visceral arteries, a code from 34842 to 34844 is chosen instead to describe the entire procedure.

Code 34845 describes endovascular repair of the visceral aorta as just mentioned, but also includes the placement of the endovascular stent into the infrarenal abdominal aorta at the same operative session, using a unibody or modular stent. If only the infrarenal abdominal aorta is treated with an endovascular stent, a code is chosen from the code series of 34800–34826. The coding notes in both these sections should be read carefully to determine the procedures that can be coded separately. Repairs done in the thoracic aorta and in the aortic arch are separately reportable.

Codes 35001–35152 include endarterectomy and preparation of the artery for anastomosis. Endarterectomy should not be coded separately because it is an integral part of these procedures.

Code 35400, Angioscopy (non-coronary vessels or grafts) during therapeutic intervention, is an add-on code. It is listed in addition to the primary procedure code.

Bypass Graft

Several add-on codes are available for veins harvested for bypass grafts. Harvesting an upper extremity vein for a lower extremity or coronary artery bypass (35500) and harvesting an upper extremity artery for coronary artery bypass (35600) are coded in addition to the primary procedure. This code would not be reported alone but, instead, along with the lower extremity bypass procedure (for example, femoral-popliteal bypass, 35556) or CABG code.

CPT codes 35501–35671 refer to bypass grafts of vein or in situ vein ("other than vein"). Each code describes the location from which the bypass graft extends and the one to which it is connected. For example, code 35556 extends from the femoral artery and is connected to the popliteal artery. The most common materials used for "other than vein" include synthetic materials such as Gore-Tex.

Three composite graft codes—35681, 35682, and 35683—are available to report harvest and anastomosis of multiple-vein segments from distant sites. These vein grafts are used as arterial bypass graft conduits.

Code 35681 is assigned when the bypass graft is composed of prosthetic material and vein; codes 35682 and 35683 are assigned for two, three, or more vein segments from two or more locations. As with all add-on codes, they cannot be reported alone but, instead, must be accompanied by a code for the primary procedure. Codes 35682 and 35683 should be used with 35556, 35566, 35570, 35571, and 35583–35587.

Vascular Injection Procedures

Careful review of the guidelines at the beginning of this subsection will help the coder select the appropriate code for vascular catheterization procedures. These services include introduction and all lesser-order selective catheterizations used in the approach.

In coding arterial catheterizations, the following definitions apply:

- Selective arterial catheterizations require that the catheter be removed, manipulated, or guided into a part of the arterial system branching from the aorta (primary, secondary, and tertiary branches) or from the vessel punctured.

- Nonselective arterial catheterizations involve placement of a catheter or needle directly into an artery, or the catheter is negotiated into the arch, thoracic, or abdominal aorta from any approach.

In coding venous catheterizations, the following definitions apply:

- Selective venous catheterizations include catheter placement in those veins that branch directly from the vena cava or the vein punctured directly (primary branches) and any subsequent (secondary) branches of the primary venous branch.

- Nonselective venous catheterizations involve direct puncture of peripheral veins (specify) or placement of the catheter in the inferior vena cava or superior vena cava from any approach.

See chapter 5 for a further discussion of interventional procedure coding.

Central Venous Access Procedures

Many therapies are now administered by various types of catheters and ports. CPT coding for catheterization procedures depends on the type and use of the catheter in question. In general, CPT codes are assigned only to catheters inserted by physicians or non-physician practitioners, not by nursing personnel. Infusion pumps and venous access ports have specific codes that should be reported when these devices are inserted. Removal of some catheters does not warrant a separate code when no surgical procedure is required and the catheter is simply pulled out. There are specific codes, such as 36589, for removal of tunneled central venous catheter, without subcutaneous port or pump.

These catheters or ports can be used for intermittent long-term IV therapies such as chemotherapy or infusions. These procedures are quite distinct from intravascular cannulization or shunt procedures, which are coded to the 36800–36861 series and involve placement of a tube between two vessels to create a shunt. The brand name of the device cannot be used to distinguish the type of catheter. In a central line catheter placement, the tip of the catheter rests within the right atrium of the heart, the inferior vena cava, the superior vena cava, and the subclavian, brachiocephalic, or iliac veins.

When assigning codes in this subsection, the coding professional will need to determine whether the access device was inserted centrally (jugular, subclavian, femoral vein, or inferior vena cava) or peripherally (basilic or cephalic vein). The access device may be an exposed catheter (external to the skin), a subcutaneous port, or a pump.

To report the appropriate code, the procedure documentation will need to state which of the following the procedure was for:

- Insertion of a newly established venous access. The age of the patient will determine the appropriate code assignment when the procedure is for insertion. An example is code 36569, Insertion of peripherally inserted central venous catheter (PICC), without subcutaneous port or pump; age 5 years or older.

- Repair of a device rather than replacement. An example is code 36576, Repair of central venous access device, with subcutaneous port or pump, central or peripheral insertion site.

- Partial replacement of only the catheter not including the port/pump. An example is code 36578, Replacement, catheter only, of central venous access device, with subcutaneous port or pump, central or peripheral insertion site.

- Complete replacement of the entire device via the same access site. An example is code 36584, Replacement, complete, of a peripherally inserted central venous catheter (PICC), without subcutaneous port or pump, through same venous access.

- Removal of the entire device. An example is code 36590, Removal of tunneled central venous access device, with subcutaneous port or pump, central or peripheral insertion.

The *CPT 2016 Professional Edition* and *CPT 2016 Standard Edition* contain a table to assist with assignment of codes for central venous access procedures. Use code 36591 for the collection of a blood specimen from a completely implantable venous access device and code 36592 for collection of blood specimen using established central or peripheral venous catheter. Both of these codes can only be used in conjunction with services from the laboratory section of CPT. Code 36593 is used to describe declotting of an implanted vascular access device or catheter.

Hemodialysis Access, Intervascular Cannulation for Extracorporeal Circulation or Shunt Insertion

The intervascular cannulization or shunt subsection contains codes for various procedures performed to open one blood vessel into another, allowing blood to pass directly from the arteries to the veins or from vein to vein without going through the capillary network. The following procedures are among those listed in this subcategory:

- Insertion of a cannula for hemodialysis, other purpose (separate procedure); vein to vein (36800)

- Insertion of a cannula for hemodialysis, other purpose (separate procedure); direct arteriovenous anastomosis (36821)

- Creation of an arteriovenous fistula by other than direct arteriovenous anastomosis (separate procedure); autogenous graft (36825)

- Creation of an arteriovenous fistula by other than direct arteriovenous anastomosis (separate procedure); nonautogenous graft (for example, biological collagen, thermoplastic graft) (36830)

Codes 36831 and 36832 indicate that these procedures for arteriovenous fistulas are open procedures. The percutaneous thrombectomy code, 36870, is not to be used with 36593, Declotting by thrombolytic agent of implanted vascular access device or catheter.

Transcatheter Procedures

This section contains codes for a variety of procedures that are performed through a catheter. These procedures include arterial or venous mechanical thrombectomy, thrombolysis, or placement of a stent or intravascular vena cava filter.

Endovascular Revascularization

Codes 37220–37235 describe *revascularization*, a surgical procedure for the provision of a new, additional, or augmented blood supply to the iliac (37220–37223), femoral and popliteal (37224–37227), tibial and peroneal (37228–37231) arteries. Codes 37232–37235 describe each additional tibial or peroneal vessel revascularization and are add-on codes to 37228–37231. These codes include the actual intervention performed as well as the work of accessing and selectively catheterizing the vessel; transversing the lesion, radiological supervision, and interpretation directly related to the intervention(s) performed; embolic protection, if used; closure of the arteriotomy by any method; and imaging performed to document completion of the intervention (AMA 2011).

The revascularization code series is built on a progressive hierarchy of codes with more intensive services inclusive of lesser intensive services. When more than one procedure in this code range is performed on the same vessel (iliac, femoral/popliteal, or tibial/peroneal), only the most intensive service provided is reported. Only one code from this code family should be reported for each lower extremity vessel treated. The hierarchy, from least intensive to most intensive is as follows:

- Transluminal angioplasty alone

- Atherectomy (includes angioplasty)

- Transluminal stent placement (includes angioplasty)

- Transluminal stent placement and atherectomy (includes angioplasty)

The iliac artery revascularization code family is slightly different because the iliac artery is the largest artery in the group and the initial vessel accessed for the revascularization procedure(s). There is no code available for atherectomy of the iliac arteries, as this vessel is normally treated with angioplasty and stents.

Code 37220 describes an initial iliac artery angioplasty and code 37221 describes an initial iliac artery angioplasty with transluminal stent placement. Add-on code 37222 describes each additional ipsilateral (same side) iliac artery angioplasty and add-on code 37223 describes each additional ipsilateral iliac angioplasty with transluminal stent placement. All codes within this section are unilateral and describe either an open or percutaneous approach. If bilateral procedures are performed, the base code is repeated for the contralateral side and modifier –59 is appended, not modifier –50. Also, for coding purposes, the tibial/peroneal trunk is considered part of the tibial/peroneal grouping.

Endovascular revascularization of arteries other than those of the lower extremity, cervical carotid, extracranial vertebral, intrathoracic carotid, intracranial or coronary with a stent, and angioplasty are coded to 37236 for the first artery and 37237 for each additional artery. Endovascular revascularization of veins using a stent and angioplasty is coded to 37238 for the first vein and 37239 for each additional vein.

The only services that are separately reportable with the revascularization codes are mechanical thrombectomy, thrombolytic infusion when delivered via a pump, ultrasound guidance for vascular access, and additional catheter access solely for diagnostic imaging purposes (without another procedure before performed at that site).

Vascular Embolization and Occlusion

The code series of 37241–37244 is used to code endovascular embolization and occlusion of arteries and veins in locations other than the central nervous system, head, and neck.

The codes include the major work of the procedure including all associated radiological supervision and interpretation, intra-procedural guidance and road mapping, and the imaging necessary to document completion of the procedure. The coding notes indicate those procedures that are separately reportable.

The coding notes also state that there may be some overlap between codes for stent placement and these embolization codes. If a stent is the only management used to treat the vessel, then a stenting code should be assigned.

Only one embolization code should be assigned for the treatment site and the surrounding area such as side branches of that vessel. If multiple surgical fields are involved including separate major areas of trauma, then separate embolization codes should be assigned.

Hemic and Lymphatic Systems

The hemic and lymphatic systems subsection includes the spleen, bone marrow transplantation services, lymph nodes and lymph channels, mediastinum, and diaphragm.

Biopsies and/or excisions of lymph nodes are coded here when they are performed separately or not included as part of a more complex surgery.

A sentinel node biopsy can be done at the same operative session as a breast biopsy (19081–19126). Location of the sentinel node is done by lymphangiography using a radioactive tracer (38792) and identification using the operative hand held gamma detector by lymphoscintigraphy where radioactive tracer is followed through the lymph node chain. The injection of radioactive tracer is included in lymphoscintigraphy and is therefore not coded separately. The node can also be located intraoperatively by the injection of a nonradioactive dye (38900). After localization, the node is excised for evaluation (38500–38542). If a subsequent lymphadenectomy is performed with a partial or radical mastectomy, combination codes may be available to describe this service. (See code series 19302–19307.)

Mediastinum and Diaphragm

The *mediastinum* is a central compartment in the thoracic cavity. It contains the heart, great vessels, esophagus, trachea, and lymph nodes of the central chest. This compartment is separate from the left and right pleura. Figure 4.15 displays the mediastinoscopy procedure coded as CPT code 39401, where a scope is introduced through a small incision just above the mediastinum to examine the space or perform a biopsy within the mediastinal cavity. CPT code 39402 is assigned when the scope is introduced to perform a lymph node biopsy.

Miscellaneous Guidelines

Following are various reporting guidelines that coders should remember when using codes from the cardiovascular system and hemic and lymphatic systems subsystems:

- When coding lymphadenectomies, it is important to locate the code for the correct body area (for example, cervical, axillary, inguinofemoral).

- Cardiac catheterization procedures are coded to the 93451–93462 series in the medicine section of the CPT code book.

Figure 4.15. Mediastinoscopy procedure

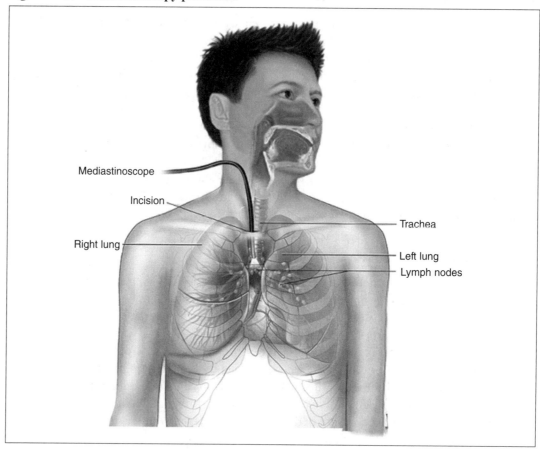

- Code 38510, Biopsy or excision of lymph node(s), open, deep cervical nodes(s), requires an approach through the platysmal muscle to gain access.

- Primary arterial and vascular procedure listings (34001–37799) include establishing both inflow and outflow by whatever procedures necessary. Also included is that portion of the operative arteriogram performed by the surgeon, as indicated. Sympathectomy, when done, is included in the listed aortic procedures.

- Procedures for direct repair of aneurysm or excision and graft insertion for aneurysm, false aneurysm, ruptured aneurysm, and associated occlusive diseases (35001–35152) include preparation of an artery for anastomosis, including endarterectomy.

- Vascular injection procedures include necessary local anesthesia, introduction of needles or catheter, injection of contrast media with or without automatic power injection, and/or necessary pre- and postcare specifically related to the injection procedure.

HCPCS Codes Used in Cardiovascular System Coding

The following HCPCS Level II codes are used with codes for surgical procedures involving the cardiovascular system:

G0269   Placement of occlusive device into either a venous or arterial access site, post surgical or interventional procedure (eg, angioseal plug, vascular plug)

G0288   Reconstruction, computed tomographic angiography of aorta for surgical planning for vascular surgery

S2205   Minimally invasive direct coronary artery bypass surgery involving mini-thoracotomy or mini-sternotomy surgery, performed under direct vision; using arterial graft(s), single coronary arterial graft

S2206   Minimally invasive direct coronary artery bypass surgery involving mini-thoracotomy or mini-sternotomy surgery, performed under direct vision; using arterial graft(s), two coronary arterial grafts

S2207   Minimally invasive direct coronary artery bypass surgery involving mini-thoracotomy or mini-sternotomy surgery, performed under direct vision; using venous graft only, single coronary venous graft

S2208   Minimally invasive direct coronary artery bypass surgery involving mini-thoracotomy or mini-sternotomy surgery, performed under direct vision; using single arterial and venous graft(s), single venous graft

S2209   Minimally invasive direct coronary artery bypass surgery involving mini-thoracotomy or mini-sternotomy surgery, performed under direct vision; using two arterial grafts and single venous graft

Exercise 4.5. Cardiovascular, Hemic, and Lymphatic Systems

Choose the best answer for each of the following questions.

1. A 3-year-old patient with leukemia is ready to start chemotherapy and requires the placement of a PICC line. How is this procedure coded?

    a. 36555
    b. 36568
    c. 36569
    d. 36580

2. The physician performs an intravenous cerebral thrombolysis for acute ischemic stroke. What is the correct surgical code assignment for this case?

    a. 36000, 37195
    b. 36011, 37212
    c. 37195
    d. 37212

3. The right common femoral artery was accessed and a catheter was inserted into the patient's abdominal aorta. The catheter was then maneuvered to the right renal artery, which was selectively catheterized. Injection and angiography were performed.

(Continued on next page)

Exercise 4.5. (Continued)

The catheter was then removed from the right renal artery and the left renal artery was selectively catheterized. Injection and angiography was performed. The catheter was then removed and manual pressure was applied until hemostasis was achieved.

a. 36245
b. 36245–50
c. 36252
d. 36254

4. CABG x3. The left internal mammary artery was anastomosed to the left anterior descending coronary artery and to the diagonal. A venous graft was placed from the aorta to the marginal circumflex artery. What is the correct surgical code assignment for this case?

a. 33512
b. 33512, 35500
c. 33524, 33510
d. 33524, 33517

Assign CPT surgery codes for the following scenarios.

5. Operative report reads: Triple coronary artery bypass (left internal mammary artery to left anterior descending; saphenous vein to diagonal; saphenous vein to right posterior descending).

_____

6. Read the following operative report and assign the appropriate CPT procedure code(s).

_____

Operative Report

Preoperative Diagnosis: DVT with inability to anticoagulate due to CVA

Postoperative Diagnosis: Same

Procedure(s):
1. Inferior venacavogram from right internal jugular vein approach
2. Vena caval Denali filter placement into the infrarenal IVC from a right internal jugular approach
3. Post procedure inferior venacavogram

Anesthesia/Meds: Fentanyl and Versed

Radiation Dose: 153.1 mGy

Fluoroscopy Time: 3.2 minutes

Contrast: 70cc Optiray 300

Operative note: The risks, benefits and alternatives of the procedure were explained to the patient, and written informed consent was then obtained.

Next, using ultrasound guidance access was gained into the right internal jugular vein with the needle seen in the patent vein by ultrasound followed by placement of a marker Omni Flush catheter into the left common iliac vein for a left common iliac venogram and inferior venacavogram to assess for any accessory IVC off of the left common vein, the size of the IVC, any thrombus in the IVC and the location of the renal veins. Next, the catheter was exchanged for the filter deployment sheath through which the filter was deployed in the infrarenal IVC. A post procedure inferior venacavogram was performed. The sheath was then removed. Hemostasis was achieved via direct pressure. The patient tolerated the procedure well including conscious sedation with no immediate complications.

Impression: Successful placement of an infrarenal IVC filter into a patent IVC

Exercise 4.5. (Continued)

7. Operative report reads: Valvuloplasty, mitral valve. Patient maintained on cardiopulmonary bypass during the procedure. How is this coded?

    _____

8. Read the following operative report and assign the appropriate CPT procedure code(s).

    _____

    Operative Report

    Preoperative Diagnosis: Advanced cardiomyopathy in a 69-year-old man

    Postoperative Diagnosis: Same

    Operation Performed: Insertion of Port-A-Cath

    Anesthesia: Local with IV sedation

    Procedure: With the patient in the supine position and the head elevated about 30 degrees, the right side of the neck and the right pectoral regions were prepared and draped in the usual manner. Anesthesia was accomplished by local infiltration of 1% Xylocaine. A small transverse incision was made in the supraclavicular fascia through skin and subcutaneous tissue, and the right external jugular vein was dissected out. A second incision was made in the subclavicular area. A space was developed for placement of the catheter. A tunnel was fashioned from this wound to the previous wound, and the catheter was passed through the tunnel. The catheter was filled with heparin solution and the jugular vein was ligated, a small venotomy was made, and the catheter was inserted. An x-ray of the chest revealed that the tip of the catheter was in the superior vena cava. The catheter was secured in place and ligated to the vein. The catheter was now transected the appropriate length, and a chamber was filled with heparin solution and attached to the catheter. The chamber was secured to the superficial fascia with two 2-0 Nylon sutures. Hemostasis was checked throughout the operative fields. The wounds were closed with interrupted 4-0 Dexon in a subcuticular layer and Steri-Strips in the skin.

    A dry sterile dressing was applied.

9. Read the following operative report and assign the appropriate CPT procedure code(s).

    _____

    Operative Report

    Preoperative Diagnosis: Pacemaker malfunction

    Postoperative Diagnosis: Same

    Anesthesia: Local

    Operation Performed: Replacement of pacemaker generator and electrode

    Procedure: The patient was positioned on the fluoroscopy table and the right chest was prepared and draped. Local anesthesia was obtained with 1% lidocaine with epinephrine. The pocket was reopened and the generator removed. Analysis of the lead showed intermittent R waves obtained. At this point, it was elected to proceed with insertion of a new lead and generator. A Medtronic lead, model #4024-52, serial number KJH124391W, was placed into the apex of the right ventricle. The lead was sutured in place using 2-0 silk and connected to a Medtronic generator. This was a DVI pacer programmed at a rate of 70. Inspection was made to be certain that hemostasis was adequate. The old lead was capped and abandoned. The wound was closed using 3-0 Vicryl for subcutaneous tissue and 3-0 nylon for skin. Dry dressings were applied, and the patient was returned to the recovery room in satisfactory condition.

(Continued on next page)

Exercise 4.5. (Continued)

10. Read the following operative report and assign the appropriate CPT procedure code(s).

Operative Report

Preoperative Diagnosis: Distal artery occlusion with severe stenosis in the left iliac artery. The patient is status post stent graft and aortofemoral bypass procedures in the past.

Postoperative Diagnosis: Distal artery occlusion with severe stenosis in the left iliac. The patient is status post stent graft and aortobifemoral bypass procedures in the past.

Operation Performed: 1. Left axillary artery to left femoral artery bypass using an 8 mm PTFE graft

Anesthesia: General
Estimated Blood Loss: Approximately 200 mL
Postoperative Condition: Stable

Procedure: After the informed consent was obtained and signed, the patient was brought to the operating room, placed in supine position. Anesthesia was administered without any complications. The appropriate time-out was performed. Preoperative antibiotics were given. We then prepped and draped the chest, abdomen, and left groin as well as the neck and the axilla in the usual sterile fashion.

We started the procedure by making an incision in the clavicular area on the left side. The incision was carried down with the Bovie device initially, then sharply we dissected the axillary vein. The vein was retracted superiorly and the subclavian artery as well as the axillary artery were dissected out and encircled with vessel loops. We achieved proximal and distal control without any complications. The adjacent structures and nerves were preserved. Next, we made a left groin incision along the previously made incision in the groin. The incision was carried down with a Bovie device. Then, we sharply dissected out the previous graft. The graft was then controlled proximally and distally with vessel loops. At this point, we used a Kelly tunneler and we tunneled the 8-mm graft. We made a tunnel underneath the pectoralis minor muscle over the chest wall where we came out the tunnel in the left axilla. Next, in the tunnel, using the Kelly tunneler, we made a tunnel in the subcutaneous area, lateral to the left common femoral artery. Umbilical tapes were placed and, at this stage, we gave the patient 5000 units of heparin. We waited three minutes and we made an arteriotomy. We controlled the subclavian axillary artery and we made an arteriotomy approximately 1 cm in length. The arteriotomy was extended with Potts scissors. At this stage, we fashioned an 8-mm graft to fit the arteriotomy, and we performed the anastomosis with the 5-0 Prolene sutures in a continuous fashion. Prior to completion of anastomosis, we flushed the anastomosis appropriately.

Next, through the preexisting tunnel underneath the pectoralis minor muscle, we tunneled the graft, ensuring the graft was not twisted into the left axilla. Next, on the left axilla we tunneled the graft all the way to the left common femoral artery. At this point, we ensured adequate length. We then controlled the graft in the common femoral artery area. Graftotomy was made with an 11 blade, and we fashioned the graft to fit the graftotomy. We performed the anastomosis with a 5-0 Prolene suture in a complex fashion. After achieving hemostasis, we then closed the groin in three layers including the skin with staples. The infraclavicular wound in the left upper chest was closed in a two-layer fashion as well. The patient had excellent signals at the end of the case. The patient was extubated and transported to the post-anesthesia recovery unit in stable condition.

Digestive System

The codes in the digestive system subsection are used to report open, endoscopic, and laparoscopic procedures performed on the mouth and related structures, the pharynx, adenoids and tonsils, esophagus, stomach, intestines, appendix, rectum, anus, liver, biliary tract, and pancreas. The codes are categorized first by body part involved and then by procedure, such as herniorrhaphy, esophagotomy, ileostomy, cholecystectomy, and hemorrhoidectomy. Figure 4.16 illustrates the parts of the digestive system.

Figure 4.16.   The digestive system

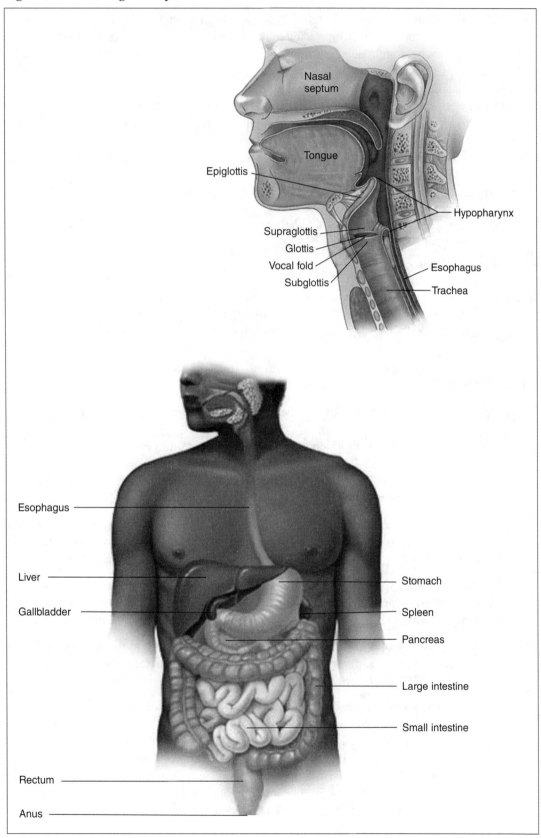

Laparoscopies

The digestive system subsection contains numerous laparoscopy codes that are distributed throughout the subsection based on various site-specific codes. When procedures are performed via laparoscopic approach, they must be distinguished from procedures performed by endoscope, open surgery, or percutaneous routes. A surgical laparoscopy always includes a diagnostic laparoscopy. When a procedure is started via a laparoscopic approach and then converted to an open procedure, the procedure should be thoroughly documented. *CPT Assistant* (March 2000) states that the open procedure should be reported with the attempted laparoscopic procedure, using the appropriate modifier.

An unlisted laparoscopy code should be assigned when a specific procedure code is not available for the applicable anatomic site.

Examples of some of the digestive system laparoscopic procedures are:

43280   Laparoscopy, surgical, esophagogastric fundoplasty (for example, Nissen, Toupet procedures)

44970   Laparoscopy, surgical, appendectomy

It is important to distinguish the laparoscopic approach from another approach, such as laparoscopic gastrostomy, code 43653, which must be distinguished from gastrostomy accomplished by open surgery (43830–43832) or percutaneous approach (43246 or 49440).

Endoscopy

Endoscopy codes specify type of instrument used, purpose of the endoscopy, and site of application.

The gastrointestinal (GI) subsection contains several guidelines involving endoscopies:

- Diagnostic endoscopies are not reported separately when performed in conjunction with a surgical endoscopy.

- When multiple procedures are performed through the endoscope, separate codes are reported for each procedure, when appropriate. The multiple procedure modifier –51 should be used for each subsequent procedure performed through the scope.

- When performing a GI endoscopy, the physician may encounter one or many lesions. Biopsies of some or all lesions may be taken. Lesion removal may be performed after a biopsy or without a biopsy. Therefore, the following guidelines should be applied:

  o When a biopsy of a lesion is taken and the remaining portion of the *same* lesion is excised during the same operative episode, a code should be assigned for the excision only (*CPT Assistant*, February 1999).

  o When one lesion is biopsied and a *different* lesion is excised, one code should be assigned for the biopsy and one for the excision. This rule is applicable unless the excision code narrative includes the phrase "with or without biopsy." In this case, only the excision code is assigned. It would be appropriate to append the biopsy code with modifier –59, Distinct Procedural Service. For patients covered by Medicare, instead of modifier –59, one of four other modifiers must be used to more clearly define a distinct procedure. The modifiers are:

    −XE: Separate encounter
    −XP: Separate practitioner
    −XS: Separate structure (or organ)
    −XU: Unusual non-overlapping service

  ○ Biopsy codes use the terminology "with biopsy, single or multiple." These codes are to be used only once, regardless of the number of biopsies taken.

  ○ Biopsy forceps may be passed through a scope to remove tissue from a suspect area; a cytology brush may be passed through the scope to obtain cells from the surface of a lesion; a suction apparatus may be used to remove foreign bodies or mucous plugs; or cell washings may be performed by instilling a solution into the esophagus or stomach and then aspirating the solution out.

Optical endomicroscopy is the evaluation of tissue by imaging in situ and without excision of a specimen or the wait for pathology results. This technique is now used with endoscopy to examine the walls of the gastrointestinal system.

Esophagoscopy

An esophagoscopy allows the physician to visualize the esophagus. Esophagoscopic photodynamic therapy is coded as an ablation procedure, code 43229, in addition to code 96570 or 96571, as appropriate.

    Esophagoscopies are coded based on the type of instrumentation used and the route used for the approach. Rigid esophagoscopy is coded to the 43191–43196 series. Transoral flexible esophagoscopy is coded to the 43200–43232 series and transnasal flexible esophagoscopy is coded to the 43197–43198 series.

Upper Gastrointestinal Endoscopies

Upper gastrointestinal endoscopies, often referred to as esophagogastroduodenoscopies (EGDs), are reported using codes 43235–43259. In these procedures, an endoscope is inserted through the mouth and down the throat to the esophagus, stomach, and either the duodenum and/or jejunum, as appropriate. Indications for these procedures include GI bleeding, ulceration, or inflammation; abdominal pain; narrowing of the esophagus; and suspected tumors or polyps.

    Figure 4.17 shows the passage of the endoscope during an upper GI endoscopy.

Lower Gastrointestinal Endoscopies

Lower GI procedures involve the small bowel, colon, and rectum. Indications for lower GI procedures include evaluation of an abnormal barium enema, lower gastrointestinal bleeding, iron deficiency anemia of unknown etiology, diarrhea, or follow-up examination after removal of a neoplastic growth.

    When coding lower gastrointestinal endoscopies, coders must distinguish among the following:

- Proctosigmoidoscopy, which is an examination of the rectum and sigmoid colon

- Sigmoidoscopy, which is an examination of the entire rectum, sigmoid colon, and may include part of the descending colon

- Colonoscopy, which is an examination of the entire colon, from rectum to cecum, with possible examination of the terminal ileum

Figure 4.17.   Stomach endoscopy

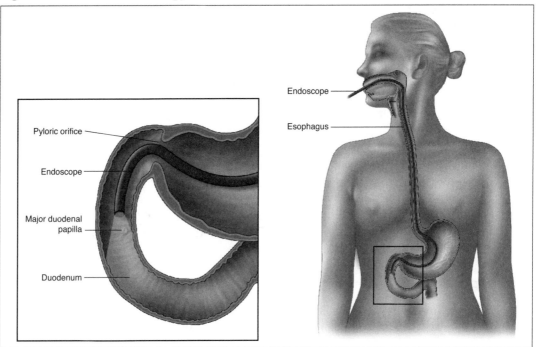

For a colonoscopy, the first step in choosing a code is to determine the route the procedure is to follow:

- Via stoma (44388–44408)

- Via rectum (45378–45398)

If a patient was scheduled and fully prepped for a colonoscopy, but the procedure was incomplete because the physician was unable to advance the colonoscope beyond the splenic flexure due to unforeseen circumstances, the colonoscopy code with modifier –53 would be reported, along with appropriate documentation.

Colonoscopies should be coded based on how far the scope was passed, not on the level where a biopsy was performed or a polyp was removed.

The following general guidelines apply to the coding of colonoscopies:

- When, during a colonoscopy, a polyp is removed and another area of the colon is biopsied, it is proper to code both procedures.

- When a biopsy of a lesion is taken and the lesion also is excised, only the excision should be coded.

- It is possible for a physician to use different techniques to remove separate polyps during the same operative episode. In this case, the appropriate CPT code is assigned to identify each technique.

If more than one procedure is performed via the endoscopy, a code must be assigned for each component.

The CPT code book recognizes the use of several techniques in performing polypectomies through a colonoscope:

- Hot biopsy forceps technique (45384), which utilizes hot biopsy forceps resembling tweezers connected to an electrosurgical unit. Grasping the polyp with the hot biopsy forceps, the physician pulls the growth away from the wall of the colon. This technique prevents bleeding, as seen with a cold biopsy, and is generally used on small polyps of 5 mm or less. A portion of the neoplasm may be removed for pathological analysis. The remaining portion is destroyed with the electrocoagulation current.

- Bipolar cautery (45384), which differs from other electrosurgery in that the electrical current flows from one jaw of the forceps through the tissue to the other jaw of the forceps.

- Snare technique (45385), in which a snare, or wire loop, slips over, or "lassos," the polyp. The stalk of the polyp is cauterized. The polyp then can be recovered in the snare itself, in a basket/net device attached to the snare, or with the aid of a suction device. This is the most successful technique in treating pedunculated polyps, midsize polyps, or large sessile polyps.

- Cold biopsy forceps technique (45380), which uses no electrocoagulation. The polyp is physically pulled from the wall of the colon.

- Laser technique (45388), which is commonly used for palliative treatment in patients who have already been diagnosed with a malignancy. Lesions of the rectum are more suitable for treatment with lasers than are lesions of the proximal colon. A device called a waveguide is used to deliver the laser beam through the scope to the area of treatment. A neodymium yttrium aluminum garnet (Nd:YAG) laser is used most commonly in the United States.

Lips

For repairs of the lip, the documentation should reflect the vertical height of the lip repair. For cleft lip/nasal deformity procedures, the supporting documentation should reflect whether the procedure is primary or secondary and whether a one- or two-stage procedure was performed.

Tongue and Floor of Mouth

CPT codes for procedures on the tongue and floor of the mouth include incision and drainage of abscess, cyst, or hematomas, and repair of lacerations. Excision of a lesion of the tongue is coded based on its location (posterior one-third or anterior two-thirds) on the tongue. When glossectomy (excision of tongue) is performed, it is important to note whether complete or partial excision was performed.

Dentoalveolar Structures

For dentoalveolar structures, it should be noted that the CPT code book does not include codes for pulling teeth because this procedure is considered a dental procedure and not a medical procedure. The American Dental Association copyrights and maintains a coding system in *Current Dental Terminology* (CDT 2016) that is used in reporting dental procedures. These dental procedures also are included in HCPCS Level II codes in the D code section and are indexed in the main HCPCS Index. See chapter 8 for an additional discussion on CDT codes.

Only a small number of codes are available in the CPT code book for dental procedures. In instances when teeth are removed for a medical problem or are incidental to another procedure performed, the only CPT code that can be used is 41899, Unlisted procedure, dentoalveolar structures. Third-party payers may not recognize HCPCS Level II dental codes for providers other than dentists but some are requiring all dental procedures be coded with HCPCS Level II. Consult the third-party payer for specifics.

Pharynx, Adenoids, and Tonsils

Tonsillectomy and adenoidectomy codes are based on type of procedure (primary or secondary) and age of the patient. *Primary* refers to the first time the tonsils and/or adenoids are removed. If the tonsils or adenoids grow back and have to be removed subsequently, this is considered *secondary* removal. Age is used in this set of codes because the level of difficulty is greater (and the patient recovery period is longer) for patients 12 years of age and older.

The February 1998 issue of *CPT Assistant* directs the coder that the tonsillectomy and adenoidectomy codes are intended to be bilateral and a modifier −50 is not appropriate with these codes. It also directs that if the procedure is performed unilaterally, a modifier −52 should be appended to the code.

Esophagus

Esophagogastric fundoplasty involves wrapping part of the upper stomach around the proximal esophagus to keep the esophagus in place below the diaphragm. Various methods are used to perform this procedure and many times this is performed in conjunction with the repair of a paraesophageal hiatal hernia. Approaches include via laparoscopy, via laparotomy, via thoracotomy, and via thoracoabdominal incision. In addition, esophageal lengthening can be performed with a fundoplasty and is coded separately, based on the approach used.

Stomach

CPT codes 43620–43641 are used to report an open gastrectomy, which is the removal of part or all of the stomach. These procedures are used to treat ulcers and malignancies. Roux-en-Y reconstruction can be performed in many different ways. This procedure involves a Y-shaped anastomosis that includes the intestines. Surgical laparoscopic procedures on the stomach are assigned to the 43644–43659 series of codes.

Codes 43760–43761 are reported for the placement, change, or repositioning of a gastrostomy tube, often referred to as a feeding tube or PEG (percutaneous endoscopic gastrostomy). For naso- or orogastric tube placement, necessitating a physician's skill, code 43752.

Introduction of Gastric and Duodenal Tubes

The codes in this section describe the various gastric and duodenal tube placement procedures. Gastric and duodenal intubation and aspiration are performed for lavage and collection of specimens. Tube placement, changes, and repositioning are coded in this section.

Bariatric Surgery

Laparoscopic bariatric surgery (gastric restrictive procedures) and later revision or removal of the adjustable band component are coded with this series. It should be noted that codes are available to revise the placement of the gastric band component but that simple postoperative adjustments to the gastric band are included in the global surgical package. Adjustments to the gastric band performed following the global period can be reported using S2083 for patients not covered by Medicare.

With this type of surgery, the patient may necessitate the removal of one or both of the component parts (gastric band component or the subcutaneous port component). Codes are available to remove one of these but if both components are removed and replaced, the coder is directed to code 43659, Unlisted laparoscopy procedure, stomach. Open gastric restrictive procedures are coded in the 43842–43848 series.

Intestines, Appendix, and Rectum

In the intestines subsection, code 44005 is used to report enterolysis, the freeing of intestinal adhesions. This is noted as a separate procedure and should ordinarily not be reported when it is part of another major procedure. According to *CPT Assistant* (January 2000), it is appropriate to code the lysis of adhesions separately when the adhesions are multiple or dense, cover the primary operative site, or add considerable time to the operative procedure and increase the risk to the patient. The coder should add modifier –22 to the surgical code. Individual payer policies may conflict with CPT policy. The ascending, transverse and descending colon are shown in figure 4.18.

Appendectomies (44950–44979) can be performed either through an open incision in the abdomen or laparoscopically. It should be noted that an incidental appendectomy (removal of a normal appendix) during another intra-abdominal surgery does not always warrant separate identification. For reporting purposes, some payers require that the

Figure 4.18. Large intestine

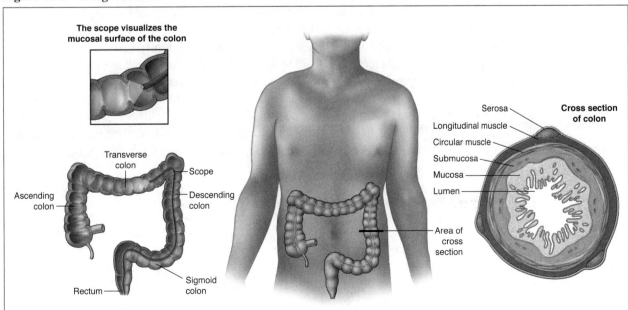

appendectomy be identified. In those cases, code 44950–52 is reported, in addition to the major abdominal procedure performed, to identify that the appendectomy was less than that usually performed. The diagnosis of a ruptured appendix also will determine the correct CPT code for an appendectomy.

CPT codes 45110–45123 describe proctectomy procedures for excising a portion of or the entire rectum. This should not be confused with prostatectomy, excision of the prostate. Thorough review of the operative report will eliminate this error. Laparoscopic procedures on the rectum are coded with the 45395–45499. This includes laparoscopic correction of rectal prolapse and complete proctectomy.

Anus

For a hemorrhoidectomy, the documentation should include the approach; whether the hemorrhoids were internal, external, or both; and whether a fissurectomy and/or fistulectomy were performed and whether more than one column/group was excised. When multiple methods are used to remove multiple hemorrhoids, each procedure can be coded separately using modifier –51. The most common hemorrhoidectomy procedure performed in a physician's office is 46221, Hemorrhoidectomy, internal, by rubber band ligations. If a single external hemorrhoid column/group is excised, the coder is directed to use code 46999.

For codes 46270–46280, the following definitions apply:

- A subcutaneous fistulectomy does not involve the sphincter muscle.

- A submuscular, or intersphincteric fistulectomy involves the division of the sphincter muscle.

Biliary Tract

A cholecystectomy can be performed either laparoscopically (47562–47564) or by open approach (47600–47620). When it is started via a laparoscope and then converted to an open procedure, the procedure should be thoroughly documented. *CPT Assistant* (March 2000) states that the open procedure should be reported with the attempted laparoscopic procedure and the appropriate modifier. Performance of an intraoperative cholangiogram and/or exploration of the common bile duct also affects code assignment.

Percutaneous procedures on the biliary tract are coded differently than endoscopic procedures. External biliary catheters drain fluid to the outside of the body and not into the intestine. An internal-external catheter drains into the intestine, to the outside of the body, or both. Percutaneous placement of these catheters is coded to 47533–47534 and removal, exchange, or conversion from one type to another is coded to 47535–47537. Stents are completely internal tubes that hold the biliary tract open and do not drain to the outside. Percutaneous placement of a stent is coded to 47538. Percutaneous dilation, biopsy or removal of calculi are coded as add-on codes with codes 47542–47544.

Abdomen, Peritoneum, and Omentum

In the abdomen, peritoneum, and omentum subsection, the exploratory laparotomy (code 49000) is a separate procedure and should not be reported when it is part of a larger procedure. This code often is used incorrectly because laparotomy is the approach to many abdominal surgeries. A laparotomy involves open surgery, whereas a laparoscopy involves only local incisions to introduce the laparoscope.

Laparoscopy codes (49320–49329) are available in the CPT code book for procedures on the abdomen, peritoneum, and omentum that are not coded to more specific laparoscopic procedures or more specific anatomic sites.

Hernia Repair

Many hernia repairs are coded in the last portion of the digestive system. An abdominal hernia occurs when internal organs, such as the intestines, break through a hole or tear in the musculature of the abdominal wall. This protrusion produces a bulge that can be seen or felt. Symptoms include burning and pain with activity. To code a hernia repair accurately, the coder must answer the following questions:

1. What is the type or site of the hernia?

   - Inguinal is a common herniation of the groin area (inguinal canal). Figure 4.19 displays the herniation of the intestine into the groin.

   - Lumbar is a rare herniation occurring in the lumbar region of the torso.

   - Incisional is a herniation at the site of a previous surgical incision.

   - Femoral is a common herniation occurring in the groin area (femoral canal).

   - Epigastric is a hernia located above the navel.

   - Umbilical is a herniation at the navel.

   - Spigelian is a herniation usually located above the inferior epigastric vessel, along the outer border of the rectus muscle.

Figure 4.19. Inguinal hernia

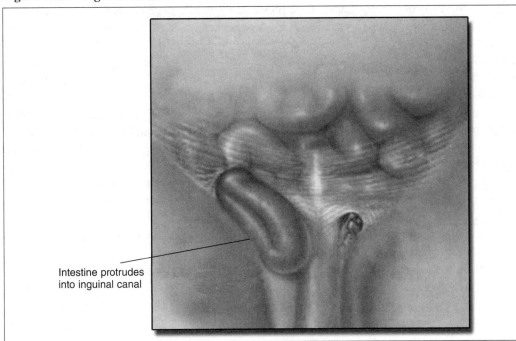

Intestine protrudes
into inguinal canal

2.   What is the age of the patient?

- Less than 37 weeks' gestation at birth, and now between birth and 50 weeks' postconception age

- Under 6 months

- Six months to under 5 years

- Age 5 years or older

3.   What is the history of the hernia?

- Initial refers to the first surgical repair of hernia

- Recurrent refers to a hernia that has been surgically repaired previously

4.   What is the clinical presentation of the hernia?

- A reducible hernia is characterized by protruding organs that can be returned to normal position by manipulation.

- A sliding hernia includes the colon or cecum as part of the hernia sac. (In some cases, the urinary bladder also may be involved.)

- An incarcerated hernia is one that cannot be reduced without surgical intervention.

- A strangulated hernia is an incarcerated hernia in which the blood supply to the contained organ is reduced. A strangulated hernia presents a medical emergency.

More than 20 million hernia repairs (herniorrhaphies) are performed worldwide each year (NYU 2013). A physician may perform one of three common types of repairs. The first type is the traditional or conventional repair. Under general anesthesia, the physician pushes the bulging tissue back into the abdominal cavity. Pulling together and stitching the surrounding muscles and ligaments closes the defect. A recovery period of four to six weeks is usually needed.

The second type of herniorrhaphy uses mesh rather than stitches to repair the abdominal defect. Because stitches are not used, the patient experiences less postoperative pain. Commonly used meshes are Marlex and Prolene. When coding a mesh repair of an incisional or ventral hernia, code 49568, Implantation of mesh or other prosthesis for incisional or ventral hernia repair, must be assigned in addition to the repair code. The use of mesh with other hernia repairs is *not* coded.

The third type of hernia repair is performed by a laparoscope. The laparoscopic repair technique (49650–49659) is used to treat inguinal, ventral and incisional hernias. Less discomfort and faster recovery are the main advantages to this approach. As with other endoscopies, a surgical laparoscopy includes a diagnostic laparoscopy.

It is important to note that diaphragmatic and hiatal hernias are not assigned to the digestive system. To identify these hernias, the coder should use codes from the 39501–39541 series in the diaphragm subsection of the CPT code book.

If the repair of a strangulated hernia includes associated repair of other organs, an additional code should be used for the other repair.

The parenthetical statement under code 54640 Orchiopexy, inguinal approach, with or without hernia repair, provides confusion to coders when coding orchiopexy and inguinal hernia repair, but *CPT Assistant* (June 2008, March 2004, and January 2004) directs the coder to code both procedures (54640) and the appropriate inguinal hernia repair if they are both performed.

Note that these codes are for unilateral repairs; bilateral hernia repairs should have the code listed twice or with the –50 modifier appended.

Points to Remember

- Identify the age of the patient and the type, clinical presentation, and history of the hernia.

- Identify the surgical approach (incisional or laparoscopic).

- Use the additional code 49568 when mesh is used to repair only an incisional or ventral hernia.

- Assign appropriate modifiers to identify laterality of hernia, such as modifier –50 for bilateral procedures.

HCPCS Codes Used in Digestive System Coding

The following HCPCS Level II codes are used with codes for surgical procedures involving the integumentary system:

G0455 Preparation with instillation of fecal microbiota by any method, including assessment of donor specimen

S2079 Laparoscopic esophagomyotomy (Heller type)

S2080 Laser-assisted uvulopalatoplasty (LAUP)

S2083 Adjustment of gastric band diameter via subcutaneous port by injection or aspiration of saline

S2102 Islet cell tissue transplant from pancreas; allogeneic

S9034 Extracorporeal shockwave lithotripsy for gall stones (if performed with ERCP, use 43265)

Exercise 4.6. Digestive System

Choose the best answer for each of the following questions.

1. The patient is taken to the endoscopy suite where the endoscope is passed into the esophagus but does not continue past the diaphragm into the stomach. Based on this documentation, what CPT code would be selected to represent this procedure?

    a. 43200
    b. 43235
    c. 43252
    d. 43260

2. Repair of bilateral strangulated recurrent inguinal hernias was performed. How is this coded?

    a. 49520–50
    b. 49351–50
    c. 49557–50
    d. 49580, 49568

(Continued on next page)

Exercise 4.6. (Continued)

3. A physician suspects that the patient has hemochromatosis and performs a needle biopsy of the liver with imaging guidance provided by the radiologist. How is this procedure coded?

    a. 10022
    b. 47000
    c. 47100
    d. 47399

4. Ultrasound reveals that the patient has a collection of fluid in the peritoneal cavity. This is drained using a laparoscope. How is this drainage procedure coded?

    a. 49020
    b. 49040
    c. 49320
    d. 49322

5. Read the following operative note and assign the appropriate CPT procedure code(s).

Operative Note

Preoperative Diagnosis: 1. Metastatic adenocarcinoma of the colon with bowel obstruction

Postoperative Diagnosis: 1. Metastatic adenocarcinoma of the colon with bowel obstruction

Procedure: Exploratory laparotomy with right hemicolectomy and ileocolonic anastomosis

Anesthesia: General

Indications for Surgery: The patient is a 38-year-old white male admitted with a bowel obstruction in the process of undergoing systemic and regional treatment for his metastatic colon cancer. The obstructive symptoms did not resolve with conservative treatment and surgery was undertaken. Potential risks were discussed. The patient understood and gave consent.

Procedure: The patient was brought to the operating room and positioned supine on the operating table. After induction of general anesthesia, the abdomen was prepped and draped in the routine sterile manner. A midline incision was made and carried down through the subcutaneous tissues. The midline fascia and peritoneum were opened, and the abdomen was explored. The patient was placed in Trendelenburg positioning, and the small bowel was packed out of the pelvis. We began by incising the peritoneal attachments, elevating the cecum out of the pelvis and rotate the ascending colon into the left upper quadrant. The duodenum was preserved and protected along its course through the dissection.

The hepatic flexure was then taken down completely, and the right colon was mobilized to the right side of the lesser sac. A suitable point of division of the terminal ileum was chosen about 5 cm proximal to the ileocecal valve. The bowel was divided at this level with a 75-mm GIA stapler. Ileocolic artery was ligated and right colic blood supply and the right branch of the middle colic blood supply was ligated. The transverse colon was divided with the GIA stapler, sending the specimen to the back table.

The blood supply to the ileum and the right transverse colon was excellent with good pulsatile flow extending all the way to the staple lines. A side-to-side functional end-to-end anastomosis was then completed between the terminal ileum and the right colon using the 75-mm GIA stapler. The enterotomies were closed in two layers with a running inner layer of 3-0 chromic followed by outer seromuscular Lembert stitches of 3-0 Vicryl. Several interrupted stitches of 3-0 Vicryl were placed at the apex of the anastomosis for reinforcement, and the mesenteric defect was closed with a running 3-0 Vicryl stitch. Upon completion of the anastomosis, it was found to be widely patent and circumferentially intact. All surgical sites were inspected for hemostasis. The small bowel was placed back in the abdomen in an anatomic fashion, and the anastomosis wrapped with the remaining normal omentum. The midline fascia was then closed with a running #2 Prolene stitch. The subcutaneous was copiously irrigated with Saline and the skin was closed with staples. At the end of the procedure, all sponge, needle and instrument counts were correct. Blood loss was 50 mL. The patient tolerated the procedure well and was transported to the PACU in stable condition.

Exercise 4.6. (Continued)

6. Read the following operative note and assign the appropriate CPT procedure code(s).

Operative Note

Preoperative Diagnosis: Morbid obesity

Postoperative Diagnosis: Morbid obesity

Procedures: Laparoscopic sleeve gastrectomy

Specimen: Resected stomach

Indication: The patient is a 34-year-old female who presented with morbid obesity. She was evaluated in a multidisciplinary evaluation for bariatric surgery and the patient was recommended to have a laparoscopic sleeve gastrectomy to which she was agreeable. Informed consent was obtained.

Procedure in Detail: The patient was brought to the operating room and placed in supine position. General anesthesia was induced. The patient was then prepped and draped in the usual sterile fashion. A time-out was completed, verifying the correct patient, procedure, site, position, prior to beginning the procedure. A supraumbilical vertical incision was made. Using a Visiport, a 12-mm trocar was placed into the abdominal cavity, and the abdomen was then insufflated and pneumoperitoneum was established. Under direct vision, two additional 12 mm trocars were placed in the left upper quadrant and two others were placed in the right upper quadrant and one was placed in the right lateral abdomen. The stomach was then decompressed using the ViSiGi 40-French tube. Using Maryland dissector attached to electrocautery, a mark was made 5 cm proximal from the pylorus along the greater curvature. Using a LigaSure, all the vessels along the greater curvature were taken down gently. This was performed along the curvature up until just lateral to the angle of His superiorly and at the level of incisura angularis inferiorly. Then, the ViSiGi tube was ensured to be along the lesser curvature. Alongside the tube, the stomach was stapled and divided sequentially in a vertical fashion, headed towards the angle of His using EndoGIA stapler with seam guard attached. There was no bleeding from the staple line. Intraoperative endoscopy was performed. This revealed no areas of stenosis or leak along the staple line nor did it reveal any bleeding into the lumen. Once the air was insufflated into the stomach, an air leak test was performed. No leak was noted. The water was suctioned out from the abdominal cavity, and the air was evacuated from the stomach endoscopically. The endoscope was then removed in its entirety and passed off the field. The lateral wall of the neo-stomach was then affixed to omentum using 2-0 Ethibond suture. The left lateral incision port was then removed. The incision site and level of the fascia were dilated. The resected stomach was then retrieved via this incision. Under visual guidance using a suture passer, the defect was approximated using a 3-0 Vicryl suture placed in a simple interrupted fashion. All the other ports and the liver retractor were removed under visual guidance. The abdomen was then desufflated. All the incision sites were closed with 4-0 Vicryl placed in a continuous subcuticular fashion. The patient tolerated the procedure well, left the operating room, was extubated, and was taken to recovery room in stable condition.

---

7. Read the following operative note and assign the appropriate CPT procedure code(s).

Operative Note

Procedure: EGD with foreign body removal

Clinical Note: This 47-year-old man experienced acute odynophagia after eating fish. The patient felt a foreign body-like sensation in his proximal esophagus. He was evaluated with lateral, C-spine films, and soft tissue films without any evidence of perforation.

Findings: After obtaining informed consent, the patient was endoscoped. He was premedicated without any complication. Under direct visualization, an Olympus Q20 was introduced orally and the esophagus was intubated without difficulty. The hypopharynx was reviewed carefully, and no abnormalities were noted. There were no foreign bodies and no lacerations to the hypopharynx. The proximal esophagus was normal. No active bleeding was noted. The endoscope was advanced farther into the esophagus, where careful review of the mucosa revealed no foreign bodies and no obstructions. However, the gastroesophageal junction did show a very small fish bone, which was removed without complications.

(Continued on next page)

Exercise 4.6. (Continued)

The endoscope was advanced into the stomach, where partially digested food was noted. The duodenum was normal. The endoscope was then removed. The patient tolerated the procedure well, and his postprocedural vital signs are stable.

8. Read the following operative note and assign the appropriate CPT procedure code(s).

Operative Note

Preoperative Diagnosis: Esophageal foreign body

Postoperative Diagnosis: Esophageal foreign body

Operation: Rigid esophagoscopy with foreign body removal

Procedure: The patient was taken to the OR, anesthesia was induced, and the patient was intubated. After a satisfactory level of anesthesia, the esophageal speculum was introduced into the right piriform sinus past the cricopharyngeus, and the following observations were made: a bony structure, by history a fish bone, was found protruding from the right posterior esophageal wall. This was grasped and removed through the esophageal speculum. Upon examination, there appeared to be a small pinpoint area where the bone had embedded itself in the esophageal wall with no significant edema. The distal esophagus was evaluated with a 6 × 30 esophagoscope, and there appeared to be no fragments or perforations. After the esophagoscope was removed, the patient was awakened from anesthesia and taken to the recovery room in good condition.

9. Read the following operative note and assign the appropriate CPT procedure code(s).

Operative Note

Preoperative Diagnosis: Symptomatic cholelithiasis

Postoperative Diagnosis: Symptomatic cholelithiasis with adhesions between the stomach wall and the gallbladder

Operation: Laparoscopic cholecystectomy and lysis of adhesions with normal intraoperative cholangiogram

Procedure: This 51-year-old woman was taken to the operating room and placed in the supine position. General endotracheal anesthesia was accomplished without complications. An infraumbilical incision was made and fascia exposed on both sides and tacked with 0-Dexon. The peritoneum was entered sharply without difficulty and the blunt Hasson trocar placed. The abdomen was insufflated with 15 cm of pressure with good pressure throughout. Initial pressure was 4. The camera was placed and a diagnostic laparoscopy performed. The liver had changes of fatty replacement, but no evidence of a tumor. The gallbladder appeared thin-walled, but there were adhesions between the liver and the anterior abdominal wall and between the falciform and the liver. Three other operative ports were placed: 10 mm in the midline, 5 mm midclavicular line, and 5 mm anterior axillary line. The gallbladder was retracted superiorly. The adhesions were taken down with sharp dissection. Careful dissection was obtained taking the stomach off the gallbladder. Cystic duct was identified and dissected down toward its juncture with the common bile duct. Cholangiogram was obtained using a taut catheter through a 14-gauge Intracath. The common duct appeared normal with no evidence of stones. There was good flow into the duodenum. The intrahepatic ducts filled poorly because of such rapid flow distally; however, we adequately visualized that intrahepatics were filling. The cystic duct was doubly clamped proximally, singly clamped distally, and divided. The gallbladder was removed from the hepatic bed with electrocautery. A bothersome oozer at the base of the gallbladder bed required the Argon beam. It was then hemostatic. It was irrigated copiously with sterile saline and inspected for hemostasis and found to be dry. The gallbladder was brought out intact with the stone in place through the upper midline port. As much of the CO2 as possible was removed. The ports were removed under direct vision after the liver had been reinspected and found to be dry. The umbilical fascia was closed with 0-Dexons. Skin wounds were closed with 4-0 Dexons and covered with Steri-Strips. The patient tolerated the procedure and was returned to the recovery room in stable condition.

Exercise 4.6. (Continued)

10. Read the following operative note and assign the appropriate CPT procedure code(s).

Operative Note

Preoperative Diagnosis: Left inguinal hernia

Postoperative Diagnosis: Same

Procedure: Left inguinal hernia repair with mesh

Anesthesia: General

Indications: The patient is a 23-year-old man who presented with several weeks' history of pain in his left groin associated with a bulge. Examination revealed that his left groin did indeed have a bulge and his right groin was normal. We discussed the procedure and the choice of anesthesia.

Operative Summary: After preoperative evaluation and clearance, the patient was brought into the operating suite and placed in a comfortable supine position on the operating room table. Monitoring equipment was attached, and general anesthesia was induced. His left groin was prepped and draped sterilely and an inguinal incision made. This was carried down through the subcutaneous tissues until the external oblique fascia was reached. This was split in a direction parallel with its fibers, and the medial aspect of the opening included the external ring. The ilioinguinal nerve was identified, and care was taken to retract this inferiorly out of the way. The cord structures were encircled and the cremasteric muscle fibers divided. At this point, we examined the floor of the inguinal canal and he did appear to have a weakness here. We then explored the cord. There was no evidence of an indirect hernia. A piece of 3 × 5 mesh was obtained and trimmed to fit. It was placed down in the inguinal canal and tacked to the pubic tubercle. It was then run inferiorly along the pelvic shelving edge until lateral to the internal ring and tacked down superiorly using interrupted sutures of 0-Prolene. A single stitch was placed lateral to the cord to recreate the internal ring. Details of the mesh were tucked underneath the external oblique fascia. The cord and the nerve were allowed to drop back into the wound, and the wound was infiltrated with 30 cc of 0.5 percent Marcaine. The external oblique fascia then was closed with a running suture of 0-Vicryl. Subcutaneous tissues were approximated with interrupted sutures of 3-0 Vicryl. The skin was closed with a running subcuticular suture of 4-0 Vicryl. Benzoin and Steri-Strips and a dry sterile dressing were applied. All sponge, needle, and instrument counts were correct at the end of the procedure. The patient tolerated the procedure well and was taken to the recovery room in stable condition.

Urinary System

The codes in the urinary system subsection are assigned to report procedures on the kidneys, ureters, bladder, and urethra. Procedures in this subsection are classified according to approach (open incision, percutaneous, endoscopic, laparoscopic) and precise anatomic site.

The urinary system subsection also contains diagnostic urodynamic procedures, such as a cystometrogram and voiding pressure studies. Transurethral prostate procedures are listed in this subsection, but the open prostatectomy codes are listed in the male genital system subsection. Figure 4.20 displays the complete urinary system.

Many procedure descriptions in the urinary system subsection are written so that the main procedure can be identified without having to list all of the minor, related functions performed during the same operation or investigative session, as in the following example:

52601 Transurethral electrosurgical resection of prostate, including control of postoperative bleeding, complete (Vasectomy, meatotomy, cystourethroscopy, urethral calibration and/or dilatation, and internal urethrotomy are included.)

Figure 4.20. The urinary system

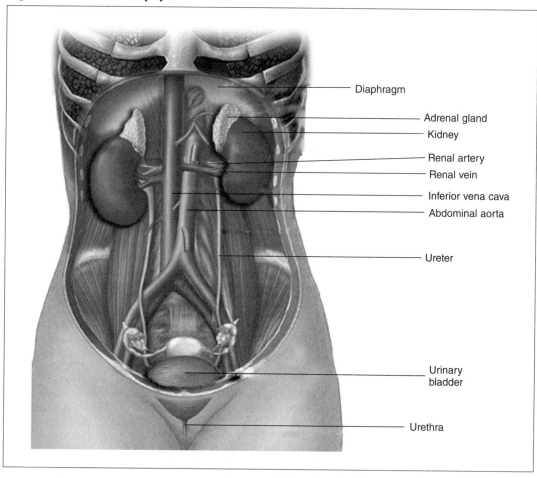

Therefore, a patient who undergoes a transurethral resection of the prostate, including internal urethrotomy and urethral calibration, is assigned only one code: 52601.

Miscellaneous Guidelines

Following are various reporting guidelines that coders should be aware of when coding procedures from the urinary system subsection:

- The urodynamics subgrouping (51725–51798) includes procedures that may be used separately or in different combinations. The coder should read the procedure report carefully to assign the appropriate codes.

- When a retrograde pyelogram (ureteropyelography) is performed by ureteral catheterization through a cystoscope, code 52005 should be assigned.

- Careful review of surgical reports is necessary prior to selecting a code. The coder must determine whether the site of the procedure was ureter or urethra. For example, code 52310 describes a cystourethroscopy with simple removal of a calculus from urethra, whereas code 52320 describes a cystourethroscopy with removal of a ureteral calculus.

- The urinary system subsection lists three headings for transurethral surgery: urethra and bladder; ureter and pelvis; and vesical neck and prostate. Thus, the coder should first identify the primary or main anatomical site for which the surgery was performed and then select a code.

- For a transurethral cystoscopy with bladder/urethra biopsy(s), code 52204 should be assigned.

Laparoscopic Codes

Laparoscopic codes are located throughout the urinary system subsection. It is important to become very familiar with the laparoscopic codes available because new codes are added every year.

When a laparoscopic approach is used, but no laparoscopic code is available for the specific procedure performed, the coder should use the unlisted laparoscopic code for the applicable site.

Codes 51990 and 51992 describe the laparoscopic repair techniques for urinary stress incontinence:

- Code 51990 describes a procedure in which sutures are placed laparoscopically into the endopelvic tissue at the bladder neck region on each side and secured to the ipsilateral Cooper's ligament to create a suspension of the bladder neck.

- Code 51992 is a variation of 51990 and often is referred to as the sling procedure. The endopelvic fascia is opened, and a tunnel is dissected between the urethra and vaginal mucosa. The sling material (cadaver or synthetic) is then passed through the tunnel and secured to Cooper's ligament bilaterally.

Kidney

In the kidney subsection, removal of urinary calculi (stones) is coded according to approach (open incision, percutaneous, endoscopic) and the anatomic site from which the stone is removed (renal pelvis; upper-, middle-, or lower-third of ureter; bladder; urethra).

Nephrolithotomy (50060–50075) describes the removal of urinary stones through an incision directly into the body of the kidney. Percutaneous nephrostolithotomy and pyelostolithotomy codes (50080–50081) are for reporting the removal of kidney stones through the creation of an artificial passageway between the skin and the kidney (that is, percutaneous technique). When the passageway (nephrostomy or pyelostomy) already exists, code 50561 is used to report removal of the stones through a renal endoscopy.

Lithotripsy is the noninvasive method of destroying urinary stones. Under radiologic guidance, sound waves are directed through a water-cushion that is placed against the patient's body at the site of the stone. The sound waves are sent in short bursts and over the course of approximately an hour, the stone is reduced to the size of fine sand. These tiny pieces pass painlessly through the urinary system with normal urination. Lithotripsy is coded as 50590, which describes a unilateral procedure. If stones are destroyed within both kidneys at the same session, a modifier –50 is appended to the code.

CPT codes 50551–50580 are used to code a renal endoscopy through an established nephrostomy or pyelostomy or through nephrotomy or pyelotomy. It should be noted that the description of these codes states "exclusive of radiologic service." When the physician also performs the radiology portion of this procedure (or when one coder is coding for both physicians' services), the coder also should refer to codes 74400–74485 and 78700–78740, depending on the procedures performed.

For nephrectomy, the documentation should include whether the procedure was partial or total, laparoscopic or open, and whether any other structures were removed. For renal transplantation, the documentation should include whether the procedure was for a donor or a recipient nephrectomy. Transplantation should indicate whether the procedure was allotransplantation or autotransplantation.

Ureter

Procedures performed on the ureter(s) are coded based on approach, such as open, endoscopic, or laparoscopic. For ureterolithotomy, the documentation should identify the portion of the ureter where the stone was removed (upper, middle, or lower one-third). Ureteral endoscopy documentation should indicate what procedure was performed through the endoscope, such as a biopsy (50955).

For surgical removal of stones from the ureter through a direct incision into the ureter, codes 50610–50630 are used. The actual code chosen is based on what part of the ureter is incised, depending on the location of the stones. When the stones are removed with a stone basket extraction through an incision in the bladder, the coder should refer to code 51065. For laparoscopic removal of ureteral stones, code 50945 should be used. This code is reported only once when multiple stones are removed from the same ureter. If stones are removed from both ureters, then modifier –50 is applied.

Percutaneous removal and/or replacement of an internally dwelling ureteral stent (a thin catheter-like tube) is coded in this section with codes 50382–50386. (A discussion of stent placement is found later in this chapter.) After conscious sedation and local anesthesia, the physician inserts a needle through the skin and into the renal calyx, then replacing the needle with a guide wire. This is done under fluoroscopic guidance. Dye is injected and the tract is dilated. A snare device is used to grab the stent and it is removed. If a new stent is required, it is deployed over the guide wire and placement is verified with fluoroscopic guidance.

Bladder

For cystectomy (excision of all or part of the urinary bladder), the documentation should identify whether the procedure was partial or complete and whether lymph nodes were removed.

Urodynamics

Urodynamics is the study of urine storage and flow through the urinary tract. It is helpful in diagnosing obstructions, altered pelvic anatomy or neuromuscular disorders (*CPT Assistant*, September 2002). Codes 51725–51798 describe urodynamic procedures that may be reported separately or in combination when more than one procedure is performed. Modifier –51 should be reported when multiple procedures are performed. These procedures are performed either by the physician or under his or her direction. The following services/supplies are considered part of the procedure and should not be reported separately: instruments, equipment, fluids, gases, probes, catheters, technicians' fees, medications, gloves, trays, tubing, and other sterile supplies.

If the physician is providing only the professional component (that is, supervision and interpretation), modifier –26 should be appended to the CPT code reported for the physician services. For example, when a physician performs a simple cystometrogram in the hospital outpatient department using hospital equipment, staff, and supplies, and interprets the results, he or she reports 51725 with a –26 modifier for the professional component of the service.

The following definitions (Rogers 1998) describing the various urodynamic procedures will help the coder assign the appropriate CPT code:

- Simple cystometrogram involves measurement of the bladder's capacity, sensation of filling, and intravesical pressure.

- Complex cystometrogram is measurement of the bladder's capacity, sensation of filling, and intravesical pressure, using a rectal probe to distinguish between intra-abdominal pressure and bladder pressure.

- Simple uroflowmetry is measurement of the volume of urine that flows out of the bladder per second. Flow is measuring using a nonautomated method.

- Complex uroflowmetry is measurement and recording of mean and peak flow and the time taken to reach peak flow during continuous urination. Flow is measured using automated equipment.

- Urethral pressure profile (UPP) is the recording of pressures along the urethra as a special catheter is slowly withdrawn.

- Electromyography studies involve the recording of muscle activity during voiding while simultaneously recording urine flow rate.

- Stimulus evoked response is the measurement of the delay time between stimulation and response of the pudendal nerve.

- Voiding pressure studies measure the urine flow rate and pressure during emptying of the bladder. Bladder voiding pressure is measured via a bladder probe and intra-abdominal voiding pressure is most often measured via rectal probe.

Endoscopy—Cystoscopy, Urethroscopy, Cystourethroscopy

In general, genitourinary endoscopies are categorized by body part involved—urethra, prostate, ureter—and specific procedure performed, such as cystourethroscopy with biopsy of the bladder or urethra, transurethral incision of prostate, cystourethroscopy with ureteral meatotomy, and cystourethroscopy with insertion of indwelling ureteral stent. The endoscopic procedures described in codes 52000–52700 are listed so that the main procedure can be identified without having to list all the minor related functions performed at the same time.

Code 52001 is reported when the reason for the cystourethroscopy is irrigation and the evacuation of multiple obstructing clots. Code 52005 is assigned when a retrograde pyelogram is done and the dye is injected through a ureteral catheter. Code 52281 is reported only when a cystoscopy with urethral calibration and/or dilatation is performed for urethral stricture or stenosis. A diagnosis of urethral stricture or stenosis must be documented by the physician before this code can be assigned appropriately.

Stents

Endoscopy guidelines in the ureter and pelvis subsection (52320–52356) clarify the reporting of temporary stents and self-retaining, indwelling stents. Insertion and removal of a temporary ureteral stent is included in codes 52320–52356 and should not be reported separately. However, the guideline states that insertion of a self-retaining, indwelling stent performed during other cystourethroscopic diagnostic or therapeutic interventions should be reported using code 52332–51, in addition to the major procedure performed. Code 52332 is considered unilateral; therefore, when an indwelling stent is placed in each ureter through the same cystoscope during the same cystourethroscopic diagnostic and/or therapeutic intervention, modifier –50, Bilateral Procedure, should be appended.

Cystourethroscopy with insertion of permanent urethral stent is coded to 52282. Cystourethroscopy with insertion of an indwelling ureteral stent is coded to 52332. For temporary prostatic urethral stent, the coder should report 53855. It is important to use caution in distinguishing ureteral procedures from urethral procedures.

Removal of Indwelling Ureteral Stent

Another common coding question is how to code removal of indwelling ureteral stents. Coding these removals can be tricky and requires specific information about the original method of stent placement. When stent removal is part of a planned or staged procedure during the associated normal postoperative follow-up period of the original procedure, code 52310 or 52315 should be reported, as appropriate, with modifier –58, Staged or Related Procedure or Service by the Same Physician during the Postoperative Period.

For example, when an indwelling stent is inserted using a ureterotomy (50605) or other procedure included in the surgical package, no additional reporting is warranted when the stent is removed during the normal postoperative follow-up period. However, when the indwelling ureteral stent is removed beyond the normal postoperative/follow-up period associated with its insertion (for example, code 50605) and no further cystourethroscopic intervention is required, removal of the indwelling ureteral stent would be reported with the appropriate level of E/M service code.

Urethra

The documentation should identify the sex of the patient because CPT code assignment varies by sex in the urinary system subsection. The diagnosis is required to assign the correct code from the excision grouping (53220–53275) within the urethra subsection. For urethroplasty (repair of the urethra), the documentation should include whether the procedure was staged and should identify the stage performed (first stage or second stage). For dilatation of urethral stricture, the coder should identify the approach, the patient's sex, and whether the procedure is an initial or subsequent dilatation.

Transurethral destruction of prostatic tissue by microwave thermotherapy is assigned to code 53850, whereas code 53852 is reported for destruction by radiofrequency thermotherapy and 55899 is reported for water-induced thermotherapy destruction, as directed by the coding notes.

HCPCS Codes Used in Urinary System Coding

The following HCPCS Level II codes are used with codes for surgical procedures involving the urinary system:

P9612   Catheterization for collection of specimen, single patient, all places of service

P9615   Catheterization for collection of specimen(s) (multiple patients)

S2070   Cystourethroscopy, with ureteroscopy and/or pyeloscopy; with endoscopic laser treatment of ureteral calculi (includes ureteral catheterization)

Exercise 4.7. Urinary System

Choose the best answer for each of the following questions.

1. The physician performs a laparoscopic radical nephrectomy with adrenalectomy. Surrounding lymph nodes are also removed. How are these procedures coded?

   a. 50545
   b. 50545, 60650
   c. 50548, 38570
   d. 50548, 60650, 38589

2. A patient with a kidney transplant has significant symptoms of rejection requiring a nephrectomy. How is this coded?

   a. 50300
   b. 50320
   c. 50340
   d. 50370

3. What is the correct code assignment for the surgical removal of kidney stones through an incision into the renal pelvis?

   a. 50060
   b. 50080
   c. 50130
   d. 50205

Assign appropriate CPT code(s) for the following scenarios.

4. A patient who is 120 days status post TURP has a second transurethral procedure for residual obstructive tissue

   _____

5. Renal cyst aspirated by percutaneous needle

   _____

6. Conversion of a nephrostomy catheter into a nephrourteral catheter through an existing hole

   _____

7. Office note: The patient is unable to void independently. A catheter is placed to extract urine from the bladder and then removed.

   _____

8. Read the following operative report and assign the appropriate CPT surgical procedure code(s).

   _____

Operative Report

Preoperative Diagnosis: Benign prostatic hyperplasia

Postoperative Diagnosis: Benign prostatic hyperplasia

Operation: 1. Cystoscopy
2. Meatotomy
3. Transurethral resection of prostate

(Continued on next page)

Exercise 4.7. (Continued)

Indications: The patient is a 69-year-old man with a history consistent with bladder outlet obstruction caused by prostate hyperplasia.

Procedure: The patient was taken to the cystoscopy suite after undergoing adequate spinal anesthesia. He was placed in the dorsolithotomy position, and prepped and draped in normal sterile manner. The 17 French cystoscope was introduced. Visualization of penile urethra was within normal limits. Prostatic urethra showed bilateral obstructing prostate, with right lobe greater than the left. The bladder showed no gross mucosal abnormalities. The ureteral orifices were of normal size and position.

At this point, it was deemed that the patient would benefit from a transurethral resection of the prostate. An attempt was made to dilate the urethra, but due to meatal stenosis, it was necessary to perform a meatotomy using a crushing clamp in the dorsal region. A small incision was made. At this point, the Van Buren sounds were easily passed. The patient was dilated using successful sounds up to 26 French.

Sounds were then removed. Then, the 24 French Iglesias resectoscope with obturator was inserted into the bladder. The obturator was removed and the lens inserted. Landmarks were observed to be ureteral orifices, bladder neck, and verumontanum. Resection was begun in the 9 o'clock position and brought down to the 6 o'clock position. Continuation then was done from the 3 o'clock position down to the 6 o'clock position, from near the 12 o'clock position to the 3 o'clock position. Hemostasis was obtained using Bovie cautery continually through the resection. These landmarks were observed to be intact.

At completion of the procedure, the clots and chips were irrigated using Ellik evacuator. The bladder was left full and the resectoscope removed. At this point, with pressure on the abdomen, a good urinary stream was noted coming through the meatus. A 24 French three-way Foley catheter was inserted and filled with 40 cc to the balloon. This was placed on traction and connected to a continuous three-way irrigation. The patient tolerated the procedure well without complications and was taken to the recovery room. Estimated blood loss was 300 cc. Specimens to pathology were the prostatic chips.

9. Read the following operative report and assign the appropriate CPT surgical procedure code(s).

Operative Report

Preoperative Diagnosis: Left ureteral calculus

Postoperative Diagnosis: Same

Operation: Cystoscopy, bilateral retrograde pyelograms, left ureteroscopy with electrohydraulic lithotripsy, and basket extraction of calculi

Procedure: The patient is brought to the cystoscopy suite where general anesthesia is induced and maintained in the usual fashion without difficulty. The patient then is placed in the dorsal lithotomy position, and the external genitalia are prepped and draped in a routine fashion. A 21-French ACMI panendoscope is assembled and inserted into the patient's bladder without difficulty. Inspection revealed the prostate to be mildly enlarged, but not particularly obstructed. The bladder itself is unremarkable. The ureteral orifices are normal. There is no efflux at all from the left side, a clear efflux from the right. Bilateral retrograde pyelograms are taken. On the left side, an obvious large stone is obstructing the middle third of the ureter. On the right side, the retrograde pyelogram is normal.

A guide wire is passed into the left ureteral orifice under fluoroscopy and can go past the stone into the renal pelvis. The guide wire is left in place. A cystoscope is now removed, and a ureteroscope is obtained and passed alongside the guide wire up to the midureter. There is some difficulty in passage, but this requires only mild dilatation with the scope. After the stone is obtained, it is fragmented with lithotripsy. Several large fragments are then extracted with a basket. The ureteroscope is passed again, and another large stone, also fragmented with lithotripsy, is encountered. A total of only about 30 shocks are needed to fragment the stone quite easily. At this point, the surgeon was able to basket the large remaining fragments, and stone extraction is completed. Very tiny fragments remain in the ureter but will pass safely.

Exercise 4.7. (Continued)

After ureteroscopy with basket extraction is completed, a cystoscope is reinserted over the guide wire into the bladder. A 7-French, 26 cm double J stent is then passed under fluoroscopy into the renal pelvis, where a good coil forms. The guide wire is then carefully removed. A coil forms in the bladder. KUB is taken confirming good positioning of the stent. The procedure is completed.

10. Read the following operative report and assign the appropriate CPT surgical procedure code(s).

Operative Report

Preoperative Diagnosis: Left renal tumor, left renal cyst

Procedure Performed: Partial nephrectomy

Indications: The patient was seen and evaluated as an outpatient, found to have a large complex cyst in the left kidney as well as a solid mass. These were all involved in the upper half of the kidney, which was to be removed. He consented for surgery.

Technique: With the patient placed on flank position under satisfactory anesthesia, an incision was made at the level of the 11th rib. The 11th rib was removed. The kidney bed was dissected. The kidney and perirenal fat were dissected all the way to pedicle. Adrenal was separated from the kidney. During this procedure, there were a couple small capsular vessels; those were all ligated. Then, the perirenal fat was removed in several places. It was a very large amount of perirenal fat. The large cyst of the upper pole was identified, and the solid mass next to it within a centimeter difference was identified. This mass was resected as a wedge resection and the large renal cyst was aspirated. This was cloudy fluid and was sent for culture and sensitivities. The cyst was unroofed. There was no evidence of malignancy in the cyst area. Then with the laser, all the endothelium of the cyst was eliminated. The resection of the mass was done with clamping of the pedicle and cooling the kidney down with ice slush. This was accomplished in a short period of time and after careful hemostasis the kidney parenchyma was approximated with 3-0 Moncryl. The kidney was packed and it was quite viable. The kidney revascularization was normal. The 12.5 grams of mannitol were given before the clamping and the 12.5 grams given after clamping. Then, a drain was left in the space and the kidney incision was closed in layers, basically three layers, and the skin was approximated with staples. The patient returned to the recovery room in excellent condition.

Male Genital System

The male genital system subsection includes procedures on the penis, testis, epididymis, tunica vaginalis, vas deferens, spermatic cord, seminal vesicles, and prostate. Figure 4.21 displays these structures.

Code assignment in the male genital subsection is determined by approach, such as incision, destruction, excision, or introduction. The reason the surgery is being performed also may affect code selection. For example, an orchiectomy (removal of testis) performed because of a testicular tumor (54530–54535) is coded differently from an orchiectomy performed prophylactically to prevent the release of hormones that may promote tumor metastasis (54520).

The coder is reminded to assign 69990 when the operating microscope is used, but not mentioned in the procedure code descriptors. Moreover, the coder should note the ranges of codes available in the CPT code book for laparoscopic procedures. It is important to review these codes, which are specific to the testes (54690–54699) and the spermatic cord (55550–55559).

Figure 4.21. The male genital system

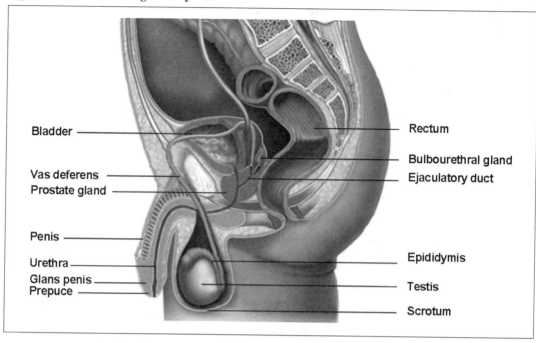

Penis

For destruction of lesion(s) (54050–54065), documentation should include the method of destruction (for example, chemical, laser surgery, or surgical excision). This selection varies from other areas in the CPT system because the amount of physician work to perform the different types of destruction varies. Code 54065 should be reported, instead of 54050 through 54060, when the physician determines that the destruction, by any method, is extensive.

For correct assignment of repair codes, the type of repair (such as plastic), the stage (second, third), and any other procedure(s) performed should be identified.

To code a circumcision, the operative report should be used to distinguish between a circumcision by clamp and/or other device or a surgical incision other than a clamp, device, or dorsal slit. In addition, correct code assignment is based on whether the patient is a newborn or other than a newborn. In cases where a revision of a past circumcision is required, CPT provides code 54162 for lysis or excision of penile postcircumcision adhesions and code 54163 for repair of an incomplete circumcision.

Coders may find coding newborn circumcision done in the hospital to be challenging. The typical service provided by a pediatrician on the second day of life is a subsequent newborn exam (not related to the circumcision), the circumcision by the chosen method, and a ring block or dorsal nerve block as regional anesthesia. If the surgical circumcision is performed, this case would be coded as:

99462–25   Subsequent hospital care, for the evaluation and management of a normal newborn, per day

54160–47   Circumcision, surgical excision other than clamp, device or dorsal slit; neonate (28 days of age or less)

64450   Injection, anesthetic agent; other peripheral nerve or branch

CPT Assistant in April and August of 2003 directs the coder to apply modifier –47 to the nerve block code and modifier –25 to the subsequent newborn exam code.

If the clamp circumcision (54150) was performed, the regional block is included in the code description and is not reported separately. Modifier –52 should be appended if the regional or ring block is not used.

Testis

For orchiectomy (excision of testis), the documentation should identify the procedure (whether simple or radical), the approach, and any additional procedures performed. For orchiopexy (suture of undescended testis), the documentation should identify the approach and additional procedures performed.

Vas Deferens

In the vas deferens subsection, a vasectomy is reported using code 55250. The code description states unilateral or bilateral; therefore, the –50 bilateral modifier is not reported for this code. This procedure includes postoperative semen examinations to determine whether the semen contains sperm. The number of semen examinations varies in each case and is determined by the physician.

Spermatic Cord

For excision or ligation of a varicocele, the documentation should distinguish between a laparoscopic approach (55550) and an abdominal approach (55535). Code 55559 is used for a laparoscopic procedure, other than a ligation for varicocele, performed on the spermatic cord.

Prostate

For prostate procedures, a prostate biopsy is reported using codes 55700–55705, depending on the type of biopsy (needle or punch, or incisional). When ultrasonic guidance is used to perform the needle biopsy, the coder should refer to code 76942. When the physician performs a needle biopsy and ultrasonic guidance, both 55700 and 76942 are coded. When stereotactic template guidance is used for saturation sampling, code 55706 is used. Code 55706 includes the imaging guidance.

When a fine needle aspiration is performed instead of a biopsy, the coder should refer to codes 10021–10022.

Reproductive System Procedures

CPT code 55920 describes the process of placing needles or catheters into pelvic organs and/ or genitalia (except the prostate) for later interstitial radioelement application.

Intersex Surgery

This section contains two codes. Code 55970 describes the process of intersex surgery from male to female and code 55980 describes intersex surgery from female to male.

Female Genital System and Maternity Care and Delivery

The female genital system subsection includes procedures on the vulva, perineum and introitus, vagina, cervix, uterus, oviducts, ovaries, and in vitro fertilization. Figure 4.22 shows the organs of the female genital system.

The procedures in the female genital system subsection are performed on women who are not pregnant. To code procedures in the female genital system accurately, the coder often must know the patient's diagnosis as well as the description of the procedure performed.

Some female genital procedures are referenced to other subsections. For example, open destruction of endometriomas is coded to the digestive subsection. All laparoscopic procedures and nonobstetrical dilatation and curettage procedure codes are located in this subsection. Biopsies of genital lesions are coded in this section but excision of lesions, both benign and malignant, are coded in the integumentary system.

Many of the procedures in this section are performed in procedure rooms within the office suite using regional anesthesia. Regional anesthesia is not part of the surgical package and should be reported separately when performed and documented. A common regional anesthesia is code 64435, Injection, anesthetic agent, paracervical (uterine) nerve. If the regional anesthesia is performed by the same physician, modifier −47 should be added to the surgical procedure code (*CPT Assistant* July 2003, 15).

Figure 4.22.   The female genital system

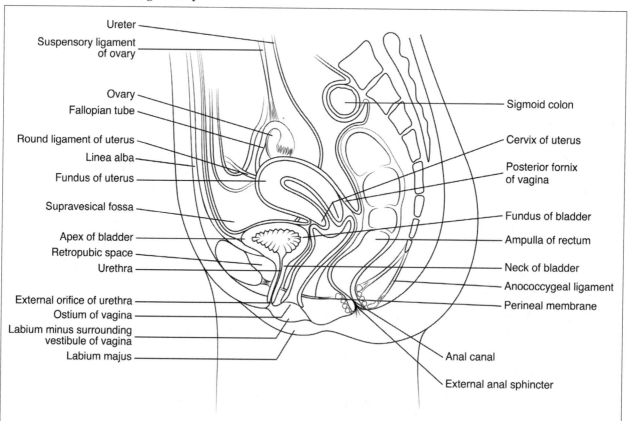

Vulva, Perineum, and Introitus

In the vulva, perineum, and introitus subsection, the coder should note the definitions for simple, radical, partial, and complete as they apply to vulvectomy (excision of the vulva). For vulvectomy (56620–56640), the documentation should state whether the procedure was simple or radical and partial or complete, and should include any additional procedure(s) performed. For destruction of vulva lesions, the physician should document whether simple or extensive destruction was performed for correct code assignment. The appropriate code is reported only once, regardless of the number of lesions removed. To report excision or fulguration of urethral caruncle, Skene's gland cyst, or abscess, the coder should refer to codes 53265 and 53270 in the urinary system subsection.

Vagina

The coder should read the code descriptions carefully in the vagina subsection because some codes include procedures that may be found in the urinary system subsection of the CPT code book. For example, when a sling operation for stress incontinence is performed via laparoscopy, code 51992 should be used from the urinary system section, not code 57288.

The appropriate code assignment for excision of the vagina (57106–57135) is determined by the extent of the excision and additional procedures performed. To assign code 57410, the documentation must state that the pelvic examination was performed under anesthesia.

In general, when the CPT description states "with or without" another procedure, it is included in the procedure and not reported separately. For example, the description for code 57240 reads "anterior colporrhaphy, repair of cystocele with or without repair of urethrocele." In this case, the repair of the urethrocele would be included when performed with an anterior colporrhaphy and should not be reported separately.

Placement of a suprapubic catheter is not included in GYN procedures but is frequently performed. When documented, catheter placement should be reported separately as CPT code 51102.

Cervix Uteri

In the cervix uteri subsection, the coder should refer to codes 57520–57522 for conization of the cervix. Conization is the removal of a cone-shaped portion of tissue. This procedure can be performed by cold knife or laser (57520) or through loop electrode excision (57522). When tissue is removed by loop electrode excision, the documentation should be reviewed carefully to ensure use of the correct code (57460 versus 57522). Conization of the cervix codes include fulguration, dilatation and curettage, and repair, when performed.

For colposcopy/vaginoscopy, the coder should refer to codes 57452–57461. This procedure is the examination of the cervix and/or vagina using a magnifying scope inserted through the vagina. The loop electrosurgical excision procedure, code 57460, is commonly referred to as the LEEP or LOOP procedure. The procedure involves the excision of tissue from the cervix with a loop electrosurgical device under colposcopic magnification. It is important to differentiate 57460 from 57522, LEEP *without* the use of the colposcopy/vaginoscopy.

Corpus Uteri

For the corpus uteri subsection, code 58120 is used to report a dilatation and curettage (D&C), diagnostic and/or therapeutic. This code description states "nonobstetrical" and should not be used when the D&C relates to pregnancy, labor, or the puerperium. When an obstetrical D&C is performed, the coder should refer to codes 59812–59870 and 59160. A D&C may be performed as a diagnostic test and, based on the findings, a more invasive procedure may be performed at the same operative setting. In these cases, the D&C would not be reported separately. Attention should be paid to the descriptors that state with or without dilatation and curettage.

Code 58152 includes the Burch procedure. Code 58340 includes the injection of dye or saline for hysterography and is used with radiology codes 74740 and 76831.

To report an abdominal hysterectomy, the coder should refer to codes 58150–58240, noting the descriptors carefully. When a total abdominal hysterectomy is performed and the tubes and/or ovaries are removed at the same time, only code 58150 is reported. Because some descriptors in this subsection state "with or without removal of tube(s), with or without removal of ovary(s)," these procedures are considered inherently bilateral and modifier –50, Bilateral Procedure, would not be appended.

For a vaginal hysterectomy, the documentation needs to state whether the procedure is performed via a laparoscope (58550–58554) or is an open procedure (58260–58294), and whether the uterus was greater or less than 250 g in size. These codes are considered inherently bilateral and modifier –50 should not be used with the hysterectomy codes.

Laparoscopy/Hysteroscopy Procedures

Laparoscopic surgery is performed by placing a viewing scope and other instrumentation through the abdominal or pelvic wall through small incisions. The cavity is filled with gas to allow viewing of internal structures. Figure 4.23 displays the surgeon performing a laparoscopic

Figure 4.23. Laparoscopic procedure

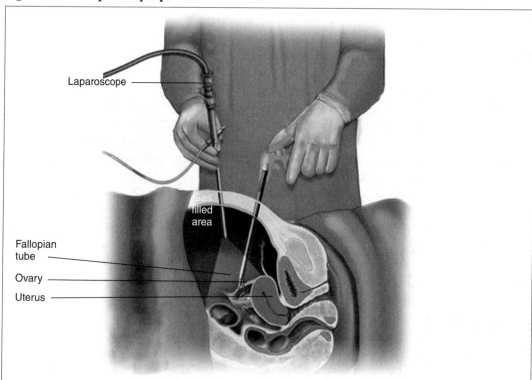

procedure on the female reproductive organs. It should be noted that a surgical laparoscopy always includes a diagnostic laparoscopy. When a procedure starts with a diagnostic laparoscopy and then a surgical procedure is performed through the laparoscope, only the surgical laparoscopic code is assigned. Code 49320 should be assigned to report a diagnostic laparoscopy when performed as a separate procedure. Code 58555 should be used to report diagnostic hysteroscopy as a separate procedure.

It also should be noted that laparoscopic fulguration of any tissue of the uterine adnexa—fallopian tubes, ovaries, pelvic viscera, and peritoneal surfaces—is coded to 58662 in the oviduct subsection, whether or not fallopian tube lesions are actually fulgurated, because their involvement is inherent in procedures on the adnexa.

If adnexal structures are removed during a surgical laparoscopy, code 58661 is used. According to *CPT Assistant* (January 2002), if either of the ovaries or the tubes are removed on both sides, modifier –50 is appended to code 58661.

A hysteroscope is a thin, telescope-like instrument that allows the physician to look inside the uterus. After insufflation of the uterine cavity with CO_2 (carbon dioxide), the hysteroscope is inserted through the cervical canal and into the uterus. This direct visualization improves the accuracy of diagnosis and treatment. Accessory instruments that may be used with a hysteroscope procedure include scissors, forceps, lasers, and various electrodes.

A D&C is commonly performed with a hysteroscopic biopsy or polypectomy (58558). Therefore, no additional code is assigned to identify the D&C because it is included in 58558.

Oviduct

The code series 58600–58770 includes procedures performed on the oviducts, or fallopian tubes. Therapeutic procedures performed by surgical laparoscopy or hysteroscopy should be distinguished from diagnostic laparoscopy.

For tubal ligation, which may be performed by ligation, transection, or other occlusion of the fallopian tubes, the coder should refer to codes 58600–58615 for abdominal or vaginal approaches. For laparoscopic tubal ligation, code 58671 is assigned. The newest procedure for achieving tubal occlusion is performed during a hysteroscopy procedure. Code 58565 describes the process of occluding the tubes by placing permanent implants.

When a postpartum tubal ligation is performed during the same hospitalization as the delivery, code 58605 should be assigned. When a tubal ligation is performed during another intra-abdominal surgery or cesarean section, code 58611 should be assigned in addition to the major procedure performed.

Codes 58700–58720 are reported for removal of fallopian tubes and/or ovaries. It should be noted that these codes are separate procedures and should not be reported when part of a larger procedure. For example, when a total abdominal hysterectomy is performed, only code 58150 is reported. Code 58700 or 58720 is included in the procedure.

Code 58740 is used to report lysis of adhesions in the fallopian tubes or ovaries by abdominal surgery. When lysis of adhesions is performed laparoscopically, the coder should refer to code 58660. When the adhesions are in another area, the coder should refer to the appropriate body site. For example, intestinal adhesions are reported using code 44005 or 44180. Lysis of adhesions often is not coded in addition to another procedure because it is classified as a separate procedure. For example, during a total abdominal hysterectomy, lysis of adhesions is performed routinely as they enter the abdomen. Only the total abdominal hysterectomy would be coded.

Ovary

Removal of one or both ovaries only, leaving the fallopian tubes intact, is called an oophorectomy, or ovariectomy. In the ovary subsection, code 58940 is used to report removal of the ovaries by open surgery, whereas code 58661 is used for laparoscopic removal of the ovaries. Code 58943 is used for an oophorectomy due to ovarian, tubal or primary peritoneal malignancy. When an ovarian malignancy is resected by performing a bilateral salpingo-oophorectomy (removal of both fallopian tubes and ovaries) and omentectomy (removal of the omentum), a code from the 58950–58952 series is selected.

When wider resection of a tumor is required, codes 58953 and 58954 are used. These include bilateral salpingo-oophorectomy with omentectomy, total abdominal hysterectomy, and radical dissection for debulking of tumors. Code 58954 adds pelvic lymphadenectomy and limited para-aortic lymphadenectomy to the description.

Maternity Care and Delivery

Many of the codes in the maternity care and delivery subsection are assigned to bill for a package of services. The physician is able to use one code rather than multiple codes to bill for the prenatal, delivery, and postpartum follow-up care of the pregnant patient. Antepartum care includes the initial and subsequent prenatal history, physical examinations, recording of weight, blood pressures, fetal heart tones, routine chemical analysis, monthly visits up to 28 weeks' gestation, biweekly visits to 36 weeks' gestation, and weekly visits until delivery. Additional visits and services beyond these are coded separately with E/M codes or other appropriate procedure codes.

Delivery services include admission to the hospital, admission history and physical examination, management of uncomplicated labor, vaginal delivery (with or without episiotomy, with or without forceps), or cesarean delivery. Medical problems complicating labor and delivery management may require additional resources. When applicable, codes in either the medicine section or the E/M section of the CPT code book should be used in addition to codes for maternity care.

Postpartum care includes hospital and office visits following vaginal or cesarean section delivery. When reporting delivery only services, report inpatient post-delivery management and discharge services using the appropriate E/M service codes. Delivery and postpartum services include delivery services and all inpatient and outpatient postpartum services. Postpartum care only services (code 59430) include office or other outpatient visits following vaginal or cesarean section delivery.

Removal of cerclage suture(s) is coded to 59871. For obstetric placement of cerclage sutures, the coder should refer to codes 59320 and 59325 and for nonobstetric placement to code 57700.

Antepartum and/or Postpartum Care Only

When the physician provides all or part of the antepartum and/or postpartum care but does not perform delivery due to termination of pregnancy by abortion or referral to another physician for delivery, the coder should refer to codes 59425–59426 and 59430. The physician assisting in the delivery would assign the appropriate delivery-only code. For example, an obstetrician is called in to perform an emergency cesarean section on a patient that is not his. He would assign code 59514 for cesarean delivery only.

Changes in the treating physician can occur for many reasons during the prenatal period, including medical complications, insurance changes, and patient relocation. To ensure proper coding, the coder should clarify exactly what services were performed and the reason they were terminated or changed. It should be noted that one to three antepartum care visits should be coded using the appropriate level of E/M code(s) based on the level of each visit. Code 59425 is used for four to six prenatal visits, and code 59426 is used for seven or more prenatal visits.

> **Example:** CPT code 59425 is for antepartum care only, four to six visits. This may be used by a family practice physician who refers a patient in the second trimester of pregnancy to an obstetrician due to a high risk of complications.

Medical and/or Surgical Complications during Pregnancy

For medical complications of pregnancy such as cardiac problems, neurological problems, diabetes, hypertension, toxemia, hyperemesis, preterm labor, or premature rupture of the membranes, the coder should refer to services in the medicine and the E/M services sections of the CPT code book. For example, when a pregnancy is complicated by gestational diabetes requiring additional office visits for blood sugar monitoring and weight and nutritional counseling, the office visits may be coded using the E/M office visit codes. The diagnosis should support the complication. In this case, gestational diabetes should be linked to the additional office visits and/or laboratory work performed.

For surgical complications occurring during pregnancy (for example, appendectomy, hernia, ovarian cyst, or Bartholin cyst), these procedures should be coded from the appropriate subsection of the surgery section.

Vaginal Birth after Cesarean Delivery

Codes for planned attempted vaginal birth after a previous cesarean delivery, referred to as a VBAC, are assigned based on whether the vaginal birth was successful or whether a repeat cesarean delivery was performed. VBACs are assigned using the code range 59610–59622. Elective repeat cesarean deliveries are coded in the cesarean delivery section.

Multiple Gestation

To report services for twins or other multiple births, the same guidelines apply and the code is based on type of delivery when the physician performed the antepartum, delivery, and postpartum services. It is challenging to code one twin as a vaginal delivery and the other as a cesarean delivery. In this case, code 59510 is used for routine obstetric care, including postpartum care, for the cesarean delivery and code 59409 is used for the vaginal delivery. Code 59400 should not be used for the vaginal delivery because the patient had only one antepartum and postpartum period. The package concept for cesarean delivery is coded because the postpartum period may be greater due to this type of delivery.

When multiple gestations are delivered by the same method and all were born vaginally, the package code would be billed once and then additional, delivery-only codes would be added for the subsequent births. *CPT Assistant* (August 2002) states that an alternate method of coding multiple gestation vaginal deliveries is to append modifier –22 to the 59400 code. It also states that if both twins of a twin birth are delivered via cesarean delivery, the code 59510 is only reported once.

Multifetal pregnancy reduction (MPR) (59866) is reported for patients with fertility treatments that result in multiple fetal development.

Abortion

Abortion treatment codes (59812–59857) are subdivided based on whether the abortion was incomplete, missed, or induced. Codes are then assigned based on variables such as method of completion and additional procedures performed at the same time. To assign a code for a missed abortion, the documentation by the physicians must be specific in identifying this as a missed abortion. A missed abortion is defined by the *Merck Manual of Diagnosis and Therapy* as "undetected death of an embryo or a fetus that is not expelled and that causes no bleeding" (Merck 2011, 2673). Missed abortions have a timeframe of less than 20 weeks 0 days gestation.

HCPCS Codes Used in the Female Genital System

The following HCPCS codes are used in the female genital system:

S2260	Induced abortion, 17 to 24 weeks
S2265	Induced abortion, 25 to 28 weeks
S2266	Induced abortion, 29 to 31 weeks
S2267	Induced abortion, 32 weeks or greater
S2400	Repair, congenital diaphragmatic hernia in the fetus, using temporary tracheal occlusion, procedure performed in utero
S2401	Repair, urinary tract obstruction in the fetus, procedure performed in utero
S2402	Repair, congenital cystic adenomatoid malformation in the fetus, procedure performed in utero
S2403	Repair, extralobar pulmonary sequestration in the fetus, procedure performed in utero
S2404	Repair, myelomeningocele in the fetus, procedure performed in utero
S2405	Repair of sacrococcygeal teratoma in the fetus, procedure performed in utero
S2409	Repair, congenital malformation of fetus, procedure performed in utero, not otherwise specified
S2411	Fetoscopic laser therapy for treatment of twin-to-twin transfusion syndrome
S4011–S4042	Various fertilization services
S4981	Insertion of levonorgestrel-releasing intrauterine system
S4989	Contraceptive intrauterine device (e.g. progestacert IUD), including implants and supplies
S9001	Home uterine monitor with or without associated nursing services
S9436–S9444	Various childbirth and parenting classes

Exercise 4.8. Male and Female Genital Systems

Choose the best answer for each of the following questions.

1. The patient undergoes a bilateral ovarian cystectomy. How is this coded?

    a. 58900–50
    b. 58920
    c. 58925
    d. 58940–50

2. Varicocele removal with laparoscopic ligation of spermatic veins. How is this coded?

    a. 55500
    b. 55520
    c. 55530
    d. 55550

3. The patient sees her physician for four prenatal visits before she transfers to a new physician in another health plan. How are these prenatal visits coded?

    a. 59425
    b. 59425, 59425, 59425, 59425
    c. No code is assigned
    d. Each coded individually with an E/M code

4. The patient requests removal of three lesions from his penis, which were diagnosed as molluscum contagiosum, each measuring 0.4 cm in size. To destroy the lesions, electrodesiccation and cryosurgery are required. How are these services coded?

    a. 17110
    b. 17270, 17270, 17270
    c. 54065
    d. 54055, 54065

Assign CPT codes for the following scenarios (include modifiers when appropriate).

5. A 55-year-old man with chronic balanitis being circumcised using a clamp. Regional dorsal penile block used for anesthesia.

    _____

6. Hysterectomy, performed vaginally, salpingectomy and repair of enterocele; uterine weight 272 g

    _____

7. Colposcopy with loop electrode biopsy

    _____

8. Read the following operative report and assign the appropriate CPT procedure code(s).

    _____

Operative Report

Preoperative Diagnoses: Enlarging fibroid uterus, symptomatic

Postoperative Diagnoses: Enlarging fibroid uterus, symptomatic

Procedures Performed: Exploratory laparotomy, Supracervical abdominal hysterectomy, bilateral salpingo-oophorectomy

Specimens: Ovaries, fallopian tubes and uterus

Description of Procedure: The patient was taken to the operating room and placed under general anesthesia. She was prepped and draped in the normal sterile fashion. A Foley was placed. Using her prior C-section incision, a Pfannenstiel skin incision was made and carried through the underlying layer of fascia. The rectus muscles were elevated and split in the midline. The peritoneum was identified, elevated, entered and stretched laterally.

(Continued on next page)

Exercise 4.8. (Continued)

The uterus revealed the enlarged uterine fibroids consistent with her preoperative exam and ultrasound. The ovaries and fallopian tubes were normal and consistent with menopause. The round ligaments were ligated, cut and held. The ureters were identified bilaterally and protected. The ovarian pedicles were free tied and stitched for excellent hemostasis. The uterine arteries were skeletonized, clamped, transected and suture ligated. The cardinal ligament was clamped, transected and suture ligated. The patient identified the desire to retain her cervix. The cervix was amputated from the uterine specimen and the specimen was handed off the table. V-lock suture was used to oversew the cervix.

The entire pelvic cavity was copiously irrigated and explored. The ureters were re-examined and were normal. The ovarian pedicles and cervical stump were dry. The peritoneum was closed with 3-0 Vicryl. The rectus muscles were brought together with a #1 interrupted and the skin was then closed in layers.

9. **Scenario:** This 21-year-old gravida 2 para 1, by Cesarean delivery last time, presented to the emergency department in active labor. She was 38 weeks' gestation, visiting her parents 250 miles from her home. Patient delivered vaginally in the elevator on the way to obstetrics. The emergency services physician, Dr. Scott, delivered the baby. An obstetrician, Dr. Dan, delivered the placenta. The patient will follow up with her obstetrician for postpartum care.

    What CPT code(s) should Dr. Scott report for the vaginal delivery?

    _____

10. In the preceding scenario, what CPT code(s) should Dr. Dan use to report delivery of the placenta?

    _____

Nervous System

The nervous system subsection includes the skull, meninges, and brain; the spine and spinal cord; and the extracranial nerves, peripheral nerves, and autonomic nervous system. The central nervous system, or CNS, includes the brain and the spinal cord. The peripheral nervous system includes the cranial nerves, the spinal nerves, and the autonomic nervous system. Figure 4.24 displays a cross section of the head, showing the cerebellum, the cerebrum, and the tentorium cerebelli, a membranous dividing line between these two parts of the brain. Figure 4.25 illustrates the spinal column, the bony protection for the spinal cord.

To assign codes accurately in the nervous system subsection, the coder must know the purpose of the procedure. Procedures such as craniectomy, craniotomy, and laminectomy are performed using various approaches and for specific purposes, such as drainage of hematomas, decompression, removal of foreign bodies, or tumor removal. Procedures on the spine are arranged by the part of the spine involved: cervical, thoracic, or lumbar.

Many procedures in the nervous system subsection require radiological supervision and interpretation. To code for both services, or for the physician performing both services, the coder also should refer to the radiology section of the CPT code book. Many codes include cross-references to specific radiology codes.

Figure 4.24. The central nervous system

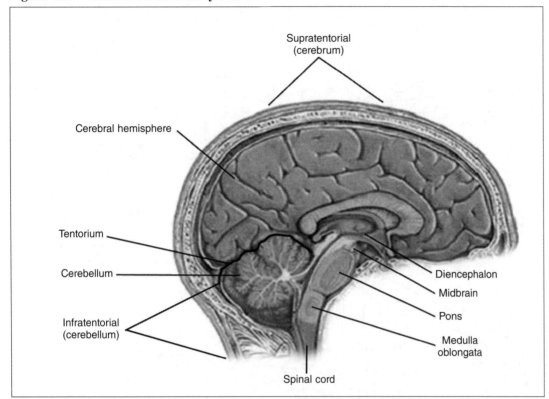

Skull, Meninges, and Brain

Twist drill hole or burr hole(s) procedures are coded based on the reason for the procedure (aspiration of hematoma or cyst) and the location (subdural or ventricular or intracerebral). Figure 4.26 shows a cut-away view of the meninges of the brain. Subdural procedures are performed below the dura mater and epidural procedures are performed at a level above the dura mater or not entering the space below the dura mater. The codes are used to describe the access (such as burr hole) and the procedure (biopsy of the brain). Do not report codes 61250 or 61253 (burr hole or trephine) if a craniotomy is performed at the same session. Some procedures not listed in this section include the burr hole(s) as part of the procedure. For example, a stereotactic biopsy or excision of intracranial lesion (code 61750) includes the burr hole approach.

Craniectomy or craniotomy procedures are reported with codes from the 61304–61576 series. When a craniectomy is performed for removal of a tumor, the type of tumor and its location should be documented. For a craniotomy with elevation of a bone flap, the indication for and/or location determines the correct code assignment. When reconstruction of the created defect is coded separately, the CPT code book refers the coder to bone reconstruction codes within the musculoskeletal subsection of CPT.

Skull Base Surgery

Skull base surgery includes the surgical management of lesions involving the skull base. These surgeries often require the skills of several surgeons from different surgical specialties working together or in tandem during the operative session. Generally, these procedures are not staged

Figure 4.25.   The spinal column

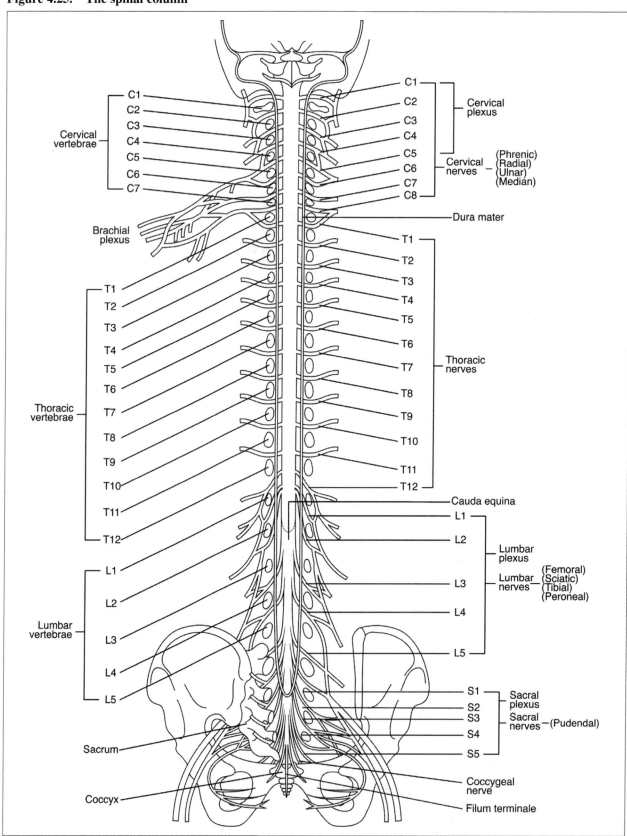

Figure 4.26. Meninges of the brain

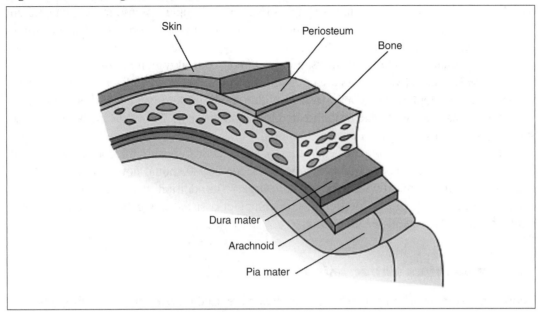

because of the need for prompt closure of the nervous system organs to prevent infection and other potential problems.

The three types of procedures employed in skull base surgery are categorized as follows:

- The approach procedure necessary to obtain adequate exposure to the lesion (pathologic entity) is described based on the anatomical area involved: anterior cranial fossa, middle cranial fossa, posterior cranial fossa, or brain stem or upper spinal cord.

- The definitive procedure(s) necessary to biopsy, excise, or otherwise treat the lesion details the repair, biopsy, resection, or excision of various lesions of the skull base and, when appropriate, primary closure of the dura, mucous membranes, and skin.

- The repair/reconstruction of the defect present following the definitive procedure(s) is reported separately only when extensive dural grafting, cranioplasty, local or regional myocutaneous pedicle flaps, or extensive skin grafts are required. When this happens, the CPT code book directs the coder to 15732 and 15756–15758 for codes describing primary closure. Secondary repair codes are included in the nervous system section.

CPT codes exist for each of the three portions of skull base surgery. Therefore, modifier –66, Surgical Team, is not appropriate with the skull base surgery codes. Rather, when multiple surgeons perform their unique part of this complex surgery, each surgeon reports the code that describes his or her contribution to the surgery. In the event that more than one procedure is performed by a single physician, modifier –51, Multiple Procedures, should be appended to the appropriate code(s).

Stereotaxis

CPT code 61751 should be used to indicate use of computed tomography (CT scans) and/or MRI guidance performed with a stereotactic biopsy procedure. The CPT code book refers the coder to the appropriate radiologic supervision and interpretation codes for each type of imaging.

Codes 61796–61799 describe stereotactic radiosurgery of cranial lesions and are coded based on whether the cranial lesion is simple or complex. Simple lesions are less than 3.5 cm and do not meet the definition of a complex lesion, which is a lesion 3.5 cm in maximum dimension or greater. In addition, the CPT coding notes state that Schwannomas, arteriovenous malformations, pituitary tumors, glomus tumors, pineal region tumors, and cavernous sinus/parasellar/petroclival tumors are complex and any lesion that is adjacent (5 mm or less) to the optic nerve/optic chasm/optic tract or within the brainstem is complex. When treating multiple lesions, and any single lesion treated is complex, use 61798. Codes 61796 and 61797 should not be coded more than once per lesion.

Application of the stereotactic headframe for stereotactic radiosurgery, code 61800, should be coded in addition to codes 61796 and 61798. Code 20660 should not be used to code the application of the frame for stereotactic radiosurgery. In addition, the code notes direct the coder to code 61781–61783 for stereotactic computer-assisted navigational guidance separately, based on the site of the procedure.

Neurostimulators (Intracranial)

Neurostimulators providing deep brain stimulation are used to treat functional disorders such as Parkinson's disease, tremors, and intractable pain.

Codes 61850–61888 describe the approach for placement of the electrodes and the actual implanting of the components. Codes 95970–95975 should be referenced to describe various aspects of neurostimulator programming. However, intraoperative microelectrode recording performed by the operating surgeon is included in the procedure. It is separately reportable if performed by another physician. Code 95961 and 95962 should be referenced for this procedure.

Patients frequently have tremors or pain on both sides of their body, necessitating placement of two electrode systems. Add-on codes for additional electrode arrays should be used to describe the second array, rather than appending modifier –50 to the first code.

The coder should take care not to confuse intracranial neurostimulators with those of the spine; the latter are found in the code range 63650–63688.

Spine and Spinal Cord

The spine and spinal cord subsection identifies percutaneous procedures on the spine, spinal injections, and other (extracranial, peripheral) nerve injections. Figure 4.27 displays a single vertebral segment, including the location of the vertebral facets. Figure 4.28 shows the spinal cord within the intervertebral foramen, also called the spinal canal.

The documentation for spinal punctures and injections should include whether the procedure is diagnostic or therapeutic, anatomic site of involvement in the spine, type of substances injected (neurolytics versus other substances), and single versus continuous injection/infusion. Spinal injections (epidural, caudal, subarachnoid, or subdural) must be distinguished from nerve root injections (for example, paravertebral facet joint nerves). In addition, the coder needs the drug classification(s) for the various agents injected or infused: anesthetic, antispasmodic, contrast media, or neurolytic substance. The placement and use of a catheter to deliver one or more epidural or subarachnoid injection on a single calendar day should be coded as if a needle had been used. If the catheter is in place for delivery of infusions over a longer

Figure 4.27.   Single vertebral segment

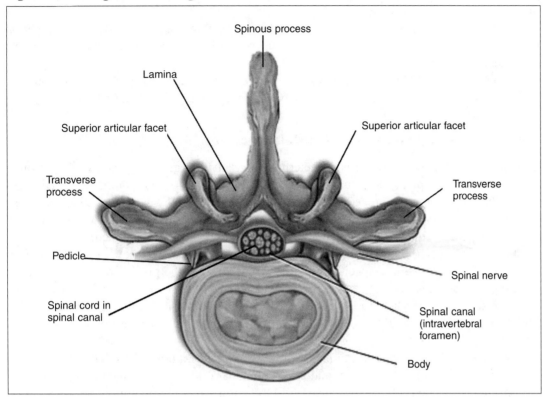

Figure 4.28.   Vertebra with spinal cord

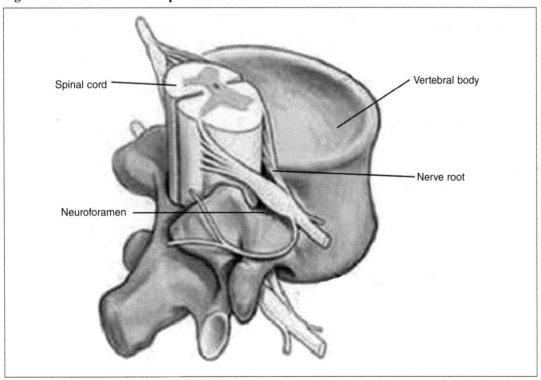

period of time, either intermittently or continuously, the coder should assign a code for injections via an indwelling catheter.

Code 62263 is reported for percutaneous lysis of epidural adhesions, by either solution injection or mechanical means. This code includes radiologic localization as well as contrast (when administered).

Codes 63620 and 62621 are used to report stereotactic radiosurgery of spinal lesions. As with cranial lesions, code 61783 should not be used with codes 63620 and 62621.

Laminectomy, Laminotomy, Hemilaminectomy

Laminotomy or laminectomy codes are determined based on surgical approach, exact anatomic location within the spine, and actual procedure(s) performed. For laminotomy (hemilaminectomy), the operative report procedure title may state laminectomy when the body of the report clearly reflects only a hemilaminectomy. Thus, careful review of the body of the operative report is imperative to ensure the accurate coding of all procedures performed.

For laminotomy (hemilaminectomy), the coder should note that the codes are based on one vertebral interspace in a specific area of the spine. When the procedure is performed on additional interspaces, the appropriate code(s) should be located in the section of the CPT code book for each additional interspace. These are considered add-on codes. Modifier –51, Multiple Procedures, should not be used to report each additional level, or interspace, for laminotomy procedures.

When reporting codes for laminectomies, the operative note should be reviewed to determine whether a facetectomy(s) and a foraminotomy(s) were performed (63045–63048). Laminectomies without the performance of a facetectomy or foraminotomy may be reported as 63001–63011 or 63015–63017. The level of the spinal column (for example, cervical or lumbar) and the indication for the procedure (for example, herniated disk) also will determine the correct code assignment.

For example, a common set of procedures is a posterior lumbar four level laminectomy with facetectomy and foraminotomy (L2-3, L3-4, L4-5, L5-S1), posterior lumbar single level arthrodesis (L4-5), posterior lumbar nonsegmental instrumentation (L4-5), local autograft bone graft. Seven CPT codes are required to correctly code this grouping of procedures:

22612   Arthrodesis, posterior or posterolateral technique, single level; (with lateral transverse technique, when performed) (L4-5)

63047–51   Laminectomy, facetectomy and foraminotomy (unilateral or bilateral with decompression of spinal cord, cauda equina and/or nerve root(s), [for example, spinal or lateral recess stenosis]), single vertebral segment; lumbar (L2-3)

63048 ×3   Each additional segment, cervical, thoracic, or lumbar (list separately in addition to code for primary procedure) (L3-4, L4-5, L5-S1)

22840   Posterior nonsegmental instrumentation (for example, Harrington rod technique, pedicle fixation across one interspace, atlantoaxial transarticular screw fixation, sublaminar wiring at C1, facet screw fixation)

20936   Autograft for spine surgery only (includes harvesting the graft); local (for example, ribs, spinous process, or laminar fragments) obtained from same incision (NASS 2007)

Spinal Injections/Infusions

When coding nerve injections for anesthetic/steroid pain relief, it is important to distinguish spinal injections (that is, epidural, subarachnoid) from paravertebral nerve/joint injections involving extracranial or peripheral nerves (64450–64484).

Nonneurolytic Injections

Epidural and subarachnoid injections of substances other than neurolytics are reported with codes 62310–62319. Nonneurolytic substances include anesthetic, antispasmodic, opioid, steroid, or other solutions. The codes for nonneurolytic spinal injections include any use of contrast. It is important to distinguish between a single (62310–62311) or continuous (62318–62319) injection and the injection site when administering substances such as an anesthetic, an antispasmodic, and a steroid.

Neurolytic Injections

Codes for spinal injection/infusion of neurolytic substances and injection for myelography and/or spinal CT are reported with codes 62280–62284. The use of any contrast is considered an inherent part of these procedures and is not reported as a separate code.

Vertebral Corpectomy, Arthrodesis

Vertebral corpectomy procedures are reported with codes 63081–63091. These procedures include discectomy above and/or below the vertebral segment. To report reconstruction of the spine, the appropriate bone graft codes, arthrodesis codes, and spinal instrumentation codes should be used in addition to the vertebral corpectomy code.

Extracranial Nerves, Peripheral Nerves, and Autonomic Nervous System

To code accurately from the extracranial nerves, peripheral nerves, and autonomic nervous system subsection, the coder must be familiar with the nerves, their grouping, and how they interact with the different body systems.

The introduction/injection codes are commonly used for pain management. The key is to determine the substance injected and what nerve was injected. The coder must identify divisions and/or branches of nerves to code correctly. For example, when an anesthetic agent is injected into the maxillary nerve, the coder should identify that this nerve is a division of the trigeminal nerve and report code 64400.

When paravertebral facet joints, or the nerve innervating that joint, require injection, imaging guidance is required to ensure that the injection is being placed correctly. Codes 64490–64492 describe the cervical or thoracic facet joint injections and include the necessary fluoroscopy or CT guidance. Codes 64493–64495 describe the lumbar or sacral facet joint injections and include the guidance. In addition, Category III codes 0213T–0218T are available to describe the same facet joint injections when they are performed using ultrasound guidance.

For destruction by neurolytic agent involving the somatic or sympathetic nerves, the coder should refer to codes 64600–64681. This procedure also is referred to as a rhizotomy.

The neurolytic agent may be chemical, thermal electrical, or percutaneous radiofrequency. These procedures are considered unilateral; modifier −50 should be appended for bilateral procedures. When more than one vertebral level is involved, the appropriate add-on code should be used for each additional level; the add-on codes are used in conjunction with the code for the primary procedure and cannot stand alone.

Neuroplasty

The neuroplasty codes include exploration, neurolysis, or nerve decompression. This includes freeing the intact nerve from scar tissue and neurolysis and transposition.

Carpal tunnel release is coded in this section. When done as an open procedure, code 64721 is assigned. When performed arthroscopically, it is coded in the musculoskeletal subsection of the CPT code book (29848).

Neurorrhaphy

Cross-references should be reviewed in the CPT code book for use of operating microscopes in neural repair (neurorrhaphy). The coder should note that use of magnifying loupes or corrected vision is not synonymous with microsurgery.

To select a code for a nerve graft (64885–64911), the coder should review the health record to determine the following:

- The site

- Whether the length of the nerve graft is less than, equal to, or greater than 4 cm

- Whether the graft involved single or multiple strands

Chemodenervation of Extremity or Trunk Muscles

Chemodenervation is the injection of a paralytic agent (such as botulinum toxin) into a muscle or muscle group to treat a spastic disorder such as multiple sclerosis tremor, motor tics, or other dystonia. Codes 64642–64645 are used to code this procedure performed in the extremity muscles. Codes 64642 and 64643 are used when 1–4 muscles are injected per extremity and codes 64644 and 64645 are coded when five or more muscles are injected per extremity. A maximum of four codes can be assigned per session when all four extremities are injected. Codes 64646–64647 are coded when trunk muscles (erector spinae, paraspinal, rectus abdominus, and oblique muscles) are injected.

HCPCS Codes Used in the Nervous System

The following HCPCS codes are used to code surgical procedures involving the nervous system:

S2340   Chemodenervation of abductor muscle(s) of vocal cord

S2341   Chemodenervation of adductor muscle(s) of vocal cord

S2348   Decompression procedure, percutaneous, of nucleus pulposus of intervertebral disc, using radiofrequency energy, single or multiple levels, lumbar

S9090   Vertebral axial decompression, per session

Exercise 4.9. Nervous System

Choose the best answer for each of the following questions.

1. The surgeon performs a discectomy of T8-T9 to decompress the nerve root, using a costovertebral approach. How is this coded?

   a. 22212
   b. 63055
   c. 63064
   d. 63077

2. The patient requires cervical facet joint injections for pain control. The physician performs these at the C3 and C4 level. How is this coded?

   a. 64490, 64490
   b. 64490, 64491
   c. 64479
   d. 64490

To complete an audit, indicate what information is missing in the documentation in order to use the code listed.

3. Code used: 61150

   Documentation: The burr hole was created 2 cm above the location of the brain cyst. Patient tolerated procedure well.

   Information missing: _____

4. Code used: 62270

   Documentation: A lumbar spinal puncture was performed.

   Information missing: _____

Assign CPT surgery codes for the following scenarios.

5. Secondary repair of dura mater due to leak of cerebrospinal fluid (CSF) of middle cranial fossa; myocutaneous flap graft

   _____

6. Revision of a cerebrospinal fluid ventriculoperitoneal shunt valve for hydrocephalus

   _____

7. Partial vertebral body resection, retroperitoneal approach, with decompression of spinal cord at T10 segment

   _____

8. Read the following operative report and assign the appropriate CPT surgical procedure code(s).

   _____

Exercise 4.9. (Continued)

Operative Report

Preoperative Diagnosis: Bilateral carpal tunnel syndrome, left greater than right

Postoperative Diagnosis: Same

Operation: Release of left carpal tunnel

Anesthesia: Axillary block

After successful axillary block was placed, the patient's left arm was prepared and draped in the usual sterile manner. A linear incision was made in the second crease in the left hand after a local anesthetic had been injected. This then was taken down through that area and curved slightly medially toward the hypothenar eminence until approximately 1 cm proximal to the wrist crease. After this was done, the incision was taken with a knife through the skin and subcutaneous tissue. Hemostasis was achieved with bipolar cautery. The ligament was identified and cut through with a scissors, starting proximally and working distally, until the whole ligament was freed up. The nerve was identified and noted to be in continuity all the way through. The nerve was freed up along the bands from this ligament. After this was done and hemostasis was achieved, a few 2-0 Dexon stitches were placed in the subcutaneous tissue and the skin was closed with interrupted 4-0 nylon. A dressing was applied, and the patient was taken to the recovery room.

9. Read the following operative report and assign the appropriate CPT surgical procedure code(s).

Operative Report

Preoperative Diagnosis: Herniated disc at L4-5, L5-S1, good relief with previous two epidural blocks

Postoperative Diagnosis: Same

Procedure: Therapeutic epidural block

The patient is kept on the left lateral side. The back is prepped with Betadine solution, and 1% Xylocaine is infiltrated at the L5-S1 interspace. Deep infiltration is carried out with a 22-gauge needle, and a 17-gauge Touhy needle is taken and the epidural performed. After careful aspiration, which was negative for blood and cerebrospinal fluid, about 80 mg of Depo-Medrol was injected along with 5 cc of 0.25% Marcaine and 1 cc of 50 mcg of Fentanyl. The injection was done in a fractionated dose in a slow fashion. The patient was examined and evaluated following the block, and was found to have excellent relief of pain. The patient is advised to continue physical therapy and to come back in 1 month for further evaluation.

10. Read the following operative report and assign the appropriate CPT surgical procedure code(s).

Operative Report

Preopertative Diagnosis: Lumbar stenosis

Postoperative Diagnosis: Lumbar stenosis

Procedure: Lumbar Laminectomy

Description of Procedure: The patient was brought to the operating room suite, and general endotracheal anesthesia was induced in standard fashion. The patient was placed prone on a Wilson frame. Care was taken to pad all pressure points. We obtained C-arm fluoroscopic views to identify the L2-L3 and L3-4 levels.

We started at the L2-L3 level. This was the worst stenosis. We started from the left side and used a spinal needle and then sequential dilators from the DePuy Spotlight system to get down to the level of the bone. We then cleared off the soft tissues and used a Kerrison rongeur and high-speed drill to

(Continued on next page)

Exercise 4.9. (Continued)

perform L2 laminectomy until the thecal sac was decompressed. We then tilted the patient away, and we performed a superior L3 laminectomy as well as right-sided L2 and L3 laminectomies to free up the thecal sac. We then achieved hemostasis, closed the fascia with UR-6 stitch, and then moved down to the L3-4 level. Of note, the patient had prior L4 through S1 fusion, so we performed an L3 laminectomy in similar fashion, dilating down to the L3 lamina, performing a laminectomy. We also did a redo L4 laminectomy to free up the thecal sac on the left side, and then tilted the patient to do it on the right side. Once the thecal sac was free, we copiously irrigated the wound. We achieved hemostasis in the epidural space with FloSeal, cleared it out, and then reapproximated the fascia with UR-6 sutures followed by 3-0 Vicryl inverted subdermal sutures followed by Dermabond.

Eye and Ocular Adnexa Systems

The eye and ocular adnexa subsection includes procedures involving the eyeball, anterior and posterior segment, ocular adnexa, and conjunctiva. The codes are categorized first by body part involved and then by type of procedure, such as retinal and choroid repair, conjunctivoplasty, cataract removal, and removal of foreign body. Figure 4.29 shows the structure of the eye.

Figure 4.29.   The structure of the eye

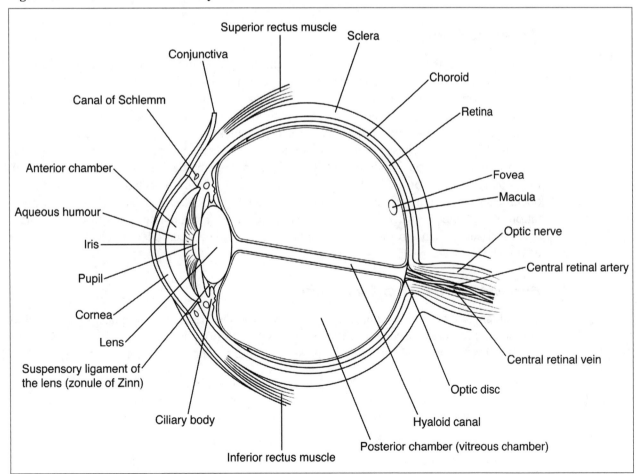

As a general rule, laterality should be indicated on all eye procedures using HCPCS modifiers –LT for left and –RT for right or the eyelid modifiers for eyelid procedures. Notes in the eye and ocular adnexa subsection inform the coder that procedures involving only the skin of the eyelid or orbit are assigned codes from the integumentary system. The CPT code book differentiates between removal of a foreign body and removal of implanted material in the eye. Codes 65205–65265 are for removal of a foreign body. The codes for removal of implanted material are:

65175   Removal of ocular implant

65920   Removal of implanted material, anterior segment eye

67120   Removal of implanted material, posterior segment; extraocular

67121   Removal of implanted material, posterior segment; intraocular

67560   Orbital implant; removal or revision

Eyeball

Procedure codes for removal of a foreign body from the external eyeball are reported based on location of the foreign body (external or intraocular), whether the object was embedded, and/or the use of a slit lamp. Repair of laceration of the eyeball (65270–65286) includes use of a conjunctival flap and restoration of the anterior chamber, by air or saline injection when indicated, and whether hospitalization was required.

Anterior Segment

The anterior segment contains two chambers, the anterior chamber and the posterior chamber. The anterior chamber is located between the cornea and the iris. The posterior chamber is located between the iris and the lens. Procedures in the anterior segment subsection include operations on the cornea, anterior chamber, anterior sclera, iris, and the lens itself.

Keratoplasty, often referred to as corneal transplant, is reported using codes from the 65710–65757 series. These procedures include the use of fresh or preserved grafts and preparation of donor material. Code 65757 is provided to describe the additional backbench work of preparation of a corneal endothelial allograft and should be reported when supported by documentation with the primary procedure of 65756. Lamellar keratoplasty refers to transplantation of the outermost layers of the cornea. Penetrating keratoplasty refers to full-thickness corneal tissue. When a refractive keratoplasty is performed, the coder should refer to codes 65760–65767.

Surgical Treatment of Glaucoma

Several procedures are available to physicians for the treatment of glaucoma, increased intraocular pressure caused by excessive fluid in the anterior chamber. All of these procedures involve differing methods of relieving pressure within the anterior chamber of the eye.

- Goniotomy (65820)—A gonioknife is used to open the angle of the ring of trabecular meshwork and increase the flow of fluid out of the anterior chamber. This procedure may also be referred to as De Vincentiis operation or Barkan's operation.

- Trabeculotomy ab externo (65850)—A trabeculotome is used in this procedure to open the trabecular meshwork. Ab externo means approaching from outside the eye.

- Trabeculoplasty using a laser (65855)—A laser is used to create extra holes in the trabecular meshwork.

- Trabeculectomy ab externo (66170–66172)—In this procedure, a scleral flap is created to form an additional reservoir to hold aqueous fluid. An iridectomy is performed (included) and a piece of trabecular meshwork is removed to allow fluid to flow out. The scleral flap reservoir holds the fluid as it is slowly reabsorbed by the body.

- Transluminal dilation of aqueous outflow canal; with or without retention of device or stent (66174–66175).

- Aqueous shunt to an extraocular reservoir (66179–66185)—A drainage tube is placed using a procedure similar to that used in a trabeculectomy. The tube drains to a reservoir that is sutured in a small open space between the extraocular muscles inside the sclera.

- Iridotomy/iridectomy by laser surgery (eg, for glaucoma) (per session) (66761).

Cataract Extraction

Cataract or lens extraction includes many auxiliary procedures, such as lateral canthotomy, iridectomy, iridotomy, anterior and posterior capsulotomy, use of viscoelastic agents, enzymatic zonulysis, pharmacologic agents, and certain injections.

The codes can include implantation of an intraocular lens prosthesis at the same time as the cataract extraction, or the insertion can be listed as a separate procedure performed subsequent to the extraction.

Codes 66830–66986 are used to report cataract procedures. It is important to note in the CPT code book that the following procedures are included in a lens extraction: lateral canthotomy, iridectomy, iridotomy, anterior capsulotomy, posterior capsulotomy, use of viscoelastic agents, enzymatic zonulysis, use of other pharmacologic agents, and subconjunctival or subtenon injections (AMA 2005).

Pertinent Definitions

Following are some definitions that are particularly useful to individuals using codes from the eye and ocular adnexa subsection:

- Extracapsular extraction is the surgical removal of the front portion and nucleus of the lens, leaving the posterior capsule in place. Generally, a posterior chamber intraocular lens is inserted after this procedure.

- Intracapsular extraction is the surgical removal of the entire lens and its capsule. Generally, an anterior chamber intraocular lens is inserted after this procedure.

- Phacoemulsification is a cataract extraction technique that uses ultrasonic waves to fragment the lens and aspirate it out of the eye.

- Phacofragmentation is a technique in which the lens is broken into fragments by a mechanical means or by ultrasound.

- Retinal detachment occurs when two layers of the retina separate from each other. This separation usually occurs when the vitreous adheres to the retina, the sensitive layer of the eye, and pulls, resulting in retinal holes and tears that may lead to retinal detachment.

The repair involves the surgical reattachment of minor or major separations of the retina from the choroid, the membranous lining inside the sclera (the white of the eye) that contains many blood vessels that supply the eye with nutrients.

- Vitrectomy is an ocular surgical procedure involving removal of the soft, jelly-like material (vitreous humor) that fills the area behind the lens of the eye (vitreous chamber) and its replacement with a clear solution. This is necessary when blood and scar tissue accumulate in the vitreous humor.

Cataract Removal and Secondary Implant(s) Procedures

Two types of lens extraction can be performed: extracapsular cataract extraction (ECCE) and intracapsular cataract extraction (ICCE). ECCE involves removal of lens material without removing the posterior capsule and is reported using codes 66840–66852, 66940, 66982, and 66984, depending on the exact procedure performed. ICCE includes removal of the lens and posterior capsule. Intracapsular procedures are reported using codes 66920, 66930, and 66983, depending on the exact procedure performed.

For purposes of definition, an ocular implant is an implant inserted inside the muscular cone; an orbital implant is an implant inserted outside the muscular cone. When an intraocular lens prosthesis (IOL) is inserted during the same operative session as the cataract removal, the coder should refer to codes 66982–66984, depending on the type of extraction. When an intraocular lens is inserted at a later date and is not associated with concurrent cataract removal, code 66985, Insertion of intraocular lens prosthesis (secondary implant), not associated with concurrent cataract removal, should be reported.

Posterior Segment

In the posterior segment subsection, a vitrectomy is reported using codes 67005–67043. To report a vitrectomy for repair of retinal detachment, the coder should refer to code 67108. The use of an operating microscope or an ophthalmic endoscope may be required to perform procedures on the posterior segment. The use of the operating microscope is included in the procedure code but the use of the ophthalmic endoscope is not (Society for Clinical Coding March 2010). The use of the endoscope (66990) should be coded separately when it is used to perform the procedures associated with codes 67036–67043 and 67113, as well as some other eye procedures.

Code 67027 describes implantation or replacement of an intravitreal drug delivery system. In addition, a HCPCS Level II code may be reported for the supply, such as J7310. For removal of the system, the coder should refer to code 67121.

For repair of retinal detachment, the coder should refer to codes 67101–67113. The code is chosen based on the method of repair. For preventative treatment to avoid retinal detachment, codes 67141–67145 should be used. These codes are considered repetitive services. The descriptors include all sessions in a treatment period defined by the physician.

Ocular Adnexa

Procedures performed on portions of the eyelid involving more than the skin are coded in this subsection. For lesion removals of the skin of the eyelid, the coder is referred to the integumentary subsection. Reconstruction of the eyelid, or blepharoplasty, involves more than the skin (for example, lid margin, tarsus, and/or palpebral conjunctiva) and may be reported with codes 67916–67924.

Modifiers to be used when performing procedures on eyelids are:

–E1   Upper left eyelid

–E2   Lower left eyelid

–E3   Upper right eyelid

–E4   Lower right eyelid

Strabismus Surgery

Strabismus surgery coding can be challenging for coders unaware of how the eye muscles are classified, how the procedure is performed, and how the codes are reported in the CPT code book. Strabismus surgery is inherently unilateral. Each code reflects the procedure performed on one eye. When the same procedure (identified by the same CPT code) is performed on both eyes, modifier –50, Bilateral Procedure, should be used.

CPT codes 67331–67340 describe conditions that indicate additional physician work is involved in the procedure because of previous eye surgery or other eye conditions. These add-on codes should be used in addition to the actual strabismus surgery performed and should not be modified with modifier –51, Multiple Procedures. Codes 67331–67340 should not be used as stand-alone codes. These codes are reported in addition to coding for the strabismus surgery performed.

The following information will assist the coder in understanding the eye muscles, as will illustrations in the professional edition of CPT:

- Six extraocular eye muscles are attached to each eye, two horizontal and four vertical. These muscles control movement and positioning of the eye.

- Two horizontal extraocular muscles—the lateral rectus muscle and the medial rectus muscle—move the eye from side to side.

- Four vertical extraocular muscles move the eye up and down: the inferior rectus muscle, the superior rectus muscle, the inferior oblique muscle, and the superior oblique muscle.

It should be noted that the CPT code book uses a separate code (67318) to identify primary strabismus surgery on the superior oblique.

CPT code 67335, Placement of adjustable suture(s) during strabismus surgery, including postoperative adjustment(s), also is considered an add-on code. When adjustable sutures are used, no matter how many sutures are placed, code 67335 should be reported once. Additionally, this code does not require the –51 modifier because it is an add-on code. When adjustable sutures are placed in both eyes, it is appropriate to use the –50 bilateral modifier.

Auditory System

The auditory system subsection includes procedures for the external ear, middle ear, inner ear, and temporal bone, and middle fossa approach. Figure 4.30 depicts the structure of the ear.

Most procedures in this subsection are considered unilateral. If a code is unilateral and bilateral, the descriptor will identify it. Code 69210 describes the removal of impacted cerumen

Figure 4.30.   The structure of the ear

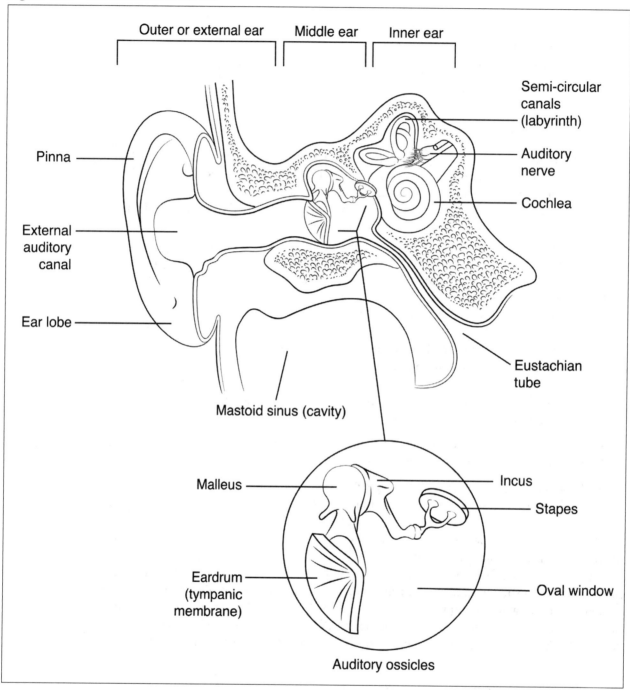

from one ear when the use of an instrument is required. When the procedure is performed bilaterally, report 69210–50. Code 69209 is used when cerumen removal is accomplished using irrigation or lavage, and is also a unilateral procedure. Assign 69209-50 when performed bilaterally. HCPCS code G0268 describes removal of impacted cerumen (one or both ears) by physician on same date of service as audiologic function testing and is required for use when cerumen is removed under these circumstances. Diagnostic services such as audiometry and vestibular testing are found in the medicine section of the CPT code book.

In patients who have had a previous radical or modified radical mastoidectomy, debridement of the mastoid cavity is required every few months. The mastoidectomy cavity is a pocket off of the ear canal that must be cleaned by a physician using a cerumen spoon, suction, or delicate forceps to remove trapped debris, sometimes requiring general anesthesia. Code 69220 is used for simple debridement and code 69222 is used for complex debridement.

One of the most commonly performed auditory surgical procedures is the tympanostomy for insertion of ventilating tubes for children with chronic ear infections. Under direct visualization with a microscope, the physician makes an incision in the eardrum (tympanum). The physician also may remove fluid from the middle ear. A ventilating tube is inserted through the opening in the tympanum. Coders may be confused by the terminology when the physician documents a "myringotomy for insertion of ventilating tubes." For coding purposes, this describes a tympanostomy (69433 or 69436).

Reconstruction procedures on the external, middle, or other portions of the ear often involve combination procedures that may require two or more codes. For example, reconstruction of the external auditory canal for congenital atresia, which also includes reconstruction of the middle ear, requires two codes.

Removal of a foreign body from the external ear, 69200 and 69205, is coded differently based on whether general anesthesia is used.

Codes from the integumentary subsection are assigned for suturing wounds or injuries of the external ear. Diagnostic services such as otoscopy under general anesthesia, audiometry, and vestibular tests are assigned codes in the medicine section of the CPT code book.

HCPCS Codes Used in the Eye and Auditory Systems

The following HCPCS codes are used to code surgical procedures involving the eye and ocular adnexal system:

G0268   Removal of impacted cerumen (one or both ears) by physician on same date of service as audiologic function testing

S2225   Myringotomy, laser-assisted

S2230   Implantation of magnetic component of semi-implantable hearing device on ossicles in middle ear

S2235   Implantation of auditory brain stem implant

Operating Microscope

Code 69990 is assigned as an additional code for surgical services using microsurgery techniques. Modifier −51 is not added to the code. The code is not used for visualization with magnifying loupes or corrective vision nor is it used when the terminology for the primary procedure includes microsurgery. This code describes the work in setting up, calibrating, positioning, and adjustment of the operating microscope. Therefore, code 69990 is reported only once per operative session, regardless of the number of procedures performed (AMA 2005). Code 69990 should not be reported in addition to procedures where the use of an operating microscope is an inclusive component.

Exercise 4.10. Eye and Ocular Adnexa, and Auditory Systems

Choose the best answer for each of the following questions.

1. The patient has a repair of a retinal detachment, completed by retinopexy. How is this coded?
   a. 67107
   b. 67108
   c. 67110
   d. 67113

2. The surgeon removes a pedunculated polyp from the patient's external auditory canal. What code describes the surgeon's work?
   a. 69145
   b. 69150
   c. 69540
   d. 69550

Assign CPT surgery codes for the following scenarios.

3. Rubeosis iridis, left eye, secondary to ischemic diabetic retinopathy; panretinal photocoagulation with argon green laser

   _____

4. Otoplasty of protruding ears

   _____

5. Tympanoplasty and mastoidectomy, radical, both ears

   _____

6. Direct closure of conjunctival laceration, right eye

   _____

7. Labyrinthectomy with mastoidectomy on right ear

   _____

8. Read the following operative report and assign the appropriate CPT surgical procedure code(s).

   _____

Operative Report

Preoperative Diagnosis: Right ear conductive hearing loss

Postoperative Diagnosis: Right ear otosclerosis

Operation: Right ear stapedectomy

Anesthesia: General

Findings: 1. Markedly thickened stapes footplate
   2. Intact eustachian tube
   3. Normal mobility of malleus and incus

Exercise 4.10. (Continued)

Procedure: The patient was prepared and draped in the normal sterile fashion, and injections were made with 1% lidocaine with 1:100,000 parts epinephrine into the external auditory canal wall.

The tympanomeatal flap was elevated from 10:00 to 6:00 in a counterclockwise fashion, using a vertical rolling knife for incision and a duckbill for elevation. The middle ear was entered at 2:00, the chorda tympani nerve identified, and the annulus lifted out of the tympanic sulcus. After elevating the tympanomeatal flap anteriorly, the ossicles were palpated. The malleus and incus moved freely, and the stapes was fixed. The posterior superior canal wall was curetted down after mobilizing the chorda tympani nerve, which was left intact. The stapes footplate was visualized easily and found to be markedly thickened. The pyramidal process was identified and the stapes tendon cut, and an IS joint knife was used to dislocate the joint between the incus and stapes. Next, small and large Buckingham mirrors were used, along with a drill, to drill out the stapes footplate. After this was done, a 0.6 × 4 mm Schuknecht piston prosthesis was placed in position. Crimping was achieved, and there was an excellent fit. The stapes footplate area then was packed with small pieces of Gelfoam. The tympanomeatal flap was put back in proper position and the middle ear packed with rayon strips of Cortisporin with a cotton ball in the middle to form a rosette. The patient was awakened in the operating room and transferred to recovery in no apparent distress.

9. Read the following operative report and assign the appropriate CPT surgical procedure code(s).

Operative Report

Preoperative Diagnosis: Cataract, left eye

Postoperative Diagnosis: Same

Operative Procedure: Phacoemulsification with intraocular lens implant, left eye

Anesthesia: Local

Procedure: On arrival in the OR, the patient's left eye was administered with Tetracine drops. Ocular akinesia was obtained with retrobulbar injection of 0.75% Sensorcaine and Wydase in the amount of 4 cc. Five minutes of intermittent digital pressure was applied. After routine preparation and draping, a small fornix-based conjunctival flap was raised superiorly. Bleeding points were cauterized. A 7-mm step incision was made above. The anterior chamber was entered under the flap with a 5531 blade. The anterior capsule was removed under Healon with a cystotome. The nucleus was emulsified in the posterior capsule. Cortex was removed with the I & A tip. The posterior capsule was vacuumed. Healon was placed in the anterior chamber and capsular bag. The wound was extended to 7 mm. A 23.5-diopter, 3161B lens was positioned in the bag horizontally. The wound was closed with a shoelace 9-0 nylon suture. After the Healon was removed from the anterior chamber with the I & A tip, intracameral Miostat was injected. The wound was tested for water tightness. Superior rectus suture was removed. Vasocidin ointment was applied along the lid margins. An eye shield was applied. The patient tolerated the procedure well and was taken to the recovery room in good condition.

10. Read the following operative report and assign the appropriate CPT surgical procedure code(s).

Operative Report

Preoperative Diagnosis(es): Left external auditory canal exostoses

Postoperative Diagnosis(es): Left external auditory canal exostoses

Operation Performed: Left canaloplasty for exostoses using microsurgery

Indications for Surgery: This is a 39-year-old male with a left side 90% canal blockage. Left canaloplasty was discussed in detail including the potential risks. After discussing the risks and benefits of surgery, the patient elected to proceed.

Operative Findings: A left transcanal excision of exostoses was performed. There was a large posterior-based lesion as well as a prominent superior exostosis that was somewhat pedunculated and extended inferiorly and a broad-based anterior exostosis.

(Continued on next page)

Exercise 4.10. (Continued)

Complete Description of Procedure: The patient was brought to the Operating Room and placed on the table in the supine position. General endotracheal anesthesia was administered. The bed was turned 180 degrees and the left ear was then prepped in the usual manner. The ear was injected with 1% lidocaine with epinephrine. Next the operating microscope was brought in for illumination, magnification, and visualization throughout the case. The tympanic membrane was visualized between the lesions and appeared to be intact. The ear was irrigated with saline and suctioned clear. The canal skin was injected with 1% lidocaine with epinephrine. A 72 Beaver blade was used to make a circumferential cut around the external auditory canal, just medial to the bony cartilaginous junction.

Next, the operating speculum was attached to the bed. Working through the operating microscope, the flap was elevated medially and the middle ear space was never entered. With the posterior lesion well exposed, it was removed using the Skeeter microdrill. Eggshell bone was created in the center of the canal. This was then fractured free with a Rosen needle. This provided additional room and the flap was elevated further. Additional exostosis was removed. The dissection was eventually brought down approaching the posterior annulus. The flap was then elevated around superiorly exposing the large pedunculated superior lesion. Working at its attachment, this was removed using the diamond burr. The lesion was carefully dissected free of the overlying skin. The lesion was then removed and sent to Pathology as a permanent specimen. The canal skin was laid back in place and covered the superior canal well. The anterior canal skin was elevated forward. The anterior lesion was then removed using a diamond burr. With this lesion removed, it was possible to remove the remaining portion of the posterior lesion. The canal had been dramatically widened with all visible lesions removed. The canal skin was intact and attached medially. It was laid back in place over the newly widened canal. The tympanic membrane was inspected and found to be intact and healthy. The canal was packed with Gelfoam soaked with ofloxacin drops. The ear was dressed with a cotton ball and bacitracin ointment.

Chapter 4 Test

Choose the appropriate answer or assign CPT surgery codes for the following scenarios.

1. A complete wrist fusion is done using a graft from the iliac crest. How is this coded?

   a. 25800
   b. 25810
   c. 25810; 20900
   d. 25825; 20900

2. Read the following operative report and assign the appropriate CPT surgical procedure code(s).

Operative Report

Preoperative Diagnosis: Retained deep foreign body, left lower extremity

Postoperative Diagnosis: Retained deep foreign body, left lower extremity

Procedure Performed: Retained deep foreign body

Operative Indications: The patient is a 37-year-old male firefighter who was admitted after he had a projectile injury to his upper leg. The patient was hit by a piece of another firefighter's ax that broke off on impact. The patient also had intractable pain. Radiograph showed a metallic foreign body in the lateral upper thigh/hip region. The risks that the patient may need specific surgery to repair or ablate a nerve were discussed. The risk of needing long term pain management was discussed. All the patient's questions were answered prior to the signing of informed consent.

Procedure in Detail: The patient was brought into the operating room and a time-out was then called with the staff. After achieving general anesthesia, the left lower extremity was then scrubbed, prepped and draped. Attention was then directed to the lateral left leg. Utilizing C-arm guidance, an incision was made over the area. This was an incision that encompassed the initial entrance wound. The incision was deepened via blunt dissection. The metallic foreign body was then located and verified on C-arm, also verifying that it had not entered the hip capsule. The area was irrigated. The area was then sutured with 4-0 Monocryl. Then, 10 mL of 0.5% Marcaine plain and 10 mL of 0.5% Marcaine with epinephrine were injected under the incision. A dry dressing was applied. The tourniquet was released.

Postoperative Plan: The patient can be readmitted to the floor. I anticipate that he can be discharged tomorrow morning. He can bear weight as tolerated.

   a. 10121
   b. 20520
   c. 27086
   d. 27372

3. The patient has a foreign body in the posterior segment of the right eye sustained at work. A flying metal fragment entered the eye while the patient was using a grinder and not wearing protective eyewear. After the eye was anesthetized, the metal shaving was retrieved using a magnet. How is this injury coded?

   a. 65205
   b. 65210
   c. 65260
   d. 65265

4. The surgeon inserts a percutaneous drainage tube of the gallbladder. How is this coded?

   a. 47490
   b. 47533
   c. 47490, 47531
   d. 47533, 47531

(Continued on next page)

Chapter 4 Test (Continued)

5. Code the following operative report:

   Preoperative Diagnoses: Right chronic sphenoid sinusitis
   Chronic cough

   Postoperative Diagnoses: Chronic sphenoid sinusitis
   Evidence of bilateral maxillary sinusitis

   Name of Procedure: Right endoscopic sphenoidotomy

   Anesthesia: General

   Indications: This patient has a long history of chronic throat clearing behavior. She has undergone allergy evaluation including a CT scan, which revealed a pacified right sphenoid sinus. Sphenoid sinus also revealed evidence of thinning of the bony wall. The chronic cough has continued despite appropriate antibiotic therapy.

   Description of Operation: The patient was brought to the operating room. General anesthesia was induced. An orotracheal tube was placed by anesthesia. The table was turned about 45 degrees. The patient was prepared and draped in the usual manner for endoscopic sinus surgery. Both sides of the nose were packed with pledgets soaked in Afrin. These were removed from the right side of the nose, and the right middle inferior turbinate and mid and posterior septum were injected with 1% Xylocaine with 1:100,000 epinephrine. The area was repacked, and the left nasal packing was removed. There were copious, thick secretions from the left middle meatus, a swab was placed in the area, and then this was sent for culture.

   The packings were removed from the right side of the nose. The area was endoscopically examined. The thick mucoid secretions were suctioned from the right middle meatus also. The middle turbinate secured approach to the sphenoid ostium and the inferior one third of the right middle turbinate was removed. A moderate amount of posterior ethmoidal air cells were removed to provide approach and the sphenoid ostium was identified. It was gradually enlarged using curette and a true cut forceps. The mucosa appeared normal. There was no significant purulent or mucoid fluid in the sphenoid sinus. The nose was suctioned copiously after irrigation, and there was no significant bleeding. The patient was awakened and brought to the recovery room in satisfactory condition.

   a. 31231, 31235
   b. 31235
   c. 31231, 31287
   d. 31287

6. Code the following operative report:

   Preoperative Diagnosis: Occluded right external iliac artery

   Postoperative Diagnosis: Same

   Indications for Operation: This is a 59-year-old white man who has undergone attempted right iliac balloon angioplasty approximately two weeks prior to this admission. We were unable to open the right external iliac artery and at this point in time, the patient presents for an elective femoral bypass graft.

   Operation: The patient was taken to the operating room and placed in the supine position. Once adequate epidural anesthesia had been obtained, the patient's lower abdomen and bilateral lower extremities were prepared and draped in the usual fashion. Incisions were made in both groins simultaneously and each common femoral and superficial femoral artery was approached using blunt dissection to the subcutaneous tissue. The common femoral artery, superficial femoral artery, and smaller arteries were then identified and isolated with ligaloops. On the left side, the common femoral artery and superficial femoral artery were palpated and noted to have an arteriosclerotic plaque posteriorly, but a soft anterior area of the artery proximal. This point was chosen for the anastomotic site. The patient was then heparinized, and after waiting an appropriate amount of time, a 1.5-cm arteriotomy was then made.

Chapter 4 Test (Continued)

The prosthetic graft was then chosen to be a ringed Gore-Tex 8 suture. A tunnel was then created from the right groin to the left through the tissue and over to the right groin. The right common femoral artery was then examined and noted to have plaque posteriorly, but was soft anteriorly. Approximately 1- to 1.5-cm arteriotomy was then made. The graft that was previously brought through the groin was then sized and the anastomosis was begun. A running #6-0 Prolene suture was used. As the anastomosis was completed, the left leg was opened and the graft was flushed to remove any clots. As distal control was released on the right superficial femoral artery, back bleeding was noted to be poor; therefore, a thrombectomy was performed using a 4-mm Fogarty catheter. Repeat back bleeding revealed good patency of the artery. The anastomosis was then completed. All ligaloops were then removed and there was noted to be good flow through both the graft and the right lower extremity with good Doppler pulses. The groin incisions were then closed in two layers and the skin was closed with interrupted nylon suture. Dressings were placed and the patient was removed from the operating room in stable condition.

   a. 35661
   b. 35661, 34201–51
   c. 34201
   d. 35661, 34151–51

7. When the patient presents with multiple lacerations that are repaired, how should the coder approach the code assignment?

   a. Code only the least complex repair
   b. Code all repairs of the same site using only the code for the most complex repair
   c. Code all wound repairs, listing the most complex repair(s) first on claim
   d. Code only the most complex repair

8. A radical nephrectomy is performed via a scope. How is this coded?

   a. 50220
   b. 50240
   c. 50543
   d. 50545

9. The physician excises a 0.8-cm cystic lesion from the floor of the patient's mouth. How is this coded?

   a. 11441
   b. 41000
   c. 41008
   d. 41116

10. Code the following operative scenario:

The patient was admitted to have a thoracoscopic lobectomy performed. The patient has a malignant neoplasm of the right middle lobe. Because of extensive pleural effusion, I was unable to complete the endoscopic procedure. We converted to an open technique, and a successful lobectomy was performed. The patient tolerated the procedure well.

   a. 32480, 32663–53
   b. 32480
   c. 32663
   d. 32440

Chapter 5

Radiology

Objectives

Upon completion of this chapter, the student should be able to do the following:

- Describe the structure of the radiology section

- Discuss the concept of radiological supervision, as opposed to interpretation only, and describe its use in the radiology section

- Identify the modifiers used in conjunction with radiology codes

- Describe the concept of component billing for professional and technical services

- Read and interpret health record documentation to identify the services provided and procedures performed

This chapter discusses coding in the radiology section of the CPT code book.

Radiology Section Format and Arrangement

The radiology section is subdivided into seven subsections, arranged by radiologic modality type, such as diagnostic imaging, guidance, or nuclear medicine.

The diagnostic radiology and diagnostic ultrasound subsections are arranged by anatomic site within the subsection. Within each site, the codes are arranged by type of test performed, for example, by plain film, magnetic resonance imaging (MRI), or angiography.

It is acceptable to code multiple procedures performed at the same session using individually appropriate codes. Each study must have a separate interpretation and report, signed by the interpreting physician. It is not appropriate to code separate codes for multiple studies when a code is available that describes the complete study. Unbundling is inappropriate in the radiology section, just as it is in the surgery section.

The radiation oncology subsection is arranged by type and method of treatment performed. Codes in the nuclear medicine subsection are subdivided based on whether the nuclear medicine was diagnostic or therapeutic.

Diagnostic Radiology

The diagnostic radiology subsection, also known as diagnostic imaging, includes services such as x-rays, computed tomography (CT) scans, magnetic resonance imaging (MRI), and other imaging procedures.

These radiology procedures may be found in the Alphabetic Index of the CPT code book by referencing the main terms of X-ray, CT Scan, Magnetic Resonance Imaging, and Magnetic Resonance Angiography. They also may be referenced under the specific site with a subterm identifying the specific procedure. For example, an x-ray of the chest is located under the main term of X-ray or the subterm of Chest. More subterms to describe the specific type of chest x-ray are located in the Index.

In the diagnostic radiology subsection, the coder must know exactly what was x-rayed and, in many cases, the number of views taken. For example, when a code description states "minimum of three views," the code is assigned as a unit of 1 for three or more views, no matter how many views are taken, as long as all the views can be described within the same code. Moreover, the coder may need to know the exact positional views taken. For example, for chest x-rays (71010–71035), the coder must know the number of views taken, the type of views, whether fluoroscopy was used, and whether special views were performed. When special views are performed in addition to another chest x-ray procedure, both can be coded. When chest fluoroscopy is performed without radiologic examination of the chest, the coder should refer to code 76000.

Contrast Materials

For both CT scans and MRI scans, the CPT code book provides different codes for radiologic procedures using contrast material consisting of radiopaque substances that obstruct the passage of x-rays. This allows the structure containing the material to appear white on the x-ray film and thus identifies abnormal growths and the contour of body structures. Contrast material may be administered orally or intravenously. Examples of contrast agents include barium or Gastrografin, iohexol, iopamidol, ioxaglate, Hypaque, and Renografin. Commonly performed radiologic examinations using contrast material include barium enema, angiography, cystogram, endoscopic retrograde cholangiopancreatogram, fistulogram, intravenous pyelogram, excretory urogram, lymphangiography, oral cholecystogram, retrograde pyelogram, and voiding cystourethrogram.

When a scan is done without contrast material, followed by contrast materials and additional scan sections, the coder should report a code specifying both with and without contrast material. For example, the coder should refer to codes 70486–70488. For a CT scan of the maxillofacial area without contrast, followed by contrast and additional CT scan sections, the coder should use code 70488. "With contrast" and "without contrast" codes should not be coded separately. It is inappropriate to report a scan of the same body area with contrast and without contrast separately. According to *CPT Assistant* (June 2001), high-resolution CT scanning is not included in a regular CT scan. To describe this procedure, it is appropriate to append modifier –22 to identify this additional evaluation. Gadolinium (gadopentetate dimeglumine) is the contrast agent most often used for MRI studies.

To code the provision of contrast material supplies, see the HCPCS section later in this chapter.

Mammography

The reporting of mammography procedures requires close attention to details. The code descriptors of 77051–77063 should be reviewed. As reported in the July 1996 issue of *CPT Assistant*, difficulty arises in deciding when to use the screening mammography code:

> Screening mammography is usually limited to two images, craniocaudal and mediolateral oblique views of each breast. It is performed to detect unsuspected cancer in an early stage in asymptomatic women, and is inherently bilateral. Occasionally, supplementary views (such as Cleopatra and Axillary views) may be necessary to adequately visualize the breast tissue. These views are not routine and are included as part of the initial screening service.

Diagnostic mammography is reported when a suspected mass or abnormality is found during a physical examination or during a previous mammography or ultrasound. The x-rays provide the physician with specific information on how to determine or rule out the suspected disease in the breast. Diagnostic mammography requires additional physician work, supervision, and interpretative skills.

In addition, *CPT* provides two codes to describe computer-aided analysis of mammogram images, with or without digitization of the images, with further physician review. Code 77051 is used for diagnostic mammography, and code 77052 is used for screening mammography. Both are add-on codes. Code 77051 should be reported with code 77055 (unilateral mammogram) or 77056 (bilateral mammogram) and 77052 with code 77057 (screening mammogram, bilateral).

Because some third-party payers interpret these codes differently, coding professionals should verify coverage issues by contacting the health plan involved. Medicare has specific guidelines for coverage of screening and diagnostic mammograms. The coder should refer to the carrier's newsletters for its reporting guidelines.

Diagnostic Ultrasound

Ultrasound is a diagnostic technique that uses high-frequency, inaudible sound waves that bounce off body tissues and then are recorded to give information about the anatomy of an internal organ. Like the procedures in the diagnostic radiology subsection, diagnostic ultrasound is structured by anatomical site, with ultrasound procedures of the head and neck, pelvis, and heart. The codes are located in the Index under the main terms of Ultrasound or Echography, with a subterm for the site of the procedure.

Four types of ultrasound are described in the CPT code book:

- **A-mode** refers to a one-dimensional ultrasonic measurement procedure.

- **M-mode** refers to a one-dimensional ultrasonic measurement procedure with movement of the trace to record amplitude and velocity of moving echo-producing structures.

- **B-scan** refers to a two-dimensional ultrasonic scanning procedure with a two-dimensional display.

- **Real-time scan** refers to a two-dimensional ultrasonic scanning procedure with display of both two-dimensional structure and motion with time.

Coding Guidelines

Coders should be aware of the following guidelines when reporting codes from the radiologic supervision and interpretation subsection:

- A common coding error occurs when the coder reports the abdominal ultrasound codes (76700–76705) for a pregnancy ultrasound. The correct obstetrical ultrasound codes can be found in the pelvis subsection codes (76801–76817), which refer to pregnant uterus. The coder should read the code description and ultrasound report carefully to choose the appropriate code.

- Another common coding issue involves needle biopsy of the prostate using ultrasonic guidance. In this case, two codes are required when the physician performs both portions of the procedure. Code 76942, Ultrasonic guidance for needle biopsy, radiological supervision, and interpretation, is used for the ultrasound guidance for the prostate needle biopsy; and code 55700, Biopsy, prostate; needle or punch, single or multiple, any approach, is used for the actual needle biopsy. Ultrasonic guidance does not include the actual procedure performed, which should always be coded separately.

The coder also should read and be guided by the extensive coding notes found in the vascular procedure subsection of radiology (75600–76499) as codes are chosen from this subsection.

Interventional Radiology

Interventional radiology is defined as the branch of medicine that diagnoses and treats a wide range of diseases using percutaneous or minimally invasive techniques under imaging guidance (*CPT Assistant*, Fall 1993). In order to accurately reflect the procedures that are performed, the coder must "component code" interventional radiology procedures. Component coding is the use of both surgical and radiological CPT codes to reflect all components of the procedure being performed rather than the assignment of one all-inclusive CPT code. Some of the component pairings are referenced within the surgery and radiology sections of the CPT code book.

Surgical component codes are found in the 10021–69999 range of the CPT code book. These surgical codes describe the procedure(s) performed (inserting catheters or needles, inflating balloons, inserting stents, and so on).

Radiological component codes are found in the radiology series of the CPT code book. These radiological codes describe the use of imaging to guide the physician who is performing the procedure. The radiological codes for these procedures are also known as supervision and interpretation (S&I) codes.

Four directional terms are commonly used during the performance of interventional radiology procedures:

- **Ipsilateral:** Situated or appearing on the same side, or affecting the same side of the body

- **Contralateral:** Pertaining to, located on, or occurring in or on the opposite side

- **Antegrade:** Extending or moving forward

- **Retrograde:** Moving backward, against the normal flow

Two separate types of catheter placement can be performed by the physician during the procedures: nonselective catheter placement and selective catheter placement.

Nonselective catheter placement is defined as placing the catheter or needle directly into an artery or vein with no further advancement into a separately identifiable branch of that vessel or placing the catheter or needle into any portion of the aorta or vena cava from any approach (SIR 2009).

Selective catheter placement means that the catheter is guided or placed into any arterial or venous vessel other than the aorta, vena cava, or the original vessel that was punctured (SIR 2009).

In order to code interventional radiology procedures correctly, the coder must have a thorough knowledge of the vascular anatomy of the human body. The arterial vasculature can be thought of as a tree and its branches. The aorta is the trunk that separates into primary branches, secondary branches, tertiary branches, and beyond. Vascular order describes the furthest point to which the catheter is placed into the branches of a vessel originating off the aorta, vena cava, or vessel punctured, if the aorta is not entered, and is referred to as the level of selectivity.

A vascular family is a group of vessels fed by a primary branch of the aorta, the vena cava, or the vessel punctured. The coder must know where the physician punctured to enter the patient's body, into what vascular family/families the physician manipulated the catheter(s), and the final position of the catheters in order to correctly assign the catheter placement codes associated with interventional radiology procedures. Appendix L of the CPT code book describes the vascular families and details the first, second, third, and beyond the third order branches of each family.

The coder must always follow five component coding rules when coding interventional radiology procedures:

1. Each vascular family must be coded separately. Each time the physician reenters the aorta to move the catheter to another branch originating off the aorta, a new vascular family is entered and should be coded independently from any other procedures that are being performed during the encounter.

2. The coder must code to the highest order of selectivity within a vascular family. The lower-order selective vessels that were manipulated through to get to the higher-order selective vessel are included in the code for the higher-order selective catheter placement.

    Example: The patient's right common femoral artery is accessed. The catheter is moved retrograde to the aortic bifurcation and then maneuvered contralaterally through the left common iliac artery to the left common femoral artery where injection and angiography is performed of the left lower extremity. The correct catheter placement surgical code assignment would be 36246 as the left common femoral artery is a second-order selective vessel. 75710 would be assigned for the left lower extremity angiography. Code 36245 is not assigned as the left common iliac artery is traversed to get to the final destination of the left common femoral artery and is included in the code for this higher-order selective vessel.

3. The code for selective catheter placement takes precedence over the code for nonselective catheter placement if done from the same puncture site. The coder would only use a code for selective catheter placement if both nonselective and selective catheter placement were performed from the same puncture site to reach the target vessel.

> **Example:** The patient's left common femoral artery is accessed. The catheter is moved retrograde to the abdominal aorta. An abdominal aortogram is performed. The catheter is then manipulated to the right superficial femoral artery where injection and lower extremity angiography is performed. Code 75625 would be coded for the abdominal aortography and code 75710 would be coded for the lower extremity angiogram. Only one catheter placement code (36247) would be correct, because the nonselective catheter placement code 36200, for placement into the abdominal aorta, is included in the selective catheter placement code 36247.

4. The coder must code each vascular access separately. If the physician performs more than one vascular access to the patient's body each site is coded independently from the others.

5. If more than one second-or third-order selective branch in the same vascular family is entered during the procedure, the additional selective catheterization must be coded as CPT code 36218 (Selective catheter placement, arterial system; additional second order, third order and beyond, thoracic or brachiocephalic branch, within a vascular family) for vessels above the diaphragm or CPT code 36248 (Selective catheter placement, arterial system; additional second order, third order and beyond, abdominal, pelvic, or lower extremity artery branch, within a vascular family) for vessels below the diaphragm.

Radiation Oncology

The radiation oncology subsection includes codes for radiation therapy to treat diseases and neoplastic tumors of various areas of the body. The extensive notes at the beginning of this subsection should be reviewed carefully before using the codes.

The CPT code book states that the listings for the radiation oncology codes provide for teletherapy (therapy from far away, or external) and brachytherapy (therapy up close, or internal), and include initial consultation, clinical treatment planning, simulation, medical radiation physics, dosimetry, treatment devices, special services, and clinical treatment management procedures. They also include normal follow-up care during the course of the treatment and for three months following its completion.

There are four unlisted service or procedure codes for this subsection that should be used when another code to describe the radiation oncology procedure is not available:

77299   Unlisted procedure, therapeutic radiology clinical treatment planning

77399   Unlisted procedure, medical radiation physics, dosimetry and treatment devices, and special services

77499   Unlisted procedure, therapeutic radiology, treatment management

77799   Unlisted procedure, clinical brachytherapy

Radiation Oncology Consultations and Treatment Planning

Codes from the E/M section may be used to reflect services such as preliminary consultation, evaluation of the patient's prior decision to treat, or full medical care, in addition to treatment management, provided by the therapeutic radiologist.

The clinical treatment planning process includes interpretation of special testing, tumor localization, treatment volume determination, treatment time/dosage determination, choice of treatment modality, and other procedures and services. This applies whether the radiation oncology is external (teletherapy) or internal (brachytherapy). The CPT code book includes detailed definitions of simple, intermediate, and complex planning.

Radiation Treatment Delivery

The radiation treatment delivery series of codes (77401–77421) describes the technical component of delivering the radiation treatment, as well as the various energy levels administered. To assign the appropriate code, the following information is needed:

- Number of treatment areas involved

- Number of ports involved

- Number of shielding blocks used

- Total million electron volts (MeV) administered

Radiation Treatment Management

Radiation treatment management is reported in units of five fractions or treatment sessions, regardless of the actual time period in which the services are furnished. The services need not be furnished on consecutive days. Multiple fractions representing two or more treatment sessions furnished on the same day may be counted as long as there has been a distinct break in therapy sessions and the fractions are of the character usually furnished on different days. Code 77427 may not be reported for one to two fractions beyond a multiple of five at the end of a course of treatment.

Hyperthermia

Hyperthermia is the use of heat to raise the temperature of a specific area of the body in an attempt to increase cell metabolism, which increases the potential for killing malignant cells. The hyperthermia treatment listed in the radiation oncology subsection includes external, interstitial, and intracavity hyperthermia. These therapies are used only as an adjunct to radiation or chemotherapy. Radiation therapy and/or chemotherapy are coded separately, when provided. The CPT code book contains more details on the sources and types of hyperthermia.

The listed treatments include physician management during the course of the therapy and for three months after the therapy is complete. Preliminary consultations are not included here but, instead, are coded using E/M codes.

Clinical Brachytherapy

Internal radiation therapy, also known as brachytherapy, involves applying a radioactive material inside the patient or in close proximity to generate local regions of high-intensity radiation. This material may be contained in various types of devices, including tubes, needles, wires, seeds, and other small containers. Common radioactive materials used in brachytherapy include radium-226, cobalt-60, cesium-137, and iodine-125. The three types of brachytherapy are as follows:

- Interstitial, which involves placing a radiation source directly into tissues

- Intracavitary, which involves the use of radiation source(s) placed in special devices and then implanted in body cavities

- Surface application, which uses radioactive material that is contained on the surface of a plaque or mold and applied directly on or close to the surface of the patient

Clinical brachytherapy requires the use of either a natural or synthetic radiation source applied into or around a treatment field of interest. The supervision of radiation sources and dose interpretation is performed only by the therapeutic radiologist. If a surgeon is needed in addition to the therapeutic radiologist, modifier –62, Two Surgeons, is used.

The clinical brachytherapy codes include initial and subsequent visits to hospitalized patients. Detailed definitions of simple, intermediate, and complex brachytherapy are listed in the CPT code book.

Coding Guidelines

Coders should be aware of the following reporting guidelines when using codes for radiation treatment management and delivery:

- When selecting a code from the radiation treatment delivery subsection (77401–77417), coders must have documentation indicating the energy level of the radiation administered.

- Codes in the radiation treatment delivery subsection recognize the technical component of radiation treatment. If the radiation oncologist does not own the radiation therapy equipment, the entity that owns the equipment should report these codes.

- Codes in the radiation treatment management subsection (77427–77499) represent a radiation oncologist's professional services provided during the course of treatment. Code 77427 describes the delivery of a unit of five radiation treatments or fractions, regardless of the time interval separating the delivery of treatments. Code 77431 describes a complete course of therapy that only requires one or two fractions.

- For both radiation treatment delivery and radiation treatment management, the professional (–26) and technical (–TC) modifiers should not be reported. These codes correctly describe the portions of the service actually provided and do not require modifiers.

- The codes for clinical brachytherapy are determined by the number of sources or ribbons.

- Clinical brachytherapy may require two or more physicians, including a therapeutic radiologist and a surgeon. The coder should append modifier –62 when two surgeons are involved or modifier –66 when a surgical team is involved. One key to using these modifiers successfully is to coordinate the reporting of services with all physicians involved. Each physician reports the services with the same CPT code and the same modifier appended.

Nuclear Medicine

The nuclear medicine subsection addresses nuclear diagnostic studies and nuclear therapeutic services. Within the diagnostic categories, the codes are assigned according to organ system. The codes can be located in the CPT Index under the main terms of Nuclear Medicine or Nuclear Imaging.

Nuclear medicine involves the administration of radioisotopes, which are radioactive elements used to diagnose diseases. The radioactive isotope deteriorates spontaneously and emits gamma rays from inside the body that enable the physician to view internal abnormalities. Some radioisotopes are absorbed selectively by tumors or specific organs in the body, making them visible on the scan.

The provision of radium or another radiation source (radiopharmaceutical product) is not a part of the nuclear medicine services codes. These supplies are coded separately using the HCPCS Level II codes in the section starting with alphabetic character "A" to specify the radiopharmaceutical agent. There are special administration codes for therapeutic nuclear medicine, from 79005–79445 based on the route of administration.

Bone and joint scan codes are found within the musculoskeletal system subsection of the diagnostic nuclear medicine codes. These scans can be used to diagnose a variety of diseases and to localize neoplasms.

The cardiovascular myocardial perfusion and cardiac blood pool imaging studies may be performed at rest and/or during stress. When these tests are performed during exercise and/or pharmacologic stress, the appropriate stress-testing code from the 93015–93018 range should be reported in addition to the appropriate code from the nuclear medicine subsection.

Applications of Nuclear Medicine Coding

Some of the more common diagnostic nuclear medicine scans are described below:

- Bone scans are performed as part of metastatic workups to identify infections such as osteomyelitis, evaluate hip prostheses, distinguish pathologic fractures from traumatic fractures, and evaluate delayed union of fractures.

- Cardiac scans are performed for diagnosis of myocardial infarction, stress testing, ejection fractures, measurement of cardiac output, and diagnosis of ventricular aneurysms.

  o The thallium 201 scan examines myocardial perfusion, with normal myocardium appearing as hot and ischemic or infarcted areas appearing as cold.

  o The technetium 99m pyrophosphate scan identifies recently damaged myocardial tissue. It is most sensitive 24 to 72 hours after an acute myocardial infarction.

  o The technetium 99m ventriculogram scan identifies abnormal wall motion, cardiac shunts, size and function of heart chambers, cardiac output, and ejection fraction. The multigated acquisition (MUGA) scan is another form of this type of study.

- Hepatobiliary scans (HIDA scans) are performed for diagnosis of biliary obstruction, acute cholecystitis, or biliary atresia.

- Lung scans (ventilation-perfusion [V/Q] scans) can reveal chronic obstructive pulmonary disease, emphysema, and other pulmonary disease. When done along with chest x-rays, these scans are important tools in evaluating pulmonary emboli.

- Renal scans are performed to evaluate the overall function of the kidneys.

- Thyroid scans are performed most commonly with technetium 99m pertechnetate and are useful in detecting nodules.

Modifiers Used in Radiology Coding

The following modifiers may be appended to codes used in reporting radiologic procedures/ services. (See chapter 9 for a complete description of CPT modifiers.)

–22   Unusual Procedural Services

–26   Professional Component: In circumstances where a radiologic procedure includes both a physician (professional) component and a technical component, modifier –26 may be reported to identify the professional component. The professional component includes supervising the procedure, reading and interpreting the results, and documenting the interpretation in a report. The technical component includes performance of the actual procedure and expenses for supplies and equipment. Usually, this service is provided by a radiologic technician at a hospital, a freestanding radiology clinic, or a physician's office. The physician reports the professional component by attaching modifier –26 to the appropriate radiologic procedure.

      Example: Code 74220, Radiologic examination of the esophagus. The physician performing the interpretation should report 74220–26. If the physician also owns the radiology equipment, no modifier is reported.

–52   Reduced Services

–53   Discontinued Procedure: Modifier –53 is appropriate in circumstances where the physician elected to terminate or discontinue a diagnostic procedure, usually because of risk to the patient's well-being. (Modifier –73 or –74 would be used for hospital outpatient reporting.)

      Example: A patient planned to have urography with KUB, which would be reported with code 74400. Because the patient fainted during the procedure, it was discontinued before completion. The physician should report 74400–53.

–59   Distinct Procedural Service: Modifier –59 may be used to identify that a procedure or service was distinct or independent from other non-E/M services provided on the same day.

For Medicare, use one of the following HCPCS modifiers to more fully describe the distinct procedural service:

        –XE: Separate encounter

        –XP: Separate practitioner

-XS: Separate structure (or organ)

-XU: Unusual non-overlapping service

-GH Diagnostic Mammogram Converted from Screening Mammogram on Same Day

-TC Technical Component: Under certain circumstances, a charge may be made for the technical component alone. Under those circumstances, the technical component charge is identified by adding modifier -TC to the usual procedure number. The technical component charge can be reported only by the actual owner of the equipment. If a physician owns the equipment and also performs the professional service involved, the usual CPT code should be reported without any modifier.

Remember that modifier -TC is not used with the radiation treatment delivery subsection of codes (77401–77418) because these codes already describe only the technical portion of the service provided.

Anatomical Modifiers

The following anatomical modifiers also may be used in reporting radiologic procedures/services:

-LT and -RT Modifiers are Level II HCPCS modifiers that should be reported when radiologic procedures are performed on a specific side of the body. In reporting these modifiers to reflect a bilateral radiologic procedure, the procedure code should be assigned twice and -LT attached to one code and -RT to the other.

> **Example:**   73650–LT and 73650–RT—Radiologic examination of the calcaneus with a minimum of two views, bilateral

Additional modifiers are available to describe the individual digits. These are summarized here:

HCPCS Level II Codes Used in Radiology Coding

Left Hand	Left Foot	Right Hand	Right Foot
-FA (Thumb)	-TA (Great toe)	-F5 (Thumb)	-T5 (Great toe)
-F1 (2nd Digit)	-T1 (2nd Digit)	-F6 (2nd Digit)	-T6 (2nd Digit)
-F2 (3rd Digit)	-T2 (3rd Digit)	-F7 (3rd Digit)	-T7 (3rd Digit)
-F3 (4th Digit)	-T3 (4th Digit)	-F8 (4th Digit)	-T8 (4th Digit)
-F4 (5th Digit)	-T4 (5th Digit)	-F9 (5th Digit)	-T9 (5th Digit)

It is not appropriate to separate out digits when the code includes all in one procedure, such as code 73140, Radiologic examination, finger(s), minimum of 2 views on the same hand.

Administration of Contrast Materials

Some of the listed procedures are commonly performed without the use of contrast materials. For procedures that may or may not be performed using contrast material, the phrase "with contrast" represents contrast material administered intravascularly. Oral and rectal contrast administration alone does not qualify as a study "with contrast."

For spinal procedures that use contrast materials, such as computed tomography, magnetic resonance imaging, and magnetic resonance angiography, the phrase "with contrast" includes intrathecal or intravascular injection.

HCPCS Codes for Contrast Material

The HCPCS code book contains codes for contrast material as well as many other supplies and medications that may be appropriate for use for radiologic services. New HCPCS codes are being developed as new supplies become available. Be sure to reference the most current HCPCS codes on the CMS website (CMS 2015a) for a complete selection of codes. Some of the HCPCS codes available for contrast material are listed below:

A4641   Supply of radiopharmaceutical diagnostic imaging agent, not otherwise classified

A4642   Indium in-111 satumomab pendetide, diagnostic, per study dose, up to 6 millicuries

A9500–A9700   Supply of various radiopharmaceutical diagnostic-imaging agents

HCPCS Codes for Diagnostic Radiology

The following HCPCS codes may be reported for diagnostic radiology:

Q0092   Set up portable x-ray equipment

R0070   Transportation of portable x-ray equipment and personnel to home or nursing home, per trip to facility or location, one patient seen

R0075   Transportation of portable x-ray equipment and personnel to home or nursing home, per trip to facility or location, more than one patient seen, per patient

HCPCS Codes for Diagnostic Ultrasound

The following HCPCS codes may be reported for diagnostic ultrasound:

S8092   Electron beam computed tomography (also known as ultrafast CT, cine CT)

S9024   Paranasal sinus ultrasound

Other HCPCS Codes for Radiology Services

Codes G0235 and G0252 provide additional codes for positron emission tomography (PET) imaging. Other HCPCS codes for radiology services include the following:

G0130   Single-energy x-ray absorptiometry (SEXA) bone density study, one or more sites; appendicular skeleton (peripheral) (for example, radius, wrist, heel)

G0202   Screening mammography, producing direct digital image, bilateral, all views

G0204   Diagnostic mammography, producing direct digital image, bilateral, all views

G0206   Diagnostic mammography, producing direct digital image, unilateral, all views

G0278   Iliac and/or femoral artery angiography, non-selective, bilateral or ipsilateral to catheter insertion, performed at the same time as cardiac catheterization and/or coronary angiography, includes positioning or placement of catheter in the distal aorta or ipsilateral femoral or iliac artery, injection of dye, production of permanent images, and radiologic supervision and interpretation and production of images (list separately in addition to primary procedure)

G0288   Reconstruction, computed tomographic angiography of aorta for surgical planning for vascular surgery

G0389   Ultrasound B-scan and/or real time with image documentation; for abdominal aortic aneurysm (AAA) screening

S8035   Magnetic source imaging

S8037   Magnetic resonance cholangiopancreatography (MRCP)

S8040   Topographic brain mapping

S8042   Magnetic resonance imaging (MRI), low-field

S8055   Ultrasound guidance for multifetal pregnancy reduction(s), technical component only

S8080   Scintimammography (radioimmunoscintigraphy) of the breast unilateral, including supply of radiopharmaceutical

S8085   Fluorine-18 fluorodeoxyglucose (F-18 FDG) imaging using dual-head coincidence detection system (non-dedicated PET scan)

Exercise 5.1. Radiology

Choose the best answer for each of the following questions.

1. When a diagnostic mammogram is completed on the same day as a screening mammogram, which modifier is used on the diagnostic mammogram code?

   a. –22
   b. –76
   c. –GA
   d. –GH

2. In clinical brachytherapy, the type of brachytherapy that involves placing a radiation source directly into the tissues is _____.

   a. Interstitial
   b. Intracavitary
   c. Surface application
   d. Teletherapy

3. Two views of the second digit on each hand, done in the physician office and read by the physician, are coded for Medicare as _____.

   a. 73130–50
   b. 73130–50, 73140–50
   c. 73140–F1, 73140–F6
   d. 73140–LT–RT

4. An intraoperative cholangiogram and pancreatogram were performed by Dr. Daniels. Dr. Kane provided radiologic supervision and interpretation for the procedure. Which code(s) would Dr. Kane report?

   a. 43260
   b. 43260, 74300
   c. 74300
   d. 76999

5. Ophthalmic ultrasound of the eye with amplitude quantification is coded as _____.

   a. 76511
   b. 76513
   c. 76516
   d. 76519

6. Which of the following statements describes a selective catheter placement?

   a. Catheter stays in the femoral artery
   b. Catheter advances into the aorta from the femoral artery
   c. Catheter stays in the vessel that was entered or in the aorta
   d. Catheter advances from the vessel entered into a branch vessel

Assign CPT codes for the following scenarios. Assume that procedures are performed in the physician office and that the physician owns the equipment.

7. Intravenous pyelogram (IVP) with kidney, ureter, and bladder (KUB) study

   _____

8. Right adrenal angiography, radiologic supervision and interpretation

   _____

Exercise 5.1. (Continued)

9. Chest x-ray, Bucky studies

_____

10. Externally generated deep hyperthermia treatment

_____

11. X-ray, forearm, anteroposterior (AP) and lateral

_____

12. CT of the heart and quantitative coronary calcium, without contrast

_____

13. AP view of pelvis and AP and oblique views of right hip

_____

14. Transvaginal real-time ultrasound at 18 weeks' gestation

_____

15. Ultrasound for amniocentesis (coding for ultrasound guidance only)

_____

Assign the appropriate codes for the following procedure(s). Include any modifiers, when applicable.

16. CT scan of the head with contrast material. Identify the appropriate code(s) and modifier the physician's office radiology department should report on the claim it submits.

_____

17. Radiologic examination (x-ray) of the forearm, AP and lateral views. What code(s) should be submitted on the claim form if the physician provided only the professional component of this procedure?

_____

18. MRI of the brain with the following interpretation by Dr. Johnson, performed at the local hospital:

Multiple sagittal images were obtained with a TR 600 and TE of 20. Multiple axial images then were obtained with a TR 2000 and TE of 30/80. In addition, coronary images with TR of 2000 and TE of 30/80 were obtained.

Findings: Sagittal images reveal effacement of sulci and heterogeneous low density in the right frontotemporal region. The cerebellar tonsils are positioned normally. The pituitary gland is normal in size.

Axial and coronal proton spin density and T2-weighted images reveal an area of generally increased density with the posterofrontal right temporal basal ganglial region. The outer margins of this high-signal finding are consistent with edema. In the center is a large mass, most likely representing glioblastoma.

There is a shift of the midline structures that include the corpus callosum and ventricles, with some compression of the right ventricular system. There is no evidence of spread across the corpus callosum by this mass.

Impression: Right basal ganglial-posterofrontal-right temporal lobe mass with surrounding edema, most compatible with a glioblastoma. There is a shift of the midline structures, but no evidence of spread across the corpus callosum to the other hemisphere.

Dr. Johnson's code(s): _____

(Continued on next page)

Exercise 5.1. (Continued)

19. X-ray of bilateral acromioclavicular joints with weights

_____

20. Dr. Smith owns the mammography equipment and contracts with Dr. Jones to read the mammograms for her practice. Code for Dr. Smith's services.

Mammogram Report

Date of Service:	8-24-09	**MRN:**	89-12-34
Primary Provider:	Smith	**Sex:**	F
Ordering Provider:	Smith	**DOB:**	09-21-45

History: Screening required per protocol

Examinations to be performed:
Bilateral screening mammograms
Left breast diagnostic mammogram

Bilateral Mammogram: Bilateral two-view film screen mammograms were performed and compared with previous bilateral mammograms from October 11, 2008, and August 11, 2006.

There are scattered fibroglandular elements that could obscure a lesion on mammography. Both breasts show no evidence of suspicious calcification. The right breast shows no suspicious masses and no significant interval change in comparison with the prior mammograms.

Diagnostic Mammogram: The left breast shows a slightly lobulated 7 × 5-mm nodule in the outer lower-to-central breast that was not definitely identified on the previous examinations. Two additional localizing views of the left breast are performed. No architectural distortion or secondary findings of malignancy are seen.

Impression:

1. Stable right breast mammogram without evidence of malignancy.
2. Left breast showing a new 7 × 5-mm slightly lobulated nodule in the outer lower to central breast. For further evaluation of this finding, a left breast ultrasound is recommended and the Radiology Department will schedule this examination.

D: 8-24-09   Mary Jones, M.D.
T: 8-25-09

CPT Code(s):_____

Chapter 5 Test

Choose the appropriate answer or assign CPT surgery codes for the following scenarios.

1. Code the following radiology procedure(s):

    History: Back pain

    Examination: Lumbosacral spine, complete

    Lumbar spine: AP, lateral and two spot lateral views are done and can be compared with a prior examination of 3 years ago.

    Vertebral body heights remain intact.

    There is marked interspace narrowing at T12–L1, L1–L2, L2–L3, and to a less extent at L4–L5, and L5–S1.

    The degree of narrowing is most marked at the L2-L3 level with associated sclerosis and spurring as well as minimal spondylolisthesis or anterior displacement of L3 relative to L2 and L2 relative to L1. I presume these findings are degenerative. These findings of spondylolisthesis and this rather marked interspace narrowing are not identified on the previous films.

    Incidental note is made of a left common iliac arterial stent in place.

    Impression:

    1. Intact lumbar vertebral body heights and a normal lordotic curvature.
    2. Multiple levels of interspace narrowing. This is most marked at the L2–L3 level and is associated with sclerosis and spurring at this level.
    3. There is a minimal spondylolisthesis of L3 relative to L2 and of L2 relative to L1. Most of the changes of interspace narrowing and spondylolisthesis are not evident on the prior examination of 3 years ago.

    a. 72100
    b. 72110
    c. 72120
    d. 72131

2. The physician's office completes x-rays of the patient's right knee including the anteroposterior, lateral and standing views, which were interpreted by the physician owner. How is this procedure coded?

    a. 73560–TC
    b. 73562
    c. 73565
    d. 73565–TC–26

3. The patient undergoes a magnetic resonance imaging at 28 weeks' gestation to assess placental placement and pelvic issues. How is this procedure coded?

    a. 72195
    b. 74712
    c. 76815
    d. 76818

4. Code the following radiology procedure(s) completed at the local hospital:

    History: Cough, dyspnea, choking sensation

    Examination: Chest CT with contrast, high-resolution CT

(Continued on next page)

Chapter 5 Test (Continued)

10-mm axial sections were obtained from the lower neck to the upper abdomen using 100 cc of Iso-vue-300. In addition, 1-mm sections at 1.0 cm intervals were obtained for the high-resolution examination.

On a few sections at the base of the neck, there is evidence of some enlargement of the thyroid gland, more so on the left side, with the trachea being displaced to the right within the lower neck and upper chest. Minimal tracheal compression cannot be excluded on the left side of the trachea. The enlarged left lobe extends into the upper chest. There is probably minimal calcification at the inferior aspect of the left thyroid lobe.

There is no evidence of hilar or mediastinal adenopathy. No axillary adenopathy. Lung window films are unremarkable with no evidence of masses, nodules, or effusion. There is minimal scarring in the left lung base. The high-resolution images are unremarkable except for minimal scarring in the left lower lobe.

A few sections through the upper abdomen demonstrate a hiatal hernia.

Impression:

1. There is evidence of an enlarged thyroid lobe, more so on the left side, with a mediastinal goiter caus-ing some displacement of the trachea to the left with perhaps minimal tracheal compression.

2. Hiatal hernia

3. Otherwise unremarkable study

    a. 71260–26
    b. 71260–22
    c. 71260–22–26
    d. 71270–22

5. The patient presents for a screening mammography examination but during the clinical breast examination, a suspicious lump is detected. Therefore, diagnostic mammography is performed. How is this service coded?

    a. 77055
    b. 77056–GH
    c. 77057
    d. 77057–GH

6. The patient received a radioelement, after which images were taken of the bones. What type of service does this represent?

    a. Clinical brachytherapy
    b. Radiation therapy
    c. Therapeutic nuclear medicine
    d. Diagnostic nuclear medicine

7. Code the following operative report:

Preoperative Diagnoses: Right nephrolithiasis, left proximal 8-mm ureteral calculus

Postoperative Diagnoses: Right nephrolithiasis, left proximal 8-mm ureteral calculus

Name of Procedures: Cystoscopy, left retrograde pyelogram, left double-J stent placement

Anesthesia: 1.5 mg Versed, 2% Xylocaine jelly

Findings: This is a very pleasant patient with a history of sarcoidosis and bilateral nephrolithiasis. Recent creatinine is 2.3. Helical CT scan revealed 8-mm left proximal ureter calculus, some hydrone-phrosis, and a 1-cm right renal pelvic stone. She is brought to the operating room for a cystoscopy, retrograde pyelogram, and double-J stent placement. She is also complaining of bilateral back pain.

Chapter 5 Test (Continued)

Description of Operation: In the lithotomy position, the patient was given 1.5 mg IV Versed sedation. Her genitals were prepared and draped in a sterile fashion. 2% Xylocaine jelly was applied per urethra. A 21 French asymmetric cystoscope was passed. The left ureteral orifice was visualized. A left retrograde pyelogram was carried out, with an 8 French long-tipped catheter. The pyelogram shows this to be a normal ureter up to proximal left ureter and at that point, there was hydronephrosis and a calculus, which was seen on preliminary films and was still evident. A 0.035 glider was passed up past the stone on fluoroscopic guidance followed by 6 × 24 Mardis double-J stent. Position was confirmed with a KUB. She tolerated the procedure well and was transferred out in stable condition.

The patient is currently on Levaquin 500 mg q. day. Urine culture was sent during the procedure after the stent was placed. One can see the left proximal ureteral calculus. She will be scheduled for left ESWL middle or end of next week. The patient understands the procedure, the risks, and benefits, and will proceed.

a. 52332
b. 52332, 74420–26
c. 52332, 74420–26, 76000
d. 52332, 76000

8. Code the following interventional radiology procedure(s):

The left external iliac artery was accessed, and a catheter was inserted into the patient's abdominal aorta and placed above the level of the renal arteries. Injection and abdominal aortography was performed. The catheter was then manipulated to the level of the aortic bifurcation where injection and angiography of the bilateral lower extremities was performed. The catheter was then removed and a vascular closure device was placed for hemostasis.

a. 36100; 75625; 75710
b. 36200; 75625; 75716
c. 36200; 75630; 75716
d. 36100; 75625; 75710–50

9. Bilateral x-rays of a patient's shoulders, both frontal and lateral, were taken in the office and read by the group's staff radiologist. How would you code these procedures to help ensure reimbursement?

a. 73020, 73020
b. 73020–50
c. 73030–LT; 73030–RT
d. 73030, 73030–51

10. Code the following interventional radiology procedure(s):

The right common femoral artery was accessed and a catheter was inserted into the patient's right superficial femoral artery. Injection and lower extremity angiography were performed. The catheter was removed and manual pressure was applied until hemostasis was achieved.

a. 36245; 75710
b. 36246; 75716
c. 36247; 75710
d. 36247; 75716

Chapter 6

Pathology and Laboratory

Objectives

Upon completion of this chapter, the student should be able to do the following:

- Describe the types of codes contained in the pathology and laboratory section of the CPT code book

- Describe the methods used to locate pathology and laboratory codes in the CPT Index

- Distinguish between the terms quantitative and qualitative in relation to pathology and laboratory codes

- Identify the modifiers that are most commonly used for pathology and laboratory coding

- Discuss the subsections of the pathology and laboratory section and specific coding guidelines for given subsections

- Discuss specific CMS guidelines for submitting panel-testing codes

- Describe HCPCS Level II codes used on a temporary basis for certain disease panel testing

This chapter discusses the codes in the pathology and laboratory section of the CPT code book. The codes in this section are used to describe procedures/services that are performed by physicians or by medical technologists under the direct supervision of a physician. The procedures include various laboratory tests such as urinalysis and blood work, and pathological examinations such as frozen sections and pap smears.

Codes within this section are assigned based on many variables such as specimen type (urine, blood sputum, and others), the type of testing method used (commercial test kit versus reagents), type of equipment used (manual versus automated), and the number of tests completed (single tests versus multiple tests in a panel). Laboratory specialists within the physician practice should be consulted to obtain answers to questions about any of these variables.

Pathology and Laboratory Section Structure and Content

The pathology and laboratory section is divided into subsections based on the type of laboratory test performed.

Alphabetic Index

Laboratory and pathology procedures/services are listed in the Alphabetic Index of the CPT code book under the following main terms:

- Specific name of the test, such as urinalysis, evocative/suppression test, and fertility test

- Specific substance/specimen/sample, such as glucose, CPK, cyanide, enterovirus, bone marrow, and nasal smear

- Specific method used, such as culture, fine needle aspiration, and microbiology

On-Site Testing versus Reference Lab Testing

When reporting laboratory services provided by the physician, the coder must determine whether the physician performed the complete procedure or only a component of it. Some physician offices and physician-owned clinics have sophisticated laboratory equipment on the premises, which enables the physicians to provide complete laboratory testing. A complete test would involve ordering the procedure/test, obtaining the sample/specimen (for example, blood, urine), handling the specimen, performing the actual procedure/test, and analyzing and interpreting the results. However, many physicians typically send the sample/specimen to a freestanding laboratory or a hospital-based laboratory for testing and analysis. In these cases, the physician should report only the collection of the specimen and a handling fee for preparation and/or transportation of the specimen and the provider performing the service should bill for the actual service. This eliminates the possibility of having a physician office laboratory submit a claim for a service that is not covered under their CLIA license. (Please refer to the discussion on CLIA later in this chapter.)

Blood Draws

Physicians may submit a code for a blood draw for any laboratory test. The CPT code book provides three codes that are routinely used in physician offices for obtaining a blood specimen from a patient:

36415   Collection of venous blood by venipuncture

36416   Collection of capillary blood specimen (that is, finger, heel, ear stick)

36600   Arterial puncture, withdrawal of blood for diagnosis

Code 36415 is used for routine venipuncture. Code 36416 is used for obtaining capillary blood in cases where this specimen type is specifically needed or where the patient is an infant and venipuncture is not practical.

Code 36600 is used for obtaining an arterial blood sample and should not be used to describe routine blood draws. Arterial blood draws require special skill and are done to examine the components of oxygen-rich arterial blood, such as arterial blood gases (ABGs). Each code should only be reported once, even when more than one blood specimen of each type is drawn during an encounter. Medicare allows only one blood draw per day.

Some physicians may refer to the drawing of blood as phlebotomy. The coder should be careful not to confuse the routine phlebotomy, or venipuncture described above, with therapeutic phlebotomy (99195). Therapeutic phlebotomy is the removal of a large volume of blood, usually one to two pints, to treat a specific medical condition, such as severely elevated hemoglobin.

Example: If a physician drew three specimens of blood for a glucose tolerance test and then sent the specimens to an outside lab for analysis, the correct code assignment would be code 36415 for the venipuncture, all three specimens.

If the physician drew the specimens and performed the test at the office, the correct code assignment would be code 36415 for the venipuncture, all three specimens, and code 82951 for the glucose tolerance test, three specimens.

Example: Dr. Reynolds performed a venipuncture to obtain a blood sample for a lipid panel. He prepared the sample for transport and sent it to an outside laboratory for testing, analysis, and interpretation.

Dr. Reynolds should report code 36415 for the venipuncture. The off-site laboratory would report code 80061 for the lipid panel.

Clinical Laboratory Improvement Amendments of 1988 (CLIA)

Physician office laboratories (POLs) are governed by the Clinical Laboratory Improvement Amendments of 1988. To be allowed to perform tests, and to bill for them, the office must be inspected by a CLIA inspector once every two years or obtain a waiver. Inspected labs receive a certification number that Medicare and Medicaid require to be on file before an office is allowed to bill for testing.

For smaller POLs that perform only basic testing, a waiver may be obtained. To obtain a waiver, the office must be performing only tests that can be performed safely by staff without formal laboratory education, using the instructions found in the package insert. This section includes tests such as dipstick urines, finger stick glucose tests, and home pregnancy testing. When reporting codes for the waived procedures that are performed by a waived laboratory, a –QW modifier must be attached to the CPT code to obtain payment from Medicare or Medicaid.

The list of tests approved for waived laboratories is updated on a periodic basis. To obtain a listing of the tests that are currently considered waived or the administrative rules of the Clinical Laboratory Improvement Act, consult the Food and Drug Administration (FDA) website or the

CMS website (CMS 2015). The 10-digit CLIA number must be present in box 23 (prior authorization number) of the CMS-1500 form (or the electronic equivalent) when billing for laboratory services.

Quantitative and Qualitative Studies

The descriptions for pathology and laboratory codes often contain the terms *qualitative* or *quantitative*. Qualitative testing seeks to determine whether or not the element is present in the specimen. Quantitative studies seek to provide results with counts of a certain element in the specimen. Often a quantitative test will be performed after a qualitative test shows that the element does indeed exist in that sample. Qualitative testing provides results as positive or negative, and quantitative testing provides results with numeric values.

The difficulty with coding procedures in the pathology and laboratory section of the CPT code book is in determining the method used to perform the tests. Often the lab report does not give the coder enough information on a test method to determine the exact code. For an example, the coder should review the code range 85004–85049.

The specific hemogram code in this series depends on whether the test was automated or manual, and the laboratory report may not specify that information. For clarification, the coder should work directly with the staff performing the test to determine the appropriate codes to report.

Guidelines Pertaining to Pathology and Laboratory Subsections

Certain subsections in the pathology and laboratory section have specific guidelines for their use, as discussed here.

Organ or Disease-Oriented Panels

The organ or disease-oriented panels subsection contains codes that are used for groups of tests commonly performed together for a given purpose, for example, one of the obstetric panels for prenatal patients. The code description indicates that the listed tests must all be performed to qualify for the use of this code. If all tests in the panel are not performed, each test completed should be coded separately. If additional tests beyond those listed in the panel are performed, they also should be coded separately.

Coders must review the exact tests listed in the panels and assign panel codes only when the tests performed match the panels exactly. Panel codes can be found using the CPT Index under Blood Tests, Panels.

Drug Procedures

There are three types of drug procedure codes identified in CPT: Drug Assay, Therapeutic Drug Assay, and Chemistry. Drug assays are divided into two types of tests, which are presumptive drug class tests and definitive drug class tests. Presumptive tests identify the presence or absence of a drug or drug class in a sample. Definitive tests are qualitative or quantitative tests to identify the presence or absence of drugs and identify the specific drugs in a sample. Therapeutic drug assays are used to monitor the clinical response to a prescribed medication and are quantitative. If no therapeutic drug assay code is found, use a code from the chemistry section of CPT.

Evocative/Suppression Testing

Evocative/suppression testing is the administration of specific agents to a patient and measurement of the agent's effect on the patient's system. Codes 80400–80440 are used to reflect the laboratory component of the procedure measuring the agent's effect. Actual administration of the agent is coded in the medicine section of the CPT code book with codes 96360, 96361, 96372–96375, and the supply of the agent is coded with the J code series of HCPCS codes. The physician's services should be reflected in an E/M code when E/M services are provided.

The code descriptions indicate the test or tests included in the code and the number of tests performed.

80436   Metyrapone panel

This panel must include the following:

Cortisol (82533 × 2)

11 deoxycortisol (82634 × 2)

Consultations in Clinical Pathology

The pathology and laboratory section of the CPT code book provides specific codes for consultation services. Consultation codes are available for both clinical pathology and anatomic pathology.

Use of the clinical pathology consultation codes requires the provision of a written report by the pathologist. An attending physician may request a clinical pathology consultation when medical interpretation of a test result is required. Code 80500 is a limited consultation without the review of patient history or medical records. Code 80502 is a comprehensive consultation for a complex diagnostic problem with the review of history and records. Neither of these codes requires face-to-face patient evaluation during the consultation. If the patient is evaluated, consultation codes from the E/M section should be used.

Chemistry

Codes from the chemistry subsection include chemical tests on any body fluid. The tests are listed alphabetically within the subsection. When an analyte is measured in multiple specimens from different sources or in specimens obtained at different times, the analyte is reported separately for each source and for each specimen. If the exact test is repeated on two different specimens on the same day, modifier –91, Repeat Clinical Diagnostic Laboratory Test, should be added to the code to avoid a claim denial as a duplicate claim.

All examinations are quantitative unless otherwise specified. Calculations in reporting test results are included in the code description. CPT provides the following note at the beginning of the chemistry section of CPT: "Clinical information derived from the results of laboratory data that is mathematically calculated (that is, free thyroxine index T7) is considered part of the test procedure and therefore is not a separately reportable service."

Hematology and Coagulation

The hematology and coagulation codes are assigned for tests such as complete blood counts (CBC), clotting tests, bone marrow procedures, and prothrombin time. Many of the code descriptions include the specific tests and methodology that are included in the code and not reported with a separate CPT code.

85007	Blood count; blood smear, microscopic examination with manual differential WBC count

Coders should note that the differential may be manual or automated. Coders should work closely with laboratory personnel to choose the appropriate code(s) in this subsection if they are unfamiliar with the equipment used and the exact procedures performed.

For bone marrow smear interpretation, code 85097 should be used. Many third-party payers previously denied the service of obtaining the bone marrow biopsy because the codes were located in the laboratory section of the CPT code book. Thus, these codes were moved to the surgical section of the book. See code 38220 for bone marrow aspiration and code 38221 for bone marrow biopsy. To code a bone biopsy, the coder should refer to codes 20220–20225.

Immunology

The immunology subsection is used for specific laboratory tests to assess the patient's immune system, or the presence of antigens and antibodies with a specimen. The CPT book categorizes the tests for the presence of antigens using codes 87260–87899 and the presence of the antibody that has been generated against the antigen with codes 86000–86804. Also included in this subsection are blood bank physician services and tissue typing. To report immunoassays by multiple-step methods, the coder should refer to codes 86602–86804. When an immunoassay is performed using a single-step method, such as reagent strip, code 86318 should be used. Many commercial test kits are read visually as positive or negative after the preparation instructions have been followed. In this case, a code for direct optic observation should be chosen.

Laboratory orders for immunology tests frequently include orders for reflex testing. Reflex testing means that the performance of subsequent tests is dependent upon the result value of the initial test. For example, when the results of a culture are positive, the positive result triggers one or more additional tests, also called reflex testing. If the culture had been negative, no further testing would take place.

Microbiology

Microbiology is the culturing of microorganisms (pathogens) and their identification. These microorganisms are also tested against a battery of drugs to determine their sensitivity to specific drugs and specific strengths of those drugs, also called susceptibility testing. These organisms can be classified as bacteria, viruses, fungi and molds or parasites. Negative cultures can frequently be coded with one CPT code. When cultures are positive and the physician has ordered reflex testing, multiple layers of coding are necessary to fully describe all the services ordered and provided.

Example: The physician orders a urine culture and colony count with reflex definitive identification and susceptibility for all positive cultures.

Step 1: If the urine culture is negative, code 87086 only.

Step 2: If the urine culture is positive, the colonies are counted, and a presumptive identification of each pathogen is done, code 87086 and 87088.

Step 3: The physician ordered definitive identification. If additional methods are required to identify an anaerobic isolate, code 87076. If additional methods are required to identify an aerobic isolate, code 87077. However, do not code presumptive ID and definitive ID together. Code only the definitive ID if both are performed.

Step 4: Some pathogens require typing, such as Salmonella. Code 87147 for this serotyping process, using a single antiserum (serum against the antigen). If multiple antisera are used, add –59 modifier to 87147 for each additional antisera used.

Step 5: The physician ordered susceptibility testing. Code for this testing based on the method used: 87184 for the disk method (Kirby Bauer test), once per plate or 87186 for the microdilution (MIC) or agar dilution method, once per plate (Ingenix 2008; Kuehn 2009a; Turegon 2007).

Anatomic Pathology

Anatomic pathology codes reflect the physician's services in cell definition.

Cytopathology

The cytopathology codes are used to describe cell identification techniques for neoplastic activity. Pap smears are coded based on several parameters. The first parameter is whether slides are prepared using a traditional method from a sample, or whether a new thin-prep method is used. The automated thin-layer preparation technique uses a special brush collection device that collects the specimen and is placed completely into a tube of preservative fluid. Special slides are then prepared from this fluid. Table 6.1 displays Pap smear codes for slides

Table 6.1. Pap smear codes: Automated thin layer preparation

Screening Type	Automated Thin Layer Preparation	
Manual screening	88142	
Automated screening		88174
Manual screening with manual rescreening	88143	
Automated screening with manual rescreening		88175
Cytopathology requiring interpretation by physician	+ 88141	+ 88141
Cytopathology—definitive hormonal evaluation	+ 88155	+ 88155

prepared using the thin-prep method. It should be noted that the word "automated" in the title "automated thin layer preparation" technique has nothing to do with whether the slides were read manually or using an automated system. "Automated" in the title refers only to the automated slide preparation technique.

The second parameter for code selection is the results reporting method. Codes 88164–88167 are used for the Bethesda reporting method, a method that reports results in a structured format, giving a statement of specimen adequacy, general categorization, and a descriptive diagnosis. Codes 88150–88154 are used to describe slides reported by any other method. Table 6.2 displays the codes used for traditional specimen slides with primary screening done manually, based on reporting method.

The third parameter used in selecting a code is the level of screening required and whether it is manual, computer-assisted, or automated. Table 6.3 shows the codes available to report smear slides with primary screening done using an automated system.

Once a code has been chosen from one of the four code families, two add-on codes are available to describe additional services that may be required. Code 88141 describes interpretation of any cytopathology slide by a physician in addition to any manual screening and rescreening that may be done. Code 88155 describes definitive hormonal evaluation of specimen material. Codes 88141 and 88155 may be reported together, in addition to a Pap smear code, if all three services are provided.

Table 6.2. Pap smear codes: Smear slides with primary screening completed manually

Screening Type	Traditional Smear Slides	
	Bethesda Reporting Method	Non-Bethesda Reporting Method
Manual screening under physician supervision	88164	88150
Manual screening and rescreening under physician supervision	88165	88153
Manual screening and computer-assisted rescreening under physician supervision	88166	88152
Manual screening and computer-assisted rescreening using cell selection under physician supervision	88167	88154
Cytopathology requiring interpretation by physician	+ 88141	+ 88141
Cytopathology—definitive hormonal evaluation	+ 88155	+ 88155

Table 6.3. Pap smear codes: Smear slides with primary screening by automated system

Screening Method	Smear Slides
Automated screening	88147
Automated screening with manual rescreening under physician supervision	88148
Cytopathology requiring interpretation by physician	+ 88141
Cytopathology—definitive hormonal evaluation	+ 88155

Manual rescreening is defined in the CPT code book as requiring a complete visual reassessment of the entire slide initially screened by either an automated or manual process. Manual review is defined as an assessment of selected cells or regions of a slide identified by initial automated review.

CPT Assistant (March 2004) directs the coders that code 88141 should not be used for negative Pap smears. It further states: "Code 88141 should be used to report physician interpretation of a Pap smear that is interpreted to be abnormal by the personnel performing the initial screening."

Cytogenetic Studies

Cytogenetic study codes describe services of cell identification for nonneoplastic disorders and chromosomal or DNA identification. Special modifiers have been developed for use with the codes in this section. The coder should refer to Appendix I of the CPT code book for a detailed listing of these modifiers.

Surgical Pathology

Codes in the first portion of the surgical pathology subsection (88300–88309) include the accession, examination, and reporting portions of the pathological examination. Other procedures covered in codes 88311–88365 and 88399 are not included and, if performed, should be coded separately. These procedures include services such as special staining, frozen-section examinations during surgery, and electron microscopy.

The unit of service for the surgical pathology codes 88300–88309 is the specimen. The CPT code book defines a specimen as a tissue or tissues submitted for individual and separate attention, requiring individual examination and pathologic diagnosis. When two or more individual specimens are submitted from a given patient, individual codes are assigned to each specimen based on the level of service for each specimen.

The codes in this group are assigned based on type of examination and specimen examined. Code 88300 is assigned when only a gross examination of any specimen is performed. Six levels of pathologic examination of specimens are identified. Codes 88302–88309 are assigned based on the specific specimen examined. The type of specimen included in each code is listed alphabetically under the code. For example, a kidney biopsy specimen examination, both gross and microscopic, is coded to 88305.

Any specimen that is not listed in any of the levels should be assigned to the code that most closely reflects the physician's work involved when compared with other specimens assigned to that code.

HCPCS contains four codes that describe a special surgical pathology service that is not reported based on an individual specimen. Code G0416 describes surgical pathology, gross and microscopic examination of prostate needle biopsy sampling.

Consultations in Anatomic Pathology

Special codes are provided to describe consultations provided on surgical specimens or during surgery. Code 88321 describes a consultation and report on slides that are referred from elsewhere (not created and originally read within the facility and sent by another pathologist or facility). Code 88323 describes a consultation and report on material that is referred from elsewhere but requires preparation of slides before evaluation. Code 88325 describes a comprehensive consultation with review of records and specimens, including a report. Codes 88329–88334 describe pathology consultations during surgery with and without frozen section(s). It should be noted that if the patient is actually examined and evaluated, consultation codes from the E/M section should be used.

Pathologists are frequently asked to provide an opinion during surgery. When the pathologist provides a consultation for another physician during the course of a surgery, but no specimen is examined under the microscope, code 88329 is reported. However, specimens are frequently submitted for immediate interpretation, to provide the surgeon with diagnostic information. This immediate interpretation is called a frozen section. It is important to understand two definitions to allow correct code assignment. A tissue block is a portion of tissue from a specimen that is frozen or encased in a support medium such as paraffin or plastic, from which sections are prepared. A section is a thin slice of tissue from a block prepared for microscopic examination.

Code 88331 is the first code assigned. This code represents the first tissue block from a specimen and any number of sections taken from the tissue block. If an additional tissue block is required from the same specimen, code 88332 is assigned in addition to 88331. Codes 88333 and 88334 can be assigned if cytologic examinations are done at the time of surgery and are reported per specimen site, not per tissue block (Kuehn 2009a).

In Vivo (eg, Transcutaneous Laboratory Procedures)

The Latin term **in vivo** means inside a living organism. The testing described in this section is performed through the patient's skin, but the tests are still considered laboratory tests. Each test in this section has a corresponding test and code that can be performed on a specimen outside of the body (**in vitro**).

Modifiers Used in Pathology and Laboratory Coding

As with other sections in the CPT code book, codes from the pathology and laboratory section may be modified to indicate that the procedure or service has been changed by some circumstance. Some of the modifiers that may be used in the pathology and laboratory section include the following:

-22 **Increased Procedural Services**: Modifier –22 is used to indicate that the service provided is greater than that normally required. Submission of a report to explain these circumstances is usually required.

-26 **Professional Component**: Modifier –26 indicates that only the physician or professional component, rather than the technical component, is being reported.

-32 **Mandated Services**: Modifier –32 indicates that the service provided has been required by a given person or organization, for example, a third-party payer or a governmental, legislative, or regulatory requirement.

-52 **Reduced Services**: Modifier –52 indicates that the service provided is less than what is normally required. A portion of the procedure may be reduced or eliminated at the physician's discretion.

-53 **Discontinued Procedure**: Modifier –53 indicates that a procedure or test was started, but not completed. Generally, this is due to circumstances where the patient's health or well-being is threatened due to development of a complication.

–59 **Distinct Procedural Service:** Modifier –59 is used when a separate and distinct service is performed on the same day for the same patient. Usually, these procedures are not reported together but in these circumstances are appropriately listed together. For Medicare, use one of the following HCPCS modifiers to more fully describe the distinct procedural service:

> –XE: Separate encounter
>
> –XP: Separate practitioner
>
> –XS: Separate structure (or organ)
>
> –XU: Unusual non-overlapping service

–90 **Reference (Outside) Laboratory:** Modifier –90 is used widely for laboratory and pathology services. It indicates that the physician does not perform the actual test or service but, instead, sends specimens to an outside laboratory.

–91 **Repeat Clinical Diagnostic Laboratory Test:** Modifier –91 may be used for laboratory test(s) performed more than once on the same day on the same patient. This modifier may not be used when tests are rerun either to confirm initial results, because of testing problems with specimens or equipment, or for any other reason when a normal, one-time, reportable result is all that is required.

–92 **Alternative Laboratory Platform Testing:** When laboratory testing is being performed using a kit or transportable instrument that wholly or in part consists of a single use, disposable analytical chamber, the service may be identified by adding modifier –92 to the usual laboratory procedure code (HIV testing 86701–86703).

–GA **Waiver of Liability Statement on File**: Refer to chapter 10 for a complete discussion of medical necessity and waivers/advance beneficiary notices.

–QW CLIA-waived test

HCPCS Codes Used in Pathology and Laboratory Coding

The following HCPCS codes may be used in reporting pathology and laboratory services/procedures. Always refer to the current HCPCS code book for the complete list of available codes.

G0123 Screening cytopathology, cervical or vaginal (any reporting system), collected in preservative fluid, automated thin-layer preparation, screening by cytotechnologist under physician supervision

G0124 Screening cytopathology, cervical or vaginal (any reporting system), collected in preservative fluid, automated thin-layer preparation, requiring interpretation by physician

G0141 Screening cytopathology smears, cervical or vaginal, performed by automated system, with manual rescreening, requiring interpretation by physician

G0143 Screening cytopathology, cervical or vaginal (any reporting system), collected in preservative fluid, automated thin-layer preparation, with manual screening and rescreening by cytotechnologist under physician supervision

G0144   Screening cytopathology, cervical or vaginal (any reporting system), collected in preservative fluid, automated thin-layer preparation, with screening by automated system under physician supervision

G0145   Screening cytopathology, cervical or vaginal (any reporting system), collected in preservative fluid, automated thin-layer preparation, with screening by automated system and manual rescreening under physician supervision

G0147   Screening cytopathology smears, cervical or vaginal, performed by automated system under physician supervision

G0148   Screening cytopathology smears, cervical or vaginal, performed by automated system with manual rescreening

G0306   Complete CBC, automated (HgB, HCT, RBC, WBC, without platelet count) and automated WBC differential count

G0307   Complete CBC, automated (HgB, HCT, RBC, WBC, without platelet count)

G0328   Colorectal cancer screening; fecal occult blood test, immunoassay, 1–3 simultaneous

G0416   Surgical pathology, gross and microscopic examination for prostate needle biopsy sampling, any method

G0431   Drug screen, qualitative, single drug class method (eg, immunoassay, enzyme assay), each drug class

G0432   Infectious agent antigen detection by enzyme immunoassay (EIA) technique, qualitative or semi-quantitative, multiple-step method, HIV-1 or HIV-2, screening

G0433   Infectious agent antigen detection by enzyme-linked immunosorbent assay (ELISA) technique, antibody, HIV-1 or HIV-2, screening

G0435   Infectious agent antigen detection by rapid antibody test of oral mucosa transudate, HIV-1 or HIV-2, screening

G0452   Molecular pathology procedure; physician interpretation and report

P2028   Cephalin floculation, blood

P2029   Congo red, blood

P2031   Hair analysis (excluding arsenic)

P2033   Thymol turbidity, blood

P2038   Mucoprotein, blood (seromucoid) (medical necessity procedure)

P3000   Screening Papanicolaou smear, cervical or vaginal, up to three smears, by technician under physician supervision

P3001   Screening Papanicolaou smear, cervical or vaginal, up to three smears, by technician requiring interpretation by physician

P7001   Culture, bacterial, urine; quantitative, sensitivity study

P9612   Catheterization for collection of specimen, single patient, all places of service

P9615   Catheterization for collection of specimen(s) (multiple patients)

Q0091   Screening Papanicolaou smear; obtaining, preparing, and conveyance of cervical or vaginal smear to laboratory

S3645   HIV-1 antibody testing of oral mucosal transudate

S3650   Saliva test, hormone level; during menopause

S3652   Saliva test, hormone level; to assess preterm labor risk

S3655   Antisperm antibodies test (immunobead)

S3708   Gastrointestinal fat absorption study

S3721   Prostate cancer antigen 3 (PCA3) testing

For physicians performing blood transfusions and providing blood products, see HCPCS codes P9010–P9060 and for gene and DNA analysis, see S3800–S3890.

Exercise 6.1. Pathology and Laboratory

Choose the best answer for each of the following questions.

1. The source of the specimen for chemistry tests coded to 82009–84999 is _____
   a. Urine
   b. Blood
   c. Sputum
   d. Any source unless otherwise specified in code descriptor

2. The pathologist completes a frozen section exam by making two tissue blocks from a specimen labeled "right kidney" and one tissue block from a specimen labeled "right ureter." How is this service coded?
   a. 88331 × 2, 88332
   b. 88305 × 2, 88331 × 2, 88332
   c. 88305 × 2
   d. 88331 × 3

3. A waived physician office laboratory performs a nonautomated urinalysis by dipstick, without microscopy. How is this service reported to Medicare?
   a. 81000
   b. 81002–GA–QW
   c. 81002–QW
   d. 81003–GA

4. The physician needs to code a pathology consultation provided during surgery. Which code series would the physician use to code this service?
   a. Consultation (Clinical Pathology) (80500–80502)
   b. Initial Inpatient Consultation (99251–99255)
   c. Office and other Outpatient Services (99201–99215)
   d. Surgical Pathology (88300–88399)

5. 10:00 a.m. Quantitative blood glucose test
   11:30 a.m. Quantitative blood glucose test, status post self-administered insulin injection
   a. 82945
   b. 82947, 82947–91
   c. 82948, 82948
   d. 82962, 82962–91

6. Hemoglobin A1C test is performed by the laboratory staff. How is this procedure coded?
   a. 83020
   b. 83026
   c. 83036
   d. 83037

Exercise 6.1. (Continued)

Assign the appropriate codes for the following pathology and laboratory procedures. Include the modifiers, when applicable.

7. *Candida* skin test

    _____

8. The following tests were performed as a group from one blood sample: Total serum cholesterol, HDL and triglycerides, carbon dioxide, chloride, potassium, and sodium

    _____

9. Quantitative testing (therapeutic drug assay) of theophylline level

    _____

10. Whole blood clot lysis time

    _____

11. Complete automated CBC with automated differential

    _____

12. Partial thromboplastin time of whole blood (PTT) and prothrombin time (PT)

    _____

13. A patient received the following laboratory tests:

    Albumin, serum   Phosphatase, alkaline
    Albumin, urine, microalbumin, quantitative   Protein, total
    Bilirubin, total   Transferase, aspartate amino
    Bilirubin, direct   Transferase, alanine amino

    _____

A pathologist examined the following specimens. Examination was both gross and microscopic unless otherwise specified. Assign CPT codes.

14. Cervical biopsy tissue

    _____

15. Three loose bodies from a joint, submitted separately

    _____

16. **Pathologic Diagnosis:** 1. Right tube and ovary—serous cystadenoma. A rare granuloma is seen in the right ovary. Fallopian tube without significant pathology.
    2. Left tube and ovary—a segment of fallopian tube and ovary with multiple small-retention cysts.

    Clinical Data: This is a 77-year-old G2P2, with pelvic mass, aortic aneurysm.

    Diagnosis: Pelvic mass, aortic aneurysm

    Specimen Source: Right tube and ovary

    Gross Description: The specimen is received in the fresh state, labeled "right tube and ovary." It was submitted for frozen section and consists of a multicystic, multiloculated ovary filled with clear fluid, measuring 7 × 4.5 × 3.5 cm in greatest dimensions. On cut surface it shows neither firm, irregular areas, nor papillary structures. Attached is a fallopian tube, apparently grossly normal measuring 6 cm

(Continued on next page)

Chapter 6.1. (Continued)

in length. The frozen-section diagnosis was reported per telephone as "ovary with multilocular cysts, no evidence of malignancy seen." This is submitted in cassette FS1. The remainder of the specimen is sampled and submitted in cassette 2 (entire fallopian tube).

Specimen 2, received fresh on the day following receipt of the first specimen, is labeled "left tube and ovary." It consists of a segment of fallopian tube measuring 5.6 cm in length and 1.1 cm in greatest outer circumference, with an attached pale-yellow ovary measuring $3.0 \times 2.0 \times 1.2$ cm in greatest dimension. The cut surface is unremarkable.

Micro: All sections are examined. Histologic findings are summarized in pathologic diagnosis. (See first paragraph of this report.)

Assign the appropriate code(s) to these procedures:

_____

17. Direct bilirubin; sample obtained in office by heel stick

_____

18. Arterial draw with evaluation of blood gases: pH, pCO_2, pO_2, CO_2, and HCO_3, done and reported by the physician.

_____

19. OB lab testing including complete CBC, Hep B antigen, ABO blood typing, Rh blood typing, RBC antigen screen, Syphilis testing, HIV testing and rubella antibody testing.

_____

20. How many sets of results must be documented for panel 80426?

_____

Chapter 6 Test

Choose the best answer for each of the following questions.

1. The physician orders a complete CBC with automated hemoglobin, hematocrit, red blood cell count, white blood cell count, and platelet count. How are these procedures coded?

   a. 80004
   b. 85025
   c. 85027
   d. 85018; 85014; 85041; 85048

2. Which of the following is the correct code assignment for the following: Fecal occult blood test, patient provided with three cards for consecutive collection?

   a. 82270
   b. 82271
   c. 82272
   d. 82274

Chapter 6 Test (Continued)

3. Urinalysis, non-automated, without microscopy is coded as:

   a. 81000
   b. 81001
   c. 81002
   d. 81003

4. Code the laboratory associated with the following office visit:

   CC: Edema

   S: This 69-year-old Medicare patient is here for follow-up of several concerns. She has been noticing more swelling of her feet recently but no shortness of breath, PND or orthopnea. Taking Lasix 60 mg b.i.d.

   O: Weight 104, BP 132/70. Lungs: Clear. Heart: Regular. Extremities: With 2+ pitting edema to the lower extremities.
   A: Edema, benign hypertension, paroxysmal atrial fibrillation, COPD and CAD.

   P: Increased her Lasix to 80 mg b.i.d. Gave scrip for potassium supplement if needed. She was also kindly seen by Dr C and had an EGD and colonoscopy, which showed gastritis and positive Helicobacter pylori. Will see him about ongoing treatment. Also had adenomatous polyps removed. Will check sodium, potassium, chloride and CO2 today. Follow up in a week.

   Blood draw done today in the office.
   Results (performed in office):

Potassium	L	3.2	(3.3–5.1) mmol/L
Sodium		139	(133–145) mmol/L
Chloride	L	92	(96–108) mmol/L
CO_2	H	32	(21–31) mmol/L

   a. 80051
   b. 80051, 36415
   c. 84132, 84295, 82435, 82374
   d. 84132, 84295, 82435, 82374, 36415

5. A Pap smear slide is read using automated screening and manual rescreening under physician supervision. How is this coded?

   a. 88142
   b. 88147
   c. 88148
   d. 88174

6. Code the following pathology report:

   Clinical History: Six-month-old with stage V retinoblastoma RE, s/p 2 course chemo Rx. No XRT.

   Gross Description: Received fresh designated Retinoblastoma—OD is a 1.6-cm superior-inferior × 1.6 cm (SP) 1.5 cm (ML) enucleated eyeball with a 4-mm long × 3 mm in diameter optic nerve stump. The pupil measures 3 mm in diameter. The specimen is trisected along the sagittal plane revealing a tan grainy mass with a base measurement of 0.8 cm, and a height of 0.3 cm, located at the posterolateral inferior quadrant. The anterior margin measures approximately 0.6 cm. and the posterior margin measures approximately 1 cm. The retina appears detached from the wall in approximately 40% of the area.

   Summary of sections: A1–optic nerve margin; A2–mid sagittal section; A3–lateral horizontal sections.

   Microscopic Description: The en face cross section of the optic nerve margin (A1) reveals nerve bundles, skeletal muscle, and loose fibrovascular tissue; there is no evidence of neoplasia in this section. Slides A2 and A3 reveal a focally detached retina with an associated largely calcified mass on the

(Continued on next page)

Chapter 6 Test (Continued)

ganglion cell layer. The loose mass consists of reactive spindle cells with only focal residual primitive retinoblastic cells present. Focal involvement of the outer layer of the retina by the retinoblastomatous cells is also present. Away from this main mass, focal nests of viable tumor cells are present on the ganglion cell layer of retina. Tumor nests do not involve the orbit wall, iris or lens.

Final Diagnosis: Eye, right, enucleation:

- Treated exophytic retinoblastoma with extensive calcifications
- Detached retina with scattered retinoblastomatous nodules on ganglion cell surface
- No evidence of tumor in the optic nerve, choroids, sclera or ciliary body

    a. 88304
    b. 88305
    c. 88307
    d. 88309

7. The physician suspects the patient may have Hepatitis C and orders an AST, ALT, alkaline phosphatase, and total bilirubin to assess hepatic function. How is this service coded?

    a. 80076
    b. 82247, 84075, 84450, 84460
    c. 82248, 84078, 84450, 84460
    d. 82247, 84078, 84450, 84460

8. Code the laboratory associated with the following office visit:

CC: Follow up Diabetes

S: Patient is a 72-year-old woman here with her neighbor. She has had an acute URI but now is feeling pretty much her usual self again. Has a mild lingering cough. It does not keep her awake at night. No fever, chills, shortness of breath or weakness. Her weight is basically stable.

Medications were reviewed. She checks her blood glucose at home but she only checks in the morning before eating. I have asked her several times to check at random times. She lives alone but is checked on by the neighbor who is with her today.

O: Examination shows a pleasant, well-nourished, well-groomed woman with occasional cough noted. Vital signs are normal. Lungs: Clear. Heart: Regular rate. Extremities: No edema or evidence of infection. Palpable popliteal pulses bilaterally intact in both feet.

A: Diabetes with resolving URI.

P: Check her A1C and glucose. She is not due for any other surveillance testing today. Did give her a scrip for Tessalon Perles #30.

Random blood draw done today in the office.

Results (performed in office):
Glucose, Random (4 hrs post-prandial)	H 183	(70–110) mg/dL
Hemoglobin A1C	H 8.8	(4.0–6.0) %

    a. 82947, 83036
    b. 82948, 83037
    c. 82948, 83036, 36415
    d. 82947, 83036, 36415

Chapter 6 Test (Continued)

9. The physician orders a therapeutic blood level of Haloperidol on a patient with Parkinsonism who has not improved with therapy. What is the proper code assignment for this test?

    a. 80301
    b. 80399
    c. 80173
    d. 84999

10. Two Cortisol determinations done on the same day, with venipuncture, for adrenal insufficiency are coded as:

    a. 82533, 82533–91, 36415 × 2
    b. 82533 × 2, 36415
    c. 80400, 36415
    d. 80400, 36415 × 2

Chapter 7

Medicine

Objectives

Upon completion of this lesson, the student should be able to do the following:

- Describe the contents and structure of the medicine section of the CPT code book

- Identify conventions specific to the immunization injections subsection

- Describe the use of specialized psychiatry codes and general E/M codes for these services

- Identify elements used in assigning dialysis codes

- Discuss the use of ophthalmology codes and the services that are included and coded separately in this subsection

- Identify the use of special otorhinolaryngologic service codes for services performed in addition to standard evaluations

- Discuss the contents and use of cardiovascular codes, including diagnostic tests such as cardiac catheterizations

- Discuss the components of noninvasive vascular diagnostic studies

- Describe the services reflected in codes for allergy and clinical immunology services

- Identify the types of services included in the codes for central nervous system assessments/tests

- Describe the use of hydration, therapeutic or diagnostic infusion/injection codes

- Discuss the chemotherapy administration codes and circumstances in which additional codes are appropriate to reflect services provided

- Describe the contents and definitions associated with codes for the physical medicine and rehabilitation, osteopathic manipulation treatment, and chiropractic manipulative treatment subsections

- Discuss the contents and limitations of codes in the special services and reports subsection

This chapter discusses the codes to be reported for a variety of specialty procedures and services in the medicine section (90281–99607) of the CPT code book. In some cases, the services listed in this section may be performed in conjunction with services or procedures listed in other sections of the code book. It may be appropriate to use multiple codes from the different sections to identify multiple services/procedures performed. For example, immunizations may be administered during an office visit for a young child. The medicine code for the immunization would be used in addition to the E/M code for the office visit.

Medicine Section Content and Structure

The medicine section includes codes for services that are primarily evaluative, diagnostic, and/or therapeutic in nature. Most of the codes in this section are for noninvasive procedures, although there are some exceptions to this. Some subsections, such as therapeutic or diagnostic injections, contain codes that are used by a wide range of specialties. Other subsections are very specific to a given specialty, such as ophthalmology. Many subsections have specific guidelines for the use of codes within that section.

Immunization Against Disease

An **immunization** (also called a vaccine or toxoid) is given prior to exposure to disease. Immune globulin (also called gamma globulin or immune serum) is given after a person is exposed to a disease to prevent infection. These two products work differently because of the body's immune response.

During the immunization process, the body recognizes a substance called an antigen as foreign. The body forms antibodies against the antigen to protect the body should the same substance be encountered again. On average, this process can take six to eight weeks. The concept of immunization involves injecting a small, relatively harmless amount of antigen into the body to start the immune response process, but not enough antigen to give the person the disease. When the antibodies are developed, the person is protected from that point forward.

Physicians have long known that antibodies obtained from one person can help protect another person. This is where immune globulin comes in. Immune globulin is composed of antibodies that have been manufactured by another person in response to a disease. The antibodies are obtained from an infected person's blood and then injected into the exposed individual. They provide immediate, short-term protection, just as though they were developed on their own. Immune globulin protection lasts for a short period of time, perhaps only two to four months. However, that time frame is sufficient to protect the patient from contracting the disease (Society for Clinical Coding 2003b).

Immune Globulins, Serum or Recombinant Products

The codes in the immune globulins subsection represent the immune globulin product only and must be reported in addition to the administration codes (96365–96368, 96372, 96374–96375), as appropriate.

Respiratory syncytial virus monoclonal antibody, recombinant, code 90378, is given to infants at risk for developing the virus. The infants are premature (born less than or equal to 35 weeks' gestation) and/or have chronic lung disease. Because there is no vaccine to help these infants develop immunity to RSV, they are given the recombinant monoclonal antibodies, one dose prior to the start of each RSV season and one dose every month during the RSV season (November through April), until they reach two years of age.

Immunization Administration for Vaccines/Toxoids

The codes in the immunization administration for vaccines/toxoids subsection are reported in addition to the code for the vaccine(s) or toxoid(s). Code 90471 is assigned for a single or combination vaccine/toxoid; code 90472 is assigned for each additional vaccine. These codes should be listed separately in addition to the code for the immunization. Codes 90473 and 90474 are used similarly for administration of intranasal or oral vaccines and are listed separately in addition to the code for the immunization.

Codes 90460–90461 describe immunization administration to patients through age 18 years via any route when the physician has counseled the patient/family regarding the vaccines. These two codes describe the work of vaccine administration based on the number of vaccines or toxoid components that are administered. (It should be noted that regardless of patient age, administration that is completed without physician face-to-face counseling should be reported using codes 90471–90474.)

A vaccine or toxoid component refers to each antigen in a vaccine that prevents disease(s) caused by one organism. Combination vaccines, such as 90707 Measles, Mumps, Rubella virus vaccine (MMR), live for subcutaneous use, contain multiple vaccine components. This code represents three components. Administration of this combination vaccine to a patient 18 years of age or younger when counseling has been provided by a physician would be coded as 90460 and 90461 × 2 (2 units).

Example: A 6-month-old receives the immunizations recommended by the Centers for Disease Control after the patient's parent receives counseling by the physician. Immunizations given were: Rotavirus, DTaP, Hepatitis B/Hib Combination, Inactivated Poliovirus, and Pneumococcal conjugate 13 valent.

Administration coding is 5 units of 90460 and 3 units of 90461 as described here:

Vaccine	Vaccine Code	Administration Code(s)
Rotavirus	90681	90460
Diphtheria, tetanus toxoids, acellular pertussis	90700	90460, 90461, 90461
Hepatitis B/Hemophilus influenza B	90748	90460, 90461
Poliovirus, inactivated	90713	90460
Pneumococcal conjugate 13 valent	90670	90460

Vaccines, Toxoids

The codes in the vaccines, toxoids subsection are assigned for the vaccine product only and must be reported in addition to the appropriate immunization administration codes.

To meet the reporting requirements of immunization registries, vaccine distribution programs, and reporting systems, the exact vaccine product administered needs to be reported. Multiple codes for a particular vaccine are provided in the CPT code book when the schedule differs for two or more products of the same vaccine type (for example, hepatitis A). Also, separate codes are available when the vaccine product is available in more than one chemical formulation, dosage, or route of administration. Many immunization codes are specific to age groups, for example, code 90657 for flu vaccine for 6 months to 35 months of age and code 90715 for Tdap for age 7 and older.

In the past several years, new immunizations have been introduced that combine vaccines in one injection to reduce the number of needle sticks required for the patient. An example of a combination immunization is code 90748, Hepatitis B and Haemophilus influenza Type b vaccine (HepB-Hib), for intramuscular use. In this case, only one code (one injection) should be reported, plus the code for the administration. When the physician uses two separate injections, one for the hepatitis B and one for the HIB, two codes should be reported.

When, in addition to the administrations code, the physician provides a service that warrants a separately identifiable E/M code, that code should be assigned in addition to the immunization product and the immunization administration code.

> **Example:** A 6-year-old established patient is seen in the physician's office for a DTaP immunization. The nurse evaluates the child's immunization history in comparison to the protocol, takes vital signs, and administers the immunization. Because the nurse provides an E/M service under the direction of a physician, the following codes are reported: 99211, 90700, and 90471.

It is important to both the reimbursement process and to public health reporting to have a CPT code in place when a vaccine is approved by the Food and Drug Administration (FDA) for use. Therefore, codes may be assigned when the vaccine is nearing the end of the approval process. The codes assigned to these vaccines are available for use as the industry prepares to use the vaccine. Codes for vaccines that are awaiting FDA approval are marked with a $\mathcal{N}$ symbol in the book and on the AMA website. These codes are listed in Appendix K of the CPT code book.

Psychiatry

Psychiatric services can be provided in any setting and the codes in this section are not setting-specific. Psychiatric diagnostic evaluations typically start the episode of psychiatric treatment. Code 90791 includes an integrated biopsychosocial assessment, including history, mental status, ordering of diagnostic studies, and recommendations. Code 90792 includes all these services and medical assessment, physical examination, prescription of necessary medications, and review and ordering of laboratory studies. Both services may include communication with family and other sources.

These codes may be reported more than once when separate diagnostic evaluations are conducted regarding the patient but with other informants, such as family members, guardians or significant others. When conducted with other informants, this service would be reported with the patient as the recipient, even though they were conducted with other individuals. In addition, codes 90791 and 90792 can be used for both diagnostic assessments and reassessments, are reported once per day, and are not reported on the same day as either E/M services or psychotherapy services.

Psychotherapy (codes 90832–90838) can be provided by a physician or other qualified healthcare professional and is the use of therapeutic communication to treat mental illness and behavioral disturbances. These services are provided face-to-face with the patient or family member as long as the patient is present for at least some of the service. Psychotherapy services provided with the family and without the patient present are reported with code 90846 for family psychotherapy.

Psychotherapy can be provided either without E/M services (codes 90832, 90834, and 90837) or with E/M services (codes 90833, 90836, and 90838). Psychotherapy with E/M service codes are add-on codes and must be reported with the E/M code that corresponds to the site of service. The timeframes listed in the psychotherapy codes should be interpreted as follows:

30 minutes = 16 to 37 minutes

45 minutes = 38 to 52 minutes

60 minutes = 53 or more minutes

Services of less than 16 minutes should not be reported with psychotherapy codes.

Example: A psychiatrist provided psychoanalysis along with E/M services in the office setting to an established patient. The office visit included an expanded problem-focused history, and an examination and medical decision making of low complexity. The following codes should be reported: 90845 and 99213.

Example: An established patient in a clinic receives individual psychotherapy for approximately 25 minutes. The physician also provides E/M services that include a problem focused history, problem-focused examination, and straightforward level of medical decision making. Codes 90833 and 99212 should be reported.

Psychiatric diagnostic evaluations and psychotherapy can be performed with interactive complexity, such as specific communication factors that complicate the delivery of communication with discordant or emotional family members, young or verbally underdeveloped or impaired patients, or those requiring an interpreter or language translator. Code 90785 is assigned as an add-on code when services are delivered in this manner. Interactive complexity requirements are met when one of four scenarios is present, as detailed in the coding notes found before code 90785 in the CPT code book. The interactive complexity code is not assigned with E/M codes when psychotherapy is not reported on the same day.

Psychotherapy for crisis is a special service provided for urgent assessment, psychotherapy, mobilization of resources to defuse the crisis, and implementation of interventions to minimize the potential for psychological trauma. The presenting problem in these cases is typically life threatening or complex and requires immediate attention; CPT code 90839 is assigned for the first 60 minutes of psychotherapy for crisis, and code 90840 is assigned as an add-on code for each additional 30 minutes of this service. Interactive complexity, code 90785, is not assigned with codes 90839 and 90840.

Other psychotherapy services involve psychoanalysis, family psychotherapy, group psychotherapy, narcosynthesis, therapeutic repetitive transcranial magnetic stimulation, electroconvulsive therapy, hypnotherapy, other evaluations of past psychiatric medical records, and pharmacologic management. Pharmacologic management includes prescription writing and review of medication(s) when performed with psychotherapy and is coded as an add-on code of 90863. It is reported with psychotherapy codes 90832, 90834, or 90837 and is not reported with the psychotherapy with E/M codes of 90833, 90836, and 90838 because the pharmacologic management is part of the E/M code that is assigned. According to the summer 1992 issue of *CPT Assistant*, narcosynthesis (90865) involves the administration of a medication that releases a patient's inhibitions and allows the patient to reveal information that had been difficult to discuss.

It should be noted that psychiatrists may choose to use any of the coding options at their discretion. They may choose from the 90785–90899 series, the E/M series, or any appropriate consultation code, if the requirements for consultation are met. It should also be noted that the 1997 Documentation Guidelines provide specific psychiatric exam criteria for use in this specialty area, which may be beneficial for reimbursement.

Biofeedback

In the biofeedback subsection, it should be noted that code 90901 is used for biofeedback training by any modality. Anorectal biofeedback training, including EMG and/or manometry, is coded using 90911. Biofeedback used in conjunction with individual psychophysiologic training is included in codes 90875 and 90876 and should not be coded separately.

Dialysis

The dialysis subsection describes services for hemodialysis, peritoneal dialysis, end-stage renal disease (ESRD), and miscellaneous dialysis procedures. Hemodialysis is defined as the process of removing metabolic waste products, toxins, and excess fluid from the blood. The coder should read the guidelines and code descriptors carefully in this section. It should be noted that E/M codes related to the ESRD that are rendered on a day when dialysis is performed, as well as all other patient care services that are rendered during the dialysis procedure, are included in the dialysis procedure. E/M services unrelated to the dialysis procedure that cannot be rendered during the dialysis session may be reported in addition to the procedure. The key to reporting E/M services in addition to dialysis is linking diagnoses to procedures on the CMS-1500 claim form. Documentation also must support the separate E/M service reported.

Within the ESRD services codes, there are three different groups of codes to describe these services. Codes 90951–90962 describe services provided in the outpatient setting for a full month. Codes 90963–90966 describe services provided for home dialysis for a full month. Codes 90967–90970 describe services provided for less than a full month and are coded per day. Codes 90951–90962 are grouped by age of the patient and further divided by the number of face-to-face physician visits performed per month. Codes 90963–90970 are subdivided by patient age. Codes for children up to 19 years of age include monitoring of the patient's nutrition, assessment of growth and development, and counseling.

Codes that describe daily services (90967–90970) can only be assigned when home dialysis is provided for less than a full month, when the patient is transient, when a partial month of services is provided with one or more visits but a complete assessment has not been done, when the patient was hospitalized before a complete assessment was furnished, when dialysis was stopped due to recovery or death, or when the patient has received a kidney transplant. The coding notes in this section provide examples to guide code selection.

The hemodialysis and peritoneal dialysis codes do not include the insertion or declotting of cannulas or catheters. These procedures are coded in the surgery section of the CPT code book. Codes describing development of a shunt, cannula, or fistula for hemodialysis also are found in the surgery section.

Dialysis is broken down further to describe the type: hemodialysis versus miscellaneous dialysis procedures.

> **Example:** Patient with renal failure is seen in the outpatient dialysis clinic for hemodialysis with evaluation of his renal condition by his physician. The following CPT code is assigned: 90935, Hemodialysis procedure with single physician evaluation.

Codes 90935 and 90937 are reported to identify the physician service(s) provided on the day of hemodialysis. Code 90935 is reported when the physician provides a single evaluation of the patient during the hemodialysis, and code 90937 is reported when the physician is required to evaluate the patient more than once during the procedure.

Peritoneal dialysis involves the insertion of a catheter into the abdominal cavity and the infusion of a fluid (dialysate) into the peritoneum that allows for diffusion between the dialyzing fluid and the body fluids containing the waste products. The fluid containing the waste products then is removed from the peritoneum through the catheter. Codes 90945 and 90947 are reported to identify the physician service(s) provided on the day of peritoneal dialysis. Code 90945 is reported when the physician provides a single evaluation of the patient during the peritoneal dialysis or other dialysis other than hemodialysis, and code 90947 is reported when the physician is required to evaluate the patient more than once during the dialysis procedure.

Home visit hemodialysis performed by a nonphysician healthcare professional is coded in the home visit procedures and services section with CPT code 99512.

Gastroenterology

The gastroenterology subsection includes codes for reporting nonsurgical gastroenterologic procedures, including a variety of esophageal and other intestinal studies. Motility studies are coded in this section. Codes 91010 and 91013 describe esophageal motility studies. Codes 91020 and 91022 describe gastric and duodenal motility studies, respectively. Code 91117 describes a colon motility study of a minimum of 6 hours of continuous reading. Codes for gastric intubation are found in the Digestive System subsection of the Surgery section of the CPT book.

Ophthalmology

The ophthalmology subsection includes general ophthalmological services, special ophthalmological services, contact lens services, and spectacles services. This subsection is unique because it is the only one in the CPT code book that has its own visit codes, similar to E/M visit codes, found under general ophthalmological services. To ensure correct reporting, the coder should review the definitions of the ophthalmology services, noting what is included in each level of service.

The general ophthalmologic E/M codes are subdivided by patient status—new or established. The definition is similar to the standard E/M code definition: A new patient is one who has not received any professional services from the physician, or another physician in the same specialty who belongs to the same group practice, within the past three years.

The complete definitions and examples provided in the CPT code book should be noted for intermediate and comprehensive ophthalmological services. Following is a summary of each:

- Intermediate services involve the evaluation of a new or existing condition complicated with a new diagnostic or management problem and include a history, general medical observation, external ocular and adnexal examination, and other diagnostic procedures, as indicated.

- Comprehensive services involve a general evaluation of the complete visual system and include a history, general medical observation, an external and ophthalmoscopic examination, gross visual fields, and a basic sensorimotor examination. Initiation of diagnostic and treatment programs is always part of a comprehensive service.

It should be noted that ophthalmologists may choose to use any of the coding options at their discretion. They may choose from the 92002–92014 series, the 99201–99215 series or any appropriate consultation code, if the requirements for consultation are met. It should also be noted that the 1997 Documentation Guidelines provide specific eye exam criteria for use in this specialty area, which may be beneficial for reimbursement.

This section also provides codes for examination under anesthesia. An ophthalmological examination performed under general anesthesia is coded to 92018 for a complete exam and 92019 for a limited exam.

When a gonioscopy with medical diagnostic evaluation is performed as a separate procedure, code 92020 should be assigned. When it is performed as part of a larger procedure, it may not be appropriate to report it separately.

Code 92025 for computerized corneal topography (CCT) is reported only when the special computerized equipment is used. Manual keratoscopy is included in the ophthalmologic service codes or single system exam in the E/M code. CCT is a three-dimensional imaging process used to map the surface power of the cornea. It is used for initial diagnosis of disease (such as keratoconus), evaluation of the progression of disease (such as pterygium) or for planning surgical intervention (such as astigmatism correction). It is also used to correctly fit rigid, gas permeable contact lenses. Code 92025 may not be reported with 65710–65771.

Special ophthalmological services include a specific evaluation of part of the visual system or special treatment that goes beyond the general ophthalmological services described above. Special services may be reported in addition to general ophthalmologic services or E/M visit codes.

HCPCS provides two codes for glaucoma screening of high-risk patients: code G0117— an optometrist or ophthalmologist performs the screening, and code G0118—the screening is performed under the supervision of an optometrist or ophthalmologist. The coder also should reference codes S0800–S0812 for various corneal procedures.

One common coding error occurs when the coder reports ophthalmoscopy when general or special ophthalmologic services are performed. The guideline under ophthalmoscopy states: "Routine ophthalmoscopy is part of general and special ophthalmologic services whenever indicated. It is a nonitemized service and is not reported separately."

Codes 92225 and 92226 are used to report extended ophthalmoscopy with retinal drawing, for example, retinal detachment.

Contact lens service is not part of the general ophthalmological services. However, follow-up of successfully fitted extended-wear lenses is reported as part of a general ophthalmological service. The prescription of spectacles, if necessary, is considered a part of code 92015, Determination of refractive state. However, fitting of the spectacles is a separately reportable service. This includes measurements, laboratory specifications, and final adjustments. The physician need not be present for this code to be reported.

The supply of materials such as an ocular prostheses, contact lenses, or spectacles is considered a separate service and should be reported using HCPCS Level II V codes.

> **Example:** An established patient is seen in his ophthalmologist's office complaining of loss of vision and some pain. A history is obtained, and a complete visual system examination is performed. Ophthalmoscopic and basic sensorimotor examinations and a gross visual fields exam are conducted, with initiation of the appropriate treatment. The following code is assigned: 92014.

> **Example:** A patient is seen for a prescription, a fitting, and a supply of a plastic custom artificial eye, with medical supervision of adaptation. The following code is assigned: V2623 (*CPT Assistant* December 2005).

Special Otorhinolaryngologic Services

E/M service codes are used to report diagnostic or treatment procedures usually included in a comprehensive otorhinolaryngologic evaluation or office visit, such as otoscopy, anterior rhinoscopy, tuning fork test, and removal of impacted cerumen. Special diagnostic and treatment services, such as laryngeal function studies or nasal function studies, usually not included in a comprehensive otorhinolaryngologic evaluation or office visit, are reported separately using codes from 92502–92700.

The subsections include:

- Vestibular function tests, with observation and evaluation by physician, without electrical recording

- Vestibular function tests, with recording and medical diagnostic evaluation

- Audiologic function tests, with medical diagnostic evaluation

- Evaluative and therapeutic services

All services include a medical diagnostic evaluation. Some technical procedures may not be performed personally by the physician; this is allowable for reporting.

Audiologic function tests are performed using calibrated equipment. All codes include the testing of both ears. If only one ear is tested, modifier –52, Reduced Services, is used.

Coders should note that code 92559 refers to an audiometric testing of groups. Additional codes to identify the specific test(s) may be assigned. All other codes for this subsection refer to individual testing.

Cardiovascular

The cardiovascular subsection includes codes for diagnostic procedures such as electrocardiograms (ECGs) and cardiac catheterizations as well as for therapeutic procedures such as percutaneous transluminal coronary angioplasty (PTCA).

Careful reading of the notes in this section is necessary to assign correct and complete codes. In addition, coders should note the cross-references used throughout the cardiovascular subsection.

Coronary Therapeutic Services and Procedures

Codes 92920–92944 describe revascularization procedures performed on the coronary arteries to treat occlusion. A hierarchy for complexity of services exists for coding percutaneous coronary interventions (PCI). The most complex procedure performed on a cardiac vessel is to place a stent into that vessel. The next most complex procedure is atherectomy on a coronary vessel, and the least complex procedure is percutaneous transluminal coronary balloon angioplasty (PTCA).

This section is designed with base codes that describe the intervention in the major coronary artery and add-on codes to describe that same intervention in additional branches of a major coronary artery. The PCI base code that includes the most intensive service provided for the target vessel should be reported. One base code is reported per vessel, and add-on codes are reported to describe interventions in additional branches of that same vessel. Treatment of bifurcation lesions would be coded as one base code and one add-on code.

These codes include the actual intervention performed as well as the work of accessing and selectively catheterizing the vessel; transversing the lesion, radiological supervision, and interpretation directly related to the intervention(s) performed, embolic protection, if used; closure of the arteriotomy by any method; and imaging performed to document completion of the intervention (AMA 2015). Diagnostic coronary angiography codes and injection codes should not be reported with PCI codes for contrast injections, roadmapping, vessel measurement, or post-PCI angiography. Diagnostic angiography at the same session as the PCI can be reported separately if no prior catheter-based angiography is available, if the patient's condition has changed since the prior study, or if there is inadequate visualization of the anatomy.

Example 1: Percutaneous transluminal coronary balloon angioplasty involving three major coronary arteries, the left main, left circumflex, and the right. Code 92920 should be reported three times, one base code for each target vessel.

Example 2: Percutaneous transluminal coronary balloon angioplasty of the right coronary artery and then stent placement at the site of the blockage. The following code should be reported: 92928.

Example 3: Percutaneous transluminal coronary balloon angioplasty of the left anterior descending artery and percutaneous transluminal coronary angioplasty of the left diagonal branch were performed. The following codes should be reported: 92920 and 92921.

In addition to the PCI codes being arranged in the hierarchy of interventions, there can be more than one base code at the same weight in the hierarchy. For descriptive purposes here, the hierarchy levels will be called tiers. Table 7.1 shows the four tiers of hierarchy with three codes composing the first tier. Code 92933 is the combination intervention of atherectomy with stent and angioplasty. Codes 92941 for treatment of an acute blockage and 92943 for treatment of a chronic total blockage are at the same weight as the combination intervention described in code 92933. The second tier is atherectomy with angioplasty or code 92924. The third tier is code 92928 for a stent with angioplasty or an intervention performed through a bypass graft, code 92937. The lowest tier is code 92920 or a coronary angioplasty without any other intervention. Table 7.1 also shows the available add-on codes for each base code. Note that reporting of the add-on codes also observes the same type of hierarchy as is used in the reporting of base codes. The add-on codes are displayed in hierarchical order. Table 7.2 displays the major coronary arteries and their recognized branches for use when coding PCI procedures in CPT.

Table 7.1. Percutaneous Coronary Intervention Hierarchy

Hierarchy Tier	Base Code (First vessel)	Brief Description	Add-on Codes in Hierarchical Order
I	92943	Chronic total occlusion (CTO), any PCI, single vessel	92944, 92934, 92925, 92929, 92921
	92941	Acute total/subtotal occlusion during MI, any PCI, single vessel	
	92933	Atherectomy with stent and angioplasty, single artery or branch	
II	92924	Atherectomy with angioplasty, single artery or branch	92944, 92925, 92921
III	92928	Stent with angioplasty, single artery or branch	92944, 92925, 92929, 92921
	92937	Through graft, any combination of stent, atherectomy or angioplasty, single vessel	92938 or 92944, 92934, 92925, 92929, 92921
IV	92920	Angioplasty, single artery or branch	92921

Table 7.2. Major Coronary Arteries and Their Recognized Branches

Major Coronary Arteries (Base Code)	Recognized Branches
Left Main (LCA or LMCA)	None
Left Circumflex (LC or LCX)	Two **obtuse marginal** branches
Left Anterior Descending (LAD)	Two **diagonal** branches
Right (RCA)	**Posterior descending** and **posterolateral** branches
Ramus Intermedius (RI)	None

Atherectomy involves debulking fat buildup along the walls of a vessel and is coded within the hierarchy of interventions. Mechanical thrombectomy involves removing clotted material from the lumen of a vessel and can be reported separately using code 92973. Other procedures that are separately reportable are brachytherapy (92974), intravascular ultrasound (92978 and 92979), and intravascular Doppler (93571 and 93572). Intravascular ultrasound codes include both diagnostic evaluation and therapeutic intervention. Intravascular ultrasound services include all transducer manipulations and repositioning within the vessel being examined, both before and after the intervention.

In reporting therapeutic services, several codes in the cardiovascular section are often misinterpreted or coded incorrectly. It should be noted that code 92950, Cardiopulmonary resuscitation, is not included in critical care services. When cardiopulmonary resuscitation is performed in addition to critical care services, both codes may be reported. Conversely, code 92953, Temporary transcutaneous pacing, is considered part of critical care and is *not* reported separately.

Code 92961 is used to report internal elective electrical cardioversion of arrhythmia. This code should not be assigned when cardioversion is performed with intraoperative pacing, EP studies, or analysis of cardioverter-defibrillator pacing because cardioversion is an integral part of these procedures. Carefully review the parenthetical note below this code regarding reporting instructions.

When coding coronary thrombolysis (92975–92977), the coder must identify the type of infusion: intracoronary or intravenous. Thrombolysis of other vessels is coded in the surgery and radiology sections of the CPT code book.

Cardiography and Cardiovascular Monitoring Services

The cardiography subsection includes codes describing electrocardiograms (ECG or EKG).

For cardiography procedures, it is important to know what services the physician performed and whether the physician used his or her own equipment. For example, if the physician interpreted the results of a 12-lead electrocardiogram and dictated a report, only code 93010 should be reported. If, however, the 12-lead electrocardiogram was performed on the physician's equipment using the practice's technician and the physician performed the test, interpreted the results, and dictated a written report, code 93000 is appropriate. This same concept is true when coding other procedures in this section, such as stress tests and Holter monitors in the Cardiovascular monitoring section.

Cardiovascular monitoring is a group of medical procedures using in-person and remote technology to monitor cardiovascular rhythm data. These technologies include Holter monitors, mobile cardiac telemetry, and event monitoring devices. Holter monitors provide monitoring over a period of up to 48 hours, with the typical testing period being approximately 24 hours. Therefore, if two 24-hour periods are recorded, codes from 93224–93227 are only reported once, because the code describes a period of up to 48 hours.

Implantable and Wearable Device Evaluations

Cardiovascular device monitoring assesses device therapy and cardiovascular physiologic data using in-person and remote technology. Device evaluations coded with codes 93279 through 93292 are coded per procedure that is performed. Pacemaker evaluation via telephone (93293) and pacemaker interrogation (93294–93296) are coded once per 90 days and not if less than 30 days. Interrogation of implantable systems (93297–93299) are to be reported once per 30 days and not if less than 10 days.

The coding notes in this section are extensive and contain thorough definitions of the terms used in this section.

Echocardiography

Echocardiography includes obtaining the ultrasound of the heart and great arteries, with two-dimensional image and color Doppler ultrasounds, and the interpretation and report. The proper coding of an echocardiography procedure often requires multiple codes from this subsection.

Code 93318 is used for echocardiography, transesophageal (TEE) for monitoring purposes, including probe placement, real-time two-dimensional image acquisition and interpretation leading to ongoing (continuous) assessment of (dynamically changing) cardiac pumping function and to therapeutic measures on an immediate time basis. This code should be used when interpretation and therapeutic measures are needed on an immediate time basis.

When interpretation is performed separately from the performance of the procedure, modifier –26, Professional Component, should be appended to the appropriate code.

Cardiac Catheterization

Cardiac catheterizations are diagnostic procedures that include the following:

- Introduction, positioning, and repositioning of catheter(s)

- Recording of intracardiac and intravascular pressure

- Final evaluation and report of procedure

Induction dilution studies (codes 93561 and 93562) are not to be used with the cardiac catheterization codes. These are assigned only when performed as a separate procedure.

Before reporting cardiac catheterization codes, the coder should review the guidelines carefully, noting what is included in the cardiac catheterization procedure and when selective injection procedures should be reported. The entire procedure report should be reviewed to determine the exact heart catheterization performed and what injection procedures were performed in conjunction with it.

Only one code is needed to correctly code most cardiac catheterization procedures performed on a heart that does not have congenital anomalies. (For coding purposes, anomalous coronary arteries, patient foramen ovale, mitral valve prolapse, and bicuspid aortic valve are to be reported as if they did not include congenital anomalies.) This combination code includes the following:

- Catheter placement

- One or more injection(s)

- The imaging supervision and interpretation

Additional codes may be required when other procedures are performed, such as right heart injection procedures, supravalvular aortography, pulmonary angiography, pharmacologic agent administration, or physiologic exercise studies.

The cardiac catheter placement codes (93530–93533) describe the insertion of catheters into the arteries, veins, or chambers of the heart. These procedures include the introduction, positioning, and repositioning of the catheters as well as the recording of the intracardiac and intravascular pressures, the collection of blood samples to measure blood gases and/or dye or other dilution curves, and the measurement of cardiac output.

A right heart catheterization is usually performed by the physician introducing the catheter into the venous system of the patient's body. The catheter is then guided through the venous system into the right atrium, right ventricle, pulmonary artery, and pulmonary wedge positions.

A left heart catheterization is usually performed by the physician introducing the catheter into the arterial system of the patient's body. The catheter is then advanced through the arterial system into the left ventricle of the heart. If the physician does not place the catheter across the aortic valve into the left ventricle and perform a pressure measurement, a left cardiac catheterization has not been performed (ZHealth 2005).

When coronary artery, arterial coronary conduit, or venous bypass graft angiography is performed without concomitant left heart cardiac catheterization, code 93454 should be used.

Codes 93451–93568 include injections and imaging procedures which are performed in the left ventricle and coronary artery bypass graft(s) (internal mammary, free arterial, or venous graft). Any injections performed to image the left or right atrium, right ventricle, supravalvular aortography, or pulmonary angiography are reported separately using codes 93565–93568.

Catheterization of a heart that has congenital defect(s) is coded differently. Codes 93530–93533 are used for this catheterization. When contrast injection(s) are performed in conjunction with cardiac catheterization for congenital anomalies, use codes 93563–93568 in addition to the primary code. Imaging supervision, interpretation, and report are included in codes 93530–93533. There is a series of tables in CPT following code 93572 that detail the heart catheterization codes and the applicable additional codes that can be assigned.

Intracardiac Electrophysiologic Procedures/Studies

Intracardiac electrophysiological procedures (EPs) may be diagnostic or therapeutic, and include the insertion and repositioning of catheters. Electrophysiologic testing is performed on patients with cardiac arrhythmias, causing palpitations, near syncope, or syncope with cardiac arrest. EP procedure codes include EP evaluation of single- or dual-chamber pacing cardioverter-defibrillators and implantable loop recorders.

Codes 93600–93612 include diagnostic EPs that provide only recording and pacing from a single site. Codes 93619–93622 describe a comprehensive electrophysiologic evaluation that may be reported when recording and pacing are performed from multiple sites.

Code 93662, Intracardiac echocardiography during therapeutic/diagnostic intervention, including imaging supervision and interpretation, should not be reported with 92961, Cardioversion, elective, electrical conversion of arrhythmia; internal. It is listed in addition to the primary procedure performed.

CPT directs the coder that modifier –51 should not be appended to 93600–93603, 93610, 93612, 93615–93618, and 93631.

Noninvasive Vascular Diagnostic Studies

The procedures in the noninvasive vascular diagnostic studies subsection include cerebrovascular arterial studies, extremity arterial and venous studies, and visceral and penile vascular studies. Handheld Doppler devices (such as those used in the emergency department) are considered part of the vascular system physical examination and, as such, are not reported separately.

The codes in this section include the patient care required to perform the studies, supervision, and interpretation of the results. This includes hard-copy output with analysis of all data, including bidirectional vascular flow or imaging when provided. If the device used does not produce hard-copy output or the record does not permit analysis of bidirectional flow, the study is considered part of the physical exam of the vascular system and is not reported separately.

A duplex scan is defined by the CPT code book to be an ultrasonic scanning procedure with display of both two-dimensional structure and motion with time and color Doppler ultrasonic signal documentation with spectral analysis and/or color flow velocity mapping or imaging.

Pulmonary

Procedures and services described in the pulmonary subsection include laboratory procedures and interpretation of test results. Spirometry is the measurement of lung function, including the amount and/or speed of air that can be inhaled and exhaled. This test can be performed with or without treatment with bronchodilating medication. It should be noted that codes 94011–94013 are a highly specialized form of spirometry, performed on an infant through the age of two years under sedation, and are not the same services described in codes 94010, 94060, and 94070 simply performed on a child younger than age two.

In coding ventilator management, separate codes exist for the first day (94002) and subsequent days (94003) for patients in the inpatient or observation setting. Code 94004 is used for ventilator management in a nursing facility, and code 94005 describes care plan oversight for home ventilator management during a calendar month.

Nebulizer treatment is coded as 94640, Pressurized or nonpressurized inhalation treatment for acute airway obstruction for therapeutic purposes and/or for diagnostic purposes. A HCPCS Level II J code also should be used with nebulizer treatments for the medication administered through the nebulizer, such as Albuterol. Code 94664 should be assigned for demonstration and/or evaluation of patient utilization of an aerosol generator, nebulizer, metered dose inhaler, or intermittent positive pressure breathing (IPPB) device. Continuous nebulizer treatment is coded as 94644. Code 94669 describes the use of mechanical chest wall oscillation using an externally-worn vest to help clear secretions from the lungs of a patient who has suffered chest wall trauma or has chronic lung disease such as cystic fibrosis or emphysema

Noninvasive pulse oximetry to determine oxygen saturation (for diagnosis of airway function) is coded as 94760. Payment for pulse oximetry in addition to an E/M service varies by payer.

Allergy and Clinical Immunology

The allergy and clinical immunology subsection includes allergy sensitivity testing and allergen immunotherapy for desensitization or hyposensitization.

Allergy Testing

Allergy testing codes are divided according to type of test. The most commonly used codes are

95004–95024	Percutaneous testing (scratch, puncture, prick) or Intradermal testing, immediate reaction (intracutaneous)
95027	Intracutaneous (intradermal) tests, sequential and incremental, with allergenic extracts for airborne allergens, immediate type reaction
95028	Intradermal testing, delayed reaction
95044	Patch or application testing
95070	Inhalation bronchial challenge testing (inhale drugs or antigens)
95076	Ingestion challenge testing (ingest food or drugs); initial 120 minutes of testing

The number of tests performed is reported in the units box in item 24G on the CMS-1500 claim form. (A copy of the CMS-1500 form and directions to the instructions are in online appendix G.) For example, if five percutaneous scratch tests with allergenic extracts were performed, code 95004 would be reported with five units listed in box 24G of the CMS-1500

273

form. The fee for skin testing should be set for an individual test. The billing software will multiply the per test fee by the number of tests performed to provide the total fee.

According to *CPT Assistant* (September 2001), code 95076, Ingestion challenge test, is the notable exception to reporting codes for the number of tests performed. Code 95076–95079 are reported based on time, regardless of the number of items tested.

Inhalation bronchial challenge testing does not include the additional pulmonary testing required to determine the effect of the inhalation. These services should be coded separately.

Allergen Immunotherapy

Immunotherapy (desensitization or hyposensitization) is the parenteral administration of allergenic extracts as antigens at periodic intervals, usually on an increasing dosage scale to reach a maintenance therapy dose level. The process of allergy immunotherapy contains two parts: preparation/provision of the allergenic extract and the actual injection of the extract. CPT provides three sets of codes to describe these processes.

There are two scenarios that describe immunotherapy:

- Scenario #1 occurs like this: After testing, the allergist prepares and provides allergenic extracts in either single- or multidose vials to begin desensitization (95144–95170). The allergenic extract vials are given or sent to the patient's primary care physician, who administers the injections based on the prescribed schedule from the allergist (95115–95117).

- Scenario #2 occurs like this: After testing, the allergist prepares and provides allergenic extracts for the patient and then administers the injections in the allergist's office based on the prescribed schedule (95120–95134).

Provision of allergenic extracts is coded based on the type of allergen being used. Separate codes are available for stinging insect venom and for whole body extract of biting insect or other arthropod (where the entire body of the insect is ground up and administered). The remaining codes are not specific to type of allergen and are generic. They can be used for any allergen.

Dust mites are a common allergen, and coding for provision of their allergen causes coding questions. *CPT Assistant* (April 2001) states that code 95170 "may appear to be the most obvious choice, as the dust mite is technically an arthropod, albeit not a biting insect. Since the allergen is not to the body of the dust mite (and it does not bite), but rather to the mite feces, code 95165 most accurately describes this type of allergen immunotherapy." Additional information is provided in *CPT Assistant* June 2005, 9.

When the code description states "specify number of vials," the units box on the claim form should state the number of doses created. A dose is defined in CPT as "the amount of antigen(s) administered in a single injection from a multiple dose vial."

Office visits may be reported in addition to the immunotherapy *only* when other identifiable services are provided at the same time. These services should be documented clearly to support that they are not related to the immunotherapy. For example, treatment of usual symptoms caused by allergies should not be reported separately, but treatment of an allergy-induced asthma attack requiring a nebulizer treatment would be coded separately.

Endocrinology

Code 95250 is reported for glucose monitoring for up to 72 hours by continuous recording and storage of glucose values from interstitial tissue fluid via a subcutaneous sensor. This code includes the hookup, calibration, patient initiation, training and recording, disconnection, and downloading with printout of data. Code 95251 is separately reported for the physician's interpretation and written report.

Neurology and Neuromuscular Procedures

This group of codes describes various electrodiagnostic medicine (EDX) studies. *CPT Assistant* (April 2002) describes EDX testing as testing "used to evaluate the integrity and function of the peripheral nervous system (most cranial nerves, spinal roots, plexi and nerves), neuromuscular junctions (NMJ), muscles, and the central nervous system (brain and spinal cord)." This testing can identify normal and abnormal areas, define the severity of abnormalities and aid in diagnosis and treatment decisions. This subsection includes sleep testing, electroencephalography (EEG), electromyography (EMG), nerve conduction studies (NCS), and neurostimulator analysis and programming. Sleep-testing codes are used to report sleep studies that are recorded unattended. Polysomnographies are coded based on the number of sleep parameters monitored and are always attended by a technologist.

In this subsection, component billing must be used if the interpreting physician does not own the equipment. Modifier –TC is attached to the code for the actual testing to create the tracing. Modifier –26 is attached to the code for the interpretation of the tracing. Normally, the muscle-testing, EMG, and nerve conduction studies are completed and interpreted as one procedure. Component billing is not required. It also should be noted that modifier –51, Multiple Procedures, does not apply to nerve conduction studies performed on multiple nerves.

The coding in this subsection is complex. Appendix J of the CPT code book provides information on electrodiagnostic medicine, including a listing of sensory, motor, and mixed nerves and their associated CPT codes (95907–95913). Electromyography is coded with 95860–95864 and 95867–95870 when no nerve conduction studies (95907–95913) are performed on the same day. Codes 95885–95887 are used for EMG services when nerve conduction studies are performed with the EMG studies on the same day.

A single nerve conduction study is defined as a sensory conduction test, a motor conduction test with or without an F wave test, or an H-reflex test. Each of these four studies (sensory, motor conduction with or without an F wave test and an H-reflex) on each nerve is considered one study when determining the number of studies to be coded with 95907–95913. Use 95885–95887 in conjunction with 95907–95913 when EMG and nerve conduction studies are performed together.

Codes 95940 and 95941 are add-on codes to report intraoperative neurophysiology testing. Code 95940 is used to code each 15 minutes of monitoring requiring personal attendance, and 95941 is used to code each hour of monitoring when performed from outside the operating room or when multiple cases are simultaneously monitored. These codes are reported in addition to other codes in this section.

Neurostimulators are classified according to whether *simple* or *complex* systems were used; whether the brain, spinal cord, and peripheral nerves or the cranial nerves were involved; whether reprogramming was performed; and how much time was required for the analysis or programming. The actual insertion or removal of the neurostimulator pulse generator is coded in the neurology subsection of the surgery section of the CPT code book.

Motion analysis codes (96000–96004) describe services performed for patients with complex movement problems, such as cerebral palsy, spina bifida, and stroke. This analysis is performed in a dedicated motion analysis laboratory.

Central Nervous System Assessments/Tests

Codes 96101–96127 are used to report the services involved in assessing the cognitive functioning of the central nervous system, including the testing of cognitive processes, visual motor responses, and abstractive abilities. Such testing is accomplished by the administration of a combination of testing procedures, and the codes include interpretation and reporting of test results. For specific therapy to develop cognitive skills, codes 97532–97533 are assigned.

Developmental services are coded with two codes, 96110 and 96111. Code 96110 is for developmental screening, such as the Developmental Screening Test II or the Early Language Milestone Screen. Office staff normally perform these tests. The testing code, code 96111, is normally performed by the physician using a variety of tools such as the Bayley Scales or the Woodcock-Johnson tests. When performed at the time of an E/M service, the E/M code would require a –25 modifier (American Academy of Pediatrics 2009). Code 96127 is used to code brief emotional or behavioral assessments such as those done for depression or attention deficit hyperactivity disorder.

Health and Behavior Assessment/Intervention

The codes in the health and behavior assessment/intervention subsection are to be reported when the assessment is focused on the biopsychosocial factors important to physical health problems and treatments. The patient requires psychiatric services but does not have a mental health diagnosis. These services are normally provided by a clinical psychologist or other non-physician practitioner. For health and behavior assessment and/or intervention performed by a physician, refer to the E/M or Preventive Medicine codes that are appropriate for the service provided. An evaluation and management service should not be reported on the same day when codes 96150–96155 are reported.

Hydration, Therapeutic, Prophylactic, Diagnostic Injections and Infusions, and Chemotherapy and Other Highly Complex Drug or Highly Complex Biologic Agent Administration

The codes in this subsection should be reported to describe injections and intravenous infusions requiring the presence or direct supervision of the physician. Many of the codes are assigned based on time. Documentation should include both the start and stop time of administration.

Hydration

These codes are used to describe administration of fluids, such as normal saline or D5W, without the addition of drugs or other substances. Code 96360 is used to report the first one hour of infusion, and code 96361 is added for each additional one hour. When hydration services are provided, the J code for the fluids administered is coded as the administered medication. For example, IV hydration with 1,000 mL of D5W administered over two hours is coded as 96360, 96361, and J7070.

Code 96361 can also be used to describe hydration given as a secondary or subsequent service after a different initial service.

Therapeutic, Prophylactic, or Diagnostic Injections and Infusions

This section covers intravenous infusions, additional sequential infusions, concurrent infusions and injections using the methods of subcutaneous, intramuscular, intra-arterial, and intravenous injections for diagnostic and/or therapeutic purposes. These codes should not be used for allergen immunotherapy injections. Code 96365 is reported for an initial infusion for a period of up to one hour. When the IV infusion is greater than one hour, code 96365 is used for the first hour and code 96366 is used for each additional hour. For example, if an IV infusion lasts three hours and 10 minutes, code 96365 is reported for the first hour and code 96366 is reported twice, once each for the second and third hours. No additional code is reported for the 10-minute interval because it has not met the requirement of greater than 30 minutes beyond the one hour increment. The advice under the code states that 96366 may be reported for infusions of greater than 30 minutes beyond the one hour. Infusions of this type may be referred to as "drip" and must list the length of time administered in the documentation.

When the physician furnishes the intravenous drug and supplies, additional codes are reported. The drugs and supplies should be reported using HCPCS Level II National Codes. The coder should review the specific payer manual to determine how to report these injections to different insurance plans.

Many medications in the J code series of HCPCS are listed in milligrams (mg) or in cubic centimeters (cc). It is important to remember that in metric equivalents, one cc equals one mL. The coder should become familiar with the medications that are provided by the physician practice. Brand names of drugs are not normally found in the HCPCS Index, and therefore coders should refer to a drug reference book to cross-reference to the generic name.

> **Example:** A patient receives 1 g of Vancomycin HCl for 2 hours. The following codes are reported: 96365, 96366, J3370, and J3370.

CPT describes sequential infusions and concurrent infusions separately from initial infusions. Some patients receive multiple drugs over a period of time and in various combinations.

Codes 96365–96366 describe the initial infusion. Once that infusion is complete, another infusion can take place through the same IV access site, called a sequential infusion. This is coded using 96367. Code 96367 should be reported in conjunction with 96365, 96374, 96409, or 96413 if provided as a secondary or subsequent service after a different initial service is administered through the same IV access. Code 96367 should be reported only once per sequential infusion of the same infusate mix.

Concurrent infusions take place at the same time as other infusions (through a different IV access site). Code 96368, an add-on code to describe any concurrent infusion, can only be coded once per encounter and can be used with 96365 and the chemotherapy infusion codes.

The prolonged service codes (99354–99357) may not be reported with this therapeutic or diagnostic injections and infusion series of codes.

Third-party payer policies vary regarding what codes and code types can be reported. The coder should check the third-party payment policies before reporting these codes.

When additional services are performed at the time of an injection, they should be reported separately. For example, if a patient receives an intramuscular (IM) penicillin injection during an established patient office visit, code 96372 is used for the IM injection, a HCPCS code is reported for the drug, and the appropriate E/M code from 99201–99215 is reported for the office visit. It should be noted that some health plans bundle the administration of injections into the E/M service.

Example: A patient is seen in the physician's office for intramuscular injection of 20 mg of Depo-Medrol without any other E/M service. The following codes are assigned:

96372, Therapeutic, prophylactic or diagnostic injection (specify substance or drug); subcutaneous or intramuscular

J1020, Injection of Methylprednisolone acetate (Depo-Medrol), 20 mg

Codes 96374–96375, Therapeutic, prophylactic, or diagnostic injection; intravenous push, single or initial substance/drug, are different from codes 96365–96368 because time is not indicated in the code description. This code is not to be used when the physician simply fails to list the time in the documentation. However, it is to be used when the documentation lists an IV push procedure or where it describes a procedure in which the IV line is inserted, the medication is administered over a short period of time (15 minutes or less), and the IV line is removed. Codes 96360–96379 should not be reported by the physician in the facility setting.

Chemotherapy Administration

The chemotherapy administration subsection is used to report the administration of antineoplastic drugs and certain other treatments for specific diseases. The administration codes are subdivided to describe the method of administration and the type of technique: subcutaneous or intramuscular, intralesional, push intravenous, infusion intravenous, push intra-arterial; infusion intra-arterial, use of a portable or implantable pump, and/or length of time for administration. Separate codes may be reported when more than one technique is used to administer the chemotherapy. Codes 96440–96450 describe the administration of chemotherapy to specific body sites: pleural or peritoneal cavity, or central nervous system. Codes 96521 and 96522 describe the maintenance and refilling of portable or implantable pumps or reservoirs.

Preparation of the chemotherapy agent is included in these codes. Provision of the actual chemotherapy drug is reported separately, using HCPCS Level II J codes, normally found between J9000 and J9999.

Example: Chemotherapy administered via intravenous infusion technique (45 minutes). Chemotherapy agent (Cisplatin solution, 10 mg) was provided by the physician's office. The following codes are assigned: 96413 and J9060.

Codes in this section are similar in use to those in the therapeutic or diagnostic injections and infusions section. Refer to the previous section on injection and infusion codes, 96360–96379 for an additional discussion, as well as the reporting guidelines under 96401–96549.

The CPT guidelines clarify when E/M services codes can be reported in addition to chemotherapy administration and when additional medications can be coded. The guidelines should be reviewed carefully. The coder also should note that surgical procedures performed to place catheters, pumps, or reservoirs may be reported from the surgery section of the CPT code book.

Regional chemotherapy infusion is reported using the codes for chemotherapy administration, intra-arterial (96420–96425). Actual placement of the intra-arterial catheter is reported using a code from the surgery section. Separate codes are assigned for each parenteral method used when chemotherapy is administered by different techniques.

If medications are administered before or after chemotherapy, they are reported separately using HCPCS Level II J codes and the appropriate administration code from the 96360–96379 series. Codes 96401–96402, 96409–96425, and 96521–96523 are not intended to be reported by the physician in the facility setting.

Photodynamic Therapy

Code 96567 is reported when photodynamic therapy is administered to destroy premalignant and/or malignant lesions of the skin, such as nonhyperkeratotic actinic keratosis lesions. Codes 96570–96571 in the photodynamic therapy subsection are add-on codes to the endoscopy codes for bronchoscopy (31641) and esophagoscopy (43229). Code 96570 is used to report the first 30 minutes of endoscopic photodynamic tissue ablation; code 96571 is reported once for each additional 15 minutes of treatment.

Special Dermatological Procedures

Photochemotherapy is found in the special dermatological procedures subsection. Photochemotherapy involves the administration of oral medication followed by treatment of the skin with long-wave ultraviolet light while the patient is seated or lying in a treatment booth. The most popular method of photochemotherapy provided in a physician's office is the PUVA (psoralens and ultraviolet A) treatment. Combination treatments also may be provided and can be coded in this area of the CPT code book.

Reflectance confocal microscopy (RCM) is a noninvasive skin examination that is performed "in vivo" without removing skin for sampling. The microscope uses infrared light to examine lesions. "As this light passes between cellular structures having different refraction indexes, it is naturally reflected, and this reflected light is then captured and recomposed into a two-dimensional gray scale image by computer software." The computerized image is then used for histologic analysis (Calzavara-Pinton 2008). CPT code 96931 describes the imaging including image acquisition, interpretation, and report for the first lesion, as well as 96934 as an add-on code for each additional lesion. Codes 96932 or 96933 are assigned when only a component of the procedure is performed, with 96935 and 96936 for each additional lesion.

Physical Medicine and Rehabilitation

To use the physical medicine and rehabilitation codes correctly, the coder should note that time documentation is important in reporting them. When time is not documented, the coder should ask the provider to clarify the amount of time spent and have the physician document it in the patient's record. If procedures are performed for more than 15 minutes, the number of 15-minute units should be indicated in box 24g of the claim form. (Refer to chapter 10 of this book for instructions on claim form completion.)

Example: Code 97760, Orthotics management and training (including assessment and fitting when not otherwise reported), upper extremity(s), lower extremity(s), and/or trunk, each 15 minutes

Example: Code 97542, Wheelchair management (eg, assessment, fitting, training), each 15 minutes

Codes in the physical medicine and rehabilitation subsection are divided according to modality and procedure. A modality is defined as any physical agent applied to produce therapeutic changes to biologic tissue. Such physical agents include thermal, acoustic, light, mechanical, and electrical energy, among others. Codes for modalities are classified in two ways:

- A supervised modality does not require direct (one-on-one) patient contact by the provider.

- A constant attendance modality requires direct (one-on-one) patient contact by the provider.

In the therapeutic procedures subgrouping, the physician or the therapist is required to have direct (one-on-one) patient contact. A therapeutic procedure involves the physician or therapist effecting functional improvement through the application of clinical skills and/or services. Code 97140 describes both manipulation and mobilization. For group therapy, code 97150 should be reported for each member of the group.

Medical Nutrition Therapy

Codes from this series may be used for "all age groups, from extremely low birth weight, premature infants to elderly individuals whose nutrition status is affected by the aging process" and chronic disease (AMA 2001). These services are typically performed by dietitians, nurses or other health educators and may be performed under the supervision of a physician.

Codes are assigned based on time. Some third-party payers may require the use of HCPCS code S9452, Nutrition classes, nonphysician provider, per session, instead of code 97804. The CPT code book directs the coder to use E/M codes when a physician performs nutrition therapy assessment and intervention.

Acupuncture

Acupuncture codes 97810–97814 are selected based on the amount of personal contact time (15-minute increments) and whether electrical stimulation was utilized. E/M codes may be reported separately if the patient's condition warrants it. The time used to provide the E/M service should not be included in the time of the acupuncture service.

Osteopathic and Chiropractic Manipulative Treatment

When coding for osteopathic manipulative treatment (OMT) or chiropractic manipulative treatment (CMT), E/M services may be reported separately by using modifier –25 if the condition requires a significant, separately identifiable E/M service not included in the usual pre- and postservice work associated with the procedure. The E/M service may be prompted by the same symptoms or condition for which the OMT or CMT service was provided. Different diagnoses are not required when reporting both codes.

OMT (98925–98929) is a form of manual treatment applied by a physician to eliminate or alleviate somatic dysfunction and related disorders. Codes are chosen based on the number of body regions manipulated. The body regions referred to are as follows:

- Head

- Cervical region

- Thoracic region

- Lumbar region

- Sacral region

- Pelvic region

- Lower extremities

- Upper extremities

- Rib cage, abdomen

- Viscera

CMT (98940–98943) is a form of manual treatment to influence joint and neurophysiological function. The codes include a premanipulation patient assessment and are assigned based on number of spinal regions involved or involvement of extraspinal regions. If the patient's condition requires a significant and separately identifiable E/M service, that code is reported with modifier –25 for E/M services on the same day of the procedure or service.

The five spinal regions are as follows:

- Cervical region, including the atlanto-occipital joint

- Thoracic region, including the costovertebral and costotransverse joints

- Lumbar region

- Sacral region

- Pelvic or sacroiliac joint region

The five extraspinal regions are as follows:

- Head, including temporomandibular joint, excluding the atlanto-occipital

- Lower extremities

- Upper extremities

- Rib cage, excluding costotransverse and costovertebral joints

- Abdomen

Education and Training for Patient Self-Management

These education and training codes are used to report services that are prescribed by a physician but delivered by a qualified nonphysician professional using a standardized curriculum. The level of nonphysician professional is not defined in the CPT code book. The notes indicate that the qualifications of the nonphysician professional must be consistent with appropriate standards. These codes are assigned based on the number of patients receiving treatment at the same time, per 30-minute period.

Non-Face-to-Face Nonphysician Services

The codes in this series for telephone calls and online medical evaluation are partner codes to those provided for physicians in the evaluation and management section, codes 99441–99444 previously discussed in chapter 2. The codes in this series are to describe work provided by nonphysician qualified practitioners and use the same rules for code assignment as the physician codes.

Special Services, Procedures, and Reports

The codes in the special services, procedures, and reports subsection are adjunct procedures and services that may be added to the basic service provided. Although the codes exist and describe services performed, they may not be reimbursed separately because payment for these procedures/services varies among insurance plans. It is important to check with payers before using these codes. Also, a more specific code may exist in HCPCS Level II. For example, supplies and materials provided by the physician or other qualified healthcare professional (CPT code 99070) can be coded instead using HCPCS Level II codes to provide specificity. Many payers, including Medicare, require the details listed in HCPCS Level II.

Qualifying Circumstances for Anesthesia

The codes in the qualifying circumstances for anesthesia subsection may be used to report additional information on patients undergoing anesthesia who show greater risk of complications. These are add-on codes to codes from the anesthesia section of the CPT code book. For example, codes describing patients of an extreme age (elderly or newborn) with total body hypothermia or controlled hypotension or with possible emergency conditions may need to be reported in addition to the code describing the anesthesia service.

Moderate (Conscious) Sedation

Codes in this subsection are used to report the conscious sedation used in a number of procedures. *CPT Assistant*, February 2006 tells the coder that the preferred term is moderate sedation, which is the drug-induced depression of consciousness during which patients respond purposefully to verbal commands, either alone or accompanied by light tactile stimulation. Spontaneous ventilation is adequate. Moderate sedation is not minimal sedation (anxiolysis), deep sedation, or monitored anesthesia care (00100–01999).

Use of these codes requires the presence of an independent, trained observer to assist the operating physician in monitoring the patient's level of consciousness and physiological status. The codes represent performance and documentation of pre-and postsedation evaluations of the patient, administration of the sedation, and monitoring of cardiorespiratory functions.

Codes 99143–99145 describe the sedation services when performed by the same physician performing the diagnostic or therapeutic procedure. Codes 99148–99150 describe the sedation services when performed by a physician other than the professional performing the procedure that the sedation supports. These codes describe services based on age of the patient and on length of intra-service time.

Other Services and Procedures

Codes in the other services and procedures subsection include procedures that do not fall naturally into any other category. Code 99170 is used to report anogenital examination with colposcopic magnification in childhood for suspected trauma. Code 99173 is used to report a screening visual acuity test (for example, Snellen chart test), when performed as a separate procedure and not part of a general ophthalmologic service or E/M service of the eye. It can be used with the preventive medicine codes from the E/M section of the CPT code book. Code 99175 is used to describe the administration of syrup of ipecac to cause emesis and empty the stomach of poison. Code 99183 describes hyperbaric oxygen therapy supervision.

Home Health Procedures/Services and Home Infusion Procedures/Services

These subsections are for reporting services by nonphysician healthcare professionals for home health procedures/services and for home infusion procedures. When physicians perform home health services, they should report their services with codes 99341–99350. The drug infused should be coded with the appropriate HCPCS level II code in addition to the home infusion procedure service code(s). Home infusion services are reported per visit based on time. Code 99601 is for a visit up to two hours with each additional hour reported with 99602.

Medication Therapy Management Services

Medication therapy management services (MTMS) is a face-to-face service provided by a pharmacist upon request. Documentation requirements include review of the patient history, prescription and nonprescription medication profile, and recommendations for improving outcomes and treatment compliance. The codes in this series are not intended to describe normal dispensing activities such as providing product information and answering questions.

Modifiers Used in Coding Medicine Services

Modifiers do not alter the definition of the main code but, rather, are used to provide additional information relating to the main code. They help express information about special circumstances or conditions surrounding the procedures. The modifiers listed here are available for use with the medicine codes. (See chapter 9 for more detailed information on the use of modifiers.)

−22   Increased Procedural Services

−26   Professional Component

−51   Multiple Procedures

−52   Reduced Services

−53   Discontinued Procedure

−59   Distinct Procedural Service

−76   Repeat Procedure by Same Physician

−77   Repeat Procedure by Another Physician

−AP   Determination of refractive state was not performed in the course of diagnostic ophthalmological examination

−AT   Acute treatment

-EJ   Subsequent claims for a defined course of treatment

-G6   ESRD patient for whom less than six dialysis sessions have been provided in a month

-TC   Technical Component

Anatomical Modifiers

Anatomical modifiers help identify exactly which digit or body area is receiving treatment. The anatomical modifiers include:

–LT Left side: Modifier –LT is used to identify procedures performed on the left side of the body.

–RT Right side: Modifier –RT is used to identify procedures performed on the right side of the body.

The modifiers assigned to each digit are summarized here:

Left Hand	Left Foot	Right Hand	Right Foot
–FA (Thumb)	–TA (Great toe)	–F5 (Thumb)	–T5 (Great toe)
–F1 (2nd Digit)	–T1 (2nd Digit)	–F6 (2nd Digit)	–T6 (2nd Digit)
–F2 (3rd Digit)	–T2 (3rd Digit)	–F7 (3rd Digit)	–T7 (3rd Digit)
–F3 (4th Digit)	–T3 (4th Digit)	–F8 (4th Digit)	–T8 (4th Digit)
–F4 (5th Digit)	–T4 (5th Digit)	–F9 (5th Digit)	–T9 (5th Digit)

HCPCS Codes Used in Coding Medicine Services

A range of HCPCS codes exists for the coding of medicine services, including immunization services, psychiatric services, cardiovascular services, pulmonary services, and special services, procedures, and reports.

Immunization Services

The following HCPCS codes may be used in reporting immunization services:

G0008   Administration of influenza virus vaccine when no physician fee schedule service on the same day

G0009   Administration of pneumococcal vaccine when no physician fee schedule service on the same day

G0010   Administration of hepatitis B vaccine when no physician fee schedule service on the same day

G0453   Continuous intraoperative neurophysiology monitoring, from outside the operating room (remote or nearby), per patient, (attention directed exclusively to one patient) each 15 minutes. (List in addition to primary procedure)

Vision Services

When vision services (the provision of frames, spectacle lenses, or contact lenses) are provided from the physician office, a durable medical equipment (DME) provider number is required when billing to Medicare.

S0500–S0590	Various prescription lens and contact lens codes
S0592	Comprehensive contact lens evaluation
S0595	Dispensing new spectacle lens for patient supplied frame
V2020	Frames, purchases
V2025	Deluxe frame

The specific lens must be recoded using a HCPCS code from the V2100–V2499 series and the specific contact lens must be recoded using a HCPCS code from the V2500–V2599 series. Prosthetic eye services are coded in HCPCS using the V2623–V2629 series of codes.

Miscellaneous eye services codes in HCPCS cover services such as balancing lenses; creating prisms in lenses; adding tint, antireflective coating, scratch-resistant, or UV coating to lenses; or creating oversized or progressive lenses.

In addition, code V2785 is available for the processing, preserving, and transporting of corneal tissue for transplantation.

Neurology and Neuromuscular Procedures

The following HCPCS codes may be used in reporting neurology procedures:

S3900	Surface electromyography (EMG)
S9015	Automated EEG monitoring

Cardiac Procedures

The following HCPCS codes may be used in reporting cardiac procedures:

G0269   Placement of occlusive device into either a venous or arterial access site, post surgical or interventional procedure (that is, angioseal plug, vascular plug)

G0278   Iliac and/or femoral artery angiography, non-selective, bilateral or ipsilateral to catheter insertion, performed at the same time as cardiac catheterization and/or coronary angiography, includes positioning or placement of the catheter in the distal aorta or ipsilateral femoral or iliac artery, injection of dye, production of permanent images, and radiologic supervision and interpretation (list separately in addition to primary procedure)

S3902   Ballistocardiogram

Pulmonary Services

The following HCPCS codes may be used in reporting pulmonary services:

S8096   Portable peak flow meter (supply)

S8110   Peak expiratory flow rate (physician services)

Special Services, Procedures, and Reports

The following HCPCS codes may be used in reporting special services, procedures, and reports:

G0108   Diabetes outpatient self-management training services, individual, per session

G0109   Diabetes outpatient self-management training services, group session, per individual

Exercise 7.1. Medicine

Choose the best answer for each of the following questions.

1. Which CPT code(s) should be reported for four injections of allergenic extracts when the extracts are not provided by the physician or other qualified healthcare professional?

   a. 95115
   b. 95115, 95117
   c. 95117
   d. 95115 × 4

2. Which CPT code(s) should be reported to a commercial insurance carrier for IV chemotherapy administration for three hours when the medication is provided by an entity other than the physician?

   a. 96409
   b. 96413, 96415, 96415
   c. 96413, 96415, 96415, and appropriate E/M code
   d. 96415 and appropriate E/M code

3. Which CPT code(s) is used to report a percutaneous transluminal coronary angioplasty of two major coronary arteries?

   a. 92920, 93454
   b. 92920, 92921
   c. 92920, 92920
   d. 92943, 92944, 93454

Assign the appropriate CPT codes (including office visit codes, if applicable) for the following scenarios.

4. A patient with hyperemesis gravidarum receives IV fluids over two hours to restore lost electrolytes.

5. The patient has an unattended sleep study that simultaneously records heart rate, oxygen saturation, airflow, and sleep time.

6. The patient undergoes a chemotherapy treatment that consists of a 2-hour infusion of one medication, followed by a 100-minute infusion of a second medication.

7. An elderly patient visits her ophthalmologist for a periodic examination for chronic open-angle glaucoma. The patient is being followed medically. A comprehensive service, along with an intermediate visual field examination, is performed. Code for the ophthalmologist's services.

8. A 2-year-old child visits the pediatrician's office for immunization with varicella virus vaccine. No other E/M service is performed and counseling was not provided that day.

9. A 46-year-old man suffers a bite from an aggressive squirrel. An expanded problem focused history and detailed examination are completed in Urgent Care. Low-level medical decision

(Continued on next page)

Exercise 7.1. (Continued)

making is used for this new patient. To protect the patient against rabies, the patient receives rabies immunoglobulin, human for intramuscular and/or subcutaneous use.

Assign the appropriate medicine section codes and modifiers, when appropriate. These exercises should be considered non-Medicare cases unless otherwise specified.

10. Physician review and interpretation of a 24-hour ambulatory blood pressure monitor

11. Hemodialysis with the physician evaluating the patient twice during the service

12. Neuropsychological testing using the Wechsler Memory Scales, administered and interpreted by a physician over 2 hours

13. Routine ECG with 15 leads, with the physician providing only the test interpretation and report

14. Percutaneous transluminal coronary angioplasty with stent placement following an atherectomy of both the left anterior descending artery and the diagonal artery.

15. Prosthetic training for 45 minutes by a physical therapist

16. Complete duplex scan of the left lower-extremity arteries

17. Chiropractic manipulation, two spinal regions involved, acute treatment

18. Device evaluation of dual-lead pacemaker system with reprogramming

19. Assign the appropriate CPT code(s) for the report shown here:

PROCEDURE: 1. Left heart catheterization

INDICATION: 1. Congestive heart failure
2. Cardiomyopathy
3. Left ventricular dysfunction

Exercise 7.1. (Continued)

DESCRIPTION OF PROCEDURE AND FINDINGS:

ACCESS: Right radial artery
COMPLICATIONS: None

The right radial artery was accessed and a 5 French sheath was placed. We then used a Jacky catheter to engage the left and right coronary arteries and also to cross the aortic valve and obtain LVEDP.

LEFT MAIN CORONARY ARTERY: Left main coronary artery is a large caliber vessel. The ostial part is angulated and appears to have a pseudolesion ostially.

LEFT ANTERIOR DESCENDING ARTERY: The left anterior descending artery is a large caliber vessel. The proximal and mid LAD tortuous were angiographically normal. Distal LAD is small caliber wrap-around vessel. The major diagonal branches were angiographically normal.

LEFT CIRCUMFLEX CORONARY ARTERY: The left circumflex coronary artery is nondominant. It has some luminal irregularities in the mid portion.

RIGHT CORONARY ARTERY: The RCA is a dominant vessel. It is angiographically normal.

LVEDP is elevated at about 28-30 mmHg.

ASSESSMENT AND PLAN:
1. Angiographically normal coronaries
2. Elevated end diastolic pressure of 30 mmHg
3. Results discussed with the patient and family
4. Continue medical therapy

20. Assign the appropriate CPT code(s) for the following diagnostic report.

_____

Diagnostic Report

Procedure: The patient was premedicated and brought to the cardiovascular laboratory, where the inguinal region was prepared and draped in the usual manner and local cutaneous anesthesia was obtained with 2% Xylocaine. An 8 French USCI sheath was inserted percutaneously into the right femoral artery, and 10,000 units of Heparin were given intravenously. The patient already had received 75 mg of lidocaine and 5 mg of verapamil intravenously, as well as 5 mg of Isordil sublingually.

We selected an 8 French Shiley JR 4 guide catheter and positioned it in the ostium of the right coronary artery. This was a large dominant vessel. In the proximal third before a point of marked angulation, there was a 70% irregular stenosis. Further distally in the mid-right coronary artery, there was a 2-cm zone of athero-sclerotic disease that was punctuated by sequential 95% and 70% narrowings.

We selected an ACS micro 3.5 XT balloon catheter and were able to advance it across both lesions. However, it did require deep seating of the guide catheter with buckling it in the aortic root. We initially brought it across the lesion in the mid-right coronary artery, where the balloon was inflated a total of seven times in an overlapping manner to a maximum of seven atmospheres of pressure for a maximum duration of 90 seconds. We then withdrew the balloon to the lesion in the proximal right coronary artery and inflated it five times to a maximum of six atmospheres of pressure for a maximum duration of 45 seconds. Repeat injections following these inflations revealed wide patency at both sites. The proximal residual stenosis was less than 30%. The lesions in the mid-right coronary artery were dilated successfully to a residual of less than 30%, as well. Distal runoff was excellent.

The patient tolerated the procedure quite well and no complications occurred. At this point the catheter was removed, but the femoral sheath was left in place and the patient was transferred back to her room with continuous intravenous heparin.

Conclusion: Successful single-vessel, double-lesion coronary angioplasty to the proximal and mid-right coronary artery for coronary arteriosclerosis.

(Continued on next page)

Chapter 7 Test

Choose the best answer for each of the following questions.

1. A 69-year-old patient receives two simultaneous intravenous antibiotics over the course of one hour. He becomes nauseated and receives an IV push of an antiemetic medication. How are the intravenous services coded?

   a. 96365, 96368, 96375
   b. 96365 × 2, 96375
   c. 96365, 96367, 96375
   d. 96365 × 2, 96368

2. Code the following operative report:

   Preoperative Diagnosis: Retinoblastoma, stage V, right eye

   Postoperative Diagnosis: Same

   Operation: Enucleation, right eye

   Anesthesia: General

   Surgical Indication: This is a 6-month-old healthy infant who was diagnosed 2 months ago with stage V retinoblastoma, right eye. The child has had two courses of chemotherapy. Because of persistent tumor, especially vitreous seeding, enucleation of the right eye was recommended. The benefits, risks, and nature of the procedure and alternative procedures were discussed in great depth with the family. The family opted for enucleation of the right eye.

   Surgical Procedure: The child was brought to the operating room after adequate preoperative medications. She was induced with facemask anesthesia, at which time an intravenous line was inserted. A cardiac monitor, blood pressure cuff, precordial stethoscope, EKG leads and pulse oximeter were attached. The child was then intubated. Both pupils were dilated with adult Kupffer solution and each retina was examined including scleral depression for 360 degrees. In the right eye there was a large tumor centered in the region between the optic nerve and macula that measured six disc diameters. It showed a typical cottage cheese pattern of regression. However, overlying this tumor was extensive particulate vitreous seeding. The segment of vitreous between the optic nerve and the equator inferiorly were filled with particulate vitreous matter. Then farther inferiorly there were gross whitish opacities in the vitreous and there were similar opacities nasally, temporally and even superiorly. In view of the extensive vitreous seeding, the decision was made to proceed with enucleation of the right eye. The left eye was examined. The disc, vessels, macula and retinal periphery were normal. No tumors were noted.

   The patient's face was then draped and prepared in the usual sterile fashion. A lid speculum was put into place on the right. A 360-degree peritomy was made with Westcott scissors and 0.12 BishopHarmon forceps. Then sequentially each of the extraocular muscles were isolated on the Stevens hook and onto a large Green's hook. A double-armed 6-0 Vicryl suture was woven through the insertion site and locked at each end respectively. The muscle was then detached from the globe and the sutures were secured to a bulldog clip. Of note, at the time of isolation of the lateral rectus muscle, the inferior oblique muscle was hooked and its insertion cleaned with sharp and blunt dissection. Its end was sutured and it was detached from the globe. Similarly, when the superior rectus muscle was accessed the superior oblique tendon was directly identified and cut.

   Once all of the extraocular muscles were detached from the globe, the stump of the medial rectus muscle was cross-clamped and the eye was proptosed. A fine tipped Metzenbaum scissors was then introduced behind the orbit from the optic nerve and then the optic nerve was cut. At this point, the globe was removed from the orbit and digital pressure was applied to the socket to obtain adequate hemostasis. Inspection of the globe revealed that it was intact. There was no extrascleral extension of tumor. A tangential portion of optic nerve was obtained measuring 7 mm at one end and 9 mm at the other end.

   After adequate hemostasis was obtained, a 14-mm prosthesis was wrapped in sclera that was secured along its seam with a 4-0 Prolene suture. The scleral-wrapped prosthesis was then inserted

Chapter 7 Test (Continued)

into the muscle cone. Each of the extraocular muscles were reattached to the sclera using the preplaced sutures. Then the overlying Tenon's was closed with nine interrupted 5-0 Vicryl sutures. The conjunctiva was then closed with a running 6-0 plain suture. Topical antibiotic ointment was then placed in the conjunctival cul-de-sac and a conformer was put into place. The eye was pressure patched with two eye pads and Tegaderm that was then secured with foam tape after the skin had been pretreated with Mastisol and the entire eye bandage was secured with an ENT head wrap. The child was then weaned from general anesthesia, extubated, and brought to the recovery room in good condition without complications.

    a. 65103–RT
    b. 65105–RT
    c. 65105–RT, 92018
    d. 65130–RT, 92018

3. A 73-year-old patient arrives for scheduled chemotherapy treatment of intravenous infusions of carboplatin for 35 minutes and Docetaxel for 60 minutes. The patient also receives ondansetron hydrochloride infused over 20 minutes as an antiemetic. All infusions are sequential. How are these intravenous services coded?

    a. 96413, 96417, 96365
    b. 96413, 96417, 96367
    c. 96413 × 2, 96365
    d. 96413 × 2, 96367

4. For moderate sedation, when does the intra-service time (calculation of time) begin?

    a. At the start of the administration of the agent
    b. At the start of the assessment
    c. When sedation is maintained
    d. At the insertion of the IV

5. The patient presents to the oncologist's office for a blood draw from a total implantable port and refilling of an implantable pump with 1,000 mg of fluorouracil to be delivered over 24 hours. How is this coded?

    a. 36591, 96416, J9190
    b. 36591, 96522, J9190 × 2
    c. 36415, 96416, J9190 × 2
    d. 36415, 96522, J9190

6. It is suspected that the patient might have an allergy to food additives and is tested. Three food items are incrementally ingested over three hours and allergy is eventually ruled out. How is this service coded?

    a. 95012
    b. 95024 × 3
    c. 95076
    d. 95076 × 2

7. How is moderate sedation coded when performed by the same physician performing the procedure) for sedation of a 3-year-old for 30 minutes?

    a. 99143
    b. 99144
    c. 99148
    d. 99149

(Continued on next page)

Chapter 7 Test (Continued)

8. Code the following procedure completed in the Stress Test Laboratory in the cardiologist's office:

    A 52-year-old man was given a stress test for recent left arm and chest pain that occurred at work while carrying a heavy object. He has hypertension and takes a mild diuretic daily. No other pertinent medical history.

    He is exercised by Bruce protocol for a duration of 7 minutes, using the treadmill. Maximum heart rate achieved was 135; 86% maximum predicted was 137. His blood pressure during the stress test was a maximum of 176/84. He denied any arm pain with this exercise.

    Following exercise, he was placed at rest. At 1 minute, he had STT wave depression and T-wave inversion in the interior and V5 and V6 leads. His blood pressure dropped to 76/40 at 5 minutes. During this time, he remained pain free and felt fine. At the 10-minute mark, the T-wave inversion resolved and the STT waves returned to normal.

    He was advised that a cardiac catheterization would be appropriate to rule out ischemic heart disease and this is scheduled.

    a. 93015
    b. 93016, 93018
    c. 93017, 93018
    d. 93018

9. Code the following operative report:

    Preoperative Diagnosis: Unstable progressive angina pectoris, markedly abnormal thallium exercise test, 95% circumflex coronary artery stenosis.

    Procedure: PTCA of left circumflex with stent placement

    Procedure Details: Following 1% Xylocaine local anesthesia in the left femoral region using the Seldinger technique, #8 French sheaths were inserted in the left femoral artery and vein. A 7 French Swan-Ganz catheter was advanced in antegrade fashion through the right heart chambers and positioned in the pulmonary artery. Selective left coronary angiography was performed with a 8Fr JL4 curved short tipped guiding catheter, after which time a 0.014" microglide exchange wire was passed down the length of the circumflex coronary artery and a 2.5-mm Shadow balloon dilatation catheter was advanced over the wire and inflated to a maximum of 9 atmospheres on multiple occasions. This balloon catheter was then removed and a 2.5-mm Cook stent was placed over a 3.0-mm. compliant balloon catheter in the circumflex main trunk. This balloon was inflated to 9 atmospheres and kept inflated for 4.0 minutes. This balloon catheter was then removed and selective angiography was performed, which demonstrated excellent flow and run-off in the circumflex and no evidence of occlusive type dissection. At this time, the arterial and venous sheaths were sutured in place and the patient was taken to the holding area of the catheterization laboratory without incident. There were no complications resulting from the procedure.

    a. 92920, 92929
    b. 92943
    c. 92928
    d. 92920, 92928

10. A child is seen on her first birthday for her first well child check at this clinic. The physician notes that the patient completed the antibiotics that she prescribed last week during an office visit and that her ears are now clear. Vaccine counseling is completed and three shots are given: Hep B-Hib combo, MMR, and IPV. How is this service coded?

    a. 99391; 90748; 90707; 90713; 90460; 90461 × 2
    b. 99392; 90744; 90648; 90707; 90713; 90460 × 4
    c. 99382; 90748; 90707; 90713; 90461 × 3
    d. 99392; 90748; 90707; 90713; 90460 × 3; 90461 × 3

Chapter 8

HCPCS Level II Coding

Objectives

Upon completion of this chapter, the student should be able to do the following:

- Define what HCPCS codes are, including their format and publishing body

- Identify when HCPCS codes are updated and where to find the updates

- Describe when HCPCS codes are used

- Explain the effect of HIPAA on HCPCS

- List the sections of HCPCS that are inappropriate for coding of professional services billed on a CMS-1500 form and explain why

- Describe the concept of HCPCS temporary codes

- Demonstrate how to assign HCPCS codes while observing the coding hierarchy

- Define which HCPCS codes can be billed to the Medicare carrier and which need to be billed to durable medical equipment (DME) contractors using a different provider number

- Describe how medications are coded using HCPCS J codes

The HCPCS (pronounced "hic-picks") Level II codes, also known as the National Codes, are created and updated quarterly by CMS. This coding system is used to bill supplies, materials, and injectable medications. It also is used to bill for certain procedures and services, such as ambulance or dental, that are not defined by the CPT code book.

National Codes are five-digit alphanumeric codes, beginning with the letters A through V, and are divided into 24 sections. Because these codes are published by CMS, a government agency, the National Codes and their descriptions are in the public domain and available online or for a nominal charge through the US Government Printing Office. Many publishing companies have reprinted the codes and arranged them into organized sections, with an index and other coding enhancements. As with the CPT coding system, it is imperative that the most current edition of HCPCS National Codes be used. To download the most recent quarterly updates of the codes, go to the HCPCS section of the CMS website (CMS 2015a).

Most publishers use the standard symbols for additions and changes that are used in the CPT code book. The bullet symbol tells of new codes and the triangle instructs the coder that the description of the code has been changed in some way from the previous year. Deleted codes are indicated with a strike-through in the text.

HCPCS Level II codes are required for claims submitted to Medicare. Most other insurers now accept these codes because of the clarity that they provide in billing. Every attempt should be made to describe services submitted to all payers using these codes.

Code Assignment Hierarchy

The use of HCPCS and CPT codes has a hierarchy. If the coding professional finds that the same procedure is coded in two levels, he or she must follow certain rules. When both a CPT code and a Level II code have virtually identical narratives for a procedure or service, the CPT code should be used. If, however, the narratives are not identical (for example, the CPT code is generic and the Level II code is specific), the Level II code should be used. For the sake of simplicity, Level I is commonly referred to as CPT and Level II is referred to as HCPCS.

Steps in HCPCS Code Assignment

- Look up the service or procedure in the Index (usually found in the front of the HCPCS book).

- For drugs, look up the drug in the Table of Drugs at the back of the book, not in the Index.

- Locate the suggested code(s) in the tabular, following any cross-referencing instructions.

- Assign the appropriate code.

- Determine whether a modifier is required to fully explain the service or supply.

- Append modifier(s), if appropriate.

Another clue to the existence of a HCPCS code is the fact that a CPT code is invalid for Medicare recipients. To determine the status of any CPT or HCPCS code, access the Medicare Physician's Fee Schedule Database, also called the Relative Value File. This file can be downloaded from CMS on the Physician Fee Schedule page (CMS 2015b). The column labeled "status code" contains an "I" for invalid on any codes that are not valid for submission to Medicare.

If the invalid code is a CPT (HCPCS Level I) code, the coder should search for a possible Level II alternative code that is valid for Medicare. For example, CPT code 90291 has a status of "I" because Level II code J0850 must be used to report the provision of Cytomegalovirus immune globulin for Medicare patients. A sample page from the Medicare Physician's Fee Schedule Database and a further discussion of this topic can be found in chapter 10.

The Effect of HIPAA on HCPCS

The Health Insurance Portability and Accountability Act (HIPAA) in the Transactions and Code Sets provision states that the code sets applicable on the date of service must be used to submit claims for those services. Therefore, CMS is now requiring the use of the current CPT codes for services rendered on or after January 1 of any year, such as 2016 codes on January 1, 2016.

HCPCS Level II Codes Inappropriate for Professional Billing

One section of Level II codes, the C codes, is inappropriate for coding and billing professional services on a CMS-1500 form. Another section, the HCPCS D codes, may be inappropriate for professional billing, depending upon the circumstances.

HCPCS C Codes

The C code section of HCPCS contains codes developed specifically to describe services, supplies, and drugs furnished in hospital outpatient departments and reimbursed under the hospital outpatient prospective payment system (OPPS). If used on a CMS-1500 claim, they will be denied.

HCPCS D Codes

The D code section of HCPCS is copyrighted by the American Dental Association (ADA) and comprises the *CDT 2016 Current Dental Terminology*. The most recent edition is effective on January 1, 2016, and is reprinted in many HCPCS books for reference only. *CDT*, complete with index, code listing with detailed descriptions, and a dental glossary, can be purchased from the ADA.

In general, physicians bill for their dental-related services using the CPT codes found in the digestive section and report them on a CMS-1500 form. In general, dentists bill for their services using HCPCS Level II D codes (CDT) and report them on an ADA Dental Claim Form. However, some commercial carriers have different requirements and both physicians and dentists should be aware of all of the codes that are available. Oromaxillofacial surgeons should carefully choose codes from both CPT and CDT that best describe all of the reconstructive work that they perform.

Temporary Codes

The HCPCS G, H, K, Q, S, and T codes are considered temporary codes. Codes in these sections are frequently added midyear in the quarterly updates decided on by the HCPCS National Panel.

Many of these codes are converted to other sections of HCPCS or to CPT codes on January 1 in the yearly comprehensive changes. For example, in 2011, G0440 described "Application of tissue cultured allogeneic skin substitute or dermal substitute for use on lower limb, includes site preparation and debridement performed, first 25 sq cm or less." This code was deleted in 2012 when the redesign of the Skin Replacement Surgery section of CPT made this code obsolete.

S and T codes are contained within the HCPCS Level II codes but are not acceptable for reporting services provided to Medicare patients. S codes are used to report services to commercial payers, and T codes are used to report services to state Medicaid agencies. The S and T series of codes are not organized well and are not indexed well in the HCPCS Index. The coder should review these sections as each new publication becomes available to become aware of all new codes.

Durable Medical Equipment Carriers

The HCPCS B, E, K, L, and V codes describe equipment or services that must be provided by a durable medical equipment (DME) provider. A special provider number is required to bill the codes in these sections, and claims processing is done by special durable medical equipment Medicare administrative contractors (DME MACs). An application to become a DME, prosthetics, orthotics, and supplies (DMEPOS) supplier can be obtained from the Medicare Provider-Supplier Enrollment page on the CMS website (CMS 2015c).

Modifiers (chapter 9) and advance beneficiary notices (chapter 10) are vitally important to accurate coding and reimbursement for DME supplies. If DME supplies are provided to Medicare beneficiaries by a non-DME provider, the beneficiaries must be told ahead of time that Medicare will not pay for the service. They must sign a waiver (advance beneficiary notice) if they want to receive the supply from a non-DME provider or they must be allowed to obtain the supply from a provider who is eligible to bill Medicare on their behalf if they want.

Drugs Administered Other Than Oral Method

HCPCS J codes describe medications that are administered by physicians. These codes should be assigned when the physician purchases the medication and administers the medication in the office setting. They should not be assigned if the medication is furnished by the patient or other source. In that case, only the administration codes should be used to describe the service of administering the medication, not the provision of the supply.

Each HCPCS J code describes a unique medication and the dosage covered by that code. For example, J0715 describes 500 mg of ceftizoxime sodium. If the physician orders 1,500 mg of ceftizoxime sodium, J0715 would be assigned and the number 3 would be placed in the Days/Units column of the CMS-1500 form. The charge for the service would be the fee for one unit of J0715 multiplied by three.

Patients may require dosages that do not match the dosage listed in the code. For example, the physician orders 400 mg of Levaquin. The coder references the Table of Drugs to locate the J code for the medication. This special Index refers the code to J1956 Levofloxacin 250 mg. The coder would assign two units of J1956 because 400 mg is between the value of one and two units. Fractions are not to be reported in the Units column of the CMS-1500 form.

Many medications in the J code series are listed in milliliters (mL) or in cubic centimeters (cc). It is important to remember that in metric equivalents, one cc equals one mL. The coder should become familiar with the medications that are stocked within the physician practice. It is also helpful to have a drug reference book available to assist in cross-referencing brand and generic names for drugs.

Exercise 8.1. HCPCS Level II Coding

Choose the best answer for each of the following questions.

1. A 36-year-old patient presents for a complete physical and requests renewal of birth control. Because of a personal history of deep vein thrombosis, the physician and the patient decide that a diaphragm is the appropriate method. A diaphragm is fitted and provided along with proper instructions on use. How is this coded?

2. After evaluating a patient and diagnosing a systemic yeast infection, the physician administers an injection of 300 mg of Diflucan for relief of symptoms. How is this medication coded on the CMS-1500 form?

    a. J1450, 1 unit
    b. J1450, 1.5 units
    c. J1450, 2 units
    d. J1450, 3 units

3. An OB-GYN office provides childbirth classes, presented by a nurse-midwife and wants to report this to commercial insurance carriers. How is this childbirth class reported?

4. A copper intrauterine device is placed for birth control when oral contraceptives are contraindicated for the patient. How is this service coded?

5. What is the correct coding assignment for casting materials for a short leg plaster cast?

6. What is the correct coding assignment for obtaining, preparing, and conveyance of cervical screening Pap smear to laboratory for a patient covered by Medicare?

7. A multispecialty clinic is equipped to provide chemotherapy services, including provision of the chemotherapeutic agents. The flow sheet for one chemotherapy visit documents the following treatment provided to a patient with colon cancer. How is this coded?

    Intravenous Push:
        Dexamethasone, 20 mg
        Zofran, 8 mg
        Normal saline, 250 cc, used to administer drug

    Chemotherapy Push:
        Leucovorin, 400 mg
        Normal saline, 250 cc, used to administer drug

    Chemotherapy infusion over 2 hours:
        Fluorouracil (5FU), 800 mg
        Normal saline, 250 cc, used to administer drug
        Port locked with heparin sodium, 600 units

8. How is a complete CBC, automated (HgB, HCT, RBC, WBC, without platelet count) and automated WBC differential count coded for Medicare?

(Continued on next page)

Exercise 8.1. (Continued)

9. The patient covered by Medicare presents for an evaluation and selection of a binaural hearing aid. Because of previous problems with excessive earwax, the physician examines the ears first and removes impacted cerumen before the test is begun. How are these services coded?

   _____

10. Surgical pathology examination for prostate needle biopsy sampling, 12 specimens is performed. How is this service coded?

   _____

Chapter 8 Test

Choose the best answer for each of the following questions.

1. A 12-year-old girl and her mother present to the clinic, stating that the mother removed a tick from the patient's upper outer thigh earlier that day due to a large red area on the skin. The tick is brought in a plastic bag for examination and the mouthparts are intact. The patient is examined and found to have a 5-cm circular lesion of cellulitis on the upper thigh. A treatment of Intravenous Rocephin is given, 1 g, push. Excluding the E/M service, how is this service coded?

   a. 96365, J0696 × 1 unit
   b. 96372, J0696 × 1 unit
   c. 96374, J0696 × 4 units
   d. 96372, J0696 × 14 units

2. A patient covered by Medicare received IV chemotherapy for 3 hours in the physician's chemotherapy suite. The prescribed dosage was 75 mg of cisplatin with 800 mg of fluorouracil. How is this service coded?

   a. J9060, J9190, 96413 × 3 units
   b. J9060 × 8 units, J9190 × 2 units, 96413, 96415 × 2 units
   c. J9060 × 8 units, J9190 × 2 units, 96409 × 3 units
   d. J9060 × 7 units, J9190, 96422, 96423 × 2 units

3. Code the following office note:

   CC: Enterocele and cystocele

   S: This patient is here for pessary placement. We placed a 2.5-cm rubber cube pessary today. If the patient can keep the pessary in for about 24 hours without increased leaking of urine, she will pass the test for correcting her enterocele and cystocele. Her predominant symptom is pressure from the enterocele and cystocele. The patient does not want to try more conservative management. I have extensively counseled her regarding Kegel exercises versus using Entex versus further urologic workup. However, the patient insisted that she would like to proceed with the surgery if it will work.

   P: I have explained to her in detail the benefits, risks, alternatives, failure rates, etc and most likely outcome of an anteroposterior colporrhaphy. This took 15 minutes of the 25-minute visit. The patient would like to proceed with this surgery. She will meet with the teaching nurse after our visit today. The patient thinks that incontinence is not a significant symptom. She leaks about once a day and does not have to wear a pad or panty liner. She is to return tomorrow to schedule surgery if the criteria are met. If not, I will reevaluate options with the patient.

Chapter 8 Test (Continued)

    a.   99213, 57160
    b.   99214, 57160, A4561
    c.   99214–25, 57160, A4561
    d.   99215–25, A4561

4.   The patient presents with an infectious disease and the physician administers 2.4 million units of Penicillin G benzathine. What is the correct coding assignment for the medication?

    a.   J2510 × 4 units
    b.   J0558 × 24 units
    c.   J0561 × 3 units
    d.   J0561 × 24 units

5.   A 35-year-old non-Medicare patient hyperextends his right thumb while at work. The physician provides a splint for the thumb. How is the splint coded?

    a.   29075–F5
    b.   29280–RT
    c.   A4570–RT
    d.   S8450–F5

6.   A 0.6-cm wound of the face is closed with Dermabond adhesive wound closure. How is this coded?

    a.   Appropriate E/M level
    b.   12011
    c.   A4649
    d.   G0168

7.   A patient with an acute exacerbation of asthma is seen by his nurse practitioner and has a detailed history taken, an expanded problem focused examination done, and low level medical decision making used. The patient expresses a desire to quit smoking and also receives 30 minutes of initial treatment in a smoking cessation program and a one-week supply of nicotine gum. How is this visit coded?

    a.   99202–25, S9453, S4990
    b.   99213–25, S9453, S4995
    c.   99213–25, 99411, S4990
    d.   99214–25, 99402, S4995

8.   The patient is a 6-year-old, newly diagnosed with asthma and is given a peak flow meter to take home. The physician demonstrated how to use the equipment. How is the peak flow meter coded?

    a.   94664
    b.   S8096
    c.   S8097
    d.   S8110

9.   A 9-year-old patient falls from the outdoor gym equipment at school and sustains a fracture of the radial shaft. At the clinic, the physician evaluates the fracture, reduces it, places the arm in a long arm fiberglass cast, and provides a sling. How is this service coded?

    a.   99212–25, 29065, A4590
    b.   99212–25, 25505, Q4008, A4565
    c.   25500, Q4007, A4565
    d.   25505, Q4008, A4565

(Continued on next page)

Chapter 8 Test (Continued)

10. The patient is seen for an injection of the ankle with 1 cc of 0.5% Sensorcaine. The injection is completed with the use of ultrasound guidance and a permanent recording and report are made. How it this coded?

    a. 20606
    b. 20606, S0020
    c. 20611
    d. 20611, S0020

Chapter 9

Modifiers

Objectives

Upon completion of this chapter, the student should be able to do the following:

- Describe what modifiers are and why they are used
- Identify where to locate the lists of modifiers
- Understand the use of the dash
- Describe the proper use of modifier –25
- Differentiate between modifiers for physician use and modifiers for hospital outpatient use
- Describe the proper use of modifier –57
- Describe the proper use of a modifier for distinct services
- Append modifiers appropriately

Modifiers are two-digit extensions to the main CPT or HCPCS code and can be alphabetic, alphanumeric, or numeric. They provide additional information about the main code but do not alter the basic definition of the code. Rather, they help describe special circumstances or conditions surrounding the procedures.

A comprehensive list of CPT modifiers is found in appendix A of the CPT code book. HCPCS Level II modifiers are usually found as an appendix in the HCPCS book and in the front and back covers of most versions. They are also available from the Medicare website on the HCPCS Release and Code Sets page (CMS 2015a).

How to Use Modifiers

Modifiers are appended to the code to provide more information or to alert the payer that a payment change is required. For example, modifier –LT is applied to code 49505 to show that an inguinal hernia is repaired on the left side. This modifier provides information to the payer but initiates no payment change. However, if modifier –50 were applied to code 49505, it would tell the payer that bilateral inguinal hernias were repaired and that additional payment is being requested.

In certain instances, more than one modifier may be called for. In such cases, the CMS-1500 form used for reporting physician services allows up to four modifiers for each service code. (See additional discussion of the CMS-1500 form in online appendix G.) In the example of a bilateral laparoscopic recurrent inguinal hernia repair, if the surgeon provided surgical care only, an additional –54 modifier would be necessary to indicate this change in service. The code would appear as 496515054 on the claim form. The claim form does not allow dashes, but instead, has faint red lines that separate the code from each of the two modifiers for ease in reading.

As you can see, code 496515054 is hard to read when not printed on the claim form. To make it easier to read, the code and modifier(s) are separated by dashes so that the code reads as 49651–50–54.

Also, it should be noted that modifiers should not be appended to unlisted codes such as 37799, Unlisted procedure, vascular surgery. These unlisted codes describe new or unclassified procedures that have no standard description. Therefore, by definition, a nonstandard description does not need modification. Supporting documentation should explain all of the unique aspects of the procedure.

Professional fee (physician services) billing has different modifiers than those used for ambulatory surgery centers or hospital outpatient reporting. Modifiers –27, –73, and –74 are not to be used on physician claims. These modifiers are reserved for facility use only.

Types of Modifiers

Both the CPT and HCPCS Level II code sets have modifiers. The CPT modifiers are numeric. The HCPCS Level II modifiers can be either alphabetic or alphanumeric. Any modifier can be appended to a code within either code set if it is appropriate to describe the coding scenario. In addition, many third-party payers have their own policies regarding the use of modifiers.

CPT Modifier Descriptions and Examples

The following modifiers are available for use on physician claims:

–22 **Increased Procedural Services:** Modifier –22 may be reported to identify that the service provided was greater than that usually required for a particular procedure, such as development of intraoperative complications requiring attention. It may be necessary to submit supporting documentation to the third-party payer to justify use of modifier –22.

> **Example:** Because of the patient's extreme obesity, the physician required an additional 30 minutes to perform a cholecystectomy. The physician should report the following: 47600–22.

–23 **Unusual Anesthesia:** Modifier –23 may be reported in circumstances when local or no anesthesia is normally needed. In cases where an unusual situation exists concerning a patient, modifier –23 describes that general anesthesia is required in this case. Examples of these situations may include extreme age, mental retardation, or psychiatric conditions.

–24 **Unrelated Evaluation and Management Service by the Same Physician or Other Qualified Health Care Professional During a Postoperative Period:** Modifier –24 can be reported with an E/M service provided during the postoperative period by the same physician who performed the original procedure. However, the E/M service must be unrelated to the condition for which the original procedure was performed.

> **Example:** An office visit is provided to a patient who is in the postoperative period for a cholecystectomy performed three weeks earlier. The patient's current complaint is a possible infection of a finger that was lacerated four days earlier. The physician may report the appropriate office visit code and attach modifier –24 to identify this activity as an unrelated service provided during the postoperative period of the cholecystectomy.

–25 **Significant, Separately Identifiable Evaluation and Management Service by the Same Physician or Other Qualified Health Care Professional on the Same Day of the Procedure or Other Service:** Appending modifier –25 tells the insurer that the patient's condition required a significant, separately identifiable E/M service on the same day as a procedure. CMS guidelines state that modifier –25 should be appended to the E/M code when reported with a minor procedure when a significant, separately identifiable service is also performed (Grider 2004). This modifier is always appended to the E/M code, never to the surgical code.

The E/M service may be prompted by the symptoms or condition for which the procedure and/or service was provided. As such, different diagnoses are not required for reporting of the E/M services on the same date.

> **Example:** An established patient well known to the physician presents to the physician office with a cut on the hand. The only service that is required is a laceration repair. In this case, there was no significant or separately identifiable E/M service provided, and no code or modifier is required.

> **Example:** A patient presents to the physician office after a syncopal episode at home in the kitchen. During the fall, she cuts her hand on a broken plate. In this case, the physician needed to evaluate the source of the syncope and repair the laceration that occurred. Modifier –25 would be appended to the E/M code for the syncope evaluation.

–26 **Professional Component:** Modifier –26 may be reported in circumstances where a procedure includes both a professional component and a technical component. The physician or other qualified health care professional attaches modifier –26 to report the professional component separately.

–32 Mandated Services: Modifier –32 is reported when someone, such as a third-party payer, mandates a service. This modifier is reported most often when a patient is sent for a second-opinion consultation.

–33 Preventive Services: When the primary purpose of the service is the delivery of an evidence based service in accordance with a US Preventive Services Task Force A or B rating in effect and other preventive services identified in preventive services mandates (legislative or regulatory), the service may be identified by adding –33 to the procedure. For separately reported services specifically identified as preventive, the modifier should not be used.

–47 Anesthesia by Surgeon: Modifier –47 may be reported to indicate that the surgeon provided regional or general (not local) anesthesia for a surgical procedure. This modifier should not be reported with the anesthesia codes.

> **Example:** An obstetrician performs emergency cesarean delivery for an out-of-town patient visiting relatives. He also administers a pudendal block (regional anesthesia). Moreover, he will provide postpartum care for the patient until she is able to return home. The physician should report the following: 59515–47 and 64430.

–50 Bilateral Procedure: Modifier –50 may be reported to identify bilateral procedures that are performed during the same operative episode.

Exception: If the description specifies the procedure as bilateral, modifier –50 should not be reported.

> **Example:** Physician performs a complex anterior packing of both nares for a nose-bleed. Physicians providing this service should report the following: 30903–50.

–51 Multiple Procedures: Modifier –51 may be reported to identify that multiple procedures were performed on the same day or during the same operative episode (excluding E/M services, Physical Medicine and Rehabilitation services or provision of supplies). The first procedure listed should identify the major or most resource-intensive procedure, which is usually paid at 100 percent of the approved amount. Subsequent or secondary procedures should be appended with modifier –51 and payment reduced according to the terms of the health plan. Policies on payment of multiple procedures vary depending on the third-party payer, so a complete understanding of each is required to ensure appropriate reimbursement.

> **Example:** Physician performed an excision of a chalazion and a dacryolith from the lacrimal passage. She should report the following: 67800 and 68530–51.

–52 Reduced Services: Modifier –52 may be reported to indicate that a service/procedure is partially reduced or eliminated at the discretion of the physician or other qualified health care professional. Although this modifier serves the purpose of identifying a reduction in the procedure/service, many physicians also use it to report a reduction in the charge for a particular procedure because the complete procedure was not performed.

–53 **Discontinued Procedure:** Modifier –53 is appropriate in circumstances where the physician or other qualified health care professional elects to terminate or discontinue a surgical or diagnostic procedure, usually because of risk to the patient's well-being. However, this modifier should not be used to report the elective cancellation of a procedure prior to the patient's surgical preparation or induction of anesthesia.

Note: Modifier –53 is not used for hospital reporting. Hospitals use modifiers –73 and –74 for reporting discontinued procedures. Modifiers –73 and –74 are not used in reporting discontinued physician services.

–54 **Surgical Care Only:** Modifier –54 may be reported to indicate that one physician or other qualified health care professional performed the surgical procedure and another provided the preoperative and postoperative care.

> **Example:** Dr. Reynolds is asked to perform an extracapsular cataract extraction with insertion of intraocular lens for his colleague, Dr. Owens, who is detained out of town. Dr. Owens provided the preoperative care and will provide postoperative care for his patient. Dr. Reynolds should report the following: 66984–54.

–55 **Postoperative Management Only:** Modifier –55 may be reported to identify that the physician or other qualified health care professional provided only postoperative care services for a particular procedure.

> **Example:** Patient sustains a fracture of the distal femur while skiing in Colorado. The physician in Colorado performed a closed treatment of the fracture with manipulation. However, the patient's postoperative care will be provided by his hometown physician, Dr. Rogers. Dr. Rogers should report the following: 27510–55.

–56 **Preoperative Management Only:** Modifier –56 may be reported to indicate that the physician or other qualified health care professional provided only preoperative care services for a particular procedure.

> **Example:** Dr. Smith provides preoperative care services including preoperative history and physical examination for his patient, who will be transferred later the same day to another hospital to undergo a lower lobectomy of the right lung by another physician who has agreed to perform the operation and provide postoperative management. Dr. Smith should report the following: 32480–56.

–57 **Decision for Surgery:** Modifier –57 may be reported when an E/M service resulted in the initial decision to perform surgery. The modifier is reported with the appropriate E/M service code.

–58 **Staged or Related Procedure or Service by the Same Physician or Other Qualified Health Care Professional During the Postoperative Period:** Modifier –58 may be reported to indicate that a staged or related procedure performed by the same physician is provided during the postoperative period. This procedure may have been planned (staged) prospectively at the time of the original procedure, or it may be more extensive than the original procedure.

Example: The patient had a radical mastectomy performed and a tissue expander was placed so that a permanent prosthesis could later be placed. The surgeon took the patient back to the operating room during the postoperative period and inserted a permanent prosthesis. The physician would report 11970–58 for the staged procedure (Grider 2004, 141).

–59 Distinct Procedural Service: Modifier –59 may be used to identify that a procedure or service was distinct or independent from other services provided on the same day. Modifier –59 should not be reported if another modifier describes the circumstance more appropriately. For Medicare, use one of the following HCPCS modifiers to more fully describe the distinct procedural service:

–XE: Separate encounter
–XP: Separate practitioner
–XS: Separate structure (or organ)
–XU: Unusual non-overlapping service

Example: Procedures 23030 and 20103 are performed on the same patient during the same operative session. Ordinarily, if these codes were reported together without a modifier, code 20103 would be denied as integral to code 23030. Because incision and drainage of the shoulder is the definitive procedure, any exploration of the area (20103) preceding this would be considered an inherent part of the more comprehensive service. If the exploration procedure was performed on a different part of the extremity, modifier –XS explains that the codes are distinct from each other and both services are eligible for reimbursement from the payer.

–62 Two Surgeons: Modifier –62 may be reported to identify that two surgeons were required to perform a particular procedure. Both physicians must report modifier –62, along with the appropriate procedure code, on their individual claim to ensure that they are reimbursed. To expedite payment, the operative note dictated by each physician should be sent to the third-party payer.

Example: Dr. Ryan and Dr. Smith perform a posterior arthrodesis of five vertebrae for a spinal deformity. Both physicians should report the following: 22800–62.

–63 Procedure Performed on Infants Less Than 4 kg: Procedures performed on neonates and infants up to a body weight of 4 kg may involve significantly increased complexity than physician work commonly associated with these patients. (To calculate kilograms, divide the number of pounds by 2.2. For example, a 7.5 lb infant [7 lbs, 8 oz] is 3.41 kg: 7.5 / 2.2 = 3.409.) Modifier –63 is intended for use with codes 20000–69979 and should not be appended to E/M, anesthesia, radiology, pathology/laboratory, or medicine codes.

–66 Surgical Team: Modifier –66 may be reported to identify a complex procedure performed by a team of physicians or other qualified health care professionals and other highly skilled personnel.

Example: Patient is admitted for a liver transplant. All the physicians involved in performing this complex procedure should report the following: 47135–66.

–76 Repeat Procedure or Service by Same Physician or Other Qualified Health Care Professional: Modifier –76 may be reported to identify a procedure that was repeated by the physician who performed the original procedure. Some third-party payers may require supporting documentation. Modifier –76 should not be appended to E/M services.

> **Example:** Patient is admitted with significant pleural effusion and congestive heart failure, and the physician performs a thoracentesis. Later in the day, the lungs again fill up with fluid, and the same physician performs a second thoracentesis. The physician or hospital should report the following: 32421 (first thoracentesis), 32421–76 (second thoracentesis identified as a repeat procedure with modifier –76).

–77 Repeat Procedure by Another Physician or Other Qualified Health Care Professional: Modifier –77 may be reported to identify a procedure that was repeated by a physician other than the one who performed the original procedure. As with modifier –76, some third-party payers may require supporting documentation. Modifier –77 should not be appended to evaluation and management services.

> **Example:** A physician performs an x-ray in the office and believes that a suspicious mass is seen. The physician sends the patient to a specialist, who performs another x-ray using different equipment. The specialist would report the x-ray code with the –77 modifier (Grider 2004, 182).

–78 Unplanned Return to the Operating/Procedure Room by the Same Physician or Other Qualified Health Care Professional Following Initial Procedure for a Related Procedure during the Postoperative Period: Modifier –78 may be used to report a related procedure performed during the postoperative period of the initial procedure.

Note: Procedures repeated on the same day as the original procedure should be reported with modifier –76.

> **Example:** Patient has a fracture of the tibia that has not healed properly. The physician who repairs the malunion should report the following: 27720–78. Reporting modifier –78 indicates to the third-party payer that the second procedure was performed during the postoperative period of the first procedure and is related to it in some way.

–79 Unrelated Procedure or Service by the Same Physician or Other Qualified Health Care Professional during the Postoperative Period: Modifier –79 may be used to report an unrelated procedure performed during the postoperative period of the initial procedure.

Note: Procedures repeated on the same day as the original procedure should be reported with modifier –76.

> **Example:** Patient had a hernia repair two weeks ago. He now returns to the hospital complaining of chills, fever, and right quadrant abdominal pain. Suspecting appendicitis, the physician admits the patient for an emergency appendectomy. To describe the appendectomy admission, the physician should report 44950–79. The appendectomy is unrelated to the initial procedure

performed (hernia repair), so modifier –79 is reported to indicate that the procedure was performed during the postoperative period but is unrelated to the initial surgery.

–80 Assistant Surgeon: Modifier –80 may be reported to indicate that the physician provided surgical assistant services for a particular procedure. The surgeon who assists another physician reports the code for the procedure that was performed, along with modifier –80. The operating surgeon should not report modifier –80.

Note: An assistant surgeon typically is present throughout the entire surgical procedure.

> **Example:** Dr. Reynolds performs a total abdominal hysterectomy with removal of fallopian tubes and ovaries. Dr. Jones provides surgical assistance. Dr. Reynolds should report 58150, and Dr. Jones should report 58150–80.

–81 Minimum Assistant Surgeon: Modifier –81 may be reported to indicate that a physician provided minimal surgical assistance when the surgeon's presence typically is not required throughout the entire procedure. The physician who provided minimal assistance reports the code for the procedure performed, along with modifier –81. As in the case of modifier –80, the operating surgeon should not report modifier –81.

–82 Assistant Surgeon (when qualified resident surgeon not available): Modifier –82 may be reported when a physician provides surgical assistance to another surgeon and a resident surgeon is unavailable. This situation occurs primarily in teaching facilities where resident surgeons often assume the role of assistant surgeon. When a qualified resident surgeon is unavailable, another physician may serve as an assistant surgeon and report the appropriate procedure code along with modifier –82. As in the case of modifiers –80 and –81, the operating surgeon should not report modifier –82.

–90 Reference (Outside) Laboratory: Modifier –90 is used widely for laboratory and pathology services. It indicates that the physician does not perform the actual test or service but, instead, sends specimens to an outside laboratory.

–91 Repeat Clinical Diagnostic Laboratory Test: Modifier –91 may be used for laboratory test(s) performed more than once on the same day on the same patient. This modifier may not be used when tests are rerun either to confirm initial results, because of testing problems with specimens or equipment, or for any other reason when a normal, one-time, reportable result is all that is required.

–92 Alternative Laboratory Platform Testing: When laboratory testing is being performed using a kit or transportable instrument that wholly or in part consists of a single use, disposable analytical chamber, the service may be identified by adding modifier –92 to the usual laboratory procedure code (HIV testing 86701–86703). The test does not require permanent dedicated space; hence by its design it may be hand-carried or transported to the vicinity of the patient for immediate testing at that site, although location of the testing is not in itself determinative of the use of this modifier.

CPT Anesthesia Physical Status Modifiers

Physical status modifiers are used to indicate the patient's condition and thus the complexity of the anesthesia service. They are consistent with the ranking system used by the American Society of Anesthesiologists (ASA).

The physical status modifiers and their definitions are as follows:

-P1   **A normal healthy patient**

-P2   **A patient with mild systemic disease**

-P3   **A patient with severe systemic disease**

-P4   **A patient with severe systemic disease that is a constant threat to life**

-P5   **A moribund patient who is not expected to survive without the operation**

-P6   **A declared brain-dead patient whose organs are being removed for donor purposes**

Not all third-party payers recognize the physical status modifiers. Thus, it is important to adhere to individual third-party payer rules and regulations when billing for anesthesia services.

HCPCS Level II Modifier Descriptions and Examples

The number of HCPCS Level II modifiers continues to grow yearly. For a complete list of HCPCS Level II modifiers, refer to the HCPCS book and the quarterly HCPCS updates on the CMS website at the HCPCS Release and Code Sets page (CMS 2015a). The following are some of the more common modifiers used in the reporting of professional services:

-AA   **Anesthesia services performed personally by an anesthesiologist**

-AD   **Medical supervision by a physician: more than four concurrent anesthesia procedures**

-AI   **Principal physician of record**

-G8   **Monitored anesthesia care (MAC) for deep complex, complicated, or markedly invasive surgical procedure**

-G9   **Monitored anesthesia care (MAC) for a patient who has history of severe cardiopulmonary condition**

-GA   **Waiver of liability statement issued, as required by payer policy**

-GC   **This service has been performed in part by a resident under the direction of a teaching physician**

-GE   **This service has been performed by a resident without the presence of a teaching physician under the primary care exception**

-GG   **Performance and payment of a screening mammogram and diagnostic mammogram on the same patient, same day**

-GH   **Diagnostic mammogram converted from screening mammogram on the same day**

-GX   **Notice of liability issued, voluntary under payer policy**

-GY   **Item or service statutorily excluded or does not meet the definition of any Medicare benefit or for non-Medicare insurers, is not a contract benefit**

-GZ   **Item or service expected to be denied as not reasonable and necessary**

-Q5   **Service furnished by a substitute physician under a reciprocal billing arrangement**

-Q6   **Service furnished by a locum tenens physician**

-QK   **Medical direction of two, three, or four concurrent anesthesia procedures involving qualified individuals**

-QS   **Monitored anesthesia care service**

-QW   **CLIA waived test**

-QX   **CRNA service: with medical direction by a physician**

-QY   **Medical direction of one certified registered nurse anesthetist (CRNA) by an anesthesiologist**

-QZ   **CRNA service: without medical direction by a physician**

-SA   **Nurse practitioner rendering service in collaboration with a physician**

-SB   **Nurse midwife**

-TC   **Technical component. Under certain circumstances, a charge may be made for the technical component alone. Under those circumstances the technical component charge is identified by adding modifier -TC to the usual procedure code.**

Anatomical Modifiers

Anatomical modifiers are HCPCS Level II modifiers that help describe exactly which digit or body area is receiving treatment. The anatomical modifiers include:

-**LT**   Modifier -LT is used to identify procedures performed on the left side of the body.

-**RT**   Modifier -RT is used to identify procedures performed on the right side of the body.

Anatomical modifiers are available to help describe the exact body location of procedures that have been performed. The -LT and -RT modifiers describe procedures performed on one side of the body when paired organs or structures exist. Also, it is common to have procedures performed on two or more fingers or two or more toes. The anatomical multiple modifiers help describe exactly which digit is receiving the treatment. The anatomical modifiers assigned to each digit (fingers and toes, not metacarpals or metatarsals) are summarized here:

Left Hand	Left Foot	Right Hand	Right Foot
–FA (Thumb)	–TA (Great toe)	–F5 (Thumb)	–T5 (Great toe)
–F1 (2nd Digit)	–T1 (2nd Digit)	–F6 (2nd Digit)	–T6 (2nd Digit)
–F2 (3rd Digit)	–T2 (3rd Digit)	–F7 (3rd Digit)	–T7 (3rd Digit)
–F3 (4th Digit)	–T3 (4th Digit)	–F8 (4th Digit)	–T8 (4th Digit)
–F4 (5th Digit)	–T4 (5th Digit)	–F9 (5th Digit)	–T9 (5th Digit)

Other anatomical modifiers help describe the exact location for procedures on the eyelids:

Left Eyelid	Right Eyelid
–E1 (Upper)	–E3 (Upper)
–E2 (Lower)	–E4 (Lower)

Modifier Index

Subject	Modifiers
72 hour rule	PD
Advanced beneficiary notice (waiver)	GA, GX, GY, GZ, KB
Agency services	H9, HU, HV, HW, HX, HY, HZ, SE, TL
Ambulance	GM, QL, QM, QN, TK, TP, TQ
Ambulatory surgery center	SG
Anatomical modifiers	E1–E4, FA–F9, LT, RT, TA–T9
Anemia	EA, EB, EC, ED, EE, GS
Anesthesia	23, 47, AA, AD, G8, G9, P1–P6, QK, QS, QX, QY, QZ
Assistant surgeon	80, 81, 82
Bilateral	50
Catastrophe/Disaster Related	CR
Category II exclusions	1P, 2P, 3P, 8P
Chiropractic services	AT
Component billing	26, TC
Coronary vessels	LC, LD, LM, RC, RI
Decision for surgery	57
Dialysis/Renal	AX, AY, CB, CD, CE, CF, EM, G1–G6
Discontinued procedure	53
Distinct procedures	59
Dressings, wounds and supplies	A1–A9, AW, JC, JD
Drug Administration Route	JA, JB, JE, JW, KD, KO, KP, RD, SH, SJ
Drugs and enteral/parenteral therapy, supplies and infusion	BA, BO, EJ, GS, JW, KD, KO, KP, KQ, KS, KT, RD, SC, SH, SJ, SK, SL, SS, SV, SY

Subject	Modifiers
Durable medical equipment	AU, AV, BP, BR, BU, EY, FB, FC, J4, K0–K4, KA, KB, KC, KE, KF, KG, KH, KI, KJ, KK, KL, KM, KN, KR, KT, KU, KV, KW, KX, KY, LL, MS, NR, NU, RA, RB, RD, RR, SC, SQ, TW, UE
Emergency services	CA, ET, GJ
Evaluation and management services	24, 25, 32, 57
Family planning	FP
Funding source	FB, HU, HV, HW, HX, HY, HZ, SE
Genetic testing	0A–9Z
Health professional shortage area (HPSA)	AQ
Hospice	GV, GW
Infants less than 4 Kg	63
Informational	AO, CC, CG, CH, CI, CJ, CK, CL, CM, CN, G1–G5, G7, GB, GD, GJ, GK, GL, KB, KX, KZ, Q4, QC, QD, QE, QF, QG, QH, QT, RE, SC, SQ, ST, SU, SY, TK, TM, TN, TR, TS, TT, TU, TV, UK, V5, V6, V7
Laboratory	90, 91, 92, BL, LR, QP, QW
Level of care	TF, TG
Location of service (VA, HPSA)	GR, SU, SS, TN
Managed care	KZ
Mandated services	32, 33, H9, Q2, SF, SM, SN
Medicaid services	EP, FP, U1–U9, UA, UB, UC, UD
Medicare Secondary Payer (MSP)	M2
Modifier –59 replacements	XE, XP, XS, XU
More than one surgeon	62, 66, 80, 81, 82
Multiple modifiers	99
Multiple procedures	51
Nonphysician services	AE, AH, AJ, AS, GF, HL, HM, HN, HO, HP, HT, QE, QF, QG, QH, SA, SB, SD, SW, TD, TE, HQ, HR, HS, QJ, SK, SY, UN, UP, UQ, UR, US
Patient identifiers	
Pharmacy services	J1, J2, J3
Physical status	P1–P6
Physician services	AF, AG, AI, AK, AM, AR, GV, HT, Q5, Q6, SU
Podiatry (foot care)	Q7, Q8, Q9
Pregnancy related	G7, TH
Prison services	QJ
Procedures in the global period	78, 79
Professional/technical components	26, TC
Program identifiers	HA, HB, HC, HD, HE, HF, HG, HH, HI, HJ, HK, HQ, HU, HV, HW, HX, HY, HZ, Q2, SE, TJ, TL, TM, TR

Subject	Modifiers
Prosthetics	AV, K0–K4, KM, KN
Radiology	26, GG, GH, PI, PS, TC
Reduced services	52
Repeat procedures	76, 77, 91
Research	Q0, Q1
Second/third opinion	SF, SM, SN
Service times	TS, UF, UG, UH, UJ
Shared services	54, 55, 56, 62, 66
Staged procedure	58, PI, PS
Surgical misadventure	PA, PB, PC
Teaching physician	GC, GE, GR
Telemedicine	GQ, GT
Therapy	GN, GO, GP
Transplant	Q3
Trauma or injury	ST
Unusual or increased procedures	22, 52, 53, 63, 76, 77
Vision services	AP, LS, LT, PL, RT, VP

Exercise 9.1. Modifiers

Choose the best answer for each of the following questions.

1. When reporting the same procedure code on two fingers of the same hand, what action should the coder take?

   a. Use a –51 modifier for the second finger
   b. Use a –LT or –RT modifier for each finger
   c. Use an anatomical modifier for each finger
   d. Use a –22 modifier for each finger

2. Modifier _____ is often confused with modifier –91.

   a. –90
   b. –77
   c. –76
   d. –59

3. A 25-year-old patient is having trouble hearing out of the right ear. The patient is given a pure tone, air only screening test of the right ear. How is this coded?

   a. 92551–RT
   b. 92551–52
   c. 92552–52
   d. 92552–RT

4. When modifier –50 is applied to a code, it means which of the following statements?

   a. The physician provided only postoperative care.
   b. A bilateral procedure was performed during the same operative session.
   c. A surgical team performed a highly complex procedure.
   d. The physician performed a repeat procedure.

5. If the provider is billing Medicare for a service that is noncovered, which modifier is the most appropriate?

   a. –GA
   b. –GB
   c. –GY
   d. –GZ

6. True or False? Modifier –59 says that the decision for surgery was made on the day of the visit. _____

7. True or False? When two surgeons perform parts of the same procedure on the same day during the same operative session, modifier –66 should be used. _____

8. True or False? Modifier –25 is appended to the E/M code. _____

9. True or False? The –53 modifier can only be used by a physician. _____

10. True or False? Modifier –TC is a HCPCS modifier used to describe the completion of the technical component. _____

Chapter 9 Test

Choose the best answer for each of the following questions.

1. If two of the same clinical laboratory tests are performed on the same calendar date, which modifier is used on the second test?

   a. –59
   b. –76
   c. –91
   d. –QW

2. Code the following operative report:

   Preoperative Diagnosis: Esotropia

   Postoperative Diagnosis: Esotropia

   Anesthesia: General

   History/Indications: This is an 8-month-old girl with a history of strabismus since early infancy. Eye muscle surgery is indicated to improve ocular alignment with anticipated functional benefits including expansion of the peripheral binocular field of vision and recovery of central binocular vision. The prognosis for binocular recovery is considered good in view of the child's early age at the time of surgery.

   Procedure: The patient was brought to the operating room and general anesthesia was induced and maintained. The regions of both eyes were prepared and draped in the usual manner for muscle surgery. The left eye was operated on first. Through an inferonasal fornix incision, the left medial rectus muscle was isolated on a hook and cleaned of its anterior fascial attachments. The tone of the muscle was moderately increased and its attachments were normal. One double-arm suture of 6-0 Vicryl was woven through the tendon just above the insertion with lock bites at each end and the muscle was disinserted from the globe. It was reattached to the sclera at a measured distance of 7 mm posterior to the original insertion using the Vicryl suture in the crossed swords fashion, with incorporation of the center of the anterior edge of the tendon into the knot for reinforcement. No suture was required for conjunctival closure. The right eye was operated on in a similar manner, again recessing the medial rectus muscle 7 mm with a single 6-0 Vicryl suture with central reinforcement. Operative findings and handling of the conjunctiva and fascia were similar to those on the left. After conclusion of the procedure, the patient was awakened in the operating room and sent to the recovery room in satisfactory condition.

   a. 67311–LT, 67311–RT
   b. 67311–50
   c. 67314–LT, 67314–RT
   d. 67314–50

3. If a test is performed in a CLIA-waived laboratory, which modifier should be appended to the test code?

   a. –GA
   b. –GZ
   c. –QP
   d. –QW

4. A patient from out of town presents through the ER, and the physician delivers twins, one vaginally and the second one via cesarean section. The physician did not provide any other OB care for the patient. How would these deliveries be coded?

   a. 59514, 59409–51
   b. 59510, 59409–59
   c. 59400, 59414–51
   d. 59899

(Continued on next page)

Chapter 9 Test (Continued)

5. The patient is a 12-year-old boy whose parents request that he undergo reconstruction of both auricles because he "can't stand being picked on because they stick out." On examination, the physician determines that an area of 0.5 cm × 0.3 cm of extra skin needs to be removed bilaterally to fix the problem. The procedure is performed in the day surgery suite. How is this surgical procedure coded?

   a. 14060, 14060–51
   b. 14061
   c. 69110–50
   d. 69300–50

6. Which of the following is used with End Stage Renal Disease services?

   a. –EC
   b. –G6
   c. –GT
   d. –SJ

7. What modifier is used with CPT Category II codes?

   a. –GW
   b. –1P
   c. –P2
   d. –26

8. Code the following operative report:

   Preoperative Diagnosis: Right hip degenerative labral tear

   Postoperative Diagnosis: Same

   Procedures:

   1. Right hip arthroscopy

   2. Labral debridement from 12 o'clock to 3 o'clock

   Indications for Procedure: Patient is a 59-year-old male with chronic hip pain. He has responded temporarily to injections, but this fails to provide significant relief. He has tried therapy and other conservative measures as well. His MRI shows possible labral tear. The plan is for hip arthroscopy and debridement.

   Complete Description of Procedure Including Findings: The patient was brought into the operating room where surgical and anesthesia time-outs were performed to verify the correct patient and procedure. The patient was then placed in a supine position under general anesthesia. The patient was positioned appropriately and well padded.

   An anterior lateral portal was then placed under C-arm guidance into the hip joint. Care was taken to avoid the labrum at all cost. I then did an air arthrogram followed by a saline arthrogram to verify that we are in the joint. I then created an anterior accessory portal lateral to the anterior superior spine line. I introduced a spinal needle into the anterior triangle of the capsule. A wire was passed and this was dilated. I then introduced another 4.5mm cannula into this portal. I then switched the camera to the accessory portal to verify the anterolateral cannula did not penetrate the labrum. I used a beaver type blade to incise the capsule only approximately 1cm around each portal to allow a diagnostic arthroscopy. A full diagnostic arthroscopy was performed. Two small partial thickness iatrogenic cartilage lesions were seen and debrided from portal insertion. The status of the articular cartilage showed that he had no significant lesions. The posterior labrum was partially torn in a degenerative pattern. The labrum was extensively torn with early cartilage delamination from 12 o'clock to 3 o'clock. The labrum was not fully disconnected. The tear was debrided to a stable border using a shaver. We released traction at approximately 40 minutes. 20cc of 1/2% marcaine was then injected around the surgery sites. The wound was irrigated and closed. Nylon was used to reapproximate the skin. The sponge and instrument count was reported to me as correct. EBL was minimal.

Chapter 9 Test (Continued)

    a.   29860–RT, 29862–RT
    b.   29862–RT, 29916–59–RT
    c.   29862–RT
    d.   29916–59–RT

9.   When a procedure is started but cannot be completed, which modifier should be assigned?

    a.   –22
    b.   –52
    c.   –53
    d.   –76

10.   What modifier(s) would best describe that the physician performed the same procedure on the third and fourth digits of the right foot?

    a.   Use –T7 on the third toe and –T8 and –51 on the fourth toe
    b.   Use a –76 modifier on the fourth toe
    c.   Use –51 and –77 modifiers on the fourth toe
    d.   Use a –22 modifier on one procedure code

Chapter 10

Reimbursement Process

Objectives

Upon completion of this chapter, the student should be able to do the following:

- Define various payment methodologies used for physician office reimbursement

- Identify ways to obtain regulatory agency and payer-specific guidelines for use in the coding and reimbursement process

- Apply payer-specific guidelines to coding principles so that codes are assigned correctly for each visit

- Define the data elements required for completing a CMS-1500—the industry-standard claim form

- Define the data elements required for a computerized internal fee schedule database

- Describe the process flow of claims generation and processing from patient visit to final payment

- Define accounts receivable management

- Describe various methods used in the process of accounts receivable management

Proper coding is only one part of achieving appropriate reimbursement. Attention must be paid to other details involved in the process, such as payment methodologies, regulatory and payer-specific guidelines, and the appropriate setting of fees. Knowledge of these areas, combined with proper coding, helps ensure payment to the physician for the services he or she provided. This chapter covers these additional areas involved in the reimbursement process.

Reimbursement Mechanisms

A number of mechanisms are available for reimbursing physicians for their services. These are discussed in the following subsections.

Standard Charges

A physician practice determines charges for medical services on the basis of a number of factors, including cost of the service provided, current market value of the service, and knowledge of who will be reimbursing the practice for the service. Standard charges, at their full-dollar value, are rarely reimbursed at 100 percent any longer. Most fees are negotiated or discounted in some way. Patients who have no insurance and must pay cash for their care may be the only parties who pay the full-dollar value.

To determine standard charges for a procedure, the physician practice may use a variety of methods. Many practices consult national fee surveys that can be adjusted for geographic cost-of-living differences. Other practices apply a percentage to the resource-based relative value scale (RBRVS) used by Medicare. (This topic is discussed in depth later in this chapter in the Fee Schedule Management section.)

Discounted Charges

Sometimes the provider agrees to see patients from a particular insurer and charge the full rate. The insurer then discounts the rate by a certain amount, usually a percentage, as the payment is made. Patients normally have no additional financial responsibility for the balance because the discount is negotiated with their insurer. This arrangement is popular with physicians because a reduced fee is exchanged for a known percentage of each charge submitted. In addition, there is no additional cost for attempting to obtain payment from a patient.

Usual and Customary Fee Profile

The usual and customary (U/C) fee profile concept is based on both the usual fee submitted by the provider for that code and the area customary fee for that code. Many large insurers maintain a database of the charges submitted for certain procedures by the physician over time. This database maintains the average charges that become the provider's fee profile.

The insurance company pays the lower of the current charges, the physician's profile amount, the area customary fee, or any schedule of benefits. A schedule of benefits may limit the amount the insurance company is required to pay for certain procedures.

> **Example:** Dr. XYZ submits a claim of $252 for CPT code 24500. In the past, he has submitted charges for this code in the amounts of $230, $240, $250, and $270, so the fee profile for code 24500 for Dr. XYZ is $247.50 (the average of his previous charge submissions). The area customary fee for code 24500 is $250. The schedule of benefits maximum lists $255. Therefore, the current claim would be paid at the lowest of all these amounts, the profile amount of $247.50.

Fee Schedule, Negotiated

A negotiated fee schedule is created between a physician and an insurance company to ensure a flat rate per procedure, visit, or service. Negotiated fees may have no relationship to normal charges and are negotiated based on supply and demand. The insurance company may be willing to pay more than the normal charge for some procedures if the physician is the only one performing that service and patient access is guaranteed. However, the payer may want a lower charge on other procedures to compensate for this one higher fee.

When a negotiated fee schedule is used, many insurance companies require that the fee received be considered payment in full. This means the practice is not allowed to balance bill the patient for any amount above the negotiated fee.

Capitation

Capitation is payment of a fixed-dollar amount for each covered person for a predetermined set of services for a specified period of time, such as a month. The physician is responsible for providing all the care needed to each of the patients for which a capitation payment is received.

With this payment arrangement, usually used by managed care organizations for their members, the physician assumes the risk for the cost and frequency of the services provided. For example, the physician may receive $25 per month for each assigned patient, whether or not the patient receives any care during the month. This is called the **per member per month** (PMPM) rate. Under capitation, claims are sent to the insurance carrier for information purposes only. The claims are not processed for payment, and bills are not sent to patients. Physicians who practice effectively can do well under this arrangement, but those who do not manage their resources well are financially at risk.

Coding is vitally important under this payment arrangement because physicians need information on how many patients were seen, how frequently, and for what reason.

RBRVS Medicare Fee Schedule

The resource-based relative value scale (RBRVS) is the national fee system used to calculate the approved amount for Medicare payments to physicians. Enacted January 1, 1992, this relative value system assigns a value unit to each CPT code. The value units are based on the work involved, practice costs, and the malpractice expense associated with the particular procedure. The Medicare conversion factors are set annually by the US Congress and are published each December in the *Federal Register* for the coming year. Many practices use the same relative value units and also use a higher conversion factor to determine their own fees.

National Physician Fee Schedule Relative Value File

This file is the electronic version of the information contained in the *Federal Register*. The file is updated quarterly and can be downloaded from the CMS website. The download process requires software that opens compressed files (such as Unzip Wizard or WinZip).

- Go to http://www.cms.gov/Medicare/Medicare-Fee-for-Service-Payment/Physician FeeSched/PFS-Relative-Value-Files.html.

- Click on RVU16A (16 represents the current year, A represents the first quarterly update) to download the file.

- In the zip folder that opens, click these three files and save the files that open:
  PPRRVU16.xlsx
  RVUPUF16.docx
  GPCI2016.xlsx

PPRRVU16.xlsx is the relative value file. Table 10.1 shows a condensed version of the 2015 file. The complete file for 2015 is almost 1,400 pages. Therefore, it is recommended that the coder use the features within the spreadsheet program to hide columns and rows that may not be needed as often.

The file contains row entries for all HCPCS and CPT codes and contains columns of data such as Part B status indicators, all RVU elements, global days, modifier indicators, and the conversation factor. The data in many columns are coded and must be translated using the information found in the RVUPUF16.docx file. The GPCI2016.xlsx file contains the geographic practice cost index information for each locality in the Medicare coverage area. Use these files to obtain the necessary data elements for RBRVS calculations.

To determine the RBRVS-approved amount, components of the relative value unit are multiplied by the corresponding components of the geographic practice cost index (GPCI), and then this figure is multiplied by a monetary conversion factor. (The GPCI is specific to the geographic area in which the practice is located.) The elements of the RBRVS formula are:

$$\begin{aligned}
W(RVU) &= \text{Work relative value unit} \\
P(RVU) &= \text{Practice expense relative value unit} \\
M(RVU) &= \text{Malpractice relative value unit (also referred to as professional liability} \\
&\quad \text{insurance [PLI] in some literature)} \\
G(W) &= \text{Work GPCI} \\
G(P) &= \text{Practice expense GPCI} \\
G(M) &= \text{Malpractice GPCI} \\
CF &= \text{Monetary conversion factor}
\end{aligned}$$

The formula is:

$$[(W(RVU) \times G(W)) + (P(RVU) \times G(P)) + (M(RVU) \times G(M))] \times CF = Payment$$

To complete the formula, look up the values associated with each component in the relative value file for the current year. Then, place the values into the formula and use standard arithmetic rules to solve the equation. The conversion factor for 2015 is \$35.9335. The 2016 conversion factor was not final at the time of publication.

For example, one geographic area of Wisconsin calculates an approved amount for 2014 of \$105.87 for code 57452:

$$[(1.5 \times 1.000) + (1.39 \times 0.955) + (0.21 \times 0.566)] = 2.94631 \times \$35.9335 = \$105.87$$

Table 10.1. Excerpt from 2015 National Physician Fee Schedule Relative Value File

HCPCS	MOD	DESCRIPTION	STATUS CODE	WORK RVU	NON-FACILITY PE RVU	FACILITY PE RVU	MP RVU	NON-FACILITY TOTAL	FACILITY TOTAL	PCTC IND	GLOB DAYS	PRE OP	INTRA OP	POST OP	MULT PROC	BILAT SURG	ASST SURG	CO-SURG	TEAM SURG	CONV FACTOR	PHYS SUPR
A4565		Slings	X	0.00	0.00	0.00	0.00	0.00	0.00	9	XXX	0.00	0.00	0.00	9	9	9	9	9	35.9335	09
A4570		Splint	I	0.00	0.00	0.00	0.00	0.00	0.00	9	XXX	0.00	0.00	0.00	9	9	9	9	9	35.9335	09
A4575		Hyperbaric o2 chamber disps	N	0.00	0.00	0.00	0.00	0.00	0.00	9	XXX	0.00	0.00	0.00	9	9	9	9	9	35.9335	09
A4580		Cast supplies (plaster)	I	0.00	0.00	0.00	0.00	0.00	0.00	9	XXX	0.00	0.00	0.00	9	9	9	9	9	35.9335	09
A4590		Special casting material	I	0.00	0.00	0.00	0.00	0.00	0.00	9	XXX	0.00	0.00	0.00	9	9	9	9	9	35.9335	09
A4595		Tens suppl 2 lead per month	X	0.00	0.00	0.00	0.00	0.00	0.00	9	XXX	0.00	0.00	0.00	9	9	9	9	9	35.9335	09
G0008		Admin influenza virus vac	X	0.00	0.00	0.00	0.00	0.00	0.00	9	XXX	0.00	0.00	0.00	9	9	9	9	9	35.9335	09
J0696		Ceftriaxone sodium injection	E	0.00	0.00	0.00	0.00	0.00	0.00	9	XXX	0.00	0.00	0.00	9	9	9	9	9	35.9335	09
J0697		Sterile cefuroxime injection	E	0.00	0.00	0.00	0.00	0.00	0.00	9	XXX	0.00	0.00	0.00	9	9	9	9	9	35.9335	09
J1100		Dexamethasone sodium phos	E	0.00	0.00	0.00	0.00	0.00	0.00	9	XXX	0.00	0.00	0.00	9	9	9	9	9	35.9335	09
11010		Debride skin at fx site	A	4.19	9.01	3.11	0.74	13.94	8.04	0	010	0.10	0.80	0.10	2	2	1	0	0	35.9335	09
11011		Debride skin musc at fx site	A	4.94	9.10	2.68	0.94	14.98	8.56	0	000	0.00	0.00	0.00	2	2	1	0	0	35.9335	09
11012		Deb skin bone at fx site	A	6.87	11.93	3.99	1.35	20.15	12.21	0	000	0.00	0.00	0.00	2	2	1	0	0	35.9335	09
27888		Amputation of foot at ankle	A	10.37	7.52	7.52	2.03	19.92	19.92	0	090	0.10	0.69	0.21	2	1	2	1	0	35.9335	09
28001		Drainage of bursa of foot	A	2.78	5.03	1.92	0.26	8.07	4.96	0	010	0.10	0.80	0.10	2	0	1	0	0	35.9335	09
33851		Remove aorta constriction	A	21.98	11.49	11.49	5.40	38.87	38.87	0	090	0.09	0.84	0.07	2	0	2	1	0	35.9335	09
33852		Repair septal defect	A	24.41	10.40	10.40	5.79	40.60	40.60	0	090	0.09	0.84	0.07	2	0	2	0	0	35.9335	09
33853		Repair septal defect	A	32.51	13.00	13.00	7.73	53.24	53.24	0	090	0.09	0.84	0.07	2	0	2	1	0	35.9335	09
57452		Exam of cervix w/scope	A	1.50	1.39	0.93	0.21	3.10	2.64	0	000	0.00	0.00	0.00	2	1	1	0	0	35.9335	09
60650		Laparoscopy adrenalectomy	A	20.73	9.58	9.58	4.08	34.39	34.39	0	090	0.09	0.84	0.07	2	1	2	1	0	35.9335	09
71250		Ct thorax w/o dye	A	1.02	3.96	3.96	0.06	5.04	5.04	1	XXX	0.00	0.00	0.00	4	0	0	0	0	35.9335	09
71250	TC	Ct thorax w/o dye	A	0.00	3.58	3.58	0.01	3.59	3.59	1	XXX	0.00	0.00	0.00	4	0	0	0	0	35.9335	01
71250	26	Ct thorax w/o dye	A	1.02	0.38	0.38	0.05	1.45	1.45	1	XXX	0.00	0.00	0.00	4	0	0	0	0	35.9335	09
80048		Metabolic panel total ca	X	0.00	0.00	0.00	0.00	0.00	0.00	9	XXX	0.00	0.00	0.00	9	9	9	9	9	35.9335	09
80050		General health panel	N	0.00	0.00	0.00	0.00	0.00	0.00	9	XXX	0.00	0.00	0.00	9	9	9	9	9	35.9335	09
80051		Electrolyte panel	X	0.00	0.00	0.00	0.00	0.00	0.00	9	XXX	0.00	0.00	0.00	9	9	9	9	9	35.9335	09
99201		Office/outpatient visit new	A	0.48	0.71	0.23	0.04	1.23	0.75	0	XXX	0.00	0.00	0.00	0	0	0	0	0	35.9335	09
99202		Office/outpatient visit new	A	0.93	1.10	0.41	0.07	2.10	1.41	0	XXX	0.00	0.00	0.00	0	0	0	0	0	35.9335	09
99203		Office/outpatient visit new	A	1.42	1.48	0.60	0.15	3.05	2.17	0	XXX	0.00	0.00	0.00	0	0	0	0	0	35.9335	09
99204		Office/outpatient visit new	A	2.43	1.99	1.02	0.22	4.64	3.67	0	XXX	0.00	0.00	0.00	0	0	0	0	0	35.9335	09
99205		Office/outpatient visit new	A	3.17	2.37	1.31	0.29	5.83	4.77	0	XXX	0.00	0.00	0.00	0	0	0	0	0	35.9335	09
99211		Office/outpatient visit est	A	0.18	0.37	0.07	0.01	0.56	0.26	0	XXX	0.00	0.00	0.00	0	0	0	0	0	35.9335	09
99212		Office/outpatient visit est	A	0.48	0.71	0.20	0.04	1.23	0.72	0	XXX	0.00	0.00	0.00	0	0	0	0	0	35.9335	09
99213		Office/outpatient visit est	A	0.97	1.01	0.40	0.06	2.04	1.43	0	XXX	0.00	0.00	0.00	0	0	0	0	0	35.9335	09
99214		Office/outpatient visit est	A	1.50	1.43	0.61	0.10	3.03	2.21	0	XXX	0.00	0.00	0.00	0	0	0	0	0	35.9335	09
99215		Office/outpatient visit est	A	2.11	1.82	0.87	0.16	4.09	3.14	0	XXX	0.00	0.00	0.00	0	0	0	0	0	35.9335	09
99217		Observation care discharge	A	1.28	0.68	0.68	0.09	2.05	2.05	0	XXX	0.00	0.00	0.00	0	0	0	0	0	35.9335	09
99218		Initial observation care	A	1.92	0.75	0.75	0.16	2.83	2.83	0	XXX	0.00	0.00	0.00	0	0	0	0	0	35.9335	09
99219		Initial observation care	A	2.60	1.05	1.05	0.18	3.83	3.83	0	XXX	0.00	0.00	0.00	0	0	0	0	0	35.9335	09
99220		Initial observation care	A	3.56	1.43	1.43	0.26	5.25	5.25	0	XXX	0.00	0.00	0.00	0	0	0	0	0	35.9335	09
99221		Initial hospital care	A	1.92	0.76	0.76	0.19	2.87	2.87	0	XXX	0.00	0.00	0.00	0	0	0	0	0	35.9335	09
99222		Initial hospital care	A	2.61	1.05	1.05	0.21	3.87	3.87	0	XXX	0.00	0.00	0.00	0	0	0	0	0	35.9335	09
99223		Initial hospital care	A	3.86	1.57	1.57	0.30	5.73	5.73	0	XXX	0.00	0.00	0.00	0	0	0	0	0	35.9335	09

CPT codes and descriptions only are copyright 2015 American Medical Association. All Rights Reserved. Applicable FARS/DFARS Apply.
Dental code (D codes) are copyright 2015 American Dental Association. All Rights Reserved.

Participating Provider Agreements

A provider that participates with an insurance plan (including Medicare) has a contractual arrangement with the plan to provide care and bill the plan directly for the services provided to plan beneficiaries. The insurance plan pays the allowed amount directly to the provider. The participating provider (PAR) adjusts off the disallowed amount and cannot bill the patient for the balance not paid by the plan.

Inherent in Medicare participation status is the agreement to accept assignment on all claims. Accepting assignment means that the payment is made directly to the provider and the provider agrees to accept the plan's allowed amount as the maximum payment that can be obtained for the service. Nonparticipation (non-PAR) means that the provider does not have an agreement with the plan and usually expects payment in full from the patient at the time of the service. The provider may accept assignment on a claim-by-claim basis at any time. However, on assigned claims from nonparticipating providers, Medicare will only pay the provider 95 percent of the approved amount. For example, if the approved amount is $100, Medicare will pay the provider $76 (95% of $80) and the patient will still responsible for the $20 (20%) coinsurance in addition to an annual Part B deductible of $166 for 2016.

For Medicare, non-PAR status also means that the provider may not bill the patient more than the Medicare limiting charge (115% of the Medicare-approved amount) on unassigned claims. For example, if the approved amount is $100, the provider may bill the patient up to $115 for the service. Medicare will pay the patient $80, and the patient is responsible for $35 out-of-pocket and the $80 Medicare payment to satisfy the $115 provider charge. Therefore, it is in the patient's best financial interest to seek a participating provider for care.

Fee Schedule Management

Fee schedule management, or setting and adjusting fees, is the lifeblood of the medical practice as well as the counterpart to correct code assignment; both must be done well so that the practice can be reimbursed properly. In today's medical practice, almost all medical fees are negotiated down in some way, so it is important to establish fees at an appropriate and fair starting level.

To manage the fee schedule, the staff must know the following:

- How the practice is reimbursed for services
- The basic value of the services provided
- The going rates of services in the marketplace
- The signals indicating that fees need adjustment
- Not to charge less than the payer will pay

There is no need to manage fees in a practice using a 100 percent negotiated fee schedule or 100 percent capitation. The fee or capitation payment is negotiated once per year, and the patient does not receive a bill. In practices where standard charges are used and reimbursed (by discount, usual and customary, or Medicare fee schedule) and patients pay all or a portion of the balance, fees must be evaluated at least annually.

Chapter 11 introduces the revenue production report. This report shows the number of times a particular procedure is coded and the total revenue produced as a result of the coding. This type of report identifies the most frequently used codes in the physician's practice and is used to develop the fee schedule management worksheet. This worksheet displays the code, description, current fee, relative value units, reimbursement from Medicare, reimbursement from Medicaid, reimbursement from several other frequently billed insurance carriers, conversion factor, and a space for the new fee. Table 10.2 provides an example of a fee schedule management worksheet.

The current fee must be evaluated to ensure that it is above the reimbursement levels allowed by the insurance carriers and to be sensitive to the demands of the patient population regarding procedures, such as preventive services, for which they frequently pay cash. These increases will be noticed immediately and could cause patient complaints. Typically, practices have fewer problems when they are sensitive to the number of times a procedure is performed as they increase fees. A small fee increase for a high volume procedure may bring a significant increase in revenue without much notice. Similarly, a larger increase in a fee for a lower volume procedure may not be seen as inappropriate. It is important to determine and enter a new fee for each procedure code into the worksheet and obtain approval for fee changes before implementation. To thoroughly evaluate the fees of a practice, consideration should be given to evaluating the codes that provide 80 percent of the revenue produced in the practice.

Throughout the year, a fee problem log organized by CPT/HCPCS code should be maintained, using either a manual log in a ring binder that is tabbed for the major sections of the CPT and HCPCS code books or, if one is available, a computerized database. Table 10.3 is an example of the page from a manual fee problem log for CPT codes 10021–19499.

An entry is made each time a problem with reimbursement on a particular code is noted:

- A patient or an insurance company alerts the office that the current fee is over the area customary fee. Make a note in the log of all information that can be obtained.

- A patient complains about the fee being higher than the fee charged by another area practice. Make note of this information, including the fee the patient has quoted.

- An insurer pays 100 percent of the charge.

A published national fee survey report is available from many vendors of practice management products. These national fee surveys show the range of fees charged for a particular code, indicating the lowest and highest fee reported in the survey as well as the 50th, 75th, and 90th percentiles of the survey. The survey should be evaluated against the current fees the practice is using to determine which level most closely approximates those fees. This survey also can be used as a reference when new procedures require fee establishment.

Table 10.2. Fee schedule management worksheet

Code	Description	Relative Fee	Value	Medicare	Medicaid	Other	Conversion Other	New Factor	Fee
12001	Wound Repair	$102.00	1.6	$56.50	$55.76	$86.50	$98.00	$70.00	$112.00

Table 10.3. Fee problem log

Code	Description	Fee	Problem	Insurer/Source	Date
12034	Wound Repair	$234.00	Paid at less than half the charge	Blue Cross	2-1-XX
17000	Lesion Destruction	$35.00	Only paid $25.00 at Dr. X's office	Patient	2-10-XX

Sources of Coding and Reimbursement Guidelines

Practices should obtain coding and reimbursement guidelines from the insurers they frequently bill. Large insurers, including all Medicare carriers, publish newsletters for physicians to help them keep current on billing and coding information. Practices that do not receive these publications should contact the insurance company's customer service center and ask to be placed on its mailing list.

Information on specific coding policies, payment rates, or payment policies is available from any Medicare carrier under the Freedom of Information Act. Requests by letter should be sent to the Medicare carrier address, marked "Attention: Freedom of Information Unit." One specific request per letter will help ensure a quick and accurate response. For example, an appropriate request might be: "Please provide the list of diagnosis codes that are acceptable for payment on CPT procedure code 88150." The Freedom of Information Unit then will send a copy of the Medicare payment policy for that particular CPT code.

When a contract is written with an insurance carrier to accept a formal discount on fees, a negotiated fee schedule, or a capitation payment, the insurance company should supply the practice with a provider manual. This manual should detail how claims should be submitted to ensure correct payment.

When a practice deals with a variety of payers with different and detailed coding and reimbursement guidelines, a full page fact sheet should be maintained for the insurance company. The fact sheet allows room to describe unique items in the contract such as participating facilities, copay arrangements, precertification requirements, and all pertinent telephone contact numbers. Figure 10.1 is an example of an insurance company fact sheet.

Payer-Specific Guidelines

Many payers have specific guidelines for coding certain procedures, supplies, and services. These payer-specific guidelines may be found in procedure manuals and in newsletters and bulletins published by the payer. Payers should be contacted to receive their guidelines. Some of the specific guidelines are discussed in the following subsections.

Medicare offers an excellent source of many educational materials found in the Medicare Learning Network catalog (CMS 2015e). The free publications found in this document explain many payer-specific guidelines for Medicare in thorough detail for any learner.

Medical Necessity and Medicare Coverage Policies

All physician offices are affected by guidelines that cover medical necessity. Payers, especially Medicare, have developed guidelines that list conditions/diagnoses (ICD-10-CM codes) they will cover for specific services (CPT codes). Medicare refers to these guidelines as national coverage determinations (NCDs) or local coverage determinations (LCDs), available on the CMS website.

Figure 10.1. Insurance company fact sheet

Insurance Company Information   Company Name:_____

Product Type: HMO   PPO   POS

Provider Identification Number used?   Y   N   #_____

Referral Information   Referral required?   Y   N

Telephone referral line: _____   Fax referral line: _____

Referral length: _____ days   months   Allowable visits/referral:_____

No referral needed for: OB/GYN Exam   Annual Eye   Pap   Mammo

Copay Information

Primary $0 $5 $10 $15 $20   Amount on card:_____

Specialty $0 $5 $10 $15 $20   Amount on card:_____

Copays include: _____ Preventive services   _____ Allergy injections

_____ Immunizations   _____ Office procedures

Other Requirements

Second opinion required for surgery/procedures?   Y   N

Precertification required for nonemergent admission?   Y   N

Precertification required for elective surgery?   Y   N

Telephone precert line: _____   Fax precert line: _____

Participating Facilities

Hospital(s): _____   Laboratory: _____

_____   _____

Radiology: _____   CT/MRI: _____

Contact Information   Timely filing limit: _____

General telephone #: _____   General fax #: _____

Contact name: _____   Telephone #: _____

Claims telephone #:_____   Claims fax #:_____

Claims submission address:

NCDs and LCDs are carrier-specific, and must be developed using a consistent format. The following 10 standard subsections must be included (Carter 2002):

- Contractor identification (who developed the NCD or LCD)

- Policy identification (title)

- Statutory and jurisdictional information (ties this NCD or LCD back to national coverage decisions)

- Policy effective date (original and revisions)

- Service description (lists specific situations for coverage)

- Service coding information (CPT/HCPCS codes)

- Diagnostic coverage and coding (ICD-10-CM codes that specifically support medical necessity and those that do not)

- Reasons for noncoverage (additional denial reasons such as cosmetic, routine, and so on)

- Billing information (specifics on claim generation such as units, POS codes, modifiers, and so on)

- Record keeping and informational background (research references, older revision dates, and any other supporting materials)

Coders who are unsure about the coding and billing requirements for a particular procedure should check for a NCD or LCD to obtain valuable information. NCDs and LCDs also list the frequency with which these services can be performed. If the service is provided for other reasons or at a different frequency than listed in the NCD or LCD, the payer will not pay for it.

Medical necessity especially affects the ordering of laboratory tests in physician practices and the way the tests are reimbursed. In the past, physicians typically ordered panels of tests because it was less expensive than ordering each individual test, and with the automation of laboratory equipment, additional results were automatic. Today, payers require a specific reason for each test and many payers will not pay for a test done for screening purposes.

Some payers allow the practice to bill the patient automatically for the service; others require the patient to sign a waiver, known as the advance beneficiary notice (ABN), in which the patient agrees to pay for the service if the payer denies the claim. The waiver/ABN must be specific to the test being performed; a blanket waiver cannot be signed. Moreover, the ABN must be signed prior to the test or service provision, not after the service has been provided. Waivers should be used when a medical necessity denial has been determined by an NCD or LCD and when tests are allowed at certain frequencies, but a prior test date is unknown (Carter 2002). Figure 10.2 is an example of the model notice developed by the Centers for Medicare and Medicaid Services (CMS) for use by Medicare patients. This form is available for download from the CMS website on the Beneficiary Notices Initiatives page (CMS 2015f).

To ensure payment when requirements of medical necessity are not met, the practice should have the patient sign such a waiver (ABN). In addition, the guideline for waivers indicates that the modifier –GA, Waiver of liability statement issued, as required by payer policy or modifier –GX, Notice of liability issued, voluntary under payer policy, must be included on the claim with the CPT code. If modifier –GA or –GX is not included on the claim and the waiver is signed, the practice still cannot bill the patient. However, it should be noted that appending modifier –GA or –GX without having the patient actually sign the waiver is fraudulent due to misrepresentation.

Figure 10.2. ABN form

A. Notifier:

B. Patient Name: C. Identification Number:

Advance Beneficiary Notice of Noncoverage (ABN)

NOTE: If Medicare doesn't pay for **D.** _____ below, you may have to pay.
Medicare does not pay for everything, even some care that you or your health care provider have
good reason to think you need. We expect Medicare may not pay for the **D.** _____ below.

D.	E. Reason Medicare May Not Pay:	F. Estimated Cost

WHAT YOU NEED TO DO NOW:
- Read this notice, so you can make an informed decision about your care.
- Ask us any questions that you may have after you finish reading.
- Choose an option below about whether to receive the **D.** _____ listed above.
  Note: If you choose Option 1 or 2, we may help you to use any other insurance
      that you might have, but Medicare cannot require us to do this.

G. OPTIONS: Check only one box. We cannot choose a box for you.

☐ **OPTION 1.** I want the **D.** _____ listed above. You may ask to be paid now, but I
also want Medicare billed for an official decision on payment, which is sent to me on a Medicare
Summary Notice (MSN). I understand that if Medicare doesn't pay, I am responsible for
payment, but **I can appeal to Medicare** by following the directions on the MSN. If Medicare
does pay, you will refund any payments I made to you, less co-pays or deductibles.

☐ **OPTION 2.** I want the **D.** _____ listed above, but do not bill Medicare. You may
ask to be paid now as I am responsible for payment. **I cannot appeal if Medicare is not billed**.

☐ **OPTION 3.** I don't want the **D.** _____ listed above. I understand with this choice I
am **not** responsible for payment, and **I cannot appeal to see if Medicare would pay.**

H. Additional Information:

This notice gives our opinion, not an official Medicare decision. If you have other questions on
this notice or Medicare billing, call **1-800-MEDICARE** (1-800-633-4227/**TTY:** 1-877-486-2048).
Signing below means that you have received and understand this notice. You also receive a copy.

I. Signature:	J. Date:

Form CMS-R-131 (03/11)   Form Approved OMB No. 0938-0566

Two additional modifiers are available and both are optional. The –GY modifier is used to indicate that a statutorily excluded service was provided. No ABN is required, but many physician practices choose to have patients sign one in this case to establish financial responsibility. Applying a –GY modifier may speed the Medicare denial so that the bill can be processed to the secondary payer or patient; however, it does create an automatic denial. Be sure that the code is a status indicator of N in the National Physician Fee Schedule Relative Value File before applying modifier –GY or the beneficiary may be charged unnecessarily for the entire fee.

The other optional modifier is the –GZ modifier. The –GZ modifier is used to tell Medicare that an ABN was not signed, perhaps in error or as an oversight. The provider still cannot bill the patient but does establish honesty in billing and reduce the "risk of a mistaken allegation of fraud or abuse" (Carter 2002). Noridian Administration Services has also issued guidance on the proper use of modifiers GY, GA, and GZ (Noridian 2009).

Diagnoses Linked to Procedures

The procedure code is approved for payment based on the diagnosis code in box 24e of the CMS-1500 claim form to which it is cross-referenced. The insurance company's claims processing software tests for medical necessity by ensuring that the procedure is cross-referenced, or linked, correctly to an acceptable diagnosis code for that service.

Example: **Diagnoses**
1. Acute tonsillitis, ICD-10-CM code J03.90
2. Painful urination, ICD-10-CM code R30.9

Procedure Code (Box 24d)	Linked Diagnosis Code (Box 24e)
99213, Office visit	A
81001, Urinalysis with microscopy	B
87070, Culture, bacterial, throat	A
87086, Culture, bacterial, urine	B

Had the coder linked all the laboratory services, including the throat culture, to the symptom of painful urination, medical necessity would not have been met for the throat culture and the claim would have been denied. To receive payment, the coder would need to resubmit the claim with the correctly linked diagnosis code.

Specific CPT or HCPCS Code Requirement

Some payers have requested that new HCPCS codes be developed to replace codes in the CPT code book. A new code could address a new method (same test, just different wording) or could be temporary until the American Medical Association (AMA) includes it in the next release of CPT.

Examples include the following (Society for Clinical Coding 2003a):

- Blood transfusions are coded in CPT with code 36430 Transfusion, blood or blood components. HCPCS provides 38 codes from P9010 to P9060 to describe the different components of blood and different formulations for transfusion.

- In accordance with the Balanced Budget Act, as of January 1998, Medicare requires that when a female patient presents for a screening pelvic examination, code G0101, Cervical or vaginal cancer screening; pelvic and clinical breast examination, must be used. Q0091 must be used for the screening Pap smear (obtaining, preparing, and conveyance of cervical or vaginal smear to laboratory). There are specific guidelines on when to use these codes. LMRPs (NCDs or LCDs) must be consulted for specifics on billing these procedures and billing the patient for the balance of the well care.

Component Billing (Modifiers –26 and –TC)

Some CPT codes may be billed based on components. The components are total, professional, or technical. They are used most often in the radiology section of the CPT code book (70010–79999). The concept of component billing is based on ownership of the technical equipment and the relationship of the professional who interprets the test to the owner of the equipment, as follows:

- The total exam can be billed when the billing entity that owns the technical equipment is owned by the professional interpreting the test (usually a physician).

    Example: The physician owns the x-ray machine, takes a chest x-ray film, interprets the film, and dictates the report. The physician can bill for the total exam by using the CPT code, such as 71010, without a modifier.

- The physician bills only the professional component of the exam by appending modifier –26 to the CPT code for the exam (for example, 71010–26) when the physician who interprets the tests and dictates the report is not the owner of the equipment. This frequently occurs when a hospital completes the x-ray exam using its equipment and then a private physician completes the interpretation and dictation of the report.

- The counterpart of the professional component is the technical component (–TC). The technical component pays for the technician's time, the overhead of performing the test, and the maintenance of the equipment. The billing entity that owns the equipment must bill for completing the test by using the CPT code with a –TC modifier, which is a HCPCS Level II modifier.

    Example: A clinic does a chest x-ray exam but sends the film to a radiologist across town for reading and dictation of the report. The clinic bills for taking the x-ray by submitting code 71010–TC. (The radiologist submits a bill for the professional component using code 71010–26.)

Medicare's National Correct Coding Initiative (NCCI) Edits

NCCI edits are pairs of CPT or HCPCS Level II codes that are not separately payable except under certain circumstances. The edits are applied to services billed by the same provider for the same beneficiary on the same date of service. CMS developed the National Correct Coding Initiative to promote national correct coding methodologies and to eliminate improper coding. The NCCI edits are developed based on coding conventions defined in the CPT code book, current standards of medical and surgical coding practice, input from specialty societies, and analysis of current coding practice. The NCCI edits are usually updated on a quarterly basis and can be downloaded from the CMS website on the National Correct Coding Initiatives Edits page (CMS 2015g).

The edits are arranged as a table. The table contains the column 1/column 2 correct coding edits (formerly known as comprehensive/component edits) and the mutually exclusive edits. The table is arranged in two columns, as represented below in table 10.4. Note that the column 2 codes in the table are not payable with the column 1 codes unless the edit permits the use of a modifier associated with NCCI.

Table 10.4. NCCI edit tables

Column 1/Column 2 Correct Coding Edits (formerly Comprehensive/Component)	
Column 1	**Column 2**
70015	36000
	36011
	36406
	36410
	76000
	76001
	77001
	77002
	77003
	96372
	96374
	96375
	96376
80061	80500
	80502
	82465
	83718
	83721
	84478

If two codes of a code pair edit are billed by the same provider for the same beneficiary for the same date of service without an appropriate modifier, the column 1 code is paid. If clinical circumstances justify appending an NCCI-associated modifier to the column 2 code of a code pair edit, payment of both codes may be allowed.

Anatomical modifiers (–E1 through –E4, –FA through –F9, –TA through –T9, –LT, and –RT), global surgery modifiers (–25, –58, –78, and –79), and modifiers –59 and –91 can be used to justify clinical circumstances that warrant separate payment.

Modifier –59 is used to indicate a distinct procedural service. For Medicare, use one of the following HCPCS modifiers to more fully describe the distinct procedural service:

–XE: Separate encounter

–XP: Separate practitioner

–XS: Separate structure (or organ)

–XU: Unusual non-overlapping service

To appropriately report these modifiers, append modifier –59 or the Medicare alternative modifier to the column 2 code to indicate that the procedure or service was independent from other services performed on the same day. The addition of this modifier indicates to the carriers or fiscal intermediaries that the procedure or service represents a distinct procedure or service from others billed on the same date of service. In other words, this may represent a different session, different anatomical site or organ system, separate incision/excision, different lesion, or different injury or area of injury (in extensive injuries). When used with a NCCI edit, modifier –59, or the Medicare alternative modifier, indicates that the procedures are different surgeries when performed at different operative areas or at different patient encounters.

Two denial messages usually alert the coder that an NCCI edit has been applied to the claim. They are: "Medicare does not pay for this service because it is part of another service that was performed at the same time," and "Payment is included in another service received on the same day."

Medicare implemented an NCCI edit called Medically Unlikely Edits (MUEs), which is based on anatomical considerations. These edits check claims for billing that is anatomically unlikely, such as procedures on more than eight fingers (excluding thumb) or more than two eyes, ears, or breasts. More information is available on the CMS website on the Medically Unlikely Edits page of the National Correct Coding Initiatives Edits topic (CMS 2015h).

Claims Submittal

The goal in claims submittal is to submit each claim as a clean claim, or containing all of the required and accurate information necessary to allow it to be processed quickly and be paid promptly. Submitting a clean claim to payers is essential in receiving timely and accurate reimbursement. This section discusses new federal regulations related to a standard format for electronic claim submission and key elements of the CMS-1500 claim form.

National Provider Identifier

The national provider identifier (NPI) is a single provider identifier, replacing the different provider numbers currently in use for individual health plans and insurers. This identifier, which implemented a requirement of the Health Insurance Portability and Accountability Act of 1996 (HIPAA), must be used by most HIPAA-covered entities, which are health plans, healthcare clearinghouses, and healthcare providers that conduct electronic transactions. The NPI replaced the current unique physician identifier number (UPIN).

All providers should have an NPI. Information can be obtained about the NPI on the CMS website on the National Provider Identifier Standard page (CMS 2015i). This site has frequently asked questions (FAQs) and other information related to the NPI and other HIPAA standards.

HIPAA Transaction and Code Sets

In October 2003, HIPAA required healthcare providers to be in compliance with the federal standards for electronic transactions, commonly referred to as the Transaction and Code Sets (TCS). (HIPAA is discussed further in chapter 12.)

Standard transactions were developed for the electronic transfer of information between health plans and healthcare providers. These standards originally included transactions for healthcare claims or equivalent encounter information, health claims attachments, health plan enrollments and disenrollments, health plan eligibility, healthcare payment and remittance advice, health plan premium payments, first report of injury, healthcare claim status, and referral certification and authorization. The Accredited Standards Committee X12 Electronic Data Interchange (ASC X12) developed the uniform standards for these transactions (LaTour et. al. 2013, 206). Standards for health claims attachments have yet to be released.

The HIPAA Transaction and Code Set requirements include the adoption of ASC X12N standards for (Amatayakul, Jorwic, and Scichilone 2003):

- Claims, encounters, and coordination of benefits (837)

- Remittance advice (835)

- Eligibility inquiry and response (270/271)

- Claim status inquiry and response (276/277)

- Precertification and referral authorization (278)

- Enrollment in a health plan (834)

- Premium payment (820)

The current format required as of January 1, 2012 is version 5010. Information about this standard is available from the Transactions and Codes Sets Standards page on the CMS website (CMS 2015j). Implementation guides are available from the Washington Publishing Company (Washington Publishing Company 2009).

CMS-1500 Claim Form

The CMS-1500 claim form is the widely accepted, standard form for submitting physician charges to insurance companies. Online appendix G of this book contains a sample of the CMS-1500 form and directions to the online instructions for its use in the paper format. Although all insurance carriers accept this form, most complete it simply by following the rules set forth by Medicare.

Electronic Claims

The CMS-1500 claim also can be submitted in an electronic format. Most practice management systems and physician billing software programs have the ability to send an electronic file to insurance companies over a modem. Using electronic data transmission saves time in several ways. First, the insurance company receives electronic claims within hours of being transmitted. Second, electronic claims are ready to be loaded into the insurance company's claims-processing system. In contrast, the data in paper claims require either optical character recognition (OCR) scanning or manual entry before they can be loaded into the claims-processing system. Moreover, the cost of paper claim forms and postage is eliminated. Detailed specifications about how electronic files must be generated can be obtained by accessing the CMS website or by contacting the local Medicare carrier or commercial insurance company for its current requirements.

Signatures

A signed agreement between the physician and the insurance company is required before claims can be submitted electronically. The physician's signature on this agreement replaces the signature required on the claim form. The patient's signature on the registration record or "signature on file" card replaces his or her signature required on the claim form. Some insurance companies may require that the patient's signature be updated annually.

Electronic Claim Submission

Electronic claims are sent via modem to the insurance carrier directly or through an organization known as a clearinghouse. The electronic claims clearinghouse processes claims from multiple healthcare organizations to many insurance companies. There are advantages to both parties when using a clearinghouse.

For physicians, the need for signature on only one agreement can save considerable time. Another advantage is that data can usually be sent in one standard format to the clearinghouse, avoiding the need for several claim formats to be maintained on the computer system.

Insurers receive more claims electronically without having to negotiate with each physician or practice separately. They also may be able to request that the clearinghouse send the data in a format that is directly compatible with their claims payment software.

In return for its services, the clearinghouse charges a fee based on the number of physicians involved, the number of batches processed, or the number of claims processed.

Submission Error Management

It should not be assumed that each claim sent electronically was received electronically. Errors in processing do occur. The data transmission software should provide a batch, or status, report on the number of claims successfully processed and the details of any claims that failed to process due to an error. Claims that have "errored out" should be investigated, corrected, and sent again as soon as possible to maximize cash flow and avoid denials based on timely filing requirements.

Other Claims-Generation Guidelines

The following guidelines apply when listing multiple surgical procedures on a claim:

- Each procedure should be listed at full value. The insurance carrier may reduce the fee, as appropriate, based on the modifier, an agreed-upon fee schedule, or its individual policies.

- The procedures should be listed in descending order by the fee amount (starting with the largest fee). Some insurance companies pay 100 percent for the first procedure, 50 percent for the second procedure, and 25 percent for any additional procedures. Listing the procedures in descending order allows the largest reduction to be taken on the lowest-priced procedure, if the insurance company uses this method.

- A fee should never be changed for a particular case unless the code is modified in some way, such as with modifier –22, Increased Procedural Services, or modifier –52, Reduced Services.

- Services on only one calendar date should be included on a claim for office services.

- Services on multiple days for the same provider should be included on a claim for hospital services.

Coders should use the birthday rule to determine primary and secondary payers when the patient is covered by two commercial insurance carriers unless state law directs otherwise. The birthday rule states that the policyholder with the birthday earliest in the calendar year carries the primary policy for dependents. If both policyholders are born on the same day, the policy that has been in force the longest is the primary policy. Some states mandate that the gender rule be used. This rule states that the insurance for the male of the household is considered primary.

All procedures must be linked to one of the diagnoses listed in box 21. The ICD indicator flag of 9 = ICD-9-CM and 0 = ICD-10-CM must be indicated. See appendix G for details on how to complete a CMS-1500 claim. The coder should enter a linking reference letter (A through L) from box 21 in box 24e. Do not use commas between letters. Use a maximum of four letters. Be sure to use the ICD indicator of 9 when resubmitting a claim with a date of service of 9-30-15 or before.

Sometimes claim attachments are necessary for supporting documents, such as a cover letter or a special report, with a paper claim form. For example, whenever an unlisted procedure code is used, the insurer will require more information before the claim is paid. Moreover, additional information may be needed with the use of certain modifiers (for example, –22). Currently, procedures are being considered to facilitate electronic attachments to minimize process delays that occur with the submission of paper claims.

A service that is unusual, variable, new, or rarely provided may require a special report for determining its medical appropriateness. Pertinent information should include an adequate definition or description of the nature, extent, and need for the procedure, and the time, effort, and equipment necessary to provide the service. Additional items that may be included are: complexity of symptoms, final diagnosis, pertinent physical findings (such as size, location, and number of lesions, if appropriate), diagnostic and therapeutic procedures (including major and supplementary surgical procedures, if appropriate), concurrent problems, and follow-up care.

Data Elements of a Computerized Internal Fee Schedule

Organizations should keep a master list of their services by CPT and HCPCS codes and the charges associated with each of the service items. This database does not have a universal name; rather, its name often comes from the software vendor being used. Examples of names include transaction code file, CPT code file, fee dictionary, and fee schedule file. The purposes of this database are to maintain charge information about CPT and HCPCS codes and to supply data on these codes when charges are entered and CMS-1500 forms are created.

The database may contain the following types of information:

- The unique service identifier is the code that is keyed to indicate the service performed. It may be the CPT code. It will correspond to a CPT or HCPCS code but may be a completely different numbering system. For example, unique identifier 123 might mean HCPCS A4565, Arm sling. This identifier is for internal use only.

- The description of service is the name of the service, supply, or product. Many systems have this loaded when purchased. If so, the description usually is the same wording found on the Medicare fee schedule. The more specific the description, the easier it is to identify the intent of the code. The number of characters that can be used in the field for the description may be limited. All abbreviated descriptions must be abbreviated in a clear and consistent manner. This description is for internal use only because no description appears on the claim form.

- The CPT code is the five-digit code that relates to the description and prints on the claim form.

- The HCPCS code is the alphanumeric code that relates to the description for supplies, drugs, and so on, and is the code that prints on the claim form.

- The standard fee is the charge for the service.

- The department is the specific department or category into which the service may be categorized for reporting purposes (for example, surgery, laboratory, x-ray, supplies, injectables).

- Place of service is the typical location where the service is performed (for example, clinic, hospital, nursing facility).

- Type of service is the categorization of the description or code into a type of service (for example, medical, diagnostic laboratory, x-ray).

- Modifiers are two-digit extensions to a code number found in the CPT and/or HCPCS code book to define a service further. When a certain service needs a modifier attached at all times, the two-digit modifier can be entered and will be present automatically on the claim when this specific code is used.

- Days or units describe the number of times a service was performed continuously or on a particular day (for example, the number of doses of a particular medication or the number of treatments given in a 24-hour period). A service code may need to be submitted with days or units. Many systems stop at data entry and ask for a days or units amount if this field is turned on. For example, if a 50 mg medication is used in a dose of 150 mg, the data-entry clerk is prompted to enter a days/units amount, and then enters 3.

- The CMS relative value units are specific to the CPT code. These data can be used when reports are generated using this database. They are not used on the CMS-1500 form.

The internal fee schedule needs to be kept current. At a minimum, updates must be made annually. The fee schedule may be maintained by the business office manager, coding supervisor, finance director, controller, facility manager, staff person in the business office or coding department, or other designated staff. A single individual may maintain the database after consultation with other staff regarding pricing or other data elements.

The Claims Process

It is important to view the claims submission process as a series of steps that begins with patient registration and ends with final payment. Failure to perform any of the steps correctly could result in denial of the claim. Although sending a corrected claim could eventually result in payment, extra time and money are needed to achieve this payment. Performing the process correctly the first time speeds up the reimbursement process.

Patient Visit through Final Payment

The following steps describe the claims process from the time the patient enters the physician's office until his or her account is finally settled to zero:

1. The patient registers and completes the registration record. If the patient has been seen before, the information is updated.

2. The receptionist generates the charge ticket.

3. The health record clerk initiates the health record if this is the first visit.

4. The patient is seen and care is provided.

5. The provider lists all of the services and the diagnoses on the charge ticket and creates appropriate health record documentation.

6. The coder codes all the services using CPT/HCPCS codes.

7. The coder codes all the diagnoses using ICD-10-CM codes.

8. The coder links all CPT/HCPCS codes to ICD-10-CM codes.

9. The data-entry clerk (or coder) enters the codes and other billing data, such as units, into the computerized encounter history database.

10. The computer program references the CMS-1500 completion requirements for the specific insurance payer, references the internal fee schedule, and attaches charges to each of the service codes.

11. The computer program generates electronic data for any insurance companies that accept electronic claims. Paper CMS-1500 forms are printed and mailed for any nonelectronic claims.

12. The insurance company processes the claim by determining: (a) that the claim is complete, or clean; (b) that the patient has coverage for the services being billed; (c) the allowable fee for the services being billed; (d) whether the patient is responsible for part of the fee (coinsurance); and (e) the final reimbursement decision (payment or denial).

13. The insurance company issues a payer remittance report, along with a check to the provider if payment is to be made.

14. The insurance company sends an explanation of benefits to the patient.

15. The data-entry clerk posts the payment to the patient's account in the provider's office. Steps 10 through 15 are repeated if the patient has a secondary insurance carrier that may be responsible for the balance of the bill.

16. The provider's office sends a statement to the patient showing the balance.

17. The patient pays any remaining balance, and the account is listed as a zero balance.

Accounts Receivable Management

Accounts receivable management is the process of collecting the amounts owed to the physician practice from a variety of sources, including commercial insurers, Medicare, Medicaid, other liability insurers, and patients. When charges are not paid in full at the time of service, the unpaid balance is posted to an account called accounts receivable (A/R) or the "to be paid later" account.

Money received later is referred to as cash, regardless of whether it was received in the form of cash, a check, or a credit card payment. When a practice agrees to accept less than its full fee for a service, a contractual allowance, sometimes called an adjustment, is made for the difference between the allowed amount and the full fee. When attempts to collect an outstanding balance are unsuccessful, it is written off (or a write-off is taken) to bring the patient's account balance to zero. If the write-off was taken from charges that were the patient's responsibility, the write-off becomes a bad debt write-off (Schraffenberger and Kuehn 2011, 460).

Days in Accounts Receivable

To track the A/R process, accountants recommend the use of a standard statistic called "Days in Accounts Receivable" or "Days in A/R" as a measure of management success. This statistic is a measure of approximately how many days it takes to collect any dollar booked into the A/R. The statistic is calculated as the A/R balance at the end of a specific period divided by the average daily revenue generated during that same period. The average revenue per day is calculated as the total A/R for the period divided by the number of days in that period.

$$\text{Days in A/R} = \frac{\text{Ending accounts receivable for the period}}{\text{Average revenue per day}}$$

Example: Ending A/R = $200,000
Total A/R for the month of April = $150,000
Days in April = 30

$$\frac{\$200,000}{\$5,000} = 40$$

The average number of days to collect money from the A/R is 40 days.

Aged Accounts Receivable

To determine how long money has been in the A/R account, accountants recommend displaying the A/R in an aged fashion, typically using 30-day increments (0–30 days, 31–60 days, and so on) with subtotals. It is best to have as much of the A/R as possible in the newest date ranges. Most computer systems produce reports listing claims from oldest to newest so that follow-up activities can be concentrated on the oldest claims first. If this is not available, a manual tickler file should be created so that claims can be followed in that manner.

Claims follow-up should include calling the insurance carrier to be sure the claim has been received, resubmitting claims that insurers say were not received, and sending corrected claims if carriers identify errors.

When a claim is denied, the process of denial management is started.

Denial Management

A well-designed denial management program can affect the financial success of the organization by improving cash flow and reducing write-offs. Denials should not be ignored or considered the final solution to the claims process. Rather, they should be managed using the following steps:

1. *Analyze the denial.* Evaluate whether the claim was coded or submitted incorrectly or whether it was processed incorrectly.

2. *Take action on the denial.* Send corrected claims for any coding or billing errors. Appeal denials if processed incorrectly. (See the following section on the appeals process.)

3. *Track the denial.* Record all actions taken in an attempt to secure payment, such as correspondence and information from telephone calls. Track denials by carrier to help recognize patterns of incorrect processing. Escalate problem claims to a supervisory level at the carrier, if necessary. Persistence sends the message that improper processing will not go uncontested.

4. *Prevent future denials.* Make system corrections based on past errors, research, or denial outcomes to reduce future denials.

The Appeals Process

Most insurance carriers have an appeals process that can be used when the initial reimbursement decision seems incorrect or unfair. The steps in the appeals process are available through insurance carrier bulletins or the company's customer service representative.

The Medicare appeals process is quite detailed and fully documented in the regulations. The appeals process is available in the *Medicare Claims Processing Manual* in Chapter 29, Section 240.

The basic steps in the Medicare appeals process are as follows:

1. When an initial determination results in a less-than-expected payment or a denial, enrollees under Part B Medicare and physicians or suppliers have the right to request a redetermination. The review must be requested within 120 days of the date of the notice of the initial determination. The request for the review must be made in writing and filed at an office of the carrier, the Social Security Administration (SSA), or CMS. The appeals process cannot resolve complaints about the Medicare fee schedule or payment policy decisions; rather, it should be made to resolve a real or perceived error in payment processing.

2. The beneficiary or the physician/supplier, if dissatisfied with the redetermination, may request a reconsideration by a qualified independent contractor (QIC). A reconsideration by a QIC must be requested 180 days from the date of receipt of the redetermination.

3. If the beneficiary or physician/supplier is dissatisfied with the results of the reconsideration and the amount in controversy is $150 or more, the beneficiary or physician/supplier may obtain an administrative law judge (ALJ) hearing. The request must be filed within 60 days from the receipt of the reconsideration notice.

4. If a party going to the ALJ hearing is dissatisfied with the ALJ's decision, the party may request a review by the Medicare Appeals Council. The request must be received within 60 days of receipt of the ALJ's decision and no set dollar amount is required.

5. If $1,460 or more is still in controversy following the Medicare Appeals Council's decision, judicial review before a federal district court judge may be requested. The request must be made within 60 days of the receipt of the Medicare Appeals Council's decision.

Regardless of insurance carrier, the right of appeal for the benefit of the physician and the patient should be asserted to ensure that all covered services are reimbursed properly.

Exercise 10.1. Reimbursement Process

Choose the best answer for each of the following questions.

1. Linking refers to which of the following?

   a. Attaching modifiers to CPT codes
   b. Substituting a HCPCS code for the appropriate CPT code
   c. Assigning a diagnosis code to a CPT code on a claim
   d. Pairing professional charges to technical charges on a claim

2. What is the function of a clearinghouse?

   a. It ensures that computer viruses are removed from billing software.
   b. It manages the process of claims appeals for Medicare.
   c. It reprices claims for a physician network.
   d. It transfers electronic claims to individual insurers.

3. Dr. Smith submitted 130 claims for code 36415 during the past year. The claim history file shows:

   36415 $8.25 — 10 claims
   36415 $8.75 — 20 claims
   36415 $9.25 — 100 claims

   What is Dr. Smith's fee profile for 36415, using U/C rules?

   a. $8.25
   b. $8.75
   c. $9.10
   d. $9.25

4. What is the approved amount for a CPT code with the following values?

   W(RVU) = 0.98
   P(RVU) = 0.95
   M(RVU) = 0.06
   G(W)   = 1.094
   G(P)   = 1.351
   G(M)   = 1.668
   CF   = $36.0666

   a. $40.18
   b. $88.57
   c. $148.34
   d. $220.11

5. If the Medicare approved amount is $400, how much is the limiting charge?

   a. $380
   b. $460
   c. $520
   d. $600

6. Work, practice cost, and malpractice cost are variables in which reimbursement methodology?

   a. Resource Based Relative Value System
   b. Discounted charges
   c. Capitation
   d. Standard charges

(Continued on next page)

Exercise 10.1 (Continued)

For items 7 through 12, match the type of information with the correct description.

a. Place of service
b. Standard fee
c. Computerized internal fee schedule

d. Modifiers
e. Unique identifier
f. Description of services

7. _____ Fee for the service is $61.

8. _____ 2-digit suffixes describing changes in code descriptions.

9. _____ The service was performed at a nursing home.

10. _____ During data entry, 2101 is keyed, which corresponds to 38220, Bone marrow; aspiration only.

11. _____ Removal foreign body, intranasal.

12. _____ Master listing of services performed, codes, and charges.

Answer true or false to the following questions.

13. True or False? The patient can pay more out-of-pocket expenses when seeing a provider that is not participating with an insurance plan. _____

14. True or False? An important management statistic regarding cash flow is called "Days in A/R." _____

15. True or False? An appeal must be filed within 6 months of initial claim determination. _____

16. True or False? "Column1/Column2 edits" are part of the NCCI. _____

Fill in the blanks.

17. The electronic version of the CMS-1500 claim form is called the _____.

18. A free source of information about the number of global surgical days assigned to a code is found in _____.

19. Modifier _____ is appended to the code when a signed ABN form is on file.

20. Review the progress note below. Code the diagnoses using ICD-10-CM and the procedures using CPT. Enter this information on the blank claim form section provided. Complete fields 21 and 24D. Be sure to link the codes.

Progress Note

S: Patient is a 58-year-old who presents to acute care today because she has had persistent problems with right hip pain. Apparently, she spoke to her regular doctor here about this at her last full physical, about 1 month ago. I've reviewed the physical for information. She has continued to have moderate to severe discomfort along the lateral part of the upper thigh and a little bit into the groin as well. Has been taking Feldene with some improvement. She reports no other muscle or joint problems. No neuro-logic problems with the right leg and no past injuries to the hip or leg. In addition to this, she thinks she may have wax in her ears, particularly on the left side, which she says "feels plugged."

Exercise 10.1 (Continued)

O: Temperature 97.6° F, pulse 88, respirations 20, weight 176 lb. EARS: Right tympanic membrane and canal are clear. The left canal is cerumen impacted. MUSC: Hip does reveal tenderness over the trochanteric bursa. She has some tenderness with internal and external rotation. Flexion and extension are normal. She walks without an antalgic gait.

A/P   1. Cerumen impaction. I curetted the ear today and was able to see the tympanic membrane, which was clear.

       2. Right hip pain. A two-view, bilateral hip x-ray was done today here at the clinic. My interpretation shows minimal degenerative changes with a small amount of degenerative spurring and perhaps some very mild joint space narrowing on the right. Left hip is normal.

       Mild localized osteoarthritis of the right hip with trochanteric bursitis. She is already on Feldene. Will refer to Orthopedics for other possible treatment plans.

Evaluation and Management Services on this visit were:

History: Expanded problem focused

Examination: Expanded problem focused

Medical Decision Making: Low complexity

21. DIAGNOSIS OR NATURE OF ILLNESS OR INJURY Relate A-L to service line below (24E)			ICD Ind.		22. RESUBMISSION CODE	ORIGINAL REF. NO.	
A.	B.	C.	D.		23. PRIOR AUTHORIZATION NUMBER		
E.	F.	G.	H.				
I.	J.	K.	L.				

24. A. DATE(S) OF SERVICE From MM DD YY	To MM DD YY	B. PLACE OF SERVICE	C. EMG	D. PROCEDURES, SERVICES, OR SUPPLIES (Explain Unusual Circumstances) CPT/HCPCS	MODIFIER	E. DIAGNOSIS POINTER	F. $ CHARGES	G. DAYS OR UNITS	H. EPSDT Family Plan	I. ID. QUAL.	J. RENDERING PROVIDER ID. #
1										NPI	
2										NPI	
3										NPI	
4										NPI	
5										NPI	
6										NPI	

PHYSICIAN OR SUPPLIER INFORMATION

Chapter 10 Test

Choose the best answer for each of the following questions.

1. Using this excerpt from the Medicare Physician Relative Value File and the following GPCI data, calculate the Medicare approved amount for draining a bursa of the shoulder.

   Work GPCI   = 1.0
   Practice Expense GPCI = 0.87
   Malpractice GPCI   = 0.779

HCPCS	DESCRIPTION	WORK RVU	PE RVU	MP RVU	TOTAL	CONV FACTOR
23020	Release shoulder joint	8.92	7.58	1.48	17.98	37.3374
23030	Drain shoulder lesion	3.42	3.01	0.51	6.94	37.3374
23031	Drain shoulder bursa	2.74	2.69	0.40	5.83	37.3374
23035	Drain shoulder bone lesion	8.60	8.51	1.44	18.55	37.3374
23040	Exploratory shoulder surgery	9.19	7.85	1.54	18.58	37.3374
23044	Exploratory shoulder surgery	7.11	6.50	1.17	14.78	37.3374
23065	Biopsy shoulder soft tissues	2.27	2.81	0.17	5.25	37.3374
23066	Biopsy shoulder tissues	4.15	5.10	0.60	9.85	37.3374
23075	Excise shoulder lesion, sq < 3 cm	2.39	2.24	0.30	4.93	37.3374

   a. $161.06
   b. $201.32
   c. $231.52
   d. $240.30

2. Using the excerpt and GPCI data provided in question #1, what is the Medicare limiting charge for removal of a shoulder lesion?

   a. There is no limiting charge
   b. $136.58
   c. $170.73
   d. $196.33

Chapter 10 Test (Continued)

3. Reference this excerpt from the Medicare Physician Relative Value File. If the physician removed a shoulder lesion 2 months ago, what modifier would the physician need to use if he performed another procedure today that required the use of the operating room?

HCPCS	DESCRIPTION	GLOBAL DAYS	PRE OP	INTRA OP	POST OP	MULT PROC	BILAT SURG
23044	Exploratory shoulder surgery	090	0.10	0.69	0.21	2	1
23065	Biopsy shoulder soft tissues	010	0.10	0.80	0.10	2	1
23066	Biopsy shoulder tissues	090	0.10	0.69	0.21	2	1
23075	Excise shoulder lesion, sq < 3 cm	010	0.10	0.80	0.10	2	1
23077	Resect shoulder tumor < 5 cm	090	0.10	0.69	0.21	2	1
23100	Biopsy of shoulder joint	090	0.10	0.69	0.21	2	1
23101	Shoulder joint surgery	090	0.10	0.69	0.21	2	1

 a. −24
 b. −76
 c. −79
 d. No modifier needed

4. Using the excerpt in question #3, what percentage of the approved amount is associated with the intraoperative work on code 23100?

 a. 0.10
 b. 0.21
 c. 0.69
 d. 0.90

5. A request for reconsideration by a qualified independent contractor must be filed within what time frame after the initial determination?

 a. 60 days
 b. 90 days
 c. 120 days
 d. 180 days

6. When multiple surgical procedures are listed on a CMS-1500 claim form, the fees for each procedure should be listed as what percentage of the full fee?

 a. 25%
 b. 50%
 c. 75%
 d. 100%

(Continued on next page)

Chapter 10 Test (Continued)

7. How often must an Advance Beneficiary Notice be signed when several instances of the same service are provided over a period of time?

   a. When requested by the patient
   b. At the time of each service
   c. Monthly
   d. Yearly

8. Which component of the RBRVS describes the value of actual physician labor?

   a. Work Relative Value Unit
   b. Practice Expense Relative Value Unit
   c. Work GPCI
   d. Conversion Factor

9. If a physician has $300,000 in outstanding A/R at the end of June and has an average daily revenue of $9,000 during the same period, what is the best action for the coder to take immediately?

   a. None, as the Days in A/R is being managed well.
   b. Investigate which payers have a longer Days in A/R and follow up.
   c. Determine where the claims processing errors are occurring.
   d. Calculate the time it takes to submit a claim and decrease it.

10. The patient sees a PAR provider and has a procedure performed after meeting the annual deductible. If the Medicare-approved amount is $200, how much is the patient's out-of-pocket expense?

   a. $0
   b. $10
   c. $20
   d. $40

Chapter 11

Coding and Reimbursement Reports and Databases

Objectives

Upon completion of this lesson, the student should be able to do the following:

- Specify the data elements required in qualitative and quantitative reports used to evaluate coding quality and completeness

- Create and evaluate a comparison graph of E/M code usage

- Use reports to identify errors in databases such as the internal fee schedule database or the encounter history database

- Recognize potential coding quality issues as reported on a payer remittance report (for example, explanation of benefits)

This chapter discusses the process of reviewing coding databases for accuracy and completeness. Coders can use a variety of reports to evaluate data in two major databases: the encounter history database and the internal fee schedule database. The chapter also describes the function of the payer remittance report.

Data Evaluation

The billing database for a physician, or a group of physicians, contains ICD-10-CM and CPT/HCPCS codes associated with specific patient dates of service. It also contains information about the specific provider of the service and the location where the service was performed. The billing database is referred to by many names, such as the encounter history database, charge history, or service records. Regardless of the name, the database contains valuable information that should be evaluated.

In a large office or a multifacility enterprise, specialized staff may perform the reviews. In a small office, the facility manager, finance department staff, lead coder, or other coder may perform these reviews.

Data can be evaluated using two methods: qualitative analysis and quantitative analysis. **Qualitative analysis** is completed on patient-specific data, such as the codes assigned to a particular service and provided by a specific provider at one encounter. These data are evaluated for correct content. **Quantitative analysis** is completed on non-patient-specific or aggregate data, usually in the form of frequency reports by diagnosis or procedure codes, and is evaluated for patterns (Kuehn 2001).

Qualitative Analysis

Two reports provide the type of organized data necessary for qualitative analysis. They are the claim(s) history (for an individual patient) and the charge summary.

Claim History

A claim history for one particular patient can provide information on situations such as potential duplicate billing or coding to a variety of different levels of specificity or accuracy. It also can pinpoint illogical claim submissions, such as billing for a nursing home visit during the dates of an actual inpatient stay. If the services in one claim history are coded by several different coders, this report can provide evidence of potential interrater reliability problems among the coders. **Interrater reliability** is established when two or more coders obtain the same coded data from the same documentation.

Figure 11.1 shows the claim history for one patient and illustrates potential coding issues demonstrated in that history. This is one type of report that was used originally by fraud investigators to identify billing problems within a particular organization or office (Burris, Houser, and Montilla 2000). Reports such as this, as well as other data mining tools continue to be used in fraud surveillance.

Charge Summary Report

Another quantitative data report is the charge summary report, which is sometimes called the office service report. This report contains a summary of all the billing data entered for the practice on one day, listing all the vital pieces of data to be included on the CMS-1500 claim form for that particular date of service. Figure 11.2 is an example of this type of report. As displayed, this report can be used to identify data-entry errors, such as a diagnosis mismatched

Figure 11.1. Claim history

Patient: Mary Jones   **ID:** 1354123   **DOB:** 7-14-43

Date	Procedure Code	Description	Fee	Linked Diagnosis	Description	Dr #	Location
9-6	99396	Prev Med Est, 40-64	$134.00	Z00.00	Health checkup	52	Office 1
9-6	85025	CBC	$27.00	Z00.00	Health checkup	52	Office 1
9-12	99203–25	Office Visit, New Pt	$66.00	C44.300	Malignant lesion	52	Office 1
9-12	11442	Excise benign lesion	$140.00	C44.300	Malignant lesion	52	Office 1
9-26	99214	Office Visit, Est Pt	$82.00	D23.9	Benign lesion	64	Office 1
9-26	71020	Two view chest x-ray	$54.00	I50.9	CHF	64	Office 1
9-26	81000	Urinalysis	$11.00	I50.9	CHF	64	Office 1
9-28	99203	Office Visit, New Pt	$84.00	E10.9	Diabetes Mellitus	64	Office 1
9-28	36415	Venipuncture	$10.00	E10.9	Diabetes Mellitus	64	Office 1
9-28	82947	Glucose test	$19.00	E10.9	Diabetes Mellitus	64	Office 1
10-2	99212	Office Visit, Est Pt	$49.00	E11.9	Diabetes Mellitus	64	Office 1
10-2	36415	Venipuncture	$10.00	E11.9	Diabetes Mellitus	64	Office 1
10-2	82947	Glucose test	$19.00	E11.9	Diabetes Mellitus	64	Office 1

Possible interrater reliability or inaccurate coding of one visit

Diagnosis/procedure mismatch

New vs established problem

349

Figure 11.2. Charge summary

Anytown Medical Group
Date of Service: 12-10

Patient	Procedure Code	Description	Fee	Linked Diagnosis	Description	Dr #	Location
Case 1							
1283112	99213–25	Office Visit, Est Pt	$66.00	D23.9	Benign lesion	52	Office 1
1283112	17000	Wart destruction	$70.00	D23.9	Benign lesion	52	Office 1
				Dx mismatch			
Case 2							
1357401	99214	Office Visit, Est Pt	$82.00	J45.901	Asthma	55	Office 1
1357401	94640	Nebulizer Treatment	$34.00	J45.901	Asthma	55	Office 1
1357401	94640	Nebulizer Treatment	$34.00	J45.901	Asthma	55	Office 1
1357401	J7611	Albuterol Concentrate	$3.00	J45.901	Asthma	55	Office 1
		Missing –76 modifier					
Case 3							
1177431	99393	Preventive Medicine	$95.00	Z00.129	Well Child	54	Hospital 1
1177431	90700	DTaP	$48.00	Z00.129	Well Child	54	Office 1
1177431	90707	MMR	$59.00	Z00.129	Well Child	54	Office 1
1177431	90471	Immun Administration	$12.00	Z00.129	Well Child	55	Office 1
		90472 missing for 2nd immunization			*Probable incorrect physician*		*Incorrect location*
Case 4							
1531892	99203	Office Visit, New Pt	$92.00	D64.9	Anemia	53	Office 1
	81000	Urinalysis w/microscopy	$12.00	R10.84	Abdominal pain	53	Office 1
	85025	CBC	$27.00	R10.84	Abdominal pain	53	Office 1
	74000	Single view abdomen	$61.00	D64.9	Anemia	53	Office 1
					Linking appears inappropriate		

to a procedure (case 1), missing data elements (case 2), incorrect physician numbers or locations (case 3), or incorrect linking of diagnoses to procedures (case 4). Any of these issues can adversely affect the amount and speed of reimbursement for the services provided.

Quantitative Analysis

It may seem that quantitative or aggregate data will not provide much valuable information. However, such data contain more information than might originally be thought.

Diagnosis Distribution

Figure 11.3 shows an excerpt from a diagnosis distribution report for the past year at Pediatric Practice, SC. This report shows three significant issues.

Figure 11.3. Diagnosis distribution—Pediatric Practice, SC 01-01 through 12-31

Code	Description	#	Code	Description	#
A08.0	Rotaviral enteritis	112	L65.9	Nonscarring hair loss	67
A09	Infectious GE and colitis	9	O80	Full-term delivery	3
A38.9	Scarlet fever	359	P07.10	Prematurity, unspecified	1471
A41.9	Sepsis, unspec organism	99	P07.16	Prematurity, 1500-1749g	5
B01.9	Varicella	344	P07.17	Prematurity, 1750-1999g	
B07	Wart	16	P07.18	Prematurity, 2000-2499g	Inappropriate to setting
B07.9	Viral warts	2121	R04.0	Epistaxis	43
B08.1	Molluscum Contagiosum	164	R06.02	Shortness of breath	3
B08.3	Fifth disease	Missing characters	R07.0	Pain in throat	1
B37.2	Candidiasis of skin, nails		R42	Dizziness and giddiness	4
D18	Hemangioma	2	R50.9	Fever	169
D18.0	Hemangioma	6	R51	Headache	41
D18.00	Hemangioma unsp site	115	R53.83	Other fatigue	27
E05	Thyrotoxicosis	1	R56.00	Simple febrile convulsions	13
E05.9	Thyrotoxicosis	2	S01.512A	Laceration, mouth, init enc	7
E05.90	Thyrotoxicosis w/o crisis	3	S09.90XA	Head injury, init enc	113
E10.9	Diabetes type 1	144	S42.009A	Fracture clavicle, init enc	61
E11	Diabetes	3	S61.509A	Laceration, wrist, init enc	10
E11.9	Diabetes type 2	45	S62.609A	Fracture phalanx, init enc	185
E66.9	Obesity, unspecified	69	T17.1XXA	Foreign body nose, init enc	43
F90.9	ADHD	188	T30.0	Burn	7
G40.909	Epilepsy	Nonspecific Coding	Z23	Immunization	15672
H65.90	Nonsuppurative OM		Z37.0	Single live birth	24
H66.90	Otitis media	788	Z38.00	Single liveborn, vaginally	372
J02.0	Strept pharyngitis	3143	Z38.01	Single liveborn, cesarean	54

The first issue noted is that the coders, or the physicians, are assigning codes without the necessary final characters. Claims containing these codes will immediately be rejected and require extra work for resubmission. The second issue concerns claims for office services that contain codes that are only appropriate for use on inpatient records, such as codes O80 and Z37.0. The third issue is a potential problem that may require additional investigation to confirm as a problem. It appears that the coders or physicians are choosing nonspecific codes when more information is probably available for coding. Unspecified otitis media (H66.90) should normally be refined to a more specific diagnosis. Similarly, unspecified prematurity (P07.10) should have the birth weight indicated because this information is normally available to the pediatrician performing the newborn exam.

Service Distribution

A frequency distribution of the services provided also can yield information about CPT/HCPCS coding patterns. Figure 11.4 displays the service distribution for the past year for Pediatric Practice, SC. This report demonstrates four problem areas in procedure coding.

The use of code 59514 for a cesarean delivery in four cases on pediatric claims is highly suggestive of error. This code is to be used by the physician who actually completed the C-section. Performing a C-section is not normally within a pediatrician's scope of work. It is more likely that code 99464, Attendance at delivery and initial stabilization of newborn, correctly describes the services provided on that date.

The second problem noted is the coding of procedures that have a low probability of being performed in the clinic setting. Code 15851, Suture removal requiring general anesthetic, probably should have been coded as an E/M service code for removal of sutures in the office. In addition, unless the office is equipped with a spirometry machine, code 94010 was likely coded in error in place of another pulmonary procedure. Coding reviewers and billing staff should be familiar with the equipment that the practice owns, as well as the scope of the services provided, to help prevent coding errors of this type.

Also noted is the use of code 99070 for medical supplies. Although HCPCS codes are only required on Medicare claims, the industry has seen a tremendous shift toward acceptance of these codes by all payers over the past few years. Use of specific HCPCS supply codes speeds up reimbursement and may eliminate the need to forward medical records to the third-party payer for review before payment is made.

The fourth issue noted is the potential problem of missing charges for supplies and medications. There were 55 cases of bladder catheterization (code 51701), but only three units of catheter supplies were coded. This discrepancy warrants investigation. Moreover, there were 29 cases last year with code 96365 for IV infusion and no HCPCS J codes for injectable medications. Unless these medications are charged separately through a providing pharmacy, significant revenue is being lost. Conversely, if the practice assigns codes for medications that are provided by a pharmacy, inappropriate billing is being created. Only supplies and medications that are actually purchased and administered by the practice can be billed for reimbursement.

A service distribution report also can be used to design new encounter form content and to complete a comparative study with inventory purchases. In completing this study, any supplies or medications that have a specific HCPCS code can be compared for utilization.

Example: On January 1, six splints are in inventory. Throughout the month of January, additional splints are ordered and received. On January 31, the ending inventory is 12. The math shows the following:

6 splints in stock + 26 splints ordered and received =
32 splints available − 12 remaining at end of period = 20 used during the period

Figure 11.4. Service distribution—pediatric practice, SC 01-01 through 12-31

Code	Description	#	Code	Description	#
99201	New Office level 1	152	15851	Suture rem, gen anesth	3
99202	New Office level 2	594	30901	Nasal Cautery	15
99203	New Office level 3	1736	36415	Blood draw	5532
99204	New Office level 4	103	51701	Catheterization, bladder	55
99205	New Office level 5	20	59514	Cesarean delivery	4
99211	Nurse Only Visit	2765	65205	Foreign body removal	6
99212	Est Office level 2	6390	69210	Ear Curettage	505
99213	Est Office level 3	69591	81002	Urinalysis w/o micro	9235
99214	Est Office level 4	3118	82948	Glucose	51
99215	Est Office level 5	699	83655	Lead, quantitative	89
99381	New physical under 1	1609	85013	HCT/Spun	1448
99382	New physical 1-4	639	85025	CBC	948
99383	New physical 5-10	622	87081	Strep culture	2538
99384	New physical 11-17	268	87880	Rapid strep	15514
99385	New physical 18-39	4	88150	Pap smear	2
99391	Est physical under 1	11619	90471	Immun admin 1st	19556
99392	Est physical 1-4	11839	90472	Immun admin addtl	28579
99393	Est physical 5-10	7552	90632	Hep A	2616
99394	Est physical 11-17	4009	90648	HIB	4002
99395	Est physical 18-39	231	90670	Pneumococcal conjugate	10427
99221	Initial hosp level 1	98	90700	DTaP	14162
99222	Initial hosp level 2	473	90707	MMR	5418
99223	Initial hosp level 3	231	90713	Injectable Polio	11510
99231	Subseq hospital level 1	315	92551	Audiometric Testing	3328
99232	Subseq hospital level 2	1020	94010	Spirometry	2
99233	Subseq hospital level 3	237	94640	Nebulizer Treatment	1793
99238	Hosp Discharge < 30 min	739	94760	Pulse Oximetry	582
99239	Hosp Discharge > 30 min	134	96365	IV Infusion	29
99460	Newborn history/exam	1363	99070	Medical Supplies	124
99462	Subsequent Newborn	246	99173	Vision Screening	3515
99463	Newborn exam/discharge	809	A4351	Catheter Supplies	3
99464	Attendance at delivery	54	J7510	Oral Prednisone	116
11740	Evac of Subungual Hema	9	J7611	Albuterol Concentrate	1789
			J????		

Inappropriate to specialty

Inappropriate to setting

Nonspecific coding

IV Meds missing

Supplies missing

The service distribution report should show that 20 splints were provided and coded during the period. If 20 splints do not appear on the report, the facility probably should determine which patients were likely candidates to have received the supply (sprains and fractures diagnosed during the month) and complete a medical record review for potential lost charges.

In evaluating inventory discrepancies, lack of charge capture is the most likely reason; however, the situations of excessive provider waste (especially in medications), employee theft, and external theft should be considered as potential causes of discrepancies.

Figure 11.4 shows a report that contains only raw numbers. In some cases, these raw numbers do not provide enough meaning to the reviewer. The most noted of these cases would be E/M codes. To fully compare these frequencies, each category of E/M codes should be evaluated separately and evaluated for its percentage of use within the category.

Figure 11.5 shows a graph comparing doctor 1's utilization of code 99222 with that of others in the practice and with national data. National usage data for each code category can be obtained from the CMS website. By converting the usage data for each code category to percentages, meaningful data comparisons can be created (Kuehn 2009).

To create a comparative graph, obtain statistics from a similar outside entity or from the CMS website. To use the CMS data, complete the following steps (Kuehn 2009):

1. Go to http://www.cms.gov/Research-Statistics-Data-and-Systems/Statistics-Trends -and-Reports/MedicareFeeforSvcPartsAB/MedicareUtilizationforPartB.html

2. Scroll down to the last set of downloads.

3. Click CY 2012 and download the PDF file. (CMS updates the files periodically, so be sure to use the most recent file available.)

4. Locate each of the E/M codes within the specialty you are interested in comparing.

Figure 11.5.   Comparative report—initial hospital visits

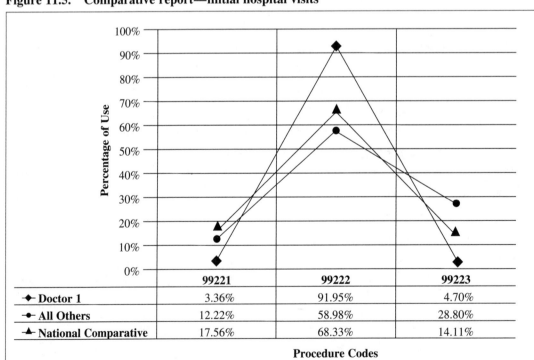

	99221	99222	99223
Doctor 1	3.36%	91.95%	4.70%
All Others	12.22%	58.98%	28.80%
National Comparative	17.56%	68.33%	14.11%

Procedure Codes

5. Convert the values in that series to percentages of the series.

6. Locate the same code series in your own facility data.

7. Convert your data to percentages of the series.

8. Compare the two sets of percentages using a graph.

The figure 11.5 comparison shows that doctor #1 has a considerably higher utilization of code 99222 than either the remainder of the practice or the national comparative data. Although this comparison alone confirms nothing, it does provide sufficient reason to initiate a medical record review of hospital charges for doctor #1 to determine whether the correct level is being assigned. Had all three distributions been similar, review efforts could have been directed elsewhere.

Service distribution reports produced for individual physicians can contain relative value unit (RVU) data as an additional element. As discussed in chapter 10, RVUs are numerical equivalents for the value of one procedure compared to another. Using RVU totals, the amount of physician labor completed by physicians of different specialties can be compared consistently using the same scale.

Example: A surgeon may perform three surgeries on one day with RVUs totaling 46. A primary care physician may see 20 patients on the same day with RVUs totaling 46. In this case, the physicians have completed the same amount of physician labor, although the services provided were totally different.

Custom Reports

Reports based on the contents of the encounter history database are valuable for evaluating the quality of coded data. Many billing systems provide the standard reports discussed previously. If standard reports are unavailable, customized reports should be requested or developed. The following reports can be helpful in assessing coding quality:

- Office service report
- Service-mix report
- Revenue production report

Office Service Report

Figure 11.6 is an example of a daily office service report for a three-physician office on May 1. It shows the services provided on that day by code number and by physician. This report is similar to the charge summary except that it adds the date of birth and sex of the patient and provides the code summary. The office service report helps the coder recognize when education may be needed, where procedures may have been forgotten, or where other errors may have occurred. For example:

Problem #1: Doctor 2501 coded 99212 as the only office visit level used.

Problem #2: Patient 65-23-19 had a joint injection with no medication coded.

Problem #3: Patient 03-75-93 had a radius and ulna fracture treated for $2,100, whereas patient 03-55-08 had a similar wrist fracture treated for $210. This raises the coder's suspicions of a data-entry error.

Figure 11.6. Office service report

	Med Rec #	D.O.B.	Sex	Doctor	D.O.S.	CPT Code	Charges	Dx	Comments
	12-56-34	10/10/44	F	2501	May-1	99212	$40.00	477.0	
	37-43-24	10/21/36	M	4401	May-1	57460	$392.25	795.00	Colp w/biopsy
	44-66-01	5/15/37	F	3701	May-1	99213	$50.00	428.0	
#2	65-23-19	8/3/35	M	3701	May-1	20600	$51.00	719.44	Injection Joint
	55-29-42	3/2/87	M	2501	May-1	27781	$470.00	823.01	Ankle fx
	55-29-42	3/2/87	M	2501	May-1	29405	$183.00	823.01	Cast
	23-23-04	8/4/40	F	2501	May-1	99212	$40.00	782.1	
	01-88-42	12/23/91	F	3701	May-1	99212	$40.00	382.9	
#3	03-75-93	11/10/66	F	2501	May-1	25565	$2,100.00	813.83	Radius & Ulna fx
	16-99-43	9/10/82	M	2501	May-1	99212	$40.00	924.11	
	12-52-76	8/4/69	F	2501	May-1	99212	$40.00	V25.49	
	12-52-76	8/4/69	F	2501	May-1	J1050	$25.00	V25.49	Injection
	02-41-78	6/15/72	F	2501	May-1	99212	$40.00	462	
	04-54-77	3/23/40	M	3701	May-1	99215	$125.00	562.10	
	03-55-08	3/5/35	M	2501	May-1	25505	$210.00	814.00	Wrist fx
	03-55-08	3/5/35	M	2501	May-1	A4580	$30.00	814.00	Cast supplies
	02-77-18	5/25/82	F	2501	May-1	99212	$40.00	461.9	
	06-52-38	4/22/72	M	3701	May-1	99215	$125.00	185	
	07-88-29	9/29/90	F	3701	May-1	99212	$40.00	380.4	
	10-45-23	4/15/57	F	4401	May-1	J1050	$47.00	V25.49	DepoProvera
	10-45-23	4/15/57	F	4401	May-1	99211	$35.00	V25.49	Visit
	10-45-23	4/15/57	F	4401	May-1	90714	$22.00	V70.0	Td
	07-43-01	2/4/94	M	3701	May-1	99212	$40.00	V20.2	
	07-43-01	2/4/94	M	3701	May-1	90700	$28.00	V06.1	Immun
	07-43-01	2/4/94	M	3701	May-1	90707	$29.00	V06.4	Immun
	07-43-01	2/4/94	M	3701	May-1	90744	$45.00	V05.3	Immun

Summary—Codes & Charges

Code	Qty	Code	Qty	Code	Qty
20600	1	57460	1	99211	1
25505	1	90700	1	99212	9
25565	1	90707	1	99213	1
27781	1	90714	1	99215	2
29405	1	90744	1	A4580	1
				J1050	2

Summary—Physician

	2501		3701		4401	
	25505	1	20600	1	57460	1
	25565	1	90700	1	J1050	1
	27781	1	90707	1	90714	1
	29405	1	90744	1	99211	1
#1	99212	6	99212	3		
	A4580	1	99213	1		
	J1050	1	99215	2		

Service-Mix Report

Figure 11.7 is an example of a service-mix report for doctor 2501. This report also could be produced to summarize the activity of a particular office within a multi-office enterprise. It is similar to the service distribution report but includes charge information.

The service-mix report provides an opportunity for discovering when procedures have not been priced consistently or when other errors have been made. For example:

Problem #1: CPT code 25565 shows an average actual charge of $1,155 with a projected average charge of $210, confirming the error suspected in the office service report.

Problem #2: CPT code 11981, Insertion, non-biodegradable drug delivery implant, was coded twice during the month, but HCPCS code J7306, Contraceptive implant supply, was coded only once, resulting in a considerable loss of revenue.

Problem #3: HCPCS code A4580, Cast material, was coded seven times during the month, whereas only four fracture care codes were indicated (25505, 25565 [twice], and 27781). The records of these patients may need to be reviewed to determine whether coding discrepancies have occurred.

Problem #4: Codes 90471 and 90472 are absent from the report, even though 43 doses of vaccine were given during the period. This results in a significant loss of revenue for the practice.

Revenue Production Report

Figure 11.8 is an excerpt from a revenue production report for the entire physician office. It is similar to the service distribution report but also contains the total revenue produced by a CPT/HCPCS code and the average reimbursement rate for that code. This report is sorted by the amount of revenue produced.

Usually, 80 percent of revenue is produced by 20 percent of the CPT codes used by the practice. Determining which codes provide the largest amount of revenue allows the evaluator to concentrate on the codes used most frequently to be sure they are coded and priced correctly.

In this revenue production report, the coder notices that CPT code 99232 is priced at $195, but the average reimbursement has been $136.50. This code should be evaluated for a possible pricing error. The coder also may project what the revenue change might be if the charge for a particular CPT code, such as 99213, was raised by only one or two dollars over the year.

Common Coding Errors Identified through Reports

Many types of coding errors can be identified using the encounter history database reports discussed above. Common errors include clustering, unbundling, missed charges, inappropriate linking, missing modifiers, and diagnosis/procedure mismatch.

Figure 11.7. Service-mix report

	Doctor	Month	CPT Code	Description	Qty	Charge	Ave Charge Actual	Ave Charge Projected
#2	2501	June	11981	Implant, drug	2	$366.00	$366.00	$366.00
	2501	June	12001	Repair, Laceration	2	$65.00	$65.00	$65.00
	2501	June	13120	Repair, Laceration	1	$168.00	$168.00	$168.00
	2501	June	20600	Small Joint Aspiration	2	$51.00	$51.00	$51.00
	2501	June	25505	Radial Fracture	1	$210.00	$210.00	$210.00
#1	2501	June	25565	Radius & Ulna Fracture	2	$210.00	$1,155.00	$210.00
	2501	June	27781	Fibular Fracture	1	$470.00	$470.00	$470.00
	2501	June	36415	Venipuncture	362	$6.00	$6.00	$6.00
	2501	June	57160	Fitting/Insertion - Pessary	1	$75.00	$75.00	$75.00
	2501	June	57452	Colposcopy	1	$106.00	$106.00	$106.00
	2501	June	57460	Colposcopy w/loop bx	2	$392.25	$392.25	$392.25
	2501	June	69210	Ear Curettage	6	$30.00	$33.33	$30.00
#4	2501	June	90700	DTaP Immunization	10	$28.00	$28.00	$28.00
	2501	June	90707	MMR Immunization	3	$22.00	$22.00	$22.00
	2501	June	90713	IPV Immunization	10	$12.00	$12.00	$12.00
	2501	June	90716	Varicella Immunization	10	$34.00	$34.00	$34.00
	2501	June	90714	Td Immunization	3	$22.00	$22.00	$22.00
	2501	June	90744	Hepatitis B	7	$65.00	$65.00	$65.00
	2501	June	96372	Injection	18	$32.00	$32.00	$32.00
	2501	June	96374	IV Injection	4	$64.00	$64.00	$64.00
	2501	June	99211	Nurse Only	118	$35.00	$35.00	$35.00
	2501	June	99212	Estab Pt Problem Foc	143	$40.00	$40.00	$40.00
	2501	June	99213	Estab Pt Expanded Pblm	262	$50.00	$50.00	$50.00
	2501	June	99214	Estab Pt Detailed	75	$80.00	$80.00	$80.00
	2501	June	99215	Estab Pt Comprehen	25	$125.00	$125.00	$125.00
	2501	June	99222	Hospital Care	3	$110.00	$110.00	$110.00
	2501	June	99223	Hospital Care	2	$125.00	$125.00	$125.00
	2501	June	99231	Hospital Care	12	$95.00	$95.00	$95.00
	2501	June	99232	Hospital Care	8	$195.00	$195.00	$195.00
	2501	June	99308	SNF Visit	6	$37.00	$37.00	$37.00
	2501	June	99309	SNF Visit	3	$53.00	$68.00	$53.00
#2	2501	June	J7306	Contraceptive Implant	1	$123.00	$123.00	$123.00
	2501	June	A4561	Pessary	1	$30.00	$30.00	$30.00
	2501	June	A4565	Sling	3	$24.00	$24.00	$24.00
#3	2501	June	A4580	Cast Material	7	$18.00	$18.00	$18.00
	2501	June	J0290	Med: Ampicillin	2	$43.00	$43.00	$43.00
	2501	June	J1050	Med: DepoProvera	6	$25.00	$36.00	$25.00
	2501	June	J1600	Med: Gold Sodium T.	5	$34.00	$34.00	$34.00
	2501	June	J1642	Med: Heparin Lock	4	$8.00	$8.00	$8.00
	2501	June	J3121	Med: Testosterone	200	$5.00	$5.00	$5.00
	2501	June	J3420	Med: Vitamin B12	5	$5.00	$5.00	$5.00
	2501	June	J7070	Med: D5W	4	$8.00	$8.00	$8.00

Figure 11.8. Revenue production report

Month	CPT Code	Description	Qty	Charge	Reimbursement	Projected Revenue (Qty × Charge)
June	J7306	Contraceptive Implant	4	$247.38	$173.22	$1,039.32
June	96372	Injection	39	$32.00	$27.00	$1,053.00
June	11981	Implant, drug	4	$366.00	$289.00	$1,156.00
June	57460	Colpscopy w/biopsy	4	$392.25	$356.12	$1,424.48
June	99232	Hospital Care	14	$195.00	$136.50	$1,911.00
June	J1050	DepoProvera 150 mg	47	$64.54	$45.18	$2,123.46
June	36415	Venipuncture	697	$6.00	$4.20	$2,927.40
June	99231	Hospital Care	42	$95.00	$91.10	$3,826.20
June	99215	Estab Pt Comprehensive	79	$125.00	$100.00	$7,900.00
June	99211	Nurse Only	334	$35.00	$24.50	$8,183.00
June	99212	Estab Pt Problem	412	$40.00	$32.00	$13,184.00
June	99214	Estab Pt Detailed	234	$80.00	$64.00	$14,976.00
June	99213	Estab Pt Expanded	759	$50.00	$40.00	$30,360.00

Clustering

Clustering is the practice of coding/charging one or two middle levels of service codes exclusively under the philosophy that, although some will be higher and some lower, the charges will average out over an extended period. In reality, this overcharges some patients and undercharges many others. If done deliberately, the practice could be considered fraudulent.

In the office service report (refer to figure 11.6), the coder noted that doctor 2501 coded all of the office visits on May 1 as 99212. This may have been a coincidence, but it also may suggest that this physician tends to cluster the office visit coding. The physician could be monitored over a period of time and, if the suspicion were confirmed, educational efforts would be needed to ensure that the coding matches the documentation and the actual service performed.

Unbundling

As discussed in chapter 4, unbundling is the practice of coding services separately that should be coded together as a package because all the parts are included within one code and, therefore, one price. Unbundling done deliberately to obtain higher reimbursement is a misrepresentation of services and can be considered insurance fraud.

In figure 11.6, doctor 2501 appears to have unbundled a service by coding an ankle fracture treatment and a cast application service for patient 55-29-42. Instructions in the CPT code book state that the cast application should be included, or bundled, into the fracture treatment.

Missed Charges

Missed charges are simply forgotten codes for services that were performed and that needed to be coded separately to obtain reimbursement. For example, in figure 11.6, the coder should have noted from the office service report that the diagnosis code 380.4, Impacted cerumen, was used for an office visit and that no code was reported for cerumen removal, which is an extremely common procedure associated with this diagnosis. Such missed charges become easier to recognize with experience.

Sources of documentation that support physician charges are discussed in chapter 1. The service-mix report can be used to verify whether charges from a variety of sources are being received. As an example, nursing home patients traditionally require a visit every 30 days. If no codes appear for nursing home visits on the monthly report, either no visits were made or no charges were submitted. Other reports can be developed to help staff monitor charge submission and watch for missing charges.

Inappropriate Linking of Diagnosis to Procedure

In figure 11.2, case 4, the coder linked the diagnosis of abdominal pain to a CBC when the diagnosis of anemia also was available for the visit. In addition, a single-view abdominal x-ray was linked to anemia instead of to the abdominal pain. Although reimbursement may be made in this case, inappropriate linking of the diagnosis to the procedure often results in lack of reimbursement.

Missing Modifiers

In figure 11.2, case 2, the coder failed to assign a –76 modifier to the second nebulizer treatment performed on the same date by the same physician. Without this modifier, the second nebulizer will likely be denied as a duplicate billing.

Diagnosis/Procedure Mismatch

Figure 11.2, case 1, shows a basic example of a specific procedure being linked to a diagnosis for a different condition. Other mismatches could be incorrect anatomical locations and benign-versus-malignant neoplasm activity.

Computerized Internal Fee Schedule Reports

As discussed in chapter 10, the computerized internal fee schedule is a database of the fees associated with particular codes and other data elements necessary to manage fees and create CMS-1500 claim forms. Reports generated from this database help to verify that codes have been entered correctly and that all entries have been developed consistently.

The fee schedule summary report in figure 11.9 shows how a coder has reviewed the report and identified multiple problems.

Problem #1: There is a discrepancy in the place of service (POS) listed for the office evaluation and management services. Each of these services should have the POS code 11 instead of 12. Only the service with unique ID 992140 is entered correctly.

Problem #2: There is both an incorrect POS code for services 992840 and 992850 and a probable pricing error for service 992850. The charge of $1,650 is high in relation to the other services in the series and could be a data-entry error.

Problem #3: Service 694361 is described as unilateral, but the modifier field entered is –50. No modifier is needed when the procedure is listed as unilateral.

Problem #4: The units entry for J33602 is incorrect. If service J33600 is Diazepam 5 mg with a unit of 1, service J33602 must be Diazepam 20 mg with a unit of 4 rather than 1.

Figure 11.9 Fee schedule summary report

	Unique ID	Description	CPT/HCPCS	Fee	POS	Modifier	Units
#1	992110	Office Visit	99211	$25.00	12		1
	992120	Office Visit	99212	$40.00	12		1
	992130	Office Visit	99213	$50.00	12		1
	992140	Office Visit	99214	$75.00	11		1
	992150	Office Visit	99215	$125.00	12		1
	A45500	Surgical Tray	A4550	$22.00	11		1
	A45800	Cast Material	A4580	$18.00	11		1
	E01100	Crutches, Pair	E0110	$26.00	11		1
	992810	ER Visit	99281	$65.00	23		1
	992820	ER Visit	99282	$85.00	23		1
	992830	ER Visit	99283	$115.00	23		1
#2	992840	ER Visit	99284	$135.00	24		1
	992850	ER Visit	99285	$1,650.00	24		1
	694360	Ear Tubes, Bilateral	69436	$425.00	22	−50	1
#3	694361	Ear Tube, Unilateral	69436	$305.00	22	−50	1
	J33600	Diazepam, 5 mg	J3360	$12.00	11		1
	J33601	Diazepam, 10 mg	J3360	$18.00	11		2
#4	J33602	Diazepam, 20 mg	J3360	$29.00	11		1
	J02900	Ampicillin, 500 mg	J0290	$7.00	11		1
	245000	Closed Rx humeral fx	24500	$240.00	11		1
	275000	Closed Rx femoral fx	27500	$380.00	11		1

Each of these errors must be investigated and corrected to ensure that the CMS-1500 form prints correctly the next time the code is used to describe a service.

Payer Remittance Report

The insurance company generates a payer remittance report to state the outcome of the claim. The report may be attached to the check for claims payment or sent as a separate mailing if the remittance is electronic. A payer remittance report is known by a number of different names, including the following:

- Explanation of benefits (EOB)
- Remittance advice (RA)
- Medicare summary notice
- Provider remittance advice
- Statement of provider claims paid
- Provider explanation of benefits
- Explanation of review
- Explanation of reimbursement

Figure 11.10 shows the information the payer remittance report contains and its format.

Each insurance company has its own format, but, in general, the summary line of the report indicates the amount to be reimbursed, the amount of patient responsibility, and the amount that has been denied.

Figure 11.10. Payer remittance report

				"Any" Insurance Company						
Prov: 123456789-01-Welby, Marcus MD										
Empl: John Doe			Patient:123456789-01—Jane Doe							
Service	Begin Date	End Date	Provider Charge	Charge Allowed	Disc Amount	Not Covered	Deductible	Copay	Co-Ins	Benefit Paid
99213	3-1-XX	3-1-XX	61.00	58.00	3.00					58.00
85025	3-1-XX	3-1-XX	25.00			50				
36415	3-1-XX	3-1-XX	16.00	4.00	12.00					4.00
Claim Totals:			102.00	62.00	15.00	25.00				62.00
Vendor Totals:			102.00	62.00	15.00	25.00				62.00
Net Payment for Claim 62.00										
Amount owed by beneficiary 0.00										

Codes and Code Edits

Code edits, or accuracy checkpoints, have been developed to identify when the CMS-1500 form may be missing information. A complete listing of the meaning of the code edits can be obtained from payers. This chapter discusses only a few that are specific to incorrect coding of the original claim. Claims should not be set aside and forgotten. Most payers have a specific time frame for resubmitting corrections, and many corrections are easy to make and resubmit.

When a service has been denied or there is an error, either a notation of "denied" or a number appears. Each insurance company and Medicare intermediary may use a different number for a similar description. Following are descriptions of potential edits:

- The diagnosis code must be present and to its most specific digit.

- The location of the service must be indicated. The place of service (POS) is a two-digit code and must match the service. For example, an initial hospital charge (99221) should not have clinic (11) as the place of service.

- A valid HCPCS or CPT procedure code must be present.

- The diagnosis code must be pointed (linked) to a service code.

- The service may be improperly bundled or unbundled.

- There may be a sex/code mismatch. For example, a procedure specific to female anatomy must pertain to a female patient.

Diagnosis codes also may cause a claim to be denied. Medical necessity and the frequency of ordering tests are becoming major deciding factors in the payment of claims. Many payers have identified specific diagnoses to indicate medical necessity for performing a service. The coder should contact payers to obtain a copy of their medical policies. Medicare has both national and local policies (reviewed in chapter 10). Some payers choose to share this information in their news bulletins instead of in a separate document.

Payers require that diagnosis codes from ICD-10-CM be submitted to their highest level of specificity. For example, right upper quadrant abdominal pain submitted as code R10.1 is incorrect because the code needs a fifth character. The coder should submit R10.11.

Other circumstances that a specific code edit may not identify include the following:

- The amount discounted is large. The coder should find out whether the discount is appropriate according to the contract or the insurer's standard practices.

- The claim is not covered. The coder should determine whether the patient should be billed for the service.

- The payment is small compared to the charge.

In researching these situations, the coder may find a coding error—usually HCPCS or CPT—that could affect payment of the claim.

A number of noncoding reasons can result in a denied claim. Following are some of the more common noncoding reasons:

- A service is ordered or referred by a physician, but the physician's name and unique physician identifier number (UPIN) do not appear on the claim.

- The provider has not been credentialed for that particular payer.

- Modifiers have not been submitted for services performed by midlevel practitioners.

- Some payers do not allow the clinic to bill for reference laboratory services.

- The incorrect primary insurance carrier is billed for services.

- Date of injury is not completed when billing for injury-specific services.

- Specific requirements for submission of a service are not followed. For example, Medicare requires a six-digit, FDA-approved, certification number for sites performing mammography.

- The payer requires report/office notes prior to determination of payment.

- The claim is filed after the filing time limit has expired.

- The service may require a prior authorization that has not been obtained.

- The claim has been paid previously.

For additional information on how to interpret explanation of benefits messages, contact your provider representative or access the carrier's website. Most carriers provide written material, upon request, regarding EOB messages.

Washington Publishing Company maintains online lookup tables of claim adjustment reason codes and remark codes. Claim adjustment reason codes are available at www.wpc -edi.com/codes/claimadjustment. Remark codes are available at www.wpc-edi.com/codes/ remittanceadvice.

Coder and Biller as a Team

When the facility's coding and billing functions are separate, teamwork is vital. Coders and billers must share the goal of claim submission and adjudication. The coder–biller team needs to look at errors as a part of the learning experience. Continuous errors of the same nature may indicate that additional training is needed in a certain area or that a process needs to be revised. They also may suggest to the payer that fraud and abuse is occurring at the site.

It is important that biller and coder not change or manipulate codes just to get the claim paid. Such an act would constitute insurance fraud. All members of the team are experts in their area. The biller is the expert on how the claim needs to look and the elements required; the coder is the expert on correct ICD-10-CM, CPT, and HCPCS codes supported by the documentation in the health record.

When a claim is returned with coding errors, the biller needs to contact the coder to review the claim. The coder may need to review the health record to determine whether the code submission is correct. After this is determined, the coder should notify the biller with the correction. Each clinic setting may have a different method of notifying the biller of changes or corrections.

Following are some examples of how changes may be communicated between biller and coder:

- Writing on the payer remittance report

- Use of the internal change form

- Conversation between coder and biller

Other areas where coder and biller can work as a team to learn from past experience are in tracking the following key indicators:

- The number of billing/coding errors per the number of bills sent. This percentage can be watched for fluctuation and improvement

- The number of "no payments" and "100 percent payments." These entries should be made in the fee problem log and investigated to determine whether they were caused by incorrect coding or billing procedures or whether the fee is inappropriately high or low

- The number of times a tracer claim needs to be sent to an insurance company to determine why a response or payment has not been received. This problem could indicate that incorrect addresses are being used or electronic data transmission problems have occurred

- The percentage of clean claims produced

Exercise 11.1. Coding and Reimbursement Reports and Databases

Identify whether the following reports are used for qualitative or quantitative review.

1. Claim history

   a. Qualitative
   b. Quantitative

2. Charge summary

   a. Qualitative
   b. Quantitative

3. Procedure/supply distribution

   a. Qualitative
   b. Quantitative

4. Diagnosis distribution

   a. Qualitative
   b. Quantitative

Use the following custom revenue production report to answer questions 5, 7, and 8.

Revenue Production Report
Small Multispecialty Group
Month: January

Code	Qty	Fee	Projected Revenue	Actual Insurance Revenue
99201	0	$50	$0	$0.00
99202	3	$75	$225	$164.10
99203	4	$90	$360	$267.94
99204	0	$120	$0	$0.00
99205	0	$150	$0	$0.00
99211	703	$28	$19,684	$14,988.32
99212	489	$47	$22,983	$18,092.65
99213	1853	$63	$116,739	$92,890.38
99214	41	$89	$3,649	$2,799.11
99215	7	$135	$945	$722.87
99241	3	$100	$300	$52.50
99242	9	$125	$1,125	$156.23
99243	27	$150	$4,050	$610.45
99244	10	$175	$1,750	$124.32
99245	1	$200	$200	$53.10

5. Which of the following is apparent to the coder about the consultation codes?

   a. The charges appear to be much lower than expected.
   b. The charges are not being paid appropriately.
   c. The consultation codes appear clustered.
   d. The consultation codes are being used more frequently than expected.

(Continued on next page)

Exercise 11.1. (Continued)

6. The coding manager has been asked to help evaluate why the cost of supplies is considerably greater this year than it was last year. What report would help the manager determine supply provision?

    a. Explanation of reimbursement
    b. Service distribution report
    c. Diagnosis distribution report
    d. Fee schedule summary

7. Which of the following statements is true regarding this report?

    a. The number of nurse visit codes is low for a practice this size.
    b. The payments received from insurance seem appropriate.
    c. The new patient codes are used less frequently than expected.
    d. The consultation codes are high for a practice this size.

8. Which coding error may be demonstrated in the report?

    a. Missed charges
    b. Clustering
    c. Overcoding
    d. Unbundling

9. "The service may be improperly bundled or unbundled" is an example of:

    a. Diagnosis distribution report
    b. A service distribution report
    c. A database review finding
    d. A code edit statement

10. What tool would the coder use to evaluate utilization patterns for E/M codes?

    a. Fee schedule report
    b. Service distribution report
    c. Comparison graph
    d. Diagnosis distribution report

11. When might an annual diagnosis distribution appropriately show codes with different numbers of digits?

    a. When a diagnosis code is subdivided as of October 1
    b. When coders use code books that are not current
    c. When physicians select nonspecific diagnoses
    d. When codes are deleted as of October 1

Use the following charge summary to answer questions 12 through 15.

Charge Summary—My Medical Group Date of Service: 10-2-20XX

CPT/HCPCS Code	Description	Fee	Linked Dx	Description	POS
Case 1. #119042 Martin, Henry					
99283–25	ER Visit	$169.00	S41.101A	Open wound, arm	22
12032	Laceration repair, arm	$210.00	S41.101A	Open wound, arm	22
Case 2. #168472 Jones, John					
99202	Office Visit, New Pt	$82.00	I10	Hypertension	11
90658	Flu injection	$14.00	Z23	Influenza Vac	11
90732	Pneumonia injection	$15.00	Z23	Pneumonia Vac	11
Case 3. #126113 Johnson, Stanley					
99244–25	Office consultation	$243.00	N94.1	Dyspareunia	11
57460	LEEP of cervix	$358.00	N87.9	Hyperplasia, cervix	11
Case 4. #168473 Albert, Maria					
99203	Office Visit, Estab Pt	$72.00	R04.0	Epistaxis	11

Exercise 11.1. (Continued)

12. Which case is likely to be rejected due to a code edit?

    a. Case 1
    b. Case 2
    c. Case 3
    d. Case 4

13. Which case appears to be coded correctly?

    a. Case 1
    b. Case 2
    c. Case 3
    d. Case 4

14. Which case displays a probable error in assigning new versus established office visits?

    a. Case 1
    b. Case 2
    c. Case 3
    d. Case 4

15. Which case displays a potential claim generation error?

    a. Case 1
    b. Case 2
    c. Case 3
    d. Case 4

Fill in the blanks.

16. Data entry errors can be identified using a _____ report.

17. The _____ report helps the manager see differences in coding among a series of visits.

18. The _____ report can be used to design new encounter form content.

Answer True or False to the following questions.

19. True or False? The bell curves associated with many medical specialties are available for download from the CMS website. _____

20. True or False? A payment for a surgical service is equal to the fee charged. This indicates that the fee should be reviewed. _____

Chapter 11 Test

Choose the best answer for each of the following questions.

1. After reviewing this Coding Summary before charge entry, what action should the coder take?

   Coding Summary
   Patient: Amanda Jacobsen, DOB: 6-10-09
   Primary Care Provider: Dr. Herbert

Date of Service	CPT Code	Description	Diagnosis
12-28-09	99382	Initial preventive medicine, early childhood, (age 1 through 4 years)	Z00.129
12-28-09	85025	Complete CBC	Z00.129
12-28-09	36416	Routine finger/heel/ear stick for collection of specimen(s)	Z00.129

   a. Verify the diagnosis with the visit documentation in the medical record.
   b. Report the codes as submitted by the primary care physician.
   c. Change the Preventive Medicine code to match the correct age grouping.
   d. Question the CPT codes for the laboratory tests, as these are included in the visit code.

2. Referring to figure 11.4 in the text, which one of the following statements is true?

   a. The number of new patient office visits is just about right when compared with established patient visits.

   b. When adding together all initial hospital and newborn history, the discharge numbers are extremely low.

   c. The number of audiometry testings and vision screening tests is appropriate for the practice.

   d. Vaccine administration codes seem to be reported correctly.

3. When investigating a patient question about possible claim inaccuracies, which report would provide the most help in the investigation?

   a. Claim history report
   b. Charge summary report
   c. Service distribution report
   d. Revenue production report

4. When reviewing the charge summary for physician work outside of the office, the coder should:

Date of Service	CPT Code	Description	Diagnosis	Charges
10/15/09	99222	Initial hospital visit	J18.9	$210.00
10/16/09	99231	Subsequent hospital visit	J18.9	$154.00
10/17/09	99309	Subsequent nursing facility care	J14	$95.00
10/18/09	99239	Hospital discharge	J14	$186.00

   a. Report the codes as they were written by the physician.
   b. Call the hospital to see if the patient was transferred to a nursing home.
   c. Question that the diagnoses changed during the episode of care.
   d. Alert the physician of a possible error on the charges.

Chapter 11 Test (Continued)

5. An office manager reviewed the coding summary on these two cases before the claims were submitted. What change, if any, should be suggested to the physician that helps ensure proper payment?

Case #	CPT Code	Description	ICD-10-CM Code	Description
1	90716	Varicella vaccine	Z23	Rubella vaccination
2	82948	Glucose, reagent strip	M79.609	Arm pain
	73090	Arm x-ray	E11.9	Diabetes mellitus

   a. Diagnoses should be selected that substantiate the procedures.
   b. Modifiers should be added on the CPT codes.
   c. Additional CPT codes are required.
   d. No change should be suggested.

6. After evaluating the graph below, what information can be determined from these data?

Established Visit Codes During 20XX

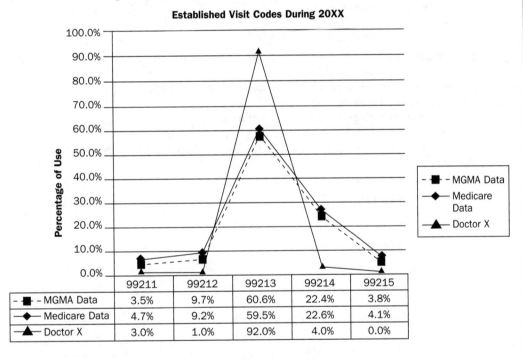

	99211	99212	99213	99214	99215
– ■ – MGMA Data	3.5%	9.7%	60.6%	22.4%	3.8%
–◆– Medicare Data	4.7%	9.2%	59.5%	22.6%	4.1%
–▲– Doctor X	3.0%	1.0%	92.0%	4.0%	0.0%

   a. Doctor X uses code 99215 less frequently than his peers.
   b. Doctor X's documentation doesn't support the codes submitted.
   c. Doctor X overutilizes code 99213 as compared with the documentation.
   d. Doctor X's overutilizes code 99212 as compared with his peers.

7. Review these hospital charges and determine the best course of action.

   Inpatient Billing Summary
   Physician: Dr. Mark Reiners
   Patient: 458963
   Name: Harry Tate
   Date of Admission: 7/20/09
   Date of Discharge: 7/23/09

(Continued on next page)

Chapter 11 Test (Continued)

Date of Service	CPT Code	Description	Diagnosis	Charge
7/20/09	99221	Initial Hospital	J18.9	$193.00
7/21/09	99221	Initial Hospital	J18.9	$193.00
7/22/09	99221	Initial Hospital	J18.9	$193.00
7/23/09	99238	Hospital Discharge	J18.9	$173.00

   a. Question that the same diagnosis was used each day.

   b. See that two daily visits are coded wrong and alert the physician.

   c. Submit the codes as the physician wrote them.

   d. Question the physician about what service was performed.

8. The outcome of a claim is listed in a report called the:

   a. Fee Problem Log

   b. Provider Explanation of Benefits

   c. Fee Schedule Summary

   d. Office Service Report

9. Which of the following surgical cases would a code editor flag as an error?

   a. Accident victim having wound debridement and an eye examination under anesthesia during same operative episode

   b. 67-year-old female patient having a dilatation and curettage

   c. 72-year-old man having a LEEP

   d. Skin grafting required following a severe burn

10. When developing or revising a charge ticket, which report would be the most helpful for the coder?

   a. Claim history report

   b. Service distribution report

   c. Service-mix report

   d. Revenue production report

Chapter 12

Evaluation of Coding Quality

Objectives

Upon completion of this lesson, the student should be able to do the following:

- Identify ways to obtain or create tools to clarify conflicting, ambiguous, or missing health record documentation and/or billing information from the physician

- Use tools designed to resolve discrepancies with physicians

- Develop assessment tools for completing internal audits to compare claim forms with health record documentation and to compare all CMS-1500 claim form data elements for consistency

- List the steps in completing an internal audit to determine whether CMS-1500 claim form data accurately describe the services documented in the health record

- Explain the concept of compliance

This chapter emphasizes the importance of maintaining and evaluating the quality of both ICD-10-CM and CPT coding. Inadequate or inappropriate coding could cause physician offices to experience financial losses as a result of claim denials or non-optimization of charges submitted. Coders should be knowledgeable of and adhere to AHIMA's Code of Ethics, provided in online appendix H.

Conflicting, ambiguous, or missing health record documentation and/or billing information submitted by the physician or individual performing the service could have an impact on the quality of coding. Moreover, it is important to audit not only the physician's documentation, but also the documentation of everyone who contributes to the record—from midlevel practitioners and nurses to laboratory and radiology staff. Finally, it is important to audit the coder to ensure that appropriate codes have been assigned to services performed (CPT) and conditions diagnosed (ICD-10-CM).

Tools for Evaluating Quality

When assessing coding quality, many different tools may be used. There are tools for collecting, analyzing, and correcting information, each with a specific purpose.

Collecting Information

The tool most commonly used to collect information is the charge ticket. The charge ticket indicates the services performed for a specific patient and, in many instances, the ICD-10-CM codes, preprinted or assigned by the coder, for a given date of service. Upon completion, this tool is routed to the charge entry or business office area for submission of charges to payers or the patient. Figures 1.4 and 1.5 (in chapter 1) are examples of collection tools.

Correcting Information

Sometimes documentation in the health record or on the charge ticket needs to be corrected or verified. Many offices develop a communication tool for use between the coder and a physician. This form can be as simple or complex as the office sees fit. Figure 12.1 is an example of a basic communication tool.

Figure 12.1.   Basic communication tool

Date:_____

Physician:_____

Please complete the following (information should be documented in the patient's chart):

_____ Diagnosis not documented

_____ Signature needed on _____

_____ Documentation does not support charge

_____ Discrepancy in dictation compared to handwritten information

_____ Reason for test not documented

_____ Other _____

Thank you,

_____

It is important to identify discrepancies when the dictation does not match a handwritten notation.

Example: Handwritten note states the patient fractured the left arm, and the dictation states a fracture of the right arm.

The communication tool in figure 12.1 should have the statement "Discrepancy in dictation compared to handwritten information" indicated with a check mark and should be returned to the physician for correction. The correction needs to be made in the appropriate place in the health record. Physicians often indicate the change on the communication tool but forget to make the correction in the health record.

Example: Record reads: "New patient. Arm pain. Sling applied. Return as needed." The physician has indicated a high-level office visit on the charge ticket.

The preceding documentation does not support a high-level office visit. The communication tool should be used to indicate to the physician that the documentation does not support the charge. An explanation may be needed to indicate why this is the case. The following reasons all indicate that the level was not supported:

- To bill a new patient office visit, the documentation must include all three key elements (history, examination, and medical decision making) of an E/M service. No examination is documented.

- The history needs to include, at a minimum, the chief complaint and a brief history of the present illness. This example only has a chief complaint (arm pain).

- Medical decision making would be implied as straightforward in this case—the lowest level of medical decision making.

Figure 12.2 shows an example of a more complex communication tool that may be used in larger offices or when more detail is needed to communicate the questions and answers between coder and physician. Either tool, shown in figure 12.1 or 12.2, can be used in any situation.

A communication tool can assist in identifying areas where further education or training may be needed. It may identify areas for individual physicians or for all of the healthcare providers within a group. By tracking the reasons the communication tool has been used, the coder can target educational programs for the most frequent areas of concern.

Analyzing Information

Many tools can be used to analyze coding information. Analyzing information is often called auditing. Internal and external audits are other beneficial ways of assessing where coding and reimbursement education needs to be heightened. (Audits are discussed in detail in the next section of this chapter.)

Figure 12.3 shows an example of a tool used to assess the quality of coding for a physician office based on the 1995 guidelines; figure 12.4 shows an alternate front page of the tool based on the 1997 guidelines. Note that page two of the tool remains the same as page two in figure 12.3. These forms should be modified to meet the needs of a particular practice setting, such as adding the bulleted elements for a particular specialty exam of the 1997 guidelines.

Figure 12.2.   Complex communication tool

Physician:_____

Patient Name: _____

Chart #: _____   Date of Service: _____ / ___ / _____

Please complete/respond to the following and return to:

Thank You

Please amend chart documentation as required.

☐   Dictation/documentation was not found for this date of service.

Charge ticket is incomplete for the following reason:

☐   No service has been indicated.

☐   No diagnosis has been indicated.

☐   Date of injury is required _____ / ___ / _____

Documentation of office visit level:

☐   Does not support the level charged

☐   Supports a higher level than charged

☐   Supports preventive visit only

☐   Supports non-well visit only

☐   Does not support an E/M charge in addition to the procedure charged

☐   Other _____

☐   Documentation for procedure _____

was not found in chart dictation/documentation.

☐   Based on documentation, procedure _____

was recoded as_____

☐   Documentation for procedure _____

is incomplete; please specify (in chart): _____

_____

☐   Documentation for diagnosis _____

was not found in chart dictation/documentation.

☐   Documentation in/on _____

is inconsistent with documentation found in/on _____

Lab tests charged require additional information:

☐   Please specify the appropriate diagnosis for_____

☐   A current order for _____

was not documented in patient's chart.

☐   Test requires waiver/ABN—was one obtained?

    ☐   Yes (please provide copy)

    ☐   No (test charge will be provider responsibility)

☐   Other:_____

Figure 12.3. Audit tool—1995 guidelines

History Component (equal to lowest category documented)	Problem Focused	Exp Problem Focused	Detailed	Comprehensive
Chief Complaint _____ HPI—History of Present Illness __ Location __ Duration __ Severity __ Quality __ Context __ Timing __ Modifying factors __ Associated signs and symptoms	Brief 1–3 HPI elements documented	Brief 1–3 HPI elements documented	Extended ≥ 4 HPI elements documented	Extended ≥ 4 HPI elements documented
ROS—Review of System(s) __ Constitutional (wt loss, etc.) __ Eyes __ GI __ Integumentary __ ENT, Mouth __ GU __ Endocrine __ Respiratory __ MS __ Hem/lymph __ Cardiovasc __ Neuro __ Allergy/Immun __ Psychiatric __ All others negative	None	Problem Specific (1 system)	Extended (2–9 systems)	Complete (Greater than 10 systems or some with all others negative)
PFSH (past medical, family and social histories) __ Previous medical (past experience with illness, injury, surgery, medical treatments, etc.) __ Family medical history (diseases which may be hereditary or with increased risk of occurrence) __ Social (relationships, diet, exercise, occupation, etc.)	None	None	Pertinent At least 1 item from at least 1 history	Complete Specifics of at least 2 history areas documented Initial = all 3

Exam Component	Problem Focused	Exp. Problem Focused	Detailed	Comprehensive
Body Areas — Organ Systems __ Head, Face __ Const. (Vitals, Gen appear) __ Neck __ Chest, Breasts __ Eyes __ GU __ Abdomen __ ENT, Mouth __ Integumentary __ Genit Groin __ Respiratory __ MS __ Back, Spine __ Cardiovasc __ Neurological __ Each Extremity __ Gastrointest __ Psychiatric __ Lymph/Hem/Immun	1 body area or system	2–4 systems incl. affected area or 2–7 basic body areas and/or organ systems	5–7 detailed systems incl. affected area or 2–7 body areas and/or organ systems with one in detail	8 or more systems

Medical Decision Making (MDM) (Highest 2 out of 3)		Straightforward	Low Complexity	Moderate Complexity	High Complexity
A	Diagnoses/Management Options	Minimal (≤1)	Limited (2)	Multiple (3)	Extensive (≥4)
B	Amount/Complexity of Data	Min/Low (≤1)	Limited (2)	Moderate (3)	Extensive (≥4)
C	Highest Risk (highest from any category)	Minimal	Low	Moderate	High

Coordination of care or counseling a factor? _____ Time documented: _____ minutes of _____ minutes of total patient encounter

Selection of E/M Level based on above components

Established Patient (requires 2 of 3 elements)

History	Exam	MDM	E/M—Office/OP Min	E/M—Office/OP Level
Min service, may not require MD			5	99211
PF	PF	SF	10	99212
EPF	EPF	Low	15	99213
Det	Det	Mod	25	99214
Comp	Comp	High	40	99215

New Patient or Consultation (requires 3 of 3 elements)

History	Exam	MDM	E/M Office/OP Min	E/M Office/OP Level	E/M OP Consult Min	E/M OP Consult Level
PF	PF	SF	10	99201	15	99241
EPF	EPF	SF	20	99202	30	99242
Det	Det	Low	30	99203	40	99243
Comp	Comp	Mod	45	99204	60	99244
Comp	Comp	High	60	99205	80	99245

Selection of E/M Level based on above components

Initial Hospital Care (requires 3 of 3 elements)

History	Exam	MDM	Initial Inpatient Min	Initial Inpatient Level	A/D Same Date Level
D/C	D/C	SF/Low	30	99221	99234
Comp	Comp	Mod	50	99222	99235
Comp	Comp	High	70	99223	99236

Subsequent Hospital (requires 2 of 3 elements)

History	Exam	MDM	Subsequent Inpatient Min	Subsequent Inpatient Level
PF	PF	SF/Low	15	99231
EPF	EPF	Mod	25	99232
Det	Det	High	35	99233

(Continued on next page)

Figure 12.3. (Continued)

A. Number of Diagnoses or Tx Options			
Categories of problem	**# × Points = Subtotal**		
Self-limited or minor (Stable, improved or worsening)		1	(max = 2)
Established problem (to examiner); stable, improved		1	
Established problem (to examiner); worsening		2	
New problem (to examiner); no additional workup planned		3	
New problem (to examiner); additional workup planned		4	
	Total		

B. Amount/Complexity of Data Reviewed	
Categories of data reviewed	
Order and/or review clinical lab tests	1
Order and/or review tests from radiology section	1
Order and/or review tests from medicine section (i.e., EKG, EMG, allergy tests, audiometry)	1
Discussion of test results with performing provider	1
Decision to obtain old records/Obtain history from other than patient/Discuss case with other provider	2
Independent visualization of image, tracing, or report	2
Total	

C. Complication Risk Factor(s) (select highest assigned to any category)

Level of Risk	Presenting Problem	Dx Procedures Ordered	Management Options Selected
Minimal	• One self-limited or minor problem	• Lab tests, x-rays, EKG, EEG	• Rest, superficial dressings, none required
Low	• Multiple self-limited or minor problems • One stable chronic illness • Acute, uncomplicated illness or injury	• Physiologic tests w/o stress • Imaging studies w/contrast • Superficial needle biopsy • Skin biopsy • Arterial blood draw	• Over-the-counter remedy • Minor surgery w/o risk factor • Physical, occupational therapy • IV fluids w/o additive
Moderate	• One or more chronic illness with exacerbation, progression, or treatment side effects • Two or more chronic stable illnesses • Undiagnosed new problem with uncertain prognosis • Acute complicated injury • Acute illness with systemic symptoms	• Stress tests • Endoscopies w/o risk factors • Cardiovascular imaging study w/o identified risk factor • Deep needle or incisional biopsy • Centesis of body cavity fluid	• Minor surgery with identified risk factors • Elective major surgery without identified risk factors • Prescription drug management • Therapeutic radiology • IV fluids with additives • Closed treatment of skeletal injury
High	• One or more chronic illnesses with severe exacerbation, progression, or treatment side effects • Acute or chronic illness or injury that may pose a threat to life or bodily functions • An abrupt change to mental status	• Cardiovascular imaging studies with identified risk factors • Cardiac electrophysiological tests • Endoscopy with identified risk factors	• Elective major surgery with identified risk factors • Emergency major surgery • Parenteral controlled substance • Drug therapy requiring intensive monitoring • DNR status

Tabulation of Medical Decision Making Elements					
A	Diagnoses/Management Options	Minimal (≤1)	Limited (2)	Multiple (3)	Extensive (≥4)
B	Amount/Complexity of Data	Min/Low (≤1)	Limited (2)	Moderate (3)	Extensive (≥4)
C	Highest Risk (from any category)	Minimal	Low	Moderate	High
	Medical Decision Making (Highest 2 of 3)	**Straightforward**	**Low Complexity**	**Moderate Complexity**	**High Complexity**

Inpatient Consultations (requires 3 of 3 elements)

History	Exam	MDM	Initial Inpatient Consult Min	Initial Inpatient Consult Level
PF	PF	SF	20	99251
EPF	EPF	SF	40	99252
Det	Det	Low	55	99253
Comp	Comp	Mod	80	99254
Comp	Comp	High	110	99255

Emergency Department Care (requires 3 of 3 elements)

History	Exam	MDM	Emergency (no minute values)
PF	PF	SF	99281
EPF	EPF	Low	99282
EPF	EPF	Mod	99283
Det	Det	Mod	99284
Comp	Comp	High	99285

Figure 12.4. Audit tool—1997 guidelines

History Component (equal to lowest category documented)	Problem Focused	Exp Problem Focused	Detailed	Comprehensive
Chief Complaint _____ HPI—History of Present Illness __ Location __ Duration __ Severity __ Quality __ Context __ Timing __ Modifying factors __ Associated signs and symptoms	Brief 1–3 HPI elements documented	Brief 1–3 HPI elements documented	Extended ≥ 4 HPI or status of ≥3 chronic conditions documented	Extended ≥ 4 HPI or status of ≥3 chronic conditions documented
ROS—Review of System(s) __ Constitutional (wt loss, etc.) __ Eyes __ GI __ Integumentary __ ENT, Mouth __ GU __ Endocrine __ Respiratory __ MS __ Hem/lymph __ Cardiovasc __ Neuro __ Allergy/Immun __ Psychiatric __ All others negative	None	Problem Specific (1 system)	Extended (2–9 systems)	Complete (Greater than 10 systems or some with all others negative)
PFSH (past medical, family and social histories) __ Previous medical (past experience with illness, injury, surgery, medical treatments, etc.) __ Family medical history (diseases which may be hereditary or with increased risk of occurrence) __ Social (relationships, diet, exercise, occupation, etc.)	None	None	Pertinent At least 1 item from at least 1 history	Complete Specifics of at least 2 history areas documented Initial = all 3

Exam Component	General Multisystem Exam	Single-Organ System Exam
Problem Focused	1–5 elements identified by a ·	1–5 elements identified by a ·
Expanded Problem Focused	≥ 6 elements identified by a ·	≥ 6 elements identified by a ·
Detailed	≥ 12 elements identified by a · from 6 areas/systems OR ≥ 12 elements identified by a · from at least 2 areas/systems	≥ 12 elements identified by a · EXCEPT ≥ 9 elements identified by a · for eye and psychiatric exams
Comprehensive	≥ 12 elements identified by a · from 9 areas/systems	Perform all elements identified by a ·; document all elements in shaded boxes; document ≥ 1 element in unshaded boxes

Medical Decision Making (MDM) (Highest 2 out of 3)		Straightforward	Low Complexity	Moderate Complexity	High Complexity
A	Diagnoses/Management Options	Minimal (≤1)	Limited (2)	Multiple (3)	Extensive (≥4)
B	Amount/Complexity of Data	Min/Low (≤1)	Limited (2)	Moderate (3)	Extensive (≥4)
C	Highest Risk (highest from any category)	Minimal	Low	Moderate	High

Coordination of care or counseling a factor? _____ Time documented: _____ minutes of _____ minutes of total patient encounter

Selection of E/M Level based on above components

Established Patient (requires 2 of 3 elements)				
History	Exam	MDM	E/M—Office/OP Min	E/M—Office/OP Level
Min service, may not require MD			5	99211
PF	PF	SF	10	99212
EPF	EPF	Low	15	99213
Det	Det	Mod	25	99214
Comp	Comp	High	40	99215

New Patient or Consultation (requires 3 of 3 elements)						
History	Exam	MDM	E/M Office/OP Min	E/M Office/OP Level	E/M OP Consult Min	E/M OP Consult Level
PF	PF	SF	10	99201	15	99241
EPF	EPF	SF	20	99202	30	99242
Det	Det	Low	30	99203	40	99243
Comp	Comp	Mod	45	99204	60	99244
Comp	Comp	High	60	99205	80	99245

Selection of E/M Level based on above components

Initial Hospital Care (requires 3 of 3 elements)					A/D Same Date Level	Subsequent Hospital (requires 2 of 3 elements)				
History	Exam	MDM	Initial Inpatient Min	Initial Inpatient Level		History	Exam	MDM	Subsequent Inpatient Min	Subsequent Inpatient Level
D / C	D / C	SF/Low	30	99221	99234	PF	PF	SF/Low	15	99231
Comp	Comp	Mod	50	99222	99235	EPF	EPF	Mod	25	99232
Comp	Comp	High	70	99223	99236	Det	Det	High	35	99233

377

Steps in Performing an Internal Audit

Several steps are involved in conducting an internal audit. The steps are very similar, if not the same, when an external person or agency performs the audit.

Identifying the Need for an Audit

Many factors indicate that an audit is necessary, including the following:

- Rejected claims indicate a pattern of possible incorrect coding

- New code rules or regulations have been implemented

- Support staff reports a suspected issue

- Physician requests an audit

- There is significant turnover in staff

- New employee or physician orientation requires a follow-up

- Payer requests a focused review

- New services have been added

Medicare has identified its own hit list of factors that can trigger an audit, which includes the following:

- Excessive use of higher-level codes, such as billing all comprehensive (99215) visits

- Excessive use of lower-level codes, such as billing problem focused (99212) visits consistently

- Billing for consultations on established patients for minor diagnoses that do not support this level of service and for referrals from providers within the same specialty

- Billing for excessive repetition of laboratory tests when results are normal

- Upcoding and overutilization billing for office visits, particularly when services rendered were deemed not medically necessary

- Billing of "incident to" services and supplies

Preparing for the Audit

Many healthcare providers or organizations consider hiring outside legal counsel to oversee their coding audits performed by external consultants. The act of doing this is considered establishing attorney–client privilege, meaning that communications are protected between client and attorney. It could be very beneficial to have attorney–client privilege when the organization believes it may have a coding compliance problem. Many organizations complete all of their coding audit functions under attorney–client privilege.

Management must understand the implications involved when considering an attorney–client privilege relationship. Although the implications and decision to enter into an attorney–client privilege are outside the scope of this book, some basic steps that will help secure the privilege are (Russo and Russo 2000):

- Execute a formal retainer agreement between the parties.

- Clarify that legal advice is being sought from outside counsel.

- Identify all documentation being forwarded or received as attorney–client privilege protected.

Conducting the Audit

Many facilities conduct an audit periodically (at least annually) to assess how things are going and to identify any issues or problems before they become uncontrollable. When establishing a regular schedule of internal audits, the person(s) being audited may not be as apprehensive about the process and begin to see the benefit of regular feedback and process improvement.

For the sake of physician revenue, it is especially important that all charge tickets are reconciled and that all supplies, all ancillary services, and all out-of-office services are billed. If any of these are missed or billed inconsistently, significant revenue can be lost.

Steps in the Audit Process

There are 10 steps in the audit process. Following these steps will help ensure that the audit flows smoothly and all work is completed and presented properly (Bowman 2008).

1. Select the audit topic.

2. Select or create an audit tool to collect data for the review.

3. Identify the audit population from which the sample will be drawn.

4. Identify the sample cases, drawn randomly from the population (or other statistically sound methodology).

5. Accumulate the required documents for each case in the sample.

6. Collect the data from the accumulated documents.

7. Summarize collected data and formulation of recommendations.

8. Present the findings and recommendations to physicians and/or practice leaders.

9. Implement the recommendations and education.

10. Assign a follow-up audit date.

Regardless of the reason for the audit, the basic tools required to complete it remain the same:

- Patient record

- Document of what has been billed (copy of the charge ticket, printout from the computer, itemized statement, or completed CMS-1500 form)

- Auditing form (Refer to figures 12.3 and 12.4 for examples of auditing forms.)

- ICD-10-CM code book

- CPT code book

- HCPCS code book

- Medical reference books (anatomy book, medical dictionary, and coding reference book), especially if auditing a less-familiar specialty

- *Federal Register* or RVU file for the listing of global surgical days

The audit sample can be determined by one of the following:

- Random sample of records per physician or other healthcare provider(s)

- All services performed on a given day

- All services performed by a specific physician for a specific time period

- Random sample of rejected claims for the same issue

A simple random sample means that every member of the population (visits, patients, physicians, etc. that were selected as the unit of measure for the sample) has an equal chance of being selected for the sample. The sample can be chosen through a random drawing or by numbering the population and making choices through the use of a random number table or a random number generator (Kuehn 2009).

A stratified random sample organizes the population into similar groups (Dr. X's patients, Dr. Y's patients, and such) or stratifies the population by a set of criteria (Orthopedic consultations, Cardiology consultations, and such). From these groups, a simple random sample is selected (Kuehn 2009). This sampling method is used when the audit must include the same number of items from each group.

Systematic sampling can also be used. "Selecting a sample systematically requires the establishment of a pattern, such as every first patient, every 10th patient, or the last patient (or some similar selection) from a given population" (Kuehn 2009).

The Office of Inspector General (OIG) recommends "five or more medical records per Federal payer (that is, Medicare, Medicaid) or five to 10 medical records per physician" (OIG 2000, 4). Some may wonder whether a five- to 10-record sample is sufficient. Although a sample size of 25 medical records per physician could provide more thorough results, lack of time and funds usually prohibits this extensive review. A compromise of 10 to 15 records per physician may meet all of the goals of the review.

In addition, the sample size can be reduced on subsequent audits for physicians who demonstrate significant mastery in code selection. For these physicians, a sample size of five to seven medical records may be sufficient. For physicians still displaying compliance problems, targeted education should be provided and the sample size should be increased on subsequent reviews.

The length of time needed to complete an audit is determined by its size and complexity and the number and efficiency of the auditors (the number of records they can audit per hour or per day).

Audit Follow-up

The results of the audit should be documented. This may be done in a detailed report or a brief overview. The style of the report depends on the purpose of the audit and the recipient of the audit results. A statistical summary should be included, indicating the total number of records/ visits reviewed and the total number of changes/errors per provider. Again, the extent of detail covered in the statistical summary may vary depending on the purpose of the audit and who sees the report.

Education is an important follow-up to an audit. The findings and recommendations need to be communicated to the appropriate people. The purpose of the audit may determine who is present at an education session. At the conclusion of many audits, the auditor sits with the coding staff and physician(s) to discuss the findings and provide guidance on how to improve. This session may include information on the following:

- Documentation requirements

- Global-day services

- Capturing missed charges

- Different processes for obtaining charges

- Possible improvements in the efficiency and accuracy of the charge ticket

Often, when a coding audit is done, other information management issues that have an impact on coding are identified, such as record flow, backlogs of loose-paper filing, unavailable records, illegible documentation, and delays in diagnostic test results. The health information management professional or a quality improvement team should address these issues to help ensure that they do not continue to hamper coding and reimbursement.

Ongoing Monitoring for Improvement

The process of monitoring involves routine spot-checking to determine if new issues have developed, if past improvements have solved problems, if error rates are stable, or if common coding errors are happening in the practice.

The practice can use current tracking mechanisms as monitors, such as the Days in A/R statistic discussed in chapter 10 or develop new tracking mechanisms to monitor the coding function. Days in A/R monitors the average length of time that it takes for claims to be paid. Decreased coding accuracy can lengthen this turnaround time and is, therefore, a monitor of potential coding problems.

New monitors might measure the time it takes for charges to be coded and billed, the time between the visit and the completed physician documentation. Either of these measures would help monitor how fast the practice is sending bills for payment.

Practices may also implement monitoring about new codes or codes that have caused significant error rates in the past. Monitors may be a sampling of records or may be a 100 percent of records for a period of time after coding changes have been made in the CPT book.

Common CPT Coding Errors

Sometimes coding errors occur because the coder does not understand the medical and surgical reports. Understanding the definitions of medical terms and the intricacies of the coding system allows any procedure or service to be coded. If a procedure cannot be located readily in the CPT code book, the coder should not assume that a code for that procedure does not exist. Medical references should be used, as needed, and the physician consulted, when necessary, for an explanation to ensure accurate coding.

Audits performed within the integumentary system subsection of surgery, for example, reveal that coders commonly make the following errors when coding the removal of skin lesions:

- Often the wrong site code is selected.

- Malignant lesions are assigned codes for benign lesions, and vice versa.

- Several lesions are removed, but only one code is reported.

- Excision codes are assigned when destruction procedures were performed.

Continuing with the integumentary system, the following common error occurs in the coding of wound repairs:

- Wound repairs are improperly coded with regard to size and type (that is, simple, intermediate, or complex).

Within the musculoskeletal system subsection of surgery, errors often are found in the coding of foot surgery. These may include the following:

- Wrong site codes frequently are selected.

- Several codes are used to describe procedures such as bunion removal or hammertoe repair when a specific code or codes are available for these procedures.

- Code 20650, Insertion of wire or pin with application of skeletal traction, including removal, should not be assigned when a wire is inserted during a bunionectomy because it is considered part of the procedure.

- Code 28285, Correction, hammertoe, should be used when the record documents hammertoe and a repair of deformed toe is performed.

Continuing with the musculoskeletal system subsection, the following point should be noted:

- Code 25290 should not be used for tenotomy, open, flexor or extensor tendon, forearm and/or wrist, single, each tendon, when release of trigger is performed. Code 26055 is correct for tendon sheath, incision for trigger finger.

Common errors within the digestive system subsection of surgery, endoscopic procedures, include the following:

- The proper site(s) is not coded. For example, colonoscopy is coded when only the rectum, sigmoid colon, and a small portion of the descending colon were viewed. For a colonoscopy, the scope must pass beyond the splenic flexure.

- A biopsy is coded instead of polyp removal, or both are coded when surgery is performed only at one site. (When a biopsy is performed and the remaining portion of the polyp is excised, only the polypectomy should be coded. When the polyp is biopsied, but not excised, only the biopsy should be coded. When multiple biopsies are taken without withdrawing the scope, the biopsy should be coded only once.)

- Colonoscopies should be coded as to how far the scope was passed, not the level at which the polyp/lesion was removed.

Audits reveal that the following common error occurs within the urinary system subsection of surgery:

- Confusion commonly arises between the ureter and the urethra. The proper site is not being selected for some procedures, such as biopsies. There are three headings for transurethral surgery, each referring to a different site. The coder must be sure he or she is under the correct subheading.

Finally, within the eye and ocular adnexa subsection of surgery, audits reveal the following common errors in the coding of cataract extractions:

- Often codes for intra- and extracapsular procedures are interchanged.

- When a patient has a diagnosis of bilateral cataracts, procedure 66983 or 66984 is recorded twice when only one cataract was extracted. Documentation must support the code selection.

- The injection of Healon or other medications used in conjunction with cataract surgery should not be coded because it is considered a part of the procedure. Frequently, code 66030 for injection of medication into the anterior segment chamber is used inappropriately.

- Neither code 66983 nor 66984 (intra- or extracapsular cataract extraction) should be used for discission of a secondary membranous cataract (after cataract). Code 66820 or 66821 should be reported, depending on the technique.

Compliance Regulations

Compliance is defined as completing or performing what is necessary to fulfill an official requirement or rule. In today's healthcare world, hardly a day goes by without hearing or seeing some reference to the term *compliance*. There are many components to compliance. Regardless of the size of the practice, coders must be in compliance with the regulations set forth by the Health Insurance Portability and Accountability Act and the Office of the Inspector General.

Health Insurance Portability and Accountability Act

In 1996, President Clinton signed into law the Health Insurance Portability and Accountability Act (HIPAA), also known as Public Law 104-191 and the Kassebaum–Kennedy law. This law contains provisions for the following (Frawley and Asmonga 1996):

- Group insurance portability, allowing individuals to take insurance from job to job

- A pilot program for medical savings accounts capped at 750,000 participants

- Prohibition on refusing or renewing coverage because of an employee's health status (preexisting conditions)

- Prohibition on using genetic information to deny insurance coverage

- An increase in the tax deductibility of health insurance for the self-employed from 30 percent to 80 percent

- Tax incentives for the purchase of long-term care insurance and other provisions relating to availability of coverage

From the viewpoint of many healthcare organizations, one of HIPAA's most significant provisions is the language pertaining to healthcare fraud and abuse, privacy, and administrative simplification. The law created the Health Care Fraud and Abuse Control Program. The intent of this program is to combat fraud and abuse in the Medicare and Medicaid programs and in the private healthcare industry.

In 1998, rules were proposed to implement several of HIPAA's provisions. Among these proposed rules were standards for electronic claims and related transactions requiring payers, providers, employers, and others to use standard formats when transmitting or accepting claims and other transactions electronically. In 2000, the final rule on administrative simplification for transactions and code sets (TCS) was issued (discussed in chapter 8). Another rule established a program for payment to individuals who provide information on Medicare fraud and abuse or other sanctionable activities.

The HIPAA privacy regulations became effective in April 2003. Protecting a patient's right to privacy of his or her health information is key to being in compliance with these regulations. Patients are allowed to exercise their rights in having access to their health information, requesting amendments to their health information, and requesting restrictions to uses and disclosures of their health information, to name only a few of their rights. The minimum necessary aspect of the regulations may affect what access a coder has to health information. Many practices and organizations are determining what access to information is allowed by job title.

Fraud and Abuse Provisions of HIPAA

The fraud and abuse provisions of HIPAA seek to toughen existing laws, stiffen penalties, and create new laws to combat fraud, particularly within the Medicare and Medicaid programs. The Medicare Integrity Program was established to conduct extensive fraud and abuse investigations. Many other private healthcare payers are beginning to look at fraud and abuse provisions more closely, as well. (See figure 12.5 for a glossary of fraud and abuse terminology.)

Fraud and abuse continues to be a high priority for the attorney general. Many organizations have been under investigation for committing fraud and have paid fines in the millions of dollars. The size of the practice neither eliminates it from scrutiny nor automatically makes it a target for a potential audit.

Investigations have uncovered a number of illegal practices, including:

- Unbundling charges to obtain higher payment than deserved

- Billing for services not rendered

- Falsifying diagnoses (billing for nonexistent covered expenses rather than the actual uncovered expense)

- Falsifying medical records to support codes, which results in increased payment

Figure 12.5. Fraud and abuse terminology

Balanced Budget Act (BBA) of 1997: A bipartisan budget deal signed on August 5, 1997, that added new penalties to the government's arsenal when fighting against fraud. These new provisions include such things as a permanent exclusion for those convicted of three healthcare-related crimes on or after the date of enactment.

Corporate integrity agreement: A mandatory agreement between the government and a healthcare provider who has entered into a settlement agreement with the government because of a fraud and abuse investigation. A corporate integrity agreement is a governmentally mandated compliance program.

Department of Health and Human Services (HHS): The Medicare program is administered by the Centers for Medicare and Medicaid Services (CMS) of the Department of Health and Human Services (HHS).

Federal False Claims Act (FCA): The FCA prohibits anyone from "knowingly" presenting a false/fraudulent claim for payment from the government, presenting a false record or statement to get a false or fraudulent claim paid by the government, conspiring to defraud the government, or using a false record or statement to conceal, avoid, or decrease an obligation to pay money or property to the government. Further, the act defines "knowingly" as either having actual knowledge of the false information, acting in deliberate ignorance of the truth or falsity of information, or acting in reckless disregard of the truth or falsity of information.

Healthcare compliance: Ensuring that a facility is providing and billing for services according to the "laws, regulations, and guidelines" that govern it.

Health Insurance Portability and Accountability Act (HIPAA): This legislation strengthens law enforcement's ability to fight healthcare fraud by broadly expanding the jurisdiction of DHHS-OIG and substantially increasing the investigative resources available to the OIG and the FBI for healthcare enforcement. Additionally, the law creates new healthcare fraud and abuse offenses and dramatically increases criminal and administrative penalties.

Office of the Inspector General (OIG): A suboffice of the HHS that is responsible for enforcing the Medicare fraud and abuse proscriptions.

Operation Restore Trust (ORT): A federal pilot program designed to combat fraud, waste, and abuse in the Medicare and Medicaid programs. ORT targets home health agencies, nursing homes, and durable medical equipment suppliers. It initially targeted the five largest Medicare states but has since been expanded to cover 12 others.

Qui tam action: A legal suit usually brought by employees naming specific activities of their employer that they believe to be fraudulent and/or abusive. These individuals are known as "relators" or "whistleblowers."

- Billing for services performed by less-qualified individuals and/or inflating the number of visits

- Inflating medical billings

Office of the Inspector General

The OIG conducts nationwide audits, investigations, and inspections. Under the False Claims Act, criminal penalties are imposed on healthcare professionals who "knowingly or willfully" attempt to execute a scheme to defraud any healthcare benefit program or to obtain, by means of false or fraudulent pretense, money or property owned by, or under the custody of, a healthcare benefit program. Criminal penalties of up to 10 years' imprisonment may be imposed. The civil monetary penalty for healthcare fraud has been increased to $10,000 for each item or service for which fraudulent payment has been received (Bowman 2008). With repayment of double or triple damages, mandatory fines are now set at $5,500 to $11,000 per incident, or per false claim filed (US Department of Justice 2009).

Coding fraud may include the following:

- Submitting services that are not medically necessary

- Unbundling services

- Assigning a code for a higher-level service than the one actually performed

- Assigning a code for a covered service when the service provided is noncovered

- Assigning codes for diagnoses that were not present

- Billing for services that were not performed

There are many prevention strategies:

- Properly trained coding staff with ongoing education

- Comprehensive, up-to-date, internal policies and procedures for coding and billing

- Internally completed coding audits to assess quality

- Evaluation of internal coding practices to ensure their consistency with coding rules and guidelines

- Education of physicians on improving documentation when documentation deficiencies are identified

Not only are physician services, hospitals, home care, and other healthcare providers being monitored for fraud and abuse, but health plans (insurance companies) also are being monitored. Health plans may be issued criminal penalties if it is found that they are not adhering to the guidelines set forth by HIPAA and CMS.

Many of the claims brought forward in relation to fraud and abuse have been initiated by means of qui tam, or whistleblower, actions. Many times, the whistleblower is an employee who knows (or thinks) that some unlawful billing practice is taking place. The person initiating the lawsuit can receive up to 25 percent of the civil penalty.

National Correct Coding Initiative

The National Correct Coding Initiative (NCCI) is Medicare's national correct coding policy. Code edits have been computerized and installed in the part B claims-processing systems of Medicare contractors. The purpose of the NCCI is to detect incorrect or inappropriate reporting of combinations of CPT codes and to promote uniformity. The edits are updated on a quarterly basis. CMS now posts the NCCI edits on their website on the National Correct Coding Initiatives Edits page (CMS 2015h). Chapter 23 of the Medicare Claims Processing Manual also discusses the concept included in the NCCI edits (CMS 2015k).

When NCCI rules are violated, the explanation of Medicare benefits shows that one or more codes are included in another service, indicating that unbundled codes were submitted. Additional information on NCCI edits appears in chapter 10.

Compliance Programs and the OIG

Compliance programs are a strategy to ensure that the physician practice obeys the law. If the practice is part of a larger organization, it may be following the corporate compliance plan.

Again, size of the practice does not matter. Regardless of the size of the practice, it is important to have a compliance program. The program can be very simple or very complex. An effective compliance program will lower a healthcare provider's risk of a lawsuit and thus the organization's financial risk.

The OIG has developed compliance program guidance documents for both individual and small group physician practices and third-party payer medical billing agencies. These program guidance documents can be downloaded from the OIG website on the Fraud Prevention and Detection page (OIG 2009).

A hotline number should be set up to allow individuals to disclose (anonymously, if preferred) procedures that may put the company at risk of being out of compliance. All hotline calls need to be followed up in a confidential manner. It is much better to handle an issue internally than to have the OIG become involved in investigating a tip. A compliance officer usually monitors the hotline.

Compliance programs should include, when applicable, the following seven elements:

- Policies and procedures

- Education and training of all employees on compliance

- Follow-up on all potential risk factors that may lead to an investigation

- Assurance that proper procedures and regulations are being followed in relation to submission of charges to health plans

- Principles of conduct

- Designation of a compliance officer or contact

- Internal monitoring and auditing

Physician offices need to look at their high-risk areas such as coding, billing, documentation, and processes (work flow). Baseline audits should be performed to begin the process of identifying problem areas. It is important to review the OIG's work plan for each year to see what areas will be the focus of the OIG. The work plan is available on the OIG website under Publications.

Exercise 12.1. Evaluation of Coding Quality

Match the type to the coding quality tool:

a. Collecting   b. Correcting   c. Analyzing

1. _____ Communication tool

2. _____ Audit form

3. _____ Charge ticket

4. After reviewing these three charge summaries, what finding might the auditor have?

Case #	CPT Code	Description	Diagnosis	Description	POS
1	15220	Full thickness graft, arm	S61.409A	Wound, hand	11
2	96374	Injection, IM	B35.3	Tinea, foot	11
3	11600	Excision, malignant lesion	D23.70	Benign lesion, lower limb	11

a. Diagnostic statements should provide the medical necessity for the procedure.
b. Some procedures may require performance in an ambulatory surgery center.
c. Additional CPT/HCPCS codes should be reported with these cases.
d. Multiple problems are present in the coding of these cases.

5. Which of the following is *not* a reason to complete a compliance audit?

a. Support staff reports a suspected issue.
b. New coding rules have been implemented.
c. There is a significant turnover in staff.
d. Revenue is less than the same month last year.

6. How is a stratified random sample selected?

a. Selecting the cases based on a pattern
b. Selecting an equal random sample from multiple groups
c. Selecting a random sample from a group of cases selected by the physician
d. Selecting the sample based on the OIG work plan recommendations

Indicate whether each statement is true or false.

7. True or false? Auditing all services performed on a given day is a valid size for an audit. _____

8. True or false? The Transaction and Code Set provisions of HIPAA have no effect on reimbursement _____

9. True or false? The OIG recommends a review of five medical records per physician, at a minimum. _____

10. True or false? Audit findings should be reported to the provider who was audited. _____

Chapter 12 Test

Choose the best answer for each of the following questions.

1. The following visit is coded as 99213–25, 26735, 73140–TC. When comparing the coding to this patient's progress note, what findings would the auditor have?

   S: A 15-year-old boy injured the left third finger in gym class five days ago. Patient states the ball jammed his finger. It has been swollen and red but is getting progressively better. Patient rested the hand last week and had the finger placed in a splint worn during a previous injury.

   O: The left third digit is positive for edema, resolving ecchymosis, and pain over the proximal phalangeal joint upon palpation. Decreased flexion with lateral deviation and decreased strength due to pain. X-ray done in the office today revealed a chip fracture over the proximal phalangeal joint.

   A: Chip fracture of the left third digit, proximal phalangeal joint.

   P: Continue with splint from home, refrain from any basketball. Use OTC drugs to decrease inflammation. Repeat visit in two weeks for follow-up.

   a. A local anesthetic should have been coded.
   b. A higher level of office visit should have been coded.
   c. The documentation does not support the codes assigned.
   d. A HCPCS Level II supply code should have been coded.

2. Where would a coder find the government's audit plan?
   a. Documentation Guidelines for E/M Services
   b. CMS website
   c. Medicare Carriers Manual
   d. OIG website

3. The patient is taken to the day surgery unit where a bronchoscopy is performed. A biopsy is taken, the trachea is dilated, and a tracheal stent is placed. If this is coded as 31631 and 31625–51, what vital piece of information would an auditor find missing?
   a. What type of stent was placed during the procedure
   b. Whether the biopsy is of bronchial tissue or from some other location
   c. Whether fluoroscopic guidance was used to perform the procedure
   d. Whether multiple biopsies were taken during the procedure

4. What finding might an auditor have if this visit was coded as 99212–25, 20611, and J1020? (Use the audit tool in figure 12.3 as a reference, if necessary).

   CC: Shoulder pain

   S: Patient is here for shoulder pain. She states that the right shoulder has been very tender and painful over the past year or so and it has gotten worse just recently. It severely limits her ability to move around and she cannot dry or curl her hair. OTC medications help only somewhat.

   O: Patient is in no acute distress. She has tenderness on palpation over the right shoulder and can abduct it only about 50 degrees. She has some restriction on external rotation as well.

   I discussed treatment options with the patient and she opts for the joint injection today. The shoulder is prepared in sterile fashion and the joint is injected with 0.5 cc of 1% lidocaine, followed by 10 mg of Depo-Medrol.

   A: Bursitis

   P: Patient is to start ibuprofen 600 mg, three times a day, being careful to watch for signs of acute stomach distress.

(Continued on next page)

Chapter 12 Test (Continued)

    a.   The E/M code is not supported by documentation.

    b.   The injection documentation does not support the use of ultrasound guidance for the procedure.

    c.   The injection code describes the incorrect joint.

    d.   The coding for the visit is fully supported by documentation.

5.   An established patient presents to the office for a follow-up on stable osteoarthritis and no other chronic problems. The physician documents a detailed interval history and a comprehensive examination. The medical decision making is calculated as Low Complexity medical decision making. The physician submitted a 99214 code for this service. What should the auditor do?

    a.   Identify an audit finding stating that medical necessity must be considered when assigning E/M codes.

    b.   Nothing. 99214 is the correct code.

    c.   Change the code to a 99212 and re-submit the claim.

    d.   Change the code to a 99213 and re-submit the claim.

6.   Which of the following is *not* an appropriate way to determine a sample size for a coding audit?

    a.   Audit those chosen by the nurse or physician

    b.   Audit all claims rejected for a particular reason

    c.   Choose a random sample of charts for a given physician

    d.   Choose all charts for a particular day of service

7.   Using the audit tool in figure 12.3 as a reference, what category and level of E/M service is substantiated here?

HPI: This patient was sent by her family physician, Dr. S. She is a 49-year-old woman who has a history of irregular bleeding. She was seen one year ago. At that time, we performed endometrial biopsy and this demonstrated a benign endometrium. Apparently, though, the patient developed bleeding on a monthly basis. I do not have a recent FSH level on the chart that would suggest her menopausal state, clinically. She was not seen by me in the interim. She did describe this as monthly cyclic bleeding, lasting three days, each month. She has been on Premarin and Provera throughout this time. She has had no other period-like symptoms. If this was truly the case, she should not have had bleeding and this would suggest a pathologic cause. She did stop bleeding between April and September, however. She recently had a normal ultrasound, showing a 6.9-mm endometrial thickness and her Pap smear in June was negative. She has had no weight fluctuation during this time. Dr. S has again sent her to have this evaluated.

EXAM: She is alert and in no acute distress. Weight is 139 lb. Blood pressure is 138/82. Abdomen: Soft and nontender. Uterus is anteverted, normal in size and nontender with no adnexal masses or tenderness.

After informed consent, an endometrial biopsy was performed. The uterus was sounded to 6 cm with minimal tissue. This will be sent for histological evaluation.

ASSESSMENT: Postmenopausal bleeding.

PLAN: I changed the patient's medication to Premarin only 0.625 mg po daily for the next three months. At that time, she'll add Prometrium 100 mg po daily. If the patient does continue with persistent bleeding problems, she will need an office hysteroscopy as the next step in her management. A copy of this note will be sent to Dr. S. FSH level ordered to be run at the hospital.

    a.   Office and Other Outpatient, New Patient, Level 2

    b.   Office and Other Outpatient, Established Patient, Level 3

    c.   Office and Other Outpatient Consultations, Level 2

    d.   Preventive Medicine Services, Established Patient, 40 to 64 years of age

Chapter 12 Test (Continued)

8. The physician submits code 99202 for the following progress note. What documentation is insufficient to support the code submitted?

New Patient Office Visit Note:

CC: Finger pain

S: Patient has suffered a contusion to his left middle finger today while playing outside.

O: The finger is tender to the touch, without paresthesias or open skin.

Follow up in four weeks for a recheck.

   a. History documentation
   b. Examination documentation
   c. Medical decision making detail
   d. Coordination of care documentation

9. A 25-year-old patient with an acute exacerbation of asthma was seen by the physician and has a detailed history taken, an expanded problem-focused examination done, and low-level medical decision making used. The patient expresses a desire to quit smoking and also receives 30 minutes of initial treatment in a smoking cessation program and a one-week supply of nicotine gum. If this visit is coded as 99214–25, G0437 and S4995, what problem would an auditor find?

   a. G0437 is always included in the E/M service.
   b. S codes are not valid for Medicare patients.
   c. The –25 modifier is not needed for this case.
   d. The E/M code is not substantiated by documentation.

10. After reviewing these three charge summaries, what recommendation might the auditor have for the physician?

Case #	CPT Code	Description	Diagnosis	Description	POS
1	95117	Allergy injections	Z23	Unspecified vaccination	11
2	12013	Laceration repair, face	S70.10xA	Contusion, thigh	11
3	20610	Aspiration, major joint	M79.673	Pain, toe	11

   a. Diagnostic statements should provide the medical necessity for the procedure.
   b. Some procedures may require performance in an ambulatory surgery center.
   c. Additional CPT codes should be reported with these cases.
   d. The use of modifiers can help ensure proper payment.

Appendix A

References and Bibliography

Accreditation Association for Ambulatory Health Care. 2015. *2015 Accreditation Handbook for Ambulatory Health Care*. Skokie, IL: Accreditation Association for Ambulatory Health Care.

Amatayakul, Margret, Teri Jorwic, and Rita Scichilone. 2003. HIPAA on the job: Ready for the transactions rule? Get started with code sets. *Journal of AHIMA* 74(7):16A–16D.

American Academy of Pediatrics. 2009. Developmental Screening/Testing Coding Fact Sheet for Primary Care Pediatricians. *Pediatric Coding Companion* 3:3–5, 7.

American Dental Association (ADA). 2016. *CDT 2016 Current Dental Terminology*. Chicago. ADA.

AHIMA Coding Products and Services Team. 2003. AHIMA Practice Brief: Managing and Improving Data Quality. *Journal of AHIMA* 74:7: 64A–C.

AHIMA House of Delegates. 2011 (October 2). AHIMA Code of Ethics. http://library.ahima.org /xpedio/groups/public/documents/ahima/bok1_024277.hcsp?dDocName=bok1_024277.

AHIMA ICD-10 webpage. 2015. http://www.ahima.org/icd10/default.aspx. Chicago: AHIMA.

American Hospital Association. 1985–2013. *Coding Clinic for ICD-9-CM*. Chicago: AHA. http://www.ahacentraloffice.org/.

American Hospital Association. 2012-2015. *Coding Clinic for ICD-10-CM/PCS*. Chicago: AHA. http://www.ahacentraloffice.org/.

American Medical Association. 2015. *CPT 2016*. Chicago: AMA.

American Medical Association. 2015a. *HCPCS 2015*. Chicago: AMA.

American Medical Association, 2015b. *CPT Assistant* Newsletter. https://catalog.ama-assn.org /Catalog/product/product_detail.jsp?productId=prod170136. Chicago: AMA.

American Medical Association. 2015c. CPT Errata. http://www.ama-assn.org/ama/pub/physician -resources/solutions-managing-your-practice/coding-billing-insurance/cpt/about-cpt/errata.page

American Medical Association. 2014. *CPT 2015*. Chicago: AMA.

American Medical Association. 2013. *CPT 2014*. Chicago: AMA.

American Medical Association. 2012. *CPT 2013*. Chicago: AMA.

American Medical Association. 2011. *CPT 2012*. Chicago: AMA.

American Medical Association. 2011. *CPT Changes 2012: An Insider's View*. Chicago: AMA.

American Medical Association. 2008. Medicare RBRVS: The Physicians' Guide. Chicago: AMA.

American Medical Association. 2005. *CPT Changes 2005: An Insider's View*. Chicago: AMA.

American Medical Association. 2001. *CPT Changes 2001: An Insider's View*. Chicago: AMA.

American Medical Association. 1992–2013. *CPT Assistant*. Chicago: AMA.

Bowman, Sue. 2008. *Health Information Management Compliance: Guidelines for Preventing Fraud and Abuse*. Chicago: AHIMA.

Burris, David, Sharon Houser, and Gary Montilla. 2000 (Sept. 23–28). Where is the government going? Proceedings of the 72nd National Convention of the AHIMA, Chicago: AHIMA.

Calzavara-Pinton, P., C. Longo, M. Venturini, R. Sala, and G. Pellacani. 2008. Reflectance Confocal Microscopy for *In Vivo* Skin Imaging. *Photochemistry and Photobiology.* 84(6): 1421–1430.

Carter, Darren. 2002. *Medicare Medical Necessity: A Guide to Accurate Reimbursement and Full Compliance.* Marblehead, MA: Opus Communications.

Centers for Disease Control. *International Classification of Diseases, Tenth Revision, Clinical Modification.* 2015. http://www.cdc.gov/nchs/icd/icd10cm.htm#10update.

Centers for Medicare and Medicaid Services. 2015. Tests Granted Waived Status Under CLIA. http://www.cms.gov/CLIA/downloads/waivetbl.pdf.

Centers for Medicare and Medicaid Services. 2015a. 2015 Alpha-Numeric HCPCS File. http://www.cms.gov/HCPCSReleaseCodeSets/ANHCPCS/list.asp#TopOfPage.

Centers for Medicare and Medicaid Services. 2015b. Physician Fee Schedule. http://www.cms.gov/PhysicianFeeSched/PFSRVF/list.asp#TopOfPage.

Centers for Medicare and Medicaid Services. 2015c. Durable Medical Equipment Supplier Application form. https://www.cms.gov/Medicare/CMS-Forms/CMS-Forms/downloads/cms855s.pdf.

Centers for Medicare and Medicaid Services. 2015d. *Medicare Claims Processing Manual,* Chapter 12: Physicians/Nonphysician Practitioners. https://www.cms.gov/Regulations-and-Guidance/Guidance/Manuals/downloads/clm104c12.pdf.

Centers for Medicare and Medicaid Services. 2015e. Medicare Learning Network. http://www.cms.gov/Outreach-and-Education/Medicare-Learning-Network-MLN/MLNProducts/index.html.

Centers for Medicare and Medicaid Services. 2015f. Beneficiary Notices Initiative. https://www.cms.gov/Medicare/Medicare-General-information/Bni/index.html.

Centers for Medicare and Medicaid Services. 2015g. National Correct Coding Initiative Edits. https://www.cms.gov/Medicare/Coding/NationalCorrectCodInitEd/index.html?redirect=/nationalcorrectcodinited/.

Centers for Medicare and Medicaid Services. 2015h. Medically Unlikely Edits. https://www.cms.gov/Medicare/Coding/NationalCorrectCodInitEd/MUE.html.

Centers for Medicare and Medicaid Services. 2015i. National Provider Identifier Standard. https://www.cms.gov/Regulations-and-Guidance/HIPAA-Administrative-Simplification/NationalProvIdentStand/index.html?redirect=/nationalprovidentstand/.

Centers for Medicare and Medicaid Services. 2015j. Transactions and Code Sets Standards. https://www.cms.gov/Regulations-and-Guidance/HIPAA-Administrative-Simplification/TransactionCodeSetsStands/index.html?redirect=/transactioncodesetsstands/02_transactionsandcodesetsregulations.asp

Centers for Medicare and Medicaid Services. 2015k. *Medicare Claims Processing Manual,* Chapter 23: Fee Schedule Administration and Coding Requirements. https://www.cms.gov/Regulations-and-Guidance/Guidance/Manuals/downloads/clm104c23.pdf.

Centers for Medicare and Medicaid Services. 2014. Quick Reference Information: Preventive Services. https://www.cms.gov/Medicare/Prevention/PrevntionGenInfo/Downloads/MPS_QuickReferenceChart_1.pdf.

Centers for Medicare and Medicaid Services. 1997 Documentation Guidelines for Evaluation and Management Services: http://www.cms.gov/Outreach-and-Education/Medicare-Learning-Network-MLN/MLNEdWebGuide/Downloads/97Docguidelines.pdf.

Centers for Medicare and Medicaid Services. 1995 Documentation Guidelines for Evaluation & Management Services: http://www.cms.gov/Outreach-and-Education/Medicare-Learning-Network-MLN/MLNEdWebGuide/Downloads/95Docguidelines.pdf.

Crow, John P. 2002 (Nov. 14). *Pediatric and Neonatal Coding 2003 at the AMA's CPT Symposium in Chicago.* Chicago: AMA.

Didier, Donna M. 2000. *Intermediate CPT/HCPCS for Physician Office Coding.* Chicago: AHIMA.

Frawley, Kathleen, and Donald Asmonga. 1996. President signs bipartisan health reform bill. *Journal of AHIMA* 67:14.

Grider, Deborah. 2004. *Coding with Modifiers: A Guide to Correct CPT and HCPCS Level II Modifier Usage.* Chicago: AMA.

Ingenix. 2008. *Coder's Desk Reference for Procedures 2009.* Salt Lake City, Utah: Ingenix.

Joint Commission. 2014. *2015 Comprehensive Accreditation Manual for Ambulatory Care (CAMAC)*. Oakbrook Terrace, IL. Joint Commission.

Jorwic, Therese M. 2000. *CPT/HCPCS for Physician Office Coding*. Chicago: AHIMA.

Joseph, Eric, Jeanne Tucker, and Leslie Fox. 1986. *Documenting Ambulatory Care*. Chicago: Care Communications.

Kuehn, Lynn. 2009. *A Practical Approach to Analyzing Healthcare Data*. Chicago: AHIMA.

Kuehn, Lynn. 2009a. Lessons 1 and 2 of "Accurate Reporting of Hospital Outpatient Laboratory and Pathology Services" Distance Education Course written for the American Health Information Management Association Distance Education Campus. Chicago: AHIMA.

Kuehn, Lynn. 2001 (Oct. 13–18). Unlock the information secrets of your billing database. Proceedings of the 73rd National Convention of the AHIMA, Miami, FL. Chicago: AHIMA.

Larimore, Walter, and Elizabeth Jordan. 1995. SOAP to SNOCAMP: improving the medical record format. *Journal of Family Practice* 41:393–98.

LaTour, Kathleen M., Shirley Eichenwald Maki, and Pamela K. Oachs, eds. 2013. *Health Information Management: Concepts, Principles, and Practice,* 4th ed. Chicago: AHIMA.

Mallett, Sherri A., and Gail I. Smith. 2000. *Basic CPT/HCPCS Coding*. Chicago: AHIMA.

New York University Lagone Medical Center General Surgery (NYU). 2013. http://surgery.med.nyu.edu/general/patient-care/hernias/overview-hernias.

Nordian Administrative Services. 2009. Proper Use of GY, GA and GZ Modifiers. https://www.noridianmedicare.com/dme/news/docs/2007/06_jun/ga_gy_gz.html.

North American Spine Society. 2007. http://www.spine.org.

Office of the Inspector General (OIG). 2009. Fraud Prevention and Detection. http://www.oig.hhs.gov/fraud.asp.

Office of the Inspector General. 2000 (Oct. 5). OIG Compliance Program for Individual and Small Group Practices. *Federal Register* 65(194).

Practice Management Information Corporation. 2001. *Reimbursement Manual for the Medical Office,* 4th ed. Los Angeles: Practice Management Information Corp.

Rogers, V.L. 1998. *Applying Inpatient Coding Skills under Prospective Payment*. Chicago: AHIMA.

Russo, Ruthann, and Joseph Russo. 2000. *Coding Compliance: A Practical Guide to the Audit Process*. Marblehead, MA: Opus Communications.

Sayles, Nanette, ed. 2014. *Health Information Management Technology: An Applied Approach,* 4th ed. Chicago: AHIMA.

Schraffenberger, Lou Ann and Lynn Kuehn. 2011. *Effective Management of Coding Services, 4th ed.* Chicago: AHIMA.

Seare, Jerry 1996. *Medical Documentation*. Salt Lake City: Medicode.

Smith, Gail. 2000. *CPT: Beyond the Basics*. Chicago: AHIMA.

Society for Clinical Coding. 2010 (March). *CodeWrite Newsletter*. Chicago: AHIMA.

Society for Clinical Coding. 2003a (June). *CodeWrite Newsletter*. Chicago: AHIMA.

Society for Clinical Coding. 2003b (August). *CodeWrite Newsletter*. Chicago: AHIMA.

Society of Interventional Radiology (SIR), the American College of Radiology. 2009. *Interventional Radiology Coding Users' Guide,* 15th ed. Reston, VA: Society of Interventional Radiology, the American College of Radiology.

The Merck Manual of Diagnosis and Therapy, 19th ed. 2011. Whitehouse Station, NJ: Merck Research Laboratories.

Turgeon, M.L. 2007. Linne and Ringsrud's Clinical Laboratory Science, 5th ed. St Louis, MO: Mosby Elsevier.

US Department of Justice, US Attorney's Office. 2009. False Claims Act Cases: Government Intervention in Qui Tam (Whistleblower) Suits, Title 31 US Code, Chapter 37, Section 3729: http://www.justice.gov/usao/pae/Documents/fcaprocess2.pdf.

Washington Publishing Company. 2009. HIPAA Products and Services: http://www.wpc-edi.com/content/view/661/393.

ZHealth Online Newsletter. 2005 (June 14). Coronary angiography without a left heart catheterization. Nashville, TN: ZHealth Publishing.

Appendix B

Review Exercises

The answer key to appendix B is available in the instructor materials located at www.ahimapress.org. Visit http://www.ahima.org/education /press for further instruction for accessing the materials. **Note:** The answer key is *not* available to anyone who is not a verified instructor.

Multiple Choice

Choose the best answer for each question.

1. The physician injects polymethylmethacrylate into the vertebrae, under fluoroscopic guidance provided by the radiologist, to help maintain the height of the vertebral bodies at L2 and L3. How are these injections coded?

   a. 22511, 22511
   b. 22511, 22512
   c. 22514, 22514
   d. 22514, 22515

2. A triangle symbol before a code number indicates that:

   a. Terminology has been changed since the last edition of CPT.
   b. This is a new code for this edition of CPT.
   c. The code has been deleted in this edition of CPT.
   d. See the beginning of the section for coding instructions.

3. A neurology patient covered by commercial insurance has been recommended for surgery. Before proceeding, his insurance company requires a second opinion. The primary care physician initiates a referral to a second physician, who performs a comprehensive history and physical examination, reviews an extensive amount of data, and considers an extensive number of treatment options. He concurs with the other physician, forwards a report to both and the surgery is scheduled. How is the second physician's encounter coded?

   a. 99215   Office E/M with comprehensive history, comprehensive examination, and high medical decision making
   b. 99245–32   Consultation E/M with comprehensive history, comprehensive examination, and high medical decision making
   c. 99254–32   Consultation E/M with comprehensive history, comprehensive examination, and moderate medical decision making
   d. 99255–32   Consultation E/M with comprehensive history, comprehensive examination, and high medical decision making

4. The patient suffered a fracture of the skull with depression of the occipital bone measuring 4.1 cm in diameter following an accidental blow to the head from a golf club of a fellow golfer. CT showed a depression of the skull fragment with two lacerations of the dura mater. The neurosurgeon repaired the defect and the lacerations. What is the proper code assignment for the surgeon's services?

   a. 62000   Elevation of depressed skull fracture; simple, extradural
   b. 62005   compound or comminuted, extradural
   c. 62010   with repair of dura and/or debridement of brain
   d. 62140   Cranioplasty for skull defect; up to 5 cm diameter

5. A two-view annual mammogram with no confirmed diagnoses or documented symptoms and no risk factors is coded as:

   a. 77053   Mammary ductogram or galactogram, single duct, radiological supervision and interpretation.
   b. 77055–50   Mammography; unilateral
   c. 77056   bilateral.
   d. 77057   Screening mammography, bilateral (2-view film study of each breast).

6. Which CPT code(s) should be reported for a fine needle aspiration of the prostate performed by a urologist?

   a. 10021
   b. 55700
   c. 55705
   d. 55700, 10021

7. A physician who is a member of a cardiology group practice treats a patient for atrial fibrillation. Two years later, a different cardiologist from the same group practice sees the same patient for new chest pain symptoms. According to CPT definitions, this patient would be considered:

   a. An established patient
   b. An observation patient
   c. A new patient
   d. An emergency department patient

8. Preoperative Diagnosis: Acute Stanford Type A Aortic Dissection

   Postoperative Diagnosis: Acute Stanford Type A Aortic Dissection

   Operations:

   1. Ascending aortic replacement with Hemashield graft

   2. Aortic arch replacement with Hemashield graft

   Indication for Surgery: Acute Stanford Type A Aortic Dissection

   Operative Procedure and Findings: The patient was taken to the operating room emergently with a diagnosis of an acute Stanford type A aortic dissection that was made after she presented here with chest pain. After informed consent was obtained from the patient, she was taken to the operating room as quickly as possible after the open heart team was assembled.

   She was induced under general endotracheal anesthesia with full hemodynamic monitoring, and a trans-esophageal echocardiogram was performed. This was reviewed and confirmed the acute type A dissection that was clearly seen in the arch, proximal descending, and distal ascending aorta. The patient was prepared and draped in the usual sterile manner after being positively identified by all team members. The right sub-clavian artery was accessed through an incision below the right clavicle. Heparin was administered. A 7 mm Hemashield graft was sutured to an arteriotomy in the right subclavian artery, and was used for inflow from the cardiopulmonary bypass unit. A sternotomy was then performed. The venous drainage was afforded with a 2-stage venous catheter placed through the right atrium. A retrograde coronary sinus cardioplegia catheter was positioned. Bypass was instituted, and the patient cooled systemically to 25 degree Centigrade. The aorta was cross clamped. There was considerable staining and hematoma throughout all the aortic tissues in the ascending arch. When we opened the aorta, there was an acute dissection with multiple tears evident. This portion of the aorta was resected. We then placed the patient in deep Trendelenburg position, and tem-porarily discontinued the heart lung machine flow while the cross clamp was released. We then repositioned this cross clamp on the proximal innominate artery so that the patient could be perfused with selective cerebral perfusion through the right subclavian artery retrograde into the right carotid and right vertebral artery. She was monitored and remained stable. Flows were adjusted by the perfusionist to assure satisfac-tory cerebral perfusion. We looked at the arch. It appeared as though the dissection started in the arch and progressed retrograde into the ascending aorta down to a level just above the coronary arteries. There was a very complex series of tears in the arch itself. The innominate artery was circumferentially dissected from the rest of the aorta. The innominate artery was separated from the rest of the arch.

   We proceeded to replace the arch with a 28-mm Hemashield woven double velour graft. A running 3-0 Prolene suture was used, reinforced with a running 4-0 Prolene suture on the inside and buttressed with felt. We then created an opening in the graft to anastomose separately the innominate artery again with a running 3-0 Prolene and with a running 4-0 Prolene suture on the inside. The flows were then temporarily diminished to allow replacement of the cross clamp from the proximal innominate artery back onto the graft proximal to the arch vessels. Warming began at this time with full flows. The ascending aorta was then replaced by placing the proximal aortic anastomosis just above the coronary arterial connection. This was conducted in a similar manner to the other suture lines with a running 3-0 Prolene suture, buttressing this with felt and using a running 4-0 Prolene suture on the inside of this. The cross clamp was released. Warming was taken to full physiologic temperatures. A needle vent site was placed in the ascending aorta with release of the cross clamp to remove any residual air from the left-sided chambers. She was defibrillated into a normal sinus rhythm. When all residual left-sided air had been evacuated and contractility was satisfactory, the patient was weaned rather easily from cardiopulmonary bypass, and the contents of the pump oxygenator were returned to her. She was decannulated in the usual manner. Protamine was used to reverse the effects of heparin. There was no surgical bleeding that could be identified. The chest was drained with a Blake drain around the back of the aortic graft and one into the right chest, which had been opened during the initial sternotomy. A 36-French Argyle catheter was placed in the anterior mediastinum. All 3 chest tubes were brought out through separate inferior incisions and fixed to the skin, and the chest reapproximated in layers with 8 sternal wires and 3 layers of Vicryl soft tissues. The right infraclavicular incision was likewise closed in layers of Vicryl after amputating the graft flush with the arteriotomy and closing it. The sponge, needle, and instrument counts were reported correct by the circulating nurse, and the patient was prepared for transfer to the intensive care unit in critical condition.

    a. 33860
    b. 33860, 33870
    c. 33864
    d. 33864, 33870

9. All of the following describe the correct use of casting or strapping codes (29000–29750) *except*:

    a. A cast to stabilize a fracture, no restorative treatment given
    b. A replacement cast
    c. Fracture reduction with initial cast application
    d. Emergency physician applies strapping and patient is transferred to another hospital

10. The Table of Risk is an important part of which evaluation and management component?

    a. History
    b. Examination
    c. Decision making
    d. Counseling

11. Preoperative Diagnosis: Post-menopausal bleeding and endometriosis

Postoperative Diagnosis: Post-menopausal bleeding and endometriosis

Procedure Performed: Laparoscopic-assisted vaginal hysterectomy and bilateral salpingo-oophorectomy

Procedure Description: The patient was taken to the operating suite where she underwent successful endotracheal anesthesia. The patient was then prepped and draped in the standard sterile manner in the dorsal lithotomy position with stirrups. A Rubin cannula was placed in the cervix. The infraumbilical area was injected with local anesthetic. A 1-cm incision was made and the Veress needle was introduced with proper placement verified by saline drop test and an opening pressure of 3 mm Hg. The abdomen was insufflated. Two additional trocar locations were injected with lidocaine and 10-mm trocars were placed in the left and right lower quadrants under direct visualization.

The pelvis was examined and the uterus was found to be grossly normal, slightly enlarged and retroverted. The tubes and ovaries appeared normal bilaterally. The left infundibulopelvic ligament was clamped and verification was made that the ureter was not within the clamp. The ligament was ligated with the Endostapler. The broad ligament was then cut through with the stapling device, after verification of the location of the ureter. The right side was transected in a similar manner using the stapler. The bladder was then elevated and the peritoneum above the bladder was transected with the Endoshears. Hemostasis was pristine and the area was dry.

Our attention then turned to the vagina. The patient was changed to high Allen stirrups. A weighted speculum was inserted, the cervix was grasped with two clamps and the mucosa of the cervix was dissected circumferentially with Bovie from the vaginal vault and removed. The bladder was dissected off the lower uterine segment and the peritoneum was entered. The posterior cul-de-sac was grasped with a Kocher clamp and elevated. Curved Mayo scissors were used to enter the posterior cul-de-sac. A speculum was then replaced. The uterosacral complex was then transected and suture-ligated with 0 Vicryl. The left uterosacral complex was transected, cut, and suture-ligated in a similar manner. The last of the remaining broad ligament was then clamped on each side, transected and suture-ligated with O Vicryl. The uterus, tubes, and ovaries were then easily removed through the vagina. Uterus weighed 315 grams. The vaginal cuff and perineum were closed together using a 2-0 Vicryl from the 12 o'clock to 6 o'clock position, tied in the midline. The uterosacral ligament pedicles had been tagged and were tied in the midline and reattached to the vaginal cuff. The vaginal cuff had good hemostasis after the sutures were placed. All instruments were removed. The patient was taken out of the stirrups, awakened, extubated, and transferred to the recovery room in stable condition.

    a.   58544

    b.   58548

    c.   58552

    d.   58554

12.   A physician performs a laryngoscopy using a laryngeal mirror and performs a biopsy through the scope. This type of laryngoscopy is coded as:

    a.   31505

    b.   31510

    c.   31535

    d.   31576

13.   Intracapsular cataract lens extraction includes which procedure(s)?

    a.   Lens exchange

    b.   Removal of lens and the posterior capsule

    c.   Removal of lens and the anterior capsule

    d.   Intraocular lens implant

14.   Preoperative Diagnosis: Right knee degenerative joint disease with varus deformity

Postoperative Diagnosis: Same

Operative Procedure: Right total knee replacement

Indication for Surgery: Severe pain, bone-on-bone x-rays, progressive pain and disability, and failure of conservative treatment

Components: Femoral component #4, tibial component #4, high density polypropylene insert 8 mm, and patellar component 38 mm

Description of Procedure: Following general anesthesia, the right lower extremity was carefully prepped and draped. A hole was cut in the waterproof drape and a Betadine-soaked Vi-Drape placed leg was elevated, wrapped with a Martin bandage, and tourniquet was applied to 300 mmHg. A midline incision was made from just above the patella to the tibial tubercle. Sharp dissection carried through skin and subcutaneous tissue, and medial and lateral flaps were made. Medial arthrotomy was produced, splitting the quadriceps longitudinally. The medial and then medial and lateral dissection was carried around the proximal tibia for exposure.

The patella was measured. A measured resection was cut, leaving a nice flat surface. The guide was used to make the three peg holes. A protective disc was placed and the patella was prepared. It was pushed in the lateral gutter. The knee was flexed. A drill hole was made up the femoral canal and enlarged. A long rod was placed up the femoral canal for the distal femoral cut which was made, leaving a nice flat surface on both condyles. The tibial external guide system was placed, adjusted, and pinned into position, and the tibial cut was made just below the low point on the tibial plateau. The bone was removed, removing the posterior cruciate ligament. The extensor gap was measured and it was perfect.

The femur was measured, and the guide was pinned into position putting in the appropriate external rotation, and chamfer cuts were made. The box cut was pinned into position and the box cut made and the femur was prepared. Trial femoral component was placed. Trial tibial component was placed with a polypropylene insert. The knee went in full extension and full flexion and was stable. The trial components were removed.

The tibia was exposed. The tibial guide was pinned into position, the stem hole and crosshatch were made, and the tibia was prepared. Surfacing were irrigated and dried. Methylmethacrylate was forced into the interstices of the bone of the tibia. The tibial component was hand pushed into position and then tapped against the bone. All cement was removed from the edges. We waited until it dried with the knee in extension.

The patella and femur were irrigated and dried. Methylmethacrylate was forced interstices of the bone of the patella. The patella component was placed, held with a clamp. All cement was removed from the edges. Methylmethacrylate was forced into the interstices of the bone of the femur. The femoral component was pushed into position and tapped against the bone. All cement was removed from the edges. The polypropylene insert was placed and the knee pushed in full extension. It was copiously, copiously irrigated, both in flexion and extension. Solcotrans drains were placed medial and lateral. The medial arthrotomy was closed with interrupted 0 Ethibond multiple interrupted sutures. The knee was tested in full flexion and full extension. The suture line was stable. The patella was stable. Subcutaneous tissue was closed with 2-0 Vicryl, 4-0 Vicryl, and skin staples. Sterile dressing applied and the procedure was terminated.

   a.   27440, 27442
   b.   27440, 27442, 27437
   c.   27445
   d.   27447

15.   What information can be obtained from the graph shown here?

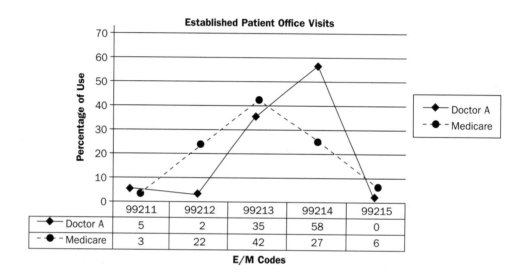

Established Patient Office Visits

E/M Codes	99211	99212	99213	99214	99215
Doctor A	5	2	35	58	0
Medicare	3	22	42	27	6

   a.   Doctor A is clustering his coding on 99214.
   b.   The Medicare percentages are calculated incorrectly.
   c.   Doctor A's failure to report 99215 skews his utilization curve.
   d.   Doctor A's patients are not as sick as the average Medicare patients.

16.   The physician completes an x-ray examination for an office patient, interprets the film, and creates a permanent report. How does the coder code for the physician's x-ray?

   a.   Code the x-ray code.
   b.   Code the x-ray code with modifier –26, Professional Component.
   c.   Code the x-ray code with modifier –TC, Technical Component.
   d.   Code the x-ray code with modifier –52, Reduced Services.

17.   What is the appropriate procedure for making corrections in the medical record?

   a.   Blacking out the error completely and signing it
   b.   Lining through the error and signing and dating it
   c.   Lining through the error and dating it
   d.   Blacking out the error and dating and timing it

18. Which CPT code(s) would be used to report the laboratory tests listed?

    Albumin, serum, plasma or whole blood (82040)
    Albumin, urine, microalbumin, quantitative (82043)
    Bilirubin, total (82247)
    Bilirubin, direct (82248)
    Phosphatase, alkaline (84075)
    Transferase, aspartate amino (84450)
    Transferase, alanine amino (84460)

    a. 80048
    b. 80076
    c. 80076, 82043
    d. 82040, 82043, 82247, 82248, 84075, 84450, 84460

19. This is a 39-year-old patient with bilateral cystic masses. Operative laparoscopy with bilateral ovarian cystectomies and lysis of adhesions is performed. What is the proper code assignment?

    a. 58662–50
    b. 58662–50, 58660
    c. 58660
    d. 49320, 58662–50, 58600

20. A patient has a left retrograde percutaneous cardiac catheterization with selective atrial angiogram. Imaging supervision and interpretation are provided. What is the proper code assignment?

    a. 93452
    b. 93452, 93567
    c. 93452, 93565
    d. 93452, 93565, 93567

21. A new patient comes to the office for evaluation and management of a recurrent urinary tract infection. A detailed history, expanded problem focused examination, and low-complexity level of decision making was included. How would this be coded?

    a. 99201   E/M with problem focused history, problem focused examination, and straight-forward medical decision making
    b. 99202   E/M with expanded problem focused history, expanded problem focused examination, and straightforward medical decision making
    c. 99203   E/M with detailed history, detailed examination, and low medical decision making
    d. 99204   E/M with comprehensive history, comprehensive examination, and moderate medical decision making

22. Which of the following indicates the need for a possible internal audit of code assignment?

    a. The staff has been with the physician for several years.
    b. Claims are being paid slowly.
    c. Claims rejections are showing a pattern of incorrect coding.
    d. A new claims supervisor decided to complete an audit.

23. A brain-dead patient whose organs are being donated is assigned which physical status modifier?

    a. P1
    b. P2
    c. P4
    d. P6

24. To complete an audit, indicate what information is missing in the documentation in order to use the code listed.

    Code used: 33270   Insertion or replacement of permanent subcutaneous implantable defibrillator system, with subcutaneous electrode, Including defibrillation threshold evaluation, induction of arrhythmia, evaluation of sensing for arrhythmia termination, and programming or reprogramming of sensing or therapeutic parameters, when performed

    Documentation: Insertion of permanent subcutaneous Implantatable system, with new electrode, threshold evaluation with arrhythmia Induction and termination

    Information missing: _____

25. To complete an audit, indicate what information is missing in the documentation in order to use the code listed.

    Code used: 63101   Vertebral corpectomy (vertebral body resection), partial or complete, lateral extracavitary approach with decompression of spinal cord and/or nerve root(s) (eg, for tumor retropulsed bone fragments); thoracic, single segment

    Documentation: Partial corpectomy of T10, decompression of nerve root

    Information missing: _____

Read the following case studies and indicate the appropriate code assignment.

26. Preoperative Diagnosis: Right inguinal hernia
    Postoperative Diagnosis: Same
    Operation: Laparoscopic right inguinal herniorrhaphy

    Indications for Surgery: 41-year-old man with an obvious right inguinal hernia, initial

    Summary of Findings: Large indirect hernia defect

    Procedure: After adequate general endotracheal anesthesia had been induced, the patient was placed in the supine position and prepared and draped in the usual sterile manner. An infraumbilical incision was made. After the patient was placed in the Trendelenburg position, the Veress needle was inserted. The abdomen was insufflated with carbon dioxide, and a 312 Auto-Suture port was placed through the infraumbilical incision. Then the laparoscope was inserted and a laparoscopic exploration was performed. The indirect hernia defect was recognized immediately. The remainder of the abdominal exploration was essentially unremarkable. Second and third ports were placed just slightly medial to the anterior axillary line and in the same plane of the infraumbilical incision on both right and left sides. Using a combination of sharp and blunt dissection with the Auto-Suture Endo-shears, the peritoneal reflection overlying the iliac vessels and cord vessels was dissected, thus developing a peritoneal flap. The vas deferens was identified and preserved carefully. The herniosac then was pulled out of the ring, and an Endo-GIA stapler was fired across the herniosac, essentially performing an extremely high ligation. A piece of Surgimesh was fashioned to the size of the floor of the canal covering both the defect and the vessels. Using the Endo-hernia stapler device, the Surgimesh was stapled into position. The peritoneal reflection then was placed over the Surgimesh and stapled in place. Meticulous hemostasis was obtained. Scopes were withdrawn. Sponge and needle counts were accurate. The patient tolerated the procedure well. Estimated blood loss less than 30 cc.

    a. 49651
    b. 49505
    c. 49650
    d. 49505, 49568

27. S: This 13-year-old boy comes in today for follow-up of long-term allergies. He has been having immunotherapy and has been feeling fairly well. He has been using his albuterol inhaler on and off, and rarely uses his steroid inhaler. He does not test his peak expiratory flow volume at home. Feels today like "a cold is coming on," but has not been wheezing, he says. No cardiac complaints. He also needs a hepatitis B shot today for school. He has a family history of allergies and asthma. No pets in the home. Has air-conditioning and attends an air-conditioned school.

    O: Weight is 221.5 lb. Temp is 98.3° F, pulse is 100, resp 20. Examination reveals no acute distress. He coughs occasionally in the room with some sound of congestion noted. No wheezing is noted, and he has no difficulty breathing. EARS: Canals patent. Tympanic membranes within normal limits. His nasal mucosa is moderately edematous, slightly paler and fuller on the left than the right. No mucus is seen. SINUSES:

Nontender to palpation in maxillary paranasal region. MOUTH AND THROAT: Pink moist mucosa. No exudate or edema. NECK: Supple with lymphadenopathy or thyromegaly. LUNGS: Clear to auscultation. No wheezes, rales, or rhonchi heard. His peak flows done today with me are 260, 260, and 270. He is obese, and I question whether this actually interferes with adequate inspiration.

A: 1. Asthma, 2. Allergies, on immunotherapy, 3. Needs #3 hepatitis B shot today

P: Use the Vanceril oral inhaler at least b.i.d. when having viral symptoms. Also, use the albuterol inhaler with wheezing. Do peak flows to establish personal best. He was given #3 hepatitis B today after obtaining consent from his mother.

History: Detailed
Exam: Detailed
Medical Decision Making: Low

    a.   99203, 90744
    b.   99213, 90746
    c.   99214, 90746, 90471
    d.   99214, S8110, 90744, 90471

28. The physician orders an ACTH stimulation test to rule out adrenal insufficiency. The patient is given an injection of 0.20 mg of cosyntropin and two cortisol level tests are drawn, 2 hours apart. How is this reported to a commercial payer?

    a.   96372, J0834, 82533, 82533-91, 36415 ×2
    b.   96372, J0834, 80400, 36415
    c.   96379, J0834 ×2, 82533 ×2, 36415 ×2
    d.   96379, J0800 ×2, 80400, 36415

29. S: This is a patient of mine who 10 days ago had a skiing accident. His ski jammed into the ice and he twisted his knee, throwing him off balance. He noticed increasing pain and significant swelling of his right knee. He used ibuprofen and an ice pack, which he did for 3 to 4 days. It was doing somewhat better but is again giving him pain and he cannot walk today without limping. There was no associated pain in the hip or the ankle or any tingling or numbness with this. He has no family history of arthritis or joint instability. No previous joint injuries or surgeries.

O: General: On exam he is alert, awake, oriented times three and in moderate distress secondary to pain. He is unable to walk without limping. RIGHT KNEE: Examination of the right knee shows medial joint line tenderness and difficulty in range of motion, especially with complete extension of the right knee. No effusion is noted. Peripheral pulsations are intact.

A: Right knee strain, most likely from skiing accident but must rule out any internal derangement.

P: The patient was asked to get an x-ray of the right knee downstairs now, which I will read. He was started on ibuprofen 800 mg 3 times per day, #60 with 1 refill, Tylenol #3, 1 to 2 tablets every 8 hours, #30 with 1 refill. Apply ice every hour and rest as much as possible. The patient was given a knee immobilizer to wear whenever he is up and around. RTC in 1 week for a recheck.

History: Detailed
Exam: Expanded problem focused
Medical Decision Making: Moderate

Knee x-ray—3 views

A knee series reveals normal mineralization. No fractures or osseous abnormalities are demonstrated. The joint spaces are well maintained. No joint effusion or soft tissue calcifications are seen.

IMPRESSION: Normal knee series

    a.   99202, 73562
    b.   99213, 73560
    c.   99214, A4570, 73562
    d.   99214, A4570, 73564

30. Preoperative Diagnosis: Incomplete spontaneous abortion

Postoperative Diagnosis: Same

Operation: Dilatation and curettage

History: This 22-year-old woman, gravida IV, para II, AB I, comes in today because of crampy abdominal pain and passing fetus on the sidewalk outside the office. Apparently, her last menstrual period was 11 weeks ago. She had been doing well; this problem just started today.

Procedure: The patient was taken to the procedure room and placed on the operating table in the lithotomy position and was prepared and draped in the usual manner. Under satisfactory intravenous sedation, the cervix was visualized by means of weighted speculum and grasped in the anterior lip with a sponge forceps. Cord was prolapsed through the cervix and vagina, and a considerable amount of placental tissue was in the vagina and cervix. This was removed. A sharp curette was used to explore the endometrial cavity, and a minimal amount of curettings was obtained. The patient tolerated the procedure well.

- a. 58120
- b. 59812
- c. 59830
- d. 59840

31. The patient is admitted for repair of a 3-cm fistula between the intestine and the abdominal wall. What is the proper coding assignment?

- a. 13101   Repair, complex, trunk; 2.6 cm to 7.5 cm
- b. 44640   Closure of intestinal cutaneous fistula
- c. 44650   Closure of enteroenteric or enterocolic fistula
- d. 44799   Unlisted procedure, intestine

32. To help ensure the best financial position for the physician practice, it is best to have the largest portion of the accounts receivable in which aging category?

- a. 0 to 30 days
- b. 31 to 60 days
- c. 61 to 90 days
- d. 91 to 120 days

33. Preoperative Diagnosis: Pacemaker malfunction

Postoperative Diagnosis: Same

Anesthesia: Local

Operation Performed: Replacement of pacemaker generator and electrode

Procedure: The patient was positioned on the fluoroscopy table and the right chest was prepared and draped. Local anesthesia was obtained with 1 percent lidocaine with epinephrine. The pocket was reopened and the generator removed. Analysis of the lead showed intermittent R waves obtained. At this point, it was elected to proceed with insertion of a new lead and generator. A Medtronic lead was placed into the apex of the right ventricle. The lead was sutured in place using 2-0 silk and connected to a new Medtronic generator. This was a single chamber pacer programmed at a rate of 70. Inspection was made to be certain that hemostasis was adequate. The old lead was capped and abandoned. The wound was closed using 3-0 Vicryl for subcutaneous tissue and 3-0 nylon for skin. Dry dressings were applied, and the patient was returned to the recovery room in satisfactory condition.

- a. 33227
- b. 33228
- c. 33229
- d. 33262

34. Which modifier is used to indicate that anesthesia was personally performed by the anesthesiologist?

- a. −AA   Anesthesia services performed personally by anesthesiologist
- b. −AD   Medical supervision by a physician; more than four concurrent anesthesia procedures
- c. −QK   Medical direction of two, three or four concurrent anesthesia procedures involving qualified individuals
- d. −QY   Medical direction of one certified registered nurse anesthetist (CRNA) by an anesthesiologist

35. Ventilating tubes are placed in a child's ears under general anesthesia. What is the proper coding assignment?

    a. 69420

    b. 69420–50

    c. 69433

    d. 69436–50

36. To calculate the Days in A/R statistic, which pair of monthly data is required?

    a. Ending accounts receivable and total contractual allowances

    b. Total accounts receivable and average cash per day

    c. Ending accounts receivable and average revenue per day

    d. Total accounts receivable and average revenue per day

37. A prostate specific antigen (PSA total) test is completed for a Medicare patient. How is this coded?

    a. G0103 Prostate cancer screening; prostate specific antigen test (PSA)

    b. 84153 Prostate specific antigen (PSA); total

    c. 84154 Prostate specific antigen (PSA); free

    d. 84999 Unlisted chemistry procedure

38. Using cardiopulmonary bypass, the patient's aortic valve is replaced with a synthetic valve. What is the proper coding assignment?

    a. 33400 Valvuloplasty, aortic valve; open, with cardiopulmonary bypass

    b. 33405 Replacement, aortic valve, with cardiopulmonary bypass; with prosthetic valve other than homograft or stentless valve

    c. 33406 with allograft valve (freehand)

    d. 33411 Replacement, aortic valve; with aortic annulus enlargement, noncoronary cusp

Refer to the following service-mix report for questions 39 and 40.

Doctor	Year	CPT Code	Description	Qty	Charge
456	20XX	59400	Total OB care	40	$2,000
456	20XX	59409	Vag delivery	3	$1,575
456	20XX	59410	Vag delivery and postpartum care	2	$1,695
456	20XX	59514	Cesarean delivery only	1	$1,995

39. If the national cesarean delivery (C-section) rate is 20 percent of an average OB physician's practice, what can the coder conclude from this service-mix report?

    a. Cesarean delivery may be overutilized in this practice.

    b. Some vaginal deliveries may have been coded incorrectly.

    c. Vaginal deliveries make up a major portion of the revenue.

    d. Postpartum care makes up a major portion of the revenue.

40. If health records indicate that 40 deliveries were done in 20XX, what conclusions can the coder draw from this information and this service-mix report?

    a. Postpartum care was missed during coding.
    b. Antepartum care was unbundled during coding.
    c. Delivery codes were unbundled during coding.
    d. Delivery codes were missed during coding.

41. The ophthalmologist measures the patient's face and writes a prescription for eyeglasses of a particular strength. They are prepared by the outside laboratory. Once the glasses arrive, the physician fits the glasses to the patient, ensuring that the bifocals are in the correct position. What is the proper coding assignment?

    a. 92002   Ophthalmological services: medical examination and evaluation with initiation of diagnostic and treatment program; intermediate, new patient
    b. 92015   Determination of refractive state
    c. 92341   Fitting of spectacles, except for aphakia; bifocal
    d. 92353   Fitting of spectacle prosthesis for aphakia; multifocal

42. A 1-year-old visits the pediatrician for a well-child checkup and a scheduled diphtheria, tetanus, and acellular pertussis injection. VIS is signed and immunization counseling is provided. What is the proper coding assignment?

    a. 99391, 90700, 90460
    b. 99392, 90700, 90460, 90461, 90461
    c. 99391, 90702, 90460
    d. 99392, 90749, 90460, 90461

43. A pathologist examined the following specimen: Products of conception, missed AB. The findings are stated as: Specimen 1: POC. Assign a CPT code.

    a. 88304   Level III—Surgical pathology, gross and microscopic examination
    b. 88305   Level IV—Surgical pathology, gross and microscopic examination
    c. 88307   Level V—Surgical pathology, gross and microscopic examination
    d. 88399   Unlisted surgical pathology procedure

44. Preoperative Diagnosis: Multivessel coronary artery disease

Postoperative Diagnosis: Same

Procedure Performed:

    1. Coronary artery bypass x5:

        One arterial graft, left internal mammary artery to left anterior descending,
        Four venous grafts, saphenous vein graft to distal left circumflex artery, sequential
        Y graft, saphenous vein to ramus, diagonal 1, and diagonal 2 artery.

    2. Endoscopic vein harvest

Description of Operation: The left internal mammary artery was harvested as a skeletonized graft. Simultaneously, a segment of the left greater saphenous vein was harvested endoscopically. We then went on cardiopulmonary bypass. First, a segment of the vein was grafted to the distal left circumflex artery. I examined the LAD system and found a second diagonal artery that was not seen on the angiogram. In addition, there was a ramus artery. I used the remaining vein and grafted first the ramus intermedius artery. The same vein was then used to perform a sequential anastomosis to a large diagonal one artery. The same vein was then used to perform another sequential anastomosis to the last diagonal artery. Lastly, the left internal mammary was grafted to the LAD. The two vein grafts were then anastomosed to the ascending aorta with a partial aortic clamp in place. The vein grafts were then de-aired. After the patient was fully rewarmed and resuscitated, we came off bypass.

The left internal mammary artery had excellent flow. The vein grafts also had good flow. Two mediastinal and one left pleural chest tubes were placed. Ventricular wires were placed. I closed the pericardium with a running 3-0 Prolene. The sternum was then closed with six interrupted steel wires. The rest of the sternal incision was then closed in layers with Vicryl followed by Monocryl for the skin.

    a. 33514
    b. 33533, 33521
    c. 33533, 33522
    d. 33536

45. According to CPT guidelines, which codes are used to report additional office visits during the first trimester to monitor weight loss due to severe vomiting and dehydration?

    a. Visits are part of the obstetrical package and not coded separately.
    b. 59899, Unlisted maternity care and delivery code
    c. Appropriate E/M office codes
    d. Appropriate E/M consultation codes

46. A general surgeon in the patient's hometown determines on 10-10-20XX that the patient requires a laparoscopic partial nephrectomy. A complete preoperative evaluation is completed, and she is referred to a nephrologist at a regional facility. The general surgeon asks that the nephrologist perform only the surgical care. This is completed on 10-11-20XX and the patient is transferred back to her hometown the next day, to the care of her general surgeon. How is the nephrologist's service coded?

    a. 50543–54
    b. 50543–58
    c. 50545–52–54
    d. 50546–58

47. How is the 10-10-20XX service of the general surgeon in question #46 coded?

    a. 50543–62
    b. 50543–56
    c. 50545–52–62
    d. 50546–58

48. A 4-year-old patient is admitted to the hospital after ingesting approximately 10 of his father's blood pressure pills over 3 hours ago. A detailed history is documented and a complete exam is performed and documented. The patient is transferred to ICU for monitoring due to his fluctuating level of consciousness. How is this physician service coded?

    a. 99221 Initial hospital care E/M with detailed or comprehensive history, detailed or comprehensive examination, and straightforward or low medical decision making
    b. 99222 Initial hospital care E/M with comprehensive history, comprehensive examination, and moderate medical decision making
    c. 99223 Initial hospital care E/M with comprehensive history, comprehensive examination, and high medical decision making
    d. 99291 Critical care, evaluation and management of the critically ill or critically injured patient; first 30 to 74 minutes

49. As the patient in question #48 improves on day 2, he is transferred to a regular pediatric bed. The physician documents an expanded problem focused history, performs a detailed examination, reviews both laboratory work and EKG tracings, and manages the patient's medication orders in preparation for discharge the following day. How is this physician service coded?

    a. 99231 Subsequent hospital care E/M with problem focused interval history, problem focused examination, and straightforward or low medical decision making
    b. 99232 Subsequent hospital care E/M with expanded problem focused interval history, expanded problem focused examination, and moderate medical decision making
    c. 99238 Hospital discharge day management; 30 minutes or less
    d. 99239 more than 30 minutes

50. On day 2 of the admission, a pediatrician managed the care of a critically ill neonate (second day of life). How is this daily care coded?

    a. 99468 Initial inpatient neonatal critical care, per day, for the evaluation and management of a critically ill neonate, 28 days of age or younger
    b. 99469 Subsequent inpatient neonatal critical care, per day, for the evaluation and management of a critically ill neonate, 28 days of age or younger
    c. 99471 Initial inpatient pediatric critical care, per day, for the evaluation and management of a critically ill infant or young child, 29 days through 24 months of age
    d. 99472 Subsequent inpatient pediatric critical care, per day, for the evaluation and management of a critically ill infant or young child, 29 days through 24 months of age

51. The patient attends a 60-minute stress management class conducted by a psychologist associated with his physician. This service is covered by his commercial insurance. How is this reported?

    a. 99404 Preventive medicine counseling and/or risk factor reduction intervention(s) provided to an individual (separate procedure); approximately 60 minutes
    b. 99412 Preventive medicine counseling and/or risk factor reduction intervention(s) provided to individuals in a group setting (separate procedure); approximately 60 minutes
    c. S9445 Patient education, not otherwise classified, nonphysician provider, individual, per-session
    d. S9454 Stress management classes, nonphysician provider, per session

52. The physician excised a salivary gland cyst from under the patient's tongue. What is the proper coding assignment?

    a. 10140 Incision and drainage of hematoma, seroma or fluid collection
    b. 42310 Drainage of abscess; submaxillary or sublingual, intraoral
    c. 42408 Excision of sublingual salivary cyst (ranula)
    d. 42450 Excision of sublingual gland

53. How much does Medicare approve for a non-PAR physician on an assigned claim?

    a. 80% of the approved amount
    b. 80% of the limiting charge
    c. 95% of a PAR provider's approved amount
    d. 115% of the approved amount

54. When completing an E/M code audit, which guidelines are the reviewer and the physician required to follow?

    a. The 1997 guidelines
    b. The 1995 guidelines
    c. The guidelines that are best for the physician
    d. None because the requirements have yet to be determined

55. The patient presents to his personal physician's office after being hurt at work. He was pushing a heavy cart, which hit a large bump on an uneven floor and "kicked back" to hit him in the right rib cage. AP and lateral x-rays taken and read by the physician reveal one broken rib. A Don-Joy rib belt is applied and pain medication is prescribed. An expanded problem focused history, expanded problem focused exam and moderate medical decision making is documented. How is this service coded?

    a. 99212, 71110, A4570
    b. 99213, 71100, A4570
    c. 99213, 71100, L0220
    d. 99214, 71110, L0220

56. A 9 lb, 4 oz newborn undergoes a repair to release pyloric stenosis. How is this procedure coded?

    a. 43520
    b. 43520–63
    c. 43800
    d. 43800–63

57. Preoperative Diagnosis: Morbid obesity

    Postoperative Diagnosis: Morbid obesity

    Procedure: Laparoscopic Roux-en-Y gastric bypass

    Indications: The patient is a 46-year-old young lady who is morbidly obese, who is admitted for elective laparoscopic Roux-en-Y gastric bypass.

    Operative Report: After identifying the patient, she was taken to the operative suite and placed in the supine position on the operating table. After induction of general anesthetic and endotracheal intubation, the patient's anterior abdomen was prepped with sterile Betadine and draped in the usual fashion. A 1.5-cm subumbilical skin incision was made. Using a Visiport trocar, a 12-mm trocar was placed through the fascia and peritoneum into the abdomen. The abdomen was insufflated with CO2 without complication. A 12-mm right and left lateral, right and left upper paramedian, and right upper quadrant trocars were placed under direct laparoscopic visualization. The transverse colon was retracted superiorly and ligament of Treitz was identified at its base. The jejunum was divided 30 cm distal to ligament of Treitz with a linear stapler. Mesenteric defect was extended with a vascular linear stapler. A 100-cm Roux limb was measured and marked. A side-to-side jejunojejunostomy was performed with the linear stapler. The enterotomy defect was oversewn using running 2-0 Surgidek suture. The mesenteric defect was then similarly repaired using running 2-0 Surgidek suture. The omentum was split down in the middle to allow passage of the Roux limb in an enterocolic intragastric fashion without creation of tension from the omentum. The lesser sac was entered on the lesser curvature side of the stomach. Distal gastrotomy was made. A suture was tied to the anvil of a 25-mm circular stapler and the anvil and suture placed into the stomach via gastrotomy. A tiny anterior gastrotomy was made at the site of the proposed anastomosis within the area of the proposed pouch. A 38 French bougie was passed through the GE junction to maintain its patency and creation of pouch. A 20 mL lesser curvature based pouch was then created with successive firings of linear stapler. The bougie was then removed. Distal gastrotomy was closed with a linear stapler. Endoscopic leak test was performed and found to be negative. The anastomosis was inspected circumferentially. There was found to be no evidence of tension on the anastomosis, and it was circumferentially intact. The left lower quadrant port site fascia was closed with a 0 Vicryl suture. The remaining ports were removed after placing a #15 Jackson-Pratt drain anterior to the anastomosis. The drain was sutured in position with 2-0 nylon suture. Remaining skin edges closed with 4-0 subcuticular Vicryl sutures. The patient tolerated the procedure well and was transferred to recovery in stable condition. All sponge, needle, and instrument counts were correct. Estimated blood loss was minimal.

a. 43644
b. 43846
c. 47741
d. 48540

58. S: The patient has had a small lump in the left inferior gluteal fold for about 7 months. Sometimes it bothers her when she sits for long periods of time. She drives for her employment. The lump has not changed during that time and consistently bothers her. She wants to have it removed today.

O: A pleasant female with a 1.5-cm lump in the skin of the gluteal fold. It was washed with iodine and then alcohol, and injected with buffered lidocaine. An ellipse was taken to include the lesion for a total excised size of 1.8 cm. It seemed to be just fatty tissue. Skin was closed with 4-0 Vicryl in an intradermal fashion. It was washed with peroxide and water, dried, and dressed with Telfa and Tegaderm.

A: Gluteal lipoma excision.

P: She was given written and verbal wound care instructions. She is to call with questions or problems. Will return only if healing is problematic.

History: Problem focused Exam: Problem focused Medical Decision Making: Straightforward

a. 99212, 11402, J2001
b. 99212–25, 11402
c. 11402, 12031
d. 11402

59. Tests performed in a physician office laboratory that holds a certification waiver from CLIA should be billed with which of these modifiers?

a. –GA   Waiver of liability on file
b. –90   Reference (outside) laboratory
c. –QP   Documentation is on file showing that the laboratory tests were ordered individually or other than automated profile codes
d. –QW   CLIA waived test

60. A 12-year-old boy sustains an unprovoked dog bite in the left thigh from an unknown dog and receives deep puncture wounds. The physician gives 820 mg of rabies immune globulin for immediate protection and the first of a series of five doses of intramuscular injections of rabies vaccine. How are these treatments coded?

a. J1562, 96372, 90675, 90471
b. J1562 ×2, 90676, 90471, 90472
c. 90375, 96372, 90675, 90471
d. 90375, 90676, 90471, 90472

Office Visit/Operative Report Exercises

Case 1—Office Note

CC: Left wrist

S: This is an 11-year-old boy who initially injured his left distal radius in April. We placed him in a long-arm cast for about 6 weeks and a short-arm cast for about 2 weeks. He was taken out of his cast last week, 7.5 weeks post-injury. Yesterday he was reaching for a ball, simply resting his weight on his extended left arm, when he felt a snap in the wrist once again. He did not sustain any specific fall. X-rays done here and read by me show a refracture at the fracture site.

O: On examination he has clinical deformity consistent with a new fracture at the old fracture site with apex dorsal angulation.

A/P: I discussed options with the patient and his dad. I discussed options for closed reduction under anesthesia versus closed reduction here in the office. He elected to try the closed reduction without any anesthesia. This was performed without difficulty and he tolerated it well. I placed a new long-arm plaster cast on the arm today. X-rays in the cast showed correction of the angular deformity on both the lateral and AP views. Precautions were given regarding the cast and neurovascular checks. He will return to see me in 5 days for a recheck.

X-ray Interpretation:

Marc Hilten, MD
Left wrist: New fracture is apparent just proximal to the old fracture site of 2 months ago. Angular deformity is present.

Marc Hilten, MD

Left wrist in plaster cast: Wrist now shows proper alignment of the distal radius.

Marc Hilten, MD

Case 1 Code(s): _____

Case 2—Operative Report

Preoperative Diagnosis: High-grade right internal carotid artery stenosis

Postoperative Diagnosis: High-grade right internal carotid artery stenosis

Procedures: Right carotid thromboendarterectomy and bovine patch angioplasty

Indications: A 61-year-old woman with high-grade stenosis detected on duplex imaging. The technique, risks, and benefits of the procedure were discussed at length with the patient and the patient agreed to proceed.

Anesthesia: General anesthesia

Findings: High-grade mixed plaque involving the carotid bulb and proximal internal carotid artery. A shunt was used throughout the reconstruction. A bovine patch was used to reconstruct the artery.

Operative Report: After informed consent was obtained, the patient was met in the procedure room. Her right neck was prepped and draped in normal sterile surgical fashion. A curvilinear neck incision was made along the anterior border of the sternocleidomastoid muscle. This was deepened down to the platysma muscle. The carotid sheath was opened and the carotid artery was circumferentially dissected and controlled. We identified the vagus and hypoglossal nerves, both of which were protected throughout the dissection. We heparinized the patient with 100 units/kg of Heparin IV. After adequate circulation time, we placed our clamps distal and then proximal. A longitudinal arteriotomy was created and a shunt was inserted. Antegrade flow was then restored through the shunt. The endarterectomy was performed in the usual fashion. We were able to obtain a nice tapered end point. Once we removed all loose intimal debris, we applied a bovine pericardial patch. A running 6-0 Prolene was used. Prior to completing anastomosis, we removed the shunt. The vessel was flushed antegrade and retrograde. Repair sutures were placed as necessary. Antegrade flow was then restored, first to the external, and then to the internal. We checked signals distally. Once we were happy with flow, we irrigated the wound copiously. Protamine 30 mg was given to partially reverse the heparinization. Gelfoam and thrombin were also used to aid with hemostasis. We irrigated the wound once again and closed in layers using Vicryl and Monocryl. All counts were correct x2 at the end of the procedure. Sterile dressings were applied and the patient transported to recovery room in satisfactory condition.

Case 2 Code(s): _____

Case 3—Operative Report

Preoperative Diagnosis: Status post amputation of left index finger with neuroma and bony prominence at distal stump

Postoperative Diagnosis: Same

Anesthesia: General

Description of Operation: The patient was prepared and draped in sterile fashion using Hibiclens solution. The digit had been preinfiltrated for a digital block with 0.25%. The extremity was exsanguinated and an upper extremity tourniquet inflated to 250 mm Hg pressure was used. An incision was made in the previous scar overlying the distal aspect of the left index finger amputation stump, which ended at the distal aspect of the proximal phalanx. This was taken down to the periosteal cuffs surrounding the distal aspect of the proximal phalanx and a subperiosteal dissection was performed. Prior to proceeding, the ulnar digital nerve was explored and it was found that there was a pacinian corpuscle that led to a neuroma-appearing tissue with irregular neural structure. This was dissected using the operating microscope and taken back to the midlevel of the proximal phalanx. The specimen was submitted to pathology. Having resected all irregular neural tissue, the amputation stump was then trimmed with a bony rongeur, noting that there were some irregularities, particularly on the ulnar aspect. This was then contoured smooth. Having completed this, the soft tissues were suspended around the distal aspect of the proximal phalanx with 4-0 Vicryl suture with adequate padding of soft tissue. The tourniquet was released and the skin was then closed with interrupted 5-0 nylon suture. A bulky hand dressing was placed. The patient was extubated and returned to the recovery area in stable condition.

Case 3 Code(s): _____

Case 4—Office Note

CC: Endometrial biopsy

S: The patient reports that her primary care physician told her she needed to come in for an endometrial biopsy. However, she thinks that the thickening that was seen had nothing to do with an abnormality, as she had miscalculated her period. Her period started 2 days following the last ultrasound. It is conceivable that because of the misinformation, the interpretation would have been made differently. We originally performed a pelvic ultrasound because of pelvic pain, which has now basically resolved.

A&P: I will complete another pelvic ultrasound today, and we can decide from there if any further testing needs to be done. I did tell her that the reason we need to follow up is because endometrial thickening can be an indicator of dysplasia or cancer. We spent 10 minutes of a 15-minute total visit counseling regarding testing options and results. No other examination was done.

Examination: Pelvic complete, Non-OB. History: Follow-up endometrial thickening

Transabdominal scanning is done showing a uterus measuring 98 mm × 55 mm with an endometrial thickness of 2.6 mm. Both ovaries are seen and are normal. There are no abnormal masses or fluid collections present. Comparison is made to the prior examination of two weeks ago, which showed an endometrial thickness of 14.1 mm.

Impression: Normal pelvic ultrasound.

Dr. C

Case 4 Code(s): _____

Case 5—Office Note

CC: Warts, right foot

S: This is a 13-year-old patient of mine who came in today because he states he has a wart on the ball of the right foot that bothers him. It has been there for a few weeks now and was not noted on his last well examination 4 months ago. He has not tried any particular treatment and has never had warts before. We did, however, just finish treatment of plantar warts for his brother.

O: Weight 134 pounds. Temperature 99.4° F. Pulse 80. Respirations 20. Examination of the right foot plantar surface reveals an approximately 4-mm verrucous papule that has been obviously scraped somewhat by the patient. Distal to this is an approximately 6-mm verrucous papule and on the plantar surface of the distal phalanx there is an approximately 3-mm verrucous papule. The left foot is clear.

A: Plantar warts, right foot.

P: The father is present today. After discussing the risks, alternatives, and benefits, the father gives consent. Cryo-cautery is utilized on each of these lesions described above. The patient tolerates the treatment well. I advised him in posttreatment care and he will follow up in 2 weeks.

Case 5 Code(s): _____

Case 6—Pathology Report

History/Clinical Dx: Sigmoid colon biopsies

Postoperative Dx: Polyps

Specimens received:
A.   Colon polyp at cecum
B.   Ascending colon polyp
C.   Distal descending colon polyp

Diagnosis:
A.   Cecum: adenomatous polyp
B.   Ascending colon: hyperplastic polyp
C.   Distal descending colon: adenomatous polyp

Gross Description:
A.   Received in formalin labeled "cecum polyp" are two pieces of tan tissue measuring up to 0.3 cm in greatest dimension. Submitted in toto in one cassette.
B.   Received in formalin labeled "ascending polyp" are multiple pieces of tan tissue measuring up to 0.4 cm in greatest dimension. Submitted in toto in one cassette.
C.   Received in formalin labeled "distal descending polyp" are two pieces of tan tissue measuring up to 0.4 cm in greatest dimension. Submitted in toto in one cassette.

Microscopic Description:
A–C. The microscopic findings support the above diagnosis.

Case 6 Code(s): _____

Case 7—Office Note

CC: Abnormal Pap smear

S: This is a 30-year-old woman who was seen last October. The patient has had abnormal Pap smears showing high-grade SIL. A LEEP was performed last August and again in February of this year. The patient continues to have high-grade lesions on her Pap smear. She is status post tubal ligation. She denies smoking. She has no past medical history to speak of. Works as an administrative assistant. She has no allergies.

She is here today to discuss a recommended cone procedure. I did speak with the patient extensively for some 20 minutes of the 35-minute visit regarding her history and the failed LEEP procedures, and certainly recommended that we perform a cone procedure. However, I was unable to convince her regarding the need for this, and the patient wanted to have just another colposcopy at this time to corroborate the prior findings. I did explain to her that as far as I was concerned it did not matter what the findings of the colposcopy showed. I would still be recommending to proceed to immediate cold cone as a day-surgery patient versus hysterectomy. But again, the patient did want to wait and see.

O: Therefore, colposcopy was performed today. I did not see any significant acetowhite tissue in the transformation zone, and there was acetowhite tissue inside the columnar cell area inside the squamocolumnar junction. However, this often and for the most part is normal as columnar tissue does turn white when you apply acetic acid. We did take representative biopsies at the 1 o'clock and 7 o'clock positions and sent them to the hospital laboratory for evaluation.

P: We will wait for the results of the tissue examination before we decide how to proceed. However, again, even if this returns normal, I would still recommend cold cone to the patient.

Case 7 Code(s): _____

Case 8—Operative Report

Preoperative Diagnosis: Small bowel obstruction

Postoperative Diagnosis: Small bowel obstruction from internal hernia

Procedure Performed: Diagnostic laparoscopy, laparoscopic enterolysis

Indications: The patient is a 67-year-old female, who has had no previous abdominal operations, who was brought into the emergency room with a small bowel obstruction. She was found on CT scan to have a swirl in the mesentery and a concern for internal hernia. Because she had a virgin abdomen, we discussed her need for surgical exploration. We elected to perform this laparoscopically. Discussed risks and benefits of procedure with the patient, and she wished to proceed.

Procedure in Detail: After correctly identifying with 2 patient identifiers, the patient was brought to the operating room, placed supine on the operating table, and the left arm was tucked. Given general endotracheal anesthesia and a Foley catheter was placed. The abdomen was then prepped and draped in normal sterile fashion. Just below the umbilicus, a small incision was made, carried down the level of fascia. The base of the umbilical stalk was grasped and elevated. The fascia was entered sharply. We placed 2 stay sutures and 0-Vicryl suture on each side of the fascia, placed Hasson trocar, insufflated the abdomen to a pressure of 15 mmHg.

We then placed a 5-mm trocar in right upper quadrant and 5-mm trocar in the right lower quadrant. Immediately upon entering the abdomen, we could see multiple dilated proximal small bowel loops with decompressed distal loops. We identified the cecum and terminal ileum and we began running the bowel proximally. In doing so, we came in the mid proximal ileum and distal jejunum. We saw this was coming underneath the band of omentum that was causing an internal hernia. It was an adhesion from the omentum to the sigmoid colon. Once we elevated this up, we divided it with the LigaSure device and this completely released it. We then were able to run the bowel proximally, pass this distended bowel up into the right upper quadrant.

We then ran the bowel again from the terminal ileum back. We saw this transition and it was completely free. There were no further adhesions. We then examined the left lower quadrant. There were several adhesions of the sigmoid colon to the anterior abdominal wall. The bowel was completely normal. There was no injury or any need for resection. We also did incidentally find jejunal diverticulum, which was not inflamed. It was completely soft and it was in a portion of the dilated bowel, but again was not at all related to the internal hernia. We then removed the trocars under direct visualization, closed the fascia and the umbilicus with #0 Vicryl sutures, placed in a figure-of-eight fashion, a total of 3 sutures were placed. Skin sites were closed with 4-0 Vicryl and covered with Dermabond. The patient was awakened from anesthesia and taken to the recovery room in stable condition.

Case 8 Code(s): _____

Case 9—Office Note

CC: Diabetes mellitus and left wrist and hand pain

S: This 70-year-old patient of mine has had left wrist pain off and on since he had a fall about a year ago. He comes in today with some discomfort mainly in the left wrist and shooting down the left hand. There is no associated tingling or numbness with that. No recent fall. He feels that he is doing well with his diabetes.

O: Alert, awake, oriented ×3, in no acute distress. Vital signs are blood pressure of 168/82, respirations are 20 and weight is 181 lb. Examination of the left wrist shows minimal soft tissue swelling with localized tenderness over the radial aspect right below the radial styloid process. There is no obvious bony deformity that I can appreciate. Extension/flexion of the left wrist is possible, but somewhat painful. The hand has good grasp. Respiratory examination revealed diminished air entry in all lung fields consistent with possible COPD. Cardiovascular revealed normal heart sounds. Neck is supple. His recent blood tests show hemoglobin A1C elevated to 8.8 and fasting blood sugar of 193 with normal electrolytes. I ordered a two-view of the hand including the wrist area.

A: Diabetes mellitus, uncontrolled
   Left wrist pain due to degenerative joint disease

P: Patient will keep regular appointments for his laboratory work and will see Orthopedics to further evaluate his wrist pain.

Mary Meier, MD

Radiology Report

Hand/wrist x-ray: Essentially all of the IP and MP joint spaces show varying degrees of degenerative change primarily manifested by joint space narrowing and some spurring. Degenerative change also involves the first carpometacarpal joint, and perhaps some cystic degenerative change within the lunate and scaphoid are present. There is bony demineralization, which may be slightly disproportionate relative to the patient's age. Arterial calcification is seen. Final impression is degenerative joint disease and bony demineralization.

Mary Meier, MD

Case 9 Code(s): _____

Case 10—Office Note

CC: Follow-up

S: This is a 1-month PCP follow-up for this 56-year-old patient who is status post bovine pericardial valve replacement per Cardiology. This was done due to severe aortic regurgitation secondary to long-standing uncontrolled hypertension. Patient actually is recovering quite well and is back to sinus rhythm from atrial fibrillation. Blood pressure now is a lot better on lisinopril 20 mg twice a day. Patient is going to have blood work today for protime, potassium, and complete blood count. He wants to go back to some 5 to 10 lb of dumbbell forearm exercise, and I think that is reasonable at this time.

O: 190.5 lb, blood pressure is 144/90, pulse rate is 60. No JVD. Clear lungs. No rub No gallop. Abdomen: Obese. Liver is not palpable. Extremities show no edema.

A: Status post bovine pericardial aortic valve replacement, doing well. Hypertension, fair control.

P: Blood count to see if we can stop the iron supplement. Protime today and continue Coumadin for another 3 weeks and then will probably change to baby aspirin. Due to the patient's previous record of misunderstanding medication, I will see him back in 2 weeks to make sure that he understands the long-term therapy that is planned. I am anticipating no further problem and will probably see him 3 times a year after I'm reassured in 2 weeks.

Blood draw done today in the office.

Results (performed in office):

Potassium		4.5	(3.3–5.1)	mmol/L
Automated Blood Count				
WBC		4.6	(3.5–10.0) 10(9)	/L
RBC	L	4.38	(4.40–6.00) 10(12)	/L
Hemoglobin		14.4	(14–17)	g/dL
Hematocrit		42.8	(41–51)	%
MCV		97.7	(80–100)	fL
MCH		32.9	(27–33)	pg
MCHC		33.7	(32–36)	g/dL
RDW		14.1	(11–15)	%
Platelet Count		177	(150–450)	10(9)/L
MPV		7.5	(6.9–10.9)	fL
Protime	H	15.4	(11.5–14.5)	sec
INR		1.22	(2.0–3.0)	
			(2.5–3.5 for mechanical prosthetic valves, prevention of recurrent MI)	

Case 10 Code(s): _____

Case 11—Office Note

Pediatric Medical Group

7–10 Years of Age	
INTERVAL HISTORY—Established Patient	NURSING NOTES
Age: 9 Female Allergies: None Medications: None Concerns: New need for glasses this year, doesn't like to wear them Immunizations: UTD Diet: likes fruit and vegetables, good variety, good appetite Sleep: 8–9 hrs Vision: corrected with glasses Urine: normal Hearing: passed screening Stools: normal School: Name:_____St. Jude_____ Year:_____4th_____ Attendance:_____Excellent_____ Learning Problems: None Sports: gymnastics, also likes piano Social Hx/Family Hx Update: Lives at home with parents and cat, no socialization issues reported. Dental: Sees dentist q 6 months	☐ Vaccine information sheets given

PHYSICAL EXAM			
Ht: 55¾" Wt: 91.5 B/P: 98/60			
	N	Variation	
Gen Appearance	✔		
Skin	✔		
Eyes: PERRL, EOMI, Fundi		New glasses this year. Helps in school but doesn't like them.	
Ears: TM's	✔		
Nose:	✔		
Mouth/Throat: tonsils, teeth	✔		
Neck: thyroid, nodes	✔		
Chest: breath	✔		
Heart: sounds, murmur, pulses	✔		
Abdomen: HSM	✔		
Genitalia: pubertal changes, testes	✔		
Extremities:	✔		
Back: scoliosis	✔		
Neuro: DTR's, CN	✔		

IMPRESSION—PROBLEMS— PLANS—FOLLOW-UP

Immunizations—Up-to-date   **Labs**—None needed at this visit

EDUCATION

Diet—3 meals/day, healthy snacks, limit junk foods
Dental—brush teeth twice a day, flossing, visit every 6 months, fluoride treatment, sealants
Behavior—prepare for puberty
Injury Prevention—seat belt in backseat, sunscreen, smoke detectors, bike helmet, guns, water safety, stranger safety, home alone, lawn mower
Guidance—encourage reading and hobbies, help child pursue talents, discourage alcohol, tobacco, drug use, TV/Computer/Internet safety

Physician's Signature: _____ John Smith, MD

Next Appointment: 1 year

Case 11 Code(s): _____

Case 12—Operative Report

Preoperative Diagnosis: Chronic Sinusitis

Postoperative Diagnosis: Chronic Sinusitis

Names of Procedures: 1. Bilateral Endoscopic Intranasal Ethmoidectomy

2. Maxillary Antrostomy

Anesthesia: General

Estimated Blood Loss: Less than 50 mL

Indication: This man has had chronic bouts of sinusitis, and we were unable to clear him unless we used prednisone and then as soon as he comes off the prednisone, his symptoms recur. He also has an accessory ostium present on a CT scan and, therefore, was brought to the operating room for above procedure.

Findings: Accessory os bilaterally that was quite large, much larger than the natural os, and mild ethmoid thickening.

Description of Operation: Under adequate general anesthesia, the nose was decongested with Afrin preoperatively. 1% lidocaine with 1:100,000 epinephrine was used to infiltrate the lateral wall of the nose, anterior to the middle turbinate, the middle turbinate, and greater palatine foramen blocks. The operation was begun on the left side with the use of the endoscope. The inferior third of the middle turbinate was removed. With this down, the accessory os was easily visible in the inferior portion of the fontanel and a shortened and malformed uncinate process also was present. This was superior to the area of his accessory os. The uncinate process was then taken down retrograde fashion and the natural ostium exposed. Then the two were connected to create one large maxillary antrostomy. The bulla ethmoidalis was identified and taken out with a microdebrider exposing the basal lamella, which was then removed back to the anterior face of the sphenoid. In this case, the anterior face of the sphenoid was opened without violating the mucous membrane of the sphenoid, and then the fovea ethmoidalis identified superiorly and the lamina papyracea laterally, and those were cleaned of ethmoid cells from a posterior to anterior direction. When this was completed, this side of the operation was deemed complete. The identical procedure was performed on the right side in a similar fashion, except on the right side, the anterior face of the sphenoid was identified and was not violated. The estimated blood loss was less than 50 mL. There was no evidence of any CSF leak or persistent bleeding from the nose. He was then awakened and taken to the recovery room in satisfactory condition.

Case 12 Code(s): _____

Case 13—Hospital Note

Arrival time: 0100 on 11/10/xx

Admitting Diagnosis: Effexor ingestion

HPI: This is a 3-year-old boy who was found by parents ingesting father's Effexor pills. Apparently only one was taken out of his mouth; the rest were scattered around him. They believe he may have taken a maximum of four tablets totaling 450 mg. Patient had been alert, active, oriented. He has been having some sniffles and a cold, but no fevers, no emesis, no diarrhea, no respiratory symptoms; otherwise has been alert and oriented.

PFSH: Medications: None

Allergies: None

Remainder is noncontributory.

In the ER, the patient was evaluated. His vitals were stable. He was given a dose of activated charcoal on the recommendation of the Poison Control Center.

EXAM: Temperature is 37° C, respiratory rate is 20, pulse is 125, blood pressure is 102/64, pulse ox is 100%.

HEENT: Normal. NECK: Is supple. CHEST: Clear to auscultation. CARDIOVASCULAR: S1 and S2 are normal, no murmurs. ABDOMEN: Soft, nontender. NEUROLOGIC: He is intact, no gross deficit.

ASSESSMENT: Effexor ingestion

0400: Currently the patient is asymptomatic. Because this is a sustained release tablet, the patient needs to be admitted for observation. We will monitor patient for tremors, seizures, agitation, and hypertension and manage accordingly. Discussed the plan with parents who agree. PCP will be notified.

DISCHARGE NOTE: 11/10/xx at 2150

Remains asymptomatic, was awake at 2015, playful in toy area of his room. Vital signs have remained WNL during the day and napped as usual. Ate appropriately and played on the unit after dinner. Discharge to parents with instructions to watch for tremors, seizures, or agitation.

Case 13 Code(s): _____

Case 14—Day Surgery

Preoperative Diagnosis: Midline dermoid cyst at the glabella

Postoperative Diagnosis: Same

Operation: Excision of dermoid cyst

Surgeons: Dr Y and Dr Z

Anesthesia: General with endotracheal tube

Indications: The patient is a 2-year-old girl with a midline mass in the region of her glabella that has been present since birth. This has grown steadily since then. CT evaluation reveals a cystic structure in the midline, approximately 0.6 cm in size.

Procedure: After obtaining informed consent from the patient's parents, the patient was anesthetized with general anesthesia and maintained with an endotracheal tube inhalant, as well as IV anesthetics. Standard monitoring was utilized. A 0.8-cm incision was made in the midline region of the glabella overlying the lesion. This was infiltrated with 0.5 cc of 0.5% lidocaine with epinephrine. Skin incision was made with a #15 Bard-Parker blade. Dissection was carried through the skin and subcutaneous tissue.

The surgical assistant was responsible for retraction, which included the use of two-prong rakes and Bishop-Harman pickups along with Ragnell retractors. Once the lesion was identified on its external surface, careful dissection was carried out starting from the superior aspect going down its side to its undersurface. This was then carried inferiorly along both lateral sides of the lesion. Once this was completed, a similar process was started from the inferior aspect. Special care was taken to make a small incision and thus the assistant needed to move the retractors in the direction of where the dissection was being performed. Once the cyst was completely free, hemostasis was obtained. The wound was closed with multiple buried interrupted 6-0 Vicryl sutures, closing the dermis and subcutaneous portions of the defect. The skin was closed with multiple interrupted 6-0 fast-absorbing plain gut sutures. Specimen sent.

The patient tolerated the procedure well and was extubated without difficulty. Her face was cleaned and Steri-Strips were positioned in anticipation of the young child potentially scratching at the wound. Antibiotic ointment was placed onto the wound area, and she was taken to the recovery room in good condition.

Case 14 Code(s): _____

Case 15—Operative Report

Preoperative Diagnosis: Peripheral arterial disease

Postoperative Diagnosis: Peripheral arterial disease

Procedure: Right femoral popliteal bypass with 6 mm PTFE

Indications: A 69-year-old man who was seen for extremely limited walking and peripheral arterial disease. He has bilateral SFA occlusions. The technique, risks, and benefits of the intervention were discussed at length with the patient and he agreed to proceed.

Anesthesia: General anesthesia

Findings: A 6 mm PTFE was tunneled deep to the sartorius muscle. End-to-side proximal and distal anastomoses were performed. The patient had palpable foot pulses at the end of the procedure.

Operative Report: After informed consent was obtained, the patient was met in the procedure room. His right leg was prepped and draped in normal sterile surgical fashion. We started by making an oblique skin incision in the right groin. This was carried down through the subcutaneous tissues. The femoral artery was circumferentially dissected and controlled. Once control was obtained of the groin, we moved down the medial thigh where longitudinal skin incision was made again and carried down through subcutaneous tissues. The popliteal artery was circumferentially controlled at this level using vessel loops. We then tunneled a 6 mm PTFE graft deep to the sartorius muscle. The patient was systemically heparinized. Clamps were placed distal and proximal in the femoral artery. A longitudinal arteriotomy was created and an end-to-side proximal anastomosis was performed using 5-0 Prolene. We back bled and forward flush through the artery to remove all air and loose debris. We then clamped and moved down to the distal anastomosis. Again, our clamps were placed distal and proximal on the popliteal artery. There was some heavily calcified plaque, which was endarterectomized down to a smooth endpoint. We then performed the distal anastomosis after beveling the graft to length. A 6-0 Prolene was used in standard running fashion. Prior to completing this anastomosis, we flushed antegrade and retrograde as well as through the graft and removed all air and loose debris. We then opened up antegrade into the foot. Palpable foot pulses were obtained during the procedure. We made sure the hemostasis was adequate at both incisions. Both wounds were irrigated copiously with Bacitracin and saline. The wounds were then closed in layers using Vicryl and Monocryl. All counts were correct x2 at the end of the procedure. Sterile dressings were applied. The patient was transported to the recovery room in satisfactory condition.

Case 15 Code(s): _____

Case 16—Day Surgery

Preoperative Diagnosis: Hemangioma, left cheek

Postoperative Diagnosis: Same

Operation: Excision of residual hemangioma, left cheek, and layered wound closure, 4 cm in length

History: This little girl presented as a baby with an enormous hemangioma on the left cheek just lateral to the commissure. This has been treated with laser and allowed to resolve. Following that, we removed a large portion of the central area of the hemangioma, placing the scar in the nasal alar crease. She is brought back today for removal of more of the residual hemangioma.

Procedure: The patient was placed on the operating table and anesthetized with endotracheal tube, prepared and draped in the usual fashion.

The old incision was now carefully opened after infiltrating with 0.5% zylocaine with adrenalin. The incision was extended upward and down just for a slight degree. The edges were now widely and extensively undermined underneath the residual hemangioma, out onto the cheek and then close to the commissure medially. A large wedge was now taken out medially and laterally, and care was taken not to take too much out to distort the commissure. The defect was now measured at 3.5 × 2 cm in diameter. The undermined edges were now carefully brought together and sutured into place with interrupted 4-0 Vicryl to the deeper layers and a running subcuticular 4-0 Monocryl to the skin. Steri-Strips and antibiotic ointment completed the procedure. She was then awakened and returned to recovery room in satisfactory condition.

Case 16 Code(s): _____

Case 17—Operative Report

Preoperative Diagnosis: Neurogenic bladder, status post Mitrofanoff and bladder augmentation with difficulty catheterizing Mitrofanoff

Postoperative Diagnosis: Mitrofanoff stenosis at the reimplant portion

Operation: Cystoscopy per Mitrofanoff and fulguration of Mitrofanoff channel and catheterization

Anesthesia: LMA

Indication: This is an 8-year-old girl with a history of spina bifida with neurogenic bowel and bladder. The patient is status post bladder augmentation and Mitrofanoff and appendiceal ACE. The patient had a Mitrofanoff revision last March and is still having difficulty inserting her catheter. The patient has had to have an indwelling catheter per her Mitrofanoff in the past several months.

Findings: On cystoscopy the patient had a dilated distal Mitrofanoff channel from the umbilicus down to her reimplant portion. There was a stenotic region at approximately 6 o'clock at the insertion into the bladder. The bladder appeared to have good capacity and no stones or tumor were noted. Bilateral ureteral orifices were visualized with reflux of clear urine.

Procedure: The patient was intubated by anesthesia and given IV Kefzol. The patient was placed in the supine position, prepared and draped in usual sterile fashion.

The Mitrofanoff channel was dilated with 12 French van Buren sounds. A 12 French cystoscope with 30-degree lens was used for intubation of the umbilicus per her Mitrofanoff channel, and we subsequently entered the bladder. Formal cystoscopy and evaluation of the Mitrofanoff under direct vision was performed. The patient had stenosis at the 6 o'clock region of her Mitrofanoff reimplant to the bladder. A 3 French Bugbee cautery set at 55 watts was used to cut this lip at 6 o'clock in her Mitrofanoff in the reimplant portion. The reimplanted region appeared to open up easily and was capacious. Cautery was then used to cauterize loose mucosa in the Mitrofanoff region at 55 watts. Good hemostasis was present.

The cystoscope sheath was subsequently removed and a 12 French silicone catheter was inserted without any problems into the bladder. The bladder was subsequently emptied and irrigated. The patient was extubated and sent in stable condition to the recovery room.

Case 17 Code(s): _____

Case 18—Operative Report

Chief Complaint: Patient requests insertion of IUD

Procedure: IUD Placement

Questions were encouraged and answered. The procedure was explained and the patient was counseled on risks in detail. Consent was obtained. Bi-manual exam was performed. Speculum was placed into the vagina and the cervix was cleaned and prepped in a sterile fashion. Tenaculum was applied to the cervix. The uterus was sounded to 7 cm. The copper IUD was inserted in typical fashion without complications. The strings were trimmed to 3 cm. Patient tolerated the procedure well and will recheck in one month.

Case 18 Code(s): _____

Case 19—Operative Report

Anesthesia: General endotracheal

Operative Indications: This man is admitted with fever, bacteremia, and sepsis. Preoperative CT of the abdomen shows a small cystic structure below the diaphragm in an area near a past surgical site. Abdominal metastasis from primary rectal CA is suspected. The patient also has significantly decreased blood flow to the lower extremities with femoral artery blockage demonstrated on preoperative arteriograms.

Operative Procedure: The patient was brought to the operating room and placed on the operating table in supine position. Following adequate induction of general endotracheal anesthesia and placement of invasive monitoring lines, the patient was prepared and draped in the usual sterile fashion. The initial procedure was creation of a right axilla to femoral to femoral extra anatomic bypass. This was done by exploring both groins through longitudinal incisions and mobilizing the common femoral, superficial femoral, and profunda femoris arteries bilaterally to the level of the inguinal ring. A tunnel was then made with blunt dissection between the two groin incisions above the external oblique fascia. The infraclavicular incision was then made in the right upper chest and the pectoralis major muscle divided along its fibers and the head of the pectoralis minor muscle was mobilized and completely divided from the coracoid process. The subclavian artery and proximal axillary artery were identified and then mobilized. The tunnel between the axillary incision and the right groin incision was made with the Garrett tunneler.

The right axilla to right femoral bypass was performed with 100-mm ringed PTFE graft. Prior to occlusion and opening of arteries, the patient received 5000 units of intravenous heparin. After 5 minutes, the axillary artery was occluded proximally and distally and then opened longitudinally. The proximal anastomosis to the axilla was performed with running 5-0 Prolene suture. Prior to completion of the anastomosis, the vessel was flushed both proximally and distally while occluding the graft. The anastomosis was completed and then blood flow was restored to the distal arm while maintaining occlusion of the graft. The graft was then trimmed to length in the right groin and arteriotomy made in the distal common femoral artery. The graft was fashioned and then the anastomosis was performed with running 6-0 Prolene suture. Prior to completion of the anastomosis, individual vessels were flushed as was the graft, and blood flow was restored first to the common femoral, then the profunda femoris artery, and finally the superficial femoral artery.

An 8-mm PTFE graft was brought through the suprapubic tunnel and the anastomosis performed in the left groin to the distal common femoral artery, again with running 6-0 Prolene suture. There was a large plaque along the medial wall of the common femoral artery, which was avoided. A small opening was left in this anastomosis for future flushing. The graft-to-graft anastomosis was then performed in the right groin in an inverted U fashion for the femoral-femoral bypass. Graftotomy was made and then the proximal graft-to-graft anastomosis performed with running 6-0 Prolene suture. The graft was flushed, the native vessels in the groin were backbled, and the anastomosis was completed. Blood flow was restored to the left leg.

Examination of the feet at this time revealed good capillary refill with warm feet. The wound was irrigated with copious amounts of neomycin solution and closed with interrupted 2-0 and 3-0 Dexon sutures and 3-0 Dermalon sutures for skin reapproximation. These wounds were then carefully dressed and excluded with Op-Site dressings.

The abdomen was then explored through an abdominal incision extending from xiphisternum to pubis. The patient had a previous and descending colon colostomy after having undergone a previous APR for rectal carcinoma. There were very few adhesions in the abdomen. Exploration, including palpation of the liver, revealed two small nodules, possibly metastatic carcinoma in the dome of the right lobe of the liver. The small bowel was reflected to the patient's right and one loop of ileum was adhesed to the sacral promontory. While mobilizing this adhesion, an old, large silk suture was encountered in the subdiaphragmatic area, which was involved in a suture abscess that contained 3 to 4 cc of pus and was drained and sent for aerobic and anaerobic cultures. The small bowel was densely adherent to this area but did not appear to have any fistula connection or defect in the integrity of the bowel wall. The retroperitoneum was densely inflamed but we were able to reclose the retroperitoneum with interrupted 3-0 and 3-0 Dexon sutures.

Wedge biopsy of the right lobe of the liver was performed in the area of the suspected metastatic disease. Hemostasis in the liver was obtained with Bovie cautery. The abdomen was then irrigated with copious amounts of neomycin solution and the abdominal fashion reapproximated with interrupted figure-of-8 #1 Prolene sutures with interrupted retention sutures of #2 Tycron. The skin was widely stapled and Betadine wound wicks placed in between the stapled areas. The patient tolerated the procedure well and was transported to the surgical intensive care unit in critical condition.

Case 19 Code(s): _____

Case 20—Operative Report

Pre-procedure Diagnoses: Paroxysmal Atrial fibrillation

Post-procedure Diagnoses: Same

Procedures: Cardioversion, elective

After obtaining informed consent, TEE ruled out intracardiac thrombus, patient was sedated by a total dose of 3 mg IV Versed and was treated by a single 170 Joule synchronized current and converted to normal sinus rhythm. During procedure, patient desaturated to 98% and developed more pulmonary congestion. At the end of the procedure, she was treated with a bolus of 80 mg IV Lasix.

Case 20 Code(s): _____

Crossword Puzzles

Reimbursement Puzzle

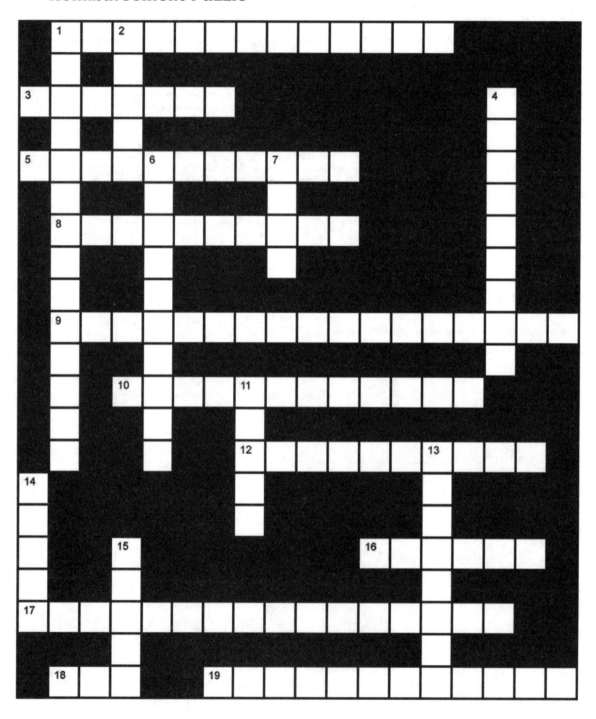

Reimbursement Puzzle Clues

Across

1. Provider status with Medicare where payment goes directly to the provider of care

3. Another term for insurance company

5. Internally, the standard charges for a practice

8. Database of the charges submitted for certain procedures by a physician over time

9. A number assigned to a procedure that describes its difficulty and expense in relationship to other procedures

10. Used to determine who is the primary payer for a claim

12. Used to track concerns about the payment of particular service codes

16. A signed statement from the patient stating the patient will pay if the claim is denied (also known as ABN)

17. Procedure must be done for an approved condition or it will not be covered

18. Federal agency that administers Medicare and publishes the standard billing form

19. The usual charge for a service by physicians of that specialty, in that geographic area

Down

1. The location where a service is performed

2. Basis for the Medicare fee schedule

4. Part of a procedure, such as technical

6. Payment of a fixed dollar amount for a covered person

7. Number replaced by the NPI that previously identified providers on claims

11. Coding system used to code supplies and drugs

13. Extra two digits used to clarify the meaning of a code for the service provided to that particular patient

14. A bill sent to an insurance company for payment

15. The number that describes the amount of service provided on a particular day, such as doses of medication

Coding Puzzle

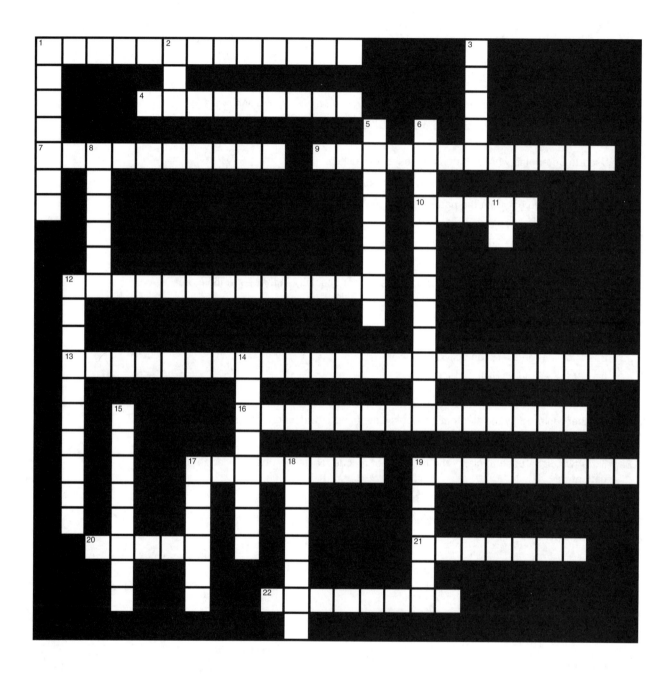

Coding Puzzle Clues

Across

1. Codes frequently replaced with G codes for Medicare
4. Included with laboratory in CPT
7. _____ and management
9. One of the components that can be billed
10. Used to start the process of coding
12. Includes the preoperative, intraoperative, and postoperative care
13. Rules for reporting physician services
16. Radiologic supervision and _____
17. Appropriately coding all the components of one procedure with one code
19. Separates main CPT entry from variable portion of description
20. Laboratory tests listed together for coding purposes
21. Sizes are added together when coding
22. Codes to be used when other codes are inadequate at describing the service

Down

1. _____ Procedural Terminology
2. Publishes CPT
3. Published by CMS
5. Helps tell the story of a particular coding event
6. Should be charged each time blood is drawn
8. Cycle on which the hard-copy CPT book is published
11. Two letters associated with physician service coding
12. Found in the front of each CPT section
14. Universal change symbol
15. _____ procedure means "not carried out as an integral component of a total service"
17. Indicates a new code in CPT
18. Matching ICD-9-CM codes to CPT codes on a claim
19. Chemistry tests are coded the same, regardless of _____ of specimen

Cross-Code Puzzle

Cross-Code Puzzle Clues

NOTE: All answers are codes and/or modifiers.

Across

1. Revision of peripheral neurostimulator pulse receiver
5. Renal vein rennin stimulation panel
6. Bilateral partial excision of turbinate
7. Mandated
8. Two blood chloride tests on same day
9. Laparoscopic cryosurgical ablation of liver tumor
13. Procedure when infants are less than 4 kg
14. Fluoroscopy by physician, of more than 1 hour to assist a nonradiologic physician
15. RS&I of shoulder arthrography procedure
18. Open treatment of radial and ulnar shaft fracture with internal fixation of ulna, done as a second procedure during the operative session
20. DTaP vaccine
22. Facial lesion, 2.1 cm, shaved
23. Capsulorrhaphy, anterior with bone block, discontinued after anesthesia
25. Destruction of lingual tonsil
26. Ureterocolon conduit on a patient with previous intestinal surgery
27. Open treatment of a rib fracture without fixation
28. Removal of maxillary tori

Down

1. Scleral buckling
2. Expanded problem focused history, expanded problem focused examination, and low medical decision making done in the home
3. Professional component of an MRI of brain without contrast
4. Exploration of orbit with removal of lesion
5. Lipoma specimen
8. Antibody, tetanus
10. Magnetic resonance spectroscopy, professional component
11. Change of dressing on small burn
12. Left hand, second digit
16. Saphenopopliteal vein anastomosis, assistant surgeon, on a related procedure requiring return to OR procedure during the postop period
17. UFR
19. Lysis of penile postcircumcision adhesions
20. External ocular photography done on the remaining eye of a patient with previous enucleation
21. One allergy injection given at the office of the allergist who provided the extract
24. T&A, age 8
27. E/M, not in the global period

Surgical Case Audit Exercise

1. Review the documentation provided for each case using the criteria on the review form provided for each case. Insert your name and the date of your review on each form.

2. Code each case and compare your codes to those on the CMS-1500 form excerpt for that case. If there are differences (variations) between the billed codes and your codes, categorize your findings using the key provided on the review form (findings A through I).

3. Document the detailed findings (results of your coding review) on the detailed findings form.

4. Document a summary of your findings (both the documentation questions and your coding review) on the summary of findings form. Enter the percentage of times the particular documentation criteria were met for each case.

Surgical Case Listing

Patient Name	MRN	Date of Service	Surgeon
Frances Zimmerman	16-42-10	3-3-XX	Martin Stengl
Michael Foltman	24-04-19	4-15-XX	Janice Kelly
John Magill	39-41-62	7-14-XX	Jeffrey Blanchard
Paul Garity	14-22-18	5-1-XX	Henry Taylor
Renee Radke	31-29-93	11-17-XX	Linda Yang

Surgical Audit—Summary of Findings

Reviewer: _____ Review Date: _____ Cases Reviewed: _____

Surgical documentation was reviewed using the established documentation criteria. The findings were as follows:

Patient identification was complete	_____
Surgical date was present	_____
Preoperative diagnosis was present	_____
Postoperative diagnosis was present	_____
Name of procedure was present	_____
Indication for procedure was present	_____
Anesthesia type was present	_____

Coding issues determined during the review:

1. _____
   _____

2. _____
   _____

3. _____
   _____

Recommendations:

1. _____
   _____

2. _____
   _____

3. _____
   _____

Surgical Audit—Detailed Findings

Reviewer: _____

Review Date: _____

Case #	Patient Name	MRN	DOS	Surgeon	Billed ICD-9-CM	Documented ICD-9-CM	Findings	Billed CPT	Documented CPT	Findings
1	Frances Zimmerman	16-42-10	3-3-XX	Martin Stengl	815.03			26615		
2	Michael Foltman	24-04-19	4-15-XX	Janice Kelly	569.89			45388		
3	John Magill	39-41-62	7-14-XX	Jeffrey Blanchard	574.10			47600 44955-51		
4	Paul Garity	14-22-18	5-1-XX	Henry Taylor	724.2 724.4			64483		
5	Renee Radke	31-29-93	11-17-XX	Linda Yang	378.31			67314		

Findings Key:

A = Inaccurate Dx code
B = Omission of Additional Dx
C = Overcoding of Dx

D = Inaccurate CPT code
E = Omission of CPT code
F = Overcoding of CPT code

G = Inaccurate Modifier
H = Omission of Modifier
I = Overcoding of Modifier

431

Case 1—Day Surgery

Patient Name: Frances Zimmerman

MRN: 16-42-10

Date of Surgery: 3-3-XX

Preoperative Diagnosis: Displaced closed right ring finger metacarpal fracture

Postoperative Diagnosis: Displaced closed right ring finger metacarpal fracture

Anesthesia: General

Surgeon: Martin Stengl, MD

Description of Procedure: The patient was taken into the operating room and draped in a normal sterile manner. General anesthesia was obtained. From there, the arm was exsanguinated and tourniquet inflated to 250 mm Hg. Once that was done, an incision was made dorsally over the metacarpal to the ring finger. The skin was retracted protecting dorsal branches of vessels and nerves. The extensor tendons were seen to be intact. They were retracted so that the fracture site could be visualized. An incision was made over the periosteum of the metacarpal. This was reflected radially and ulnarly. The fracture site was visualized and was irrigated to remove any coagulum or debris. The fracture was reduced. Two 1.5-mm lag screws were placed in the usual fashion. Periosteum was closed over the metacarpal. The skin was closed using 4-0 interrupted chromic catgut suture for the subcutaneous layer and 4-0 running and interrupted nylon sutures for the skin. Local anesthetic was placed in the area of the fracture and incision to aid in comfort during recovery.

Signature: Martin Stengl, MD

21. DIAGNOSIS OR NATURE OF ILLNESS OR INJURY Relate A-L to service line below (24E)		ICD Ind.		22. RESUBMISSION CODE		ORIGINAL REF. NO.
A. _____ B. _____	C. _____ D. _____					
E. _____ F. _____	G. _____ H. _____			23. PRIOR AUTHORIZATION NUMBER		
I. _____ J. _____	K. _____ L. _____					

24. A. DATE(S) OF SERVICE From — To		B. PLACE OF SERVICE	C. EMG	D. PROCEDURES, SERVICES, OR SUPPLIES (Explain Unusual Circumstances) CPT/HCPCS | MODIFIER	E. DIAGNOSIS POINTER	F. $ CHARGES	G. DAYS OR UNITS	H. EPSDT Family Plan	I. ID. QUAL.	J. RENDERING PROVIDER ID. #
MM DD YY | MM DD YY										
1									NPI	
2									NPI	
3									NPI	
4									NPI	
5									NPI	
6									NPI	

Case 1: Surgical Audit Review Form

MRN: _____ Date of Service: _____

Patient Name: _____ Reviewer: _____

Report Evaluation:

Documentation Criteria	Yes	No	N/A
Patient identification complete?	_____	_____	_____
Surgical date present?	_____	_____	_____
Preoperative diagnosis present?	_____	_____	_____
Postoperative diagnosis present?	_____	_____	_____
Name of procedure present?	_____	_____	_____
Indication for procedure present?	_____	_____	_____
Anesthesia type present?	_____	_____	_____
Surgeon(s) and assistant(s) present?	_____	_____	_____
Procedure details present?	_____	_____	_____
Specimen(s) sent?	_____	_____	_____
Blood loss present?	_____	_____	_____
Complications present?	_____	_____	_____
Signature present?	_____	_____	_____

Coding Evaluation:

		Claim Codes	Reviewer Codes	Findings*
ICD-10-CM Dx Codes	1	_____	_____	_____
	2	_____	_____	_____
	3	_____	_____	_____
	4	_____	_____	_____
CPT/HCPCS Codes (Include modifier[s] with code)	1	_____	_____	_____
	2	_____	_____	_____
	3	_____	_____	_____
	4	_____	_____	_____
	5	_____	_____	_____
	6	_____	_____	_____

*Findings Key:

A = Inaccurate Dx code   D = Inaccurate CPT code   G = Inaccurate modifier
B = Omission of additional Dx   E = Omission of CPT code   H = Omission of modifier
C = Overcoding of Dx   F = Overcoding of CPT code   I = Overcoding of modifier

Comments:

_____

_____

_____

Recommendations:

_____

_____

_____

Case 2—Operative Report

Patient Name: Michael Foltman

MRN: 24-04-19

Date of Procedure: 4-15-XX

Procedure: Colonoscopy

Indications: The patient is a 26-year-old with a history of abdominal pain, bloody stools, and CT results consistent with inflammatory bowel disease. Consent obtained.

Anesthesia: General

Surgeon: Janice Kelly, MD

Procedure Note: Following adequate sedation, the patient was positioned for colonoscopy. The colonoscope was placed in the anus and advanced to the terminal ileum. Biopsies from the terminal ileum, cecum, ascending, descending, transverse, and rectosigmoid areas were obtained. Mucosa through the colon looked normal. Mucosa in the terminal ileum appeared erythematous with three small areas of white plaque. Biopsies were obtained and the areas of plaque were ablated. The scope was withdrawn and the patient tolerated the procedure well with no complications.

Assessment: Lesions within the terminal ileum.

Signature: Janice Kelly, MD

21. DIAGNOSIS OR NATURE OF ILLNESS OR INJURY Relate A-L to service line below (24E)			ICD Ind.	22. RESUBMISSION CODE	ORIGINAL REF. NO.
A.	B.	C.	D.		
E.	F.	G.	H.	23. PRIOR AUTHORIZATION NUMBER	
I.	J.	K.	L.		

24. A. DATE(S) OF SERVICE From MM DD YY To MM DD YY	B. PLACE OF SERVICE	C. EMG	D. PROCEDURES, SERVICES, OR SUPPLIES (Explain Unusual Circumstances) CPT/HCPCS | MODIFIER	E. DIAGNOSIS POINTER	F. $ CHARGES	G. DAYS OR UNITS	H. EPSDT Family Plan	I. ID. QUAL.	J. RENDERING PROVIDER ID. #
1								NPI	
2								NPI	
3								NPI	
4								NPI	
5								NPI	
6								NPI	

Case 2: Surgical Audit Review Form

MRN: _____ Date of Service: _____

Patient Name: _____ Reviewer: _____

Report Evaluation:

Documentation Criteria	Yes	No	N/A
Patient identification complete?	_____	_____	_____
Surgical date present?	_____	_____	_____
Preoperative diagnosis present?	_____	_____	_____
Postoperative diagnosis present?	_____	_____	_____
Name of procedure present?	_____	_____	_____
Indication for procedure present?	_____	_____	_____
Anesthesia type present?	_____	_____	_____
Surgeon(s) and assistant(s) present?	_____	_____	_____
Procedure details present?	_____	_____	_____
Specimen(s) sent?	_____	_____	_____
Blood loss present?	_____	_____	_____
Complications present?	_____	_____	_____
Signature present?	_____	_____	_____

Coding Evaluation:

		Claim Codes	Reviewer Codes	Findings*
ICD-10-CM Dx Codes	1	_____	_____	_____
	2	_____	_____	_____
	3	_____	_____	_____
	4	_____	_____	_____
CPT/HCPCS Codes (Include modifier[s] with code)	1	_____	_____	_____
	2	_____	_____	_____
	3	_____	_____	_____
	4	_____	_____	_____
	5	_____	_____	_____
	6	_____	_____	_____

*Findings Key:

A = Inaccurate Dx code	D = Inaccurate CPT code	G = Inaccurate modifier
B = Omission of additional Dx	E = Omission of CPT code	H = Omission of modifier
C = Overcoding of Dx	F = Overcoding of CPT code	I = Overcoding of modifier

Comments:

_____

_____

_____

Recommendations:

_____

_____

_____

Case 3—Operative Report

Patient Name: John Magill

MRN: 39-41-62

Date of Surgery: 7-14-XX

Preoperative Diagnosis: Cholelithiasis and chronic cholecystitis

Postoperative Diagnosis: Same

Anesthesia: General

Operation: Cholecystectomy

Surgeon: Jeffrey Blanchard, MD

Procedure: Under general anesthesia and after Betadine preparation and drape, a right subcostal incision was made.

The muscles were cut with electrocautery. The abdomen was opened, entered, and explored. The gallbladder had a number of adhesions and palpable stones. The adhesions were taken down. The wound was packed off. The cystic artery was long and anterior to the common duct. It was doubly clipped and transected near the entrance to the gallbladder. The cystic duct was quite long. It was dissected for a portion, and then the gallbladder was removed

in an antegrade manner. The base of the liver bed was then electrocauterized dry. The cystic duct was dissected down to the junction of the common duct where it was triply clipped, transected, and submitted. The wound was irrigated clean and dry. No drain was used. Packings were removed. The cecum was exteriorized, and the appendix was taken down between hemostats on the mesoappendix and tied with #2-0 silk. The base was encircled with #3-0 silk, cross-clamped, tied with #2-0 chromic catgut suture, inverted in the pursestring, and reinforced with additional Lembert sutures. The wound was then closed using #0 Dexon clips, irrigation in all layers with Kantrex solution, #3-0 Dexon subcutaneously. Marcaine 20 cc was then used in the muscle and subcutaneous space. Skin staples closed the skin. Dressings were applied. The patient returned to the recovery room in satisfactory condition.

Specimens sent: Gallbladder and appendix

Signature: Jeffrey Blanchard, MD

21. DIAGNOSIS OR NATURE OF ILLNESS OR INJURY Relate A-L to service line below (24E) ICD Ind.						22. RESUBMISSION CODE ORIGINAL REF. NO.					
A. ___ B. ___ C. ___ D. ___											
E. ___ F. ___ G. ___ H. ___						23. PRIOR AUTHORIZATION NUMBER					
I. ___ J. ___ K. ___ L. ___											
24. A. DATE(S) OF SERVICE			B. PLACE OF SERVICE	C. EMG	D. PROCEDURES, SERVICES, OR SUPPLIES (Explain Unusual Circumstances) CPT/HCPCS | MODIFIER	E. DIAGNOSIS POINTER	F. $ CHARGES	G. DAYS OR UNITS	H. EPSDT Family Plan	I. ID. QUAL.	J. RENDERING PROVIDER ID. #
From MM DD YY	To MM DD YY										
1										NPI	
2										NPI	
3										NPI	
4										NPI	
5										NPI	
6										NPI	

Case 3: Surgical Audit Review Form

MRN: _____ Date of Service: _____

Patient Name: _____ Reviewer: _____

Report Evaluation:

Documentation Criteria	Yes	No	N/A
Patient identification complete?	_____	_____	_____
Surgical date present?	_____	_____	_____
Preoperative diagnosis present?	_____	_____	_____
Postoperative diagnosis present?	_____	_____	_____
Name of procedure present?	_____	_____	_____
Indication for procedure present?	_____	_____	_____
Anesthesia type present?	_____	_____	_____
Surgeon(s) and assistant(s) present?	_____	_____	_____
Procedure details present?	_____	_____	_____
Specimen(s) sent?	_____	_____	_____
Blood loss present?	_____	_____	_____
Complications present?	_____	_____	_____
Signature present?	_____	_____	_____

Coding Evaluation:

		Claim Codes	Reviewer Codes	Findings*
ICD-10-CM Dx Codes	1	_____	_____	_____
	2	_____	_____	_____
	3	_____	_____	_____
	4	_____	_____	_____
CPT/HCPCS Codes (Include modifier[s] with code)	1	_____	_____	_____
	2	_____	_____	_____
	3	_____	_____	_____
	4	_____	_____	_____
	5	_____	_____	_____
	6	_____	_____	_____

*Findings Key:

A = Inaccurate Dx code	D = Inaccurate CPT code	G = Inaccurate modifier
B = Omission of additional Dx	E = Omission of CPT code	H = Omission of modifier
C = Overcoding of Dx	F = Overcoding of CPT code	I = Overcoding of modifier

Comments:

_____

_____

_____

Recommendations:

_____

_____

_____

Case 4—Operative Report

Patient Name: Paul Garity

MRN: 14-12-18

Date of Surgery: 5-1-XX

Preoperative Diagnosis: Low back pain with radiculopathy

Postoperative Diagnosis: Same

Anesthesia: 1% lidocaine

Surgeon: Henry Taylor, MD

Discussion: The patient had his first lumbar epidural steroid injection in April. Following that injection, he had approximately 36 hours of very good relief of painful symptoms. He then resumed full normal activity, possibly increased somewhat because he felt so good, and by the end of the next 24 hours he had return of most of the preprocedure symptoms. In the ensuing days, the pain has continued to be moderately severe. He has had no new numbness or weakness. After discussing the procedure, alternatives, and expectations and strongly encouraging him to resume normal activity much more judiciously, the patient agrees to his second lumbar epidural steroid injection.

Description of Operation: In a sitting position, after Betadine preparation and under sterile technique, 1% preservative-free lidocaine was used to inject the skin and deeper tissues over the L4-L5 interspace. An 18-gauge Tuohy epidural needle was used to identify the epidural space at a depth of 6 cm. No CSF, blood, or paraesthesias were noted. Methylprednisolone 100 mg and 1% preservative-free lidocaine, 2.5 cc were injected slowly. After 20 minutes of bed rest, the patient was able to ambulate without difficulty and was discharged home to be followed by telephone.

Signature: Henry Taylor, MD

21. DIAGNOSIS OR NATURE OF ILLNESS OR INJURY Relate A-L to service line below (24E)				ICD Ind.		22. RESUMISSION CODE	ORIGINAL REF. NO.
A. ___	B. ___	C. ___	D. ___				
E. ___	F. ___	G. ___	H. ___			23. PRIOR AUTHORIZATION NUMBER	
I. ___	J. ___	K. ___	L. ___				

24. A. DATE(S) OF SERVICE From MM DD YY To MM DD YY	B. PLACE OF SERVICE	C. EMG	D. PROCEDURES, SERVICES, OR SUPPLIES (Explain Unusual Circumstances) CPT/HCPCS | MODIFIER	E. DIAGNOSIS POINTER	F. $ CHARGES	G. DAYS OR UNITS	H. EPSDT Family Plan	I. ID. QUAL.	J. RENDERING PROVIDER ID. #
1								NPI	
2								NPI	
3								NPI	
4								NPI	
5								NPI	
6								NPI	

Case 4: Surgical Audit Review Form

MRN: _____ Date of Service: _____

Patient Name: _____ Reviewer: _____

Report Evaluation:

Documentation Criteria	Yes	No	N/A
Patient identification complete?	_____	_____	_____
Surgical date present?	_____	_____	_____
Preoperative diagnosis present?	_____	_____	_____
Postoperative diagnosis present?	_____	_____	_____
Name of procedure present?	_____	_____	_____
Indication for procedure present?	_____	_____	_____
Anesthesia type present?	_____	_____	_____
Surgeon(s) and assistant(s) present?	_____	_____	_____
Procedure details present?	_____	_____	_____
Specimen(s) sent?	_____	_____	_____
Blood loss present?	_____	_____	_____
Complications present?	_____	_____	_____
Signature present?	_____	_____	_____

Coding Evaluation:

		Claim Codes	Reviewer Codes	Findings*
ICD-10-CM Dx Codes	1	_____	_____	_____
	2	_____	_____	_____
	3	_____	_____	_____
	4	_____	_____	_____
CPT/HCPCS Codes (Include modifier[s] with code)	1	_____	_____	_____
	2	_____	_____	_____
	3	_____	_____	_____
	4	_____	_____	_____
	5	_____	_____	_____
	6	_____	_____	_____

*Findings Key:

A = Inaccurate Dx code
B = Omission of additional Dx
C = Overcoding of Dx

D = Inaccurate CPT code
E = Omission of CPT code
F = Overcoding of CPT code

G = Inaccurate modifier
H = Omission of modifier
I = Overcoding of modifier

Comments:

_____
_____
_____

Recommendations:

_____
_____
_____

Case 5—Operative Report

Patient Name: Renee Radke

MRN: 31-29-93

Date of Surgery: 11-17-XX

Preoperative Diagnosis: Hypertropia

Postoperative Diagnosis: Same

Procedure: Recess right superior rectus muscle 5.0 mm

Anesthesia: General by LMA

Complications: None

Surgeon: Linda Yang, MD

Description of Procedure: The patient was taken to the operating room and given general anesthesia by LMA. The right eye was prepared and draped in a normal sterile ophthalmic fashion. A lid speculum was placed in the right eye and traction sutures placed with the eye rotated down and out. The right superior rectus muscle was then isolated from a Formix approach with care taken to make sure that the entire muscle was incorporated on the hook. A double-armed 6-0 Vicryl suture was then woven through the distal muscle tendon in locking fashion and the muscle disinserted from the globe. Hemostasis was obtained with bipolar cautery. The needles were then passed through superficial sclera 5.0 mm posterior to the original insertion and the muscle tied down firmly into this position. The conjunctival wound was closed with interrupted 7-0 Vicryl sutures. Erythromycin ointment was applied to the right eye. The patient was awakened and taken to the recovery room in good condition.

Signature: Linda Yang, MD

21. DIAGNOSIS OR NATURE OF ILLNESS OR INJURY Relate A-L to service line below (24E)					ICD Ind.		22. RESUBMISSION CODE		ORIGINAL REF. NO.	
A.	B.	C.	D.							
E.	F.	G.	H.				23. PRIOR AUTHORIZATION NUMBER			
I.	J.	K.	L.							

24. A. DATE(S) OF SERVICE From MM DD YY To MM DD YY	B. PLACE OF SERVICE	C. EMG	D. PROCEDURES, SERVICES, OR SUPPLIES (Explain Unusual Circumstances) CPT/HCPCS | MODIFIER	E. DIAGNOSIS POINTER	F. $ CHARGES	G. DAYS OR UNITS	H. EPSDT Family Plan	I. ID. QUAL.	J. RENDERING PROVIDER ID. #
1								NPI	
2								NPI	
3								NPI	
4								NPI	
5								NPI	
6								NPI	

Case 5: Surgical Audit Review Form

MRN: _____ Date of Service: _____

Patient Name: _____ Reviewer: _____

Report Evaluation:

Documentation Criteria	Yes	No	N/A
Patient identification complete?	_____	_____	_____
Surgical date present?	_____	_____	_____
Preoperative diagnosis present?	_____	_____	_____
Postoperative diagnosis present?	_____	_____	_____
Name of procedure present?	_____	_____	_____
Indication for procedure present?	_____	_____	_____
Anesthesia type present?	_____	_____	_____
Surgeon(s) and assistant(s) present?	_____	_____	_____
Procedure details present?	_____	_____	_____
Specimen(s) sent?	_____	_____	_____
Blood loss present?	_____	_____	_____
Complications present?	_____	_____	_____
Signature present?	_____	_____	_____

Coding Evaluation:

		Claim Codes	Reviewer Codes	Findings*
ICD-10-CM Dx Codes	1	_____	_____	_____
	2	_____	_____	_____
	3	_____	_____	_____
	4	_____	_____	_____
CPT/HCPCS Codes (Include modifier[s] with code)	1	_____	_____	_____
	2	_____	_____	_____
	3	_____	_____	_____
	4	_____	_____	_____
	5	_____	_____	_____
	6	_____	_____	_____

*Findings Key:

A = Inaccurate Dx code	D = Inaccurate CPT code	G = Inaccurate modifier
B = Omission of additional Dx	E = Omission of CPT code	H = Omission of modifier
C = Overcoding of Dx	F = Overcoding of CPT code	I = Overcoding of modifier

Comments:

_____

_____

_____

Recommendations:

_____

_____

_____

Evaluation and Management Audit Exercise

1. Review the documentation provided for each case using the 1995 E/M Documentation Guidelines and the form provided.

2. Code each case and compare code(s) to those on the attached CMS-1500 excerpt for that case.

3. Document the detailed findings and summary for your audit on the health record audit summary form. Summarize your findings and provide recommendations based on review.

Health Record Audit
Audit Details

Case #	CPT Code(s) Submitted	History	Exam	Medical Decision Making	Reviewer CPT Code(s)
1	99202				
2	99242–25 59200				
3	99215				
4	99243				
5	99212 81000				

Audit Summary

_____ E/M documentation appears to support the code submitted.

_____ E/M documentation appears to support a lower level of service than the code submitted.

_____ E/M documentation appears to support a higher level of service than the code submitted.

_____ Consultation does not meet established criteria.

_____ Other issues noted:

_____

_____

_____

_____

Accuracy Rate: _____%

Recommendations for improvement:

_____

_____

_____

Audit Case #1—Visit Note

CC: Right knee pain

S: The patient notes he has had pain in the knee on the right side for a couple of weeks. Sometimes he will get a shot of pain and have the knee give way, but this is more from his discomfort than functional difficulty with the knee. The left knee hurts a bit anteriorly. The right knee generally hurts in the biceps tendons more medially than laterally. The patient has taken occasional anti-inflammatory medication for it, but nothing regularly. No injuries and no effusion have been reported.

O: This is a pleasant 48-year-old man who is new to my practice. Weight is 200 lb. Normal vital signs. No distress. Range of motion of the knee is good. Good muscular tone to the legs. No palpable tenderness anteriorly, no effusion. He is tender to medial and lateral biceps tendons of the right knee. Negative Lachman's, negative drawer sign, no McMurray testing. X-rays requested by me and taken at the hospital today were called back to me, showing minimal degenerative changes.

A: Right femoral biceps tendonitis

P: Naprosyn 500 mg b.i.d. routinely for 5 days as well as heat to the area, p.r.n. thereafter. Follow up if not improving. If necessary, will consider orthopedic evaluation at that time.

Answer:

History: _____

Examination: _____

Medical Decision Making: _____

E/M Code: _____

CMS-1500 Excerpt: _____

21. DIAGNOSIS OR NATURE OF ILLNESS OR INJURY Relate A-L to service line below (24E) ICD Ind.			22. RESUBMISSION CODE ORIGINAL REF. NO.
A. ____ B. ____ C. ____ D. ____			
E. ____ F. ____ G. ____ H. ____			23. PRIOR AUTHORIZATION NUMBER
I. ____ J. ____ K. ____ L. ____			

24. A. DATE(S) OF SERVICE From MM DD YY / To MM DD YY	B. PLACE OF SERVICE	C. EMG	D. PROCEDURES, SERVICES, OR SUPPLIES (Explain Unusual Circumstances) CPT/HCPCS | MODIFIER	E. DIAGNOSIS POINTER	F. $ CHARGES	G. DAYS OR UNITS	H. EPSDT Family Plan	I. ID. QUAL.	J. RENDERING PROVIDER ID. #
1			99202					NPI	
2								NPI	
3								NPI	
4								NPI	
5								NPI	
6								NPI	

Audit Case #2—Visit Note

Requested by Dr. Harting

CC: Fetal demise on ultrasound

S: This is a 33-year-old caucasian female, gravida 5, para 3-0-1-3, now 16-1/7 weeks pregnant. She was seen yesterday by her family practice physician, Dr. Harting, for a normal prenatal appointment. The patient has not felt fetal movement as of yet. The ultrasound in Dr. Harting's office showed fetal demise at 16.1 weeks. Dr. Harting could not find fetal heart tones by Doppler. The patient did have a second trimester pregnancy lost last year with Prostin induction in Labor and Delivery, transferred to my care at that time. This fetus did demonstrate triploidy. She has no history of asthma or any medical problems. She is Rh positive. Her pregnancy, otherwise, has been uncomplicated.

O: Vital signs are normal. I discussed in detail the treatment plan. I gave her the option of being admitted for a D&E. I explained to her in detail what D&E involved. However, the patient wanted to be admitted for Prostin pellet induction. She understands the risks of this. I placed *Laminaria*, a midthick piece into the cervical os. The uterus is about 15-week size. It is nontender. The os is closed.

A: Fetal demise at 16+ weeks

P: The patient will be admitted tomorrow to the Labor and Delivery unit. We will give her a 20-mg Prostin induction in the morning after *Laminaria* is removed. The patient was advised to report immediately to the hospital for admission if she had any problems during the night. She understands the risks of retained placenta and that the potential for D&C is necessary. We will send fetal tissue for cytogenetics. I will continue to see this patient in follow-up and will provide care for any future pregnancies, treating her in our high-risk program.

Answer:

History: _____

Examination: _____

Medical Decision Making: _____

E/M Code: _____

CMS-1500 Excerpt: _____

21. DIAGNOSIS OR NATURE OF ILLNESS OR INJURY Relate A-L to service line below (24E)			ICD Ind.	22. RESUBMISSION CODE	ORIGINAL REF. NO.
A.	B.	C.	D.		
E.	F.	G.	H.	23. PRIOR AUTHORIZATION NUMBER	
I.	J.	K.	L.		

24. A. DATE(S) OF SERVICE From / To MM DD YY MM DD YY	B. PLACE OF SERVICE	C. EMG	D. PROCEDURES, SERVICES, OR SUPPLIES (Explain Unusual Circumstances) CPT/HCPCS	MODIFIER	E. DIAGNOSIS POINTER	F. $ CHARGES	G. DAYS OR UNITS	H. EPSDT Family Plan	I. ID. QUAL.	J. RENDERING PROVIDER ID. #
1			99242	25					NPI	
2			59200						NPI	
3									NPI	
4									NPI	
5									NPI	
6									NPI	

Audit Case #3—Visit Note

CC: Discuss test results

S: This 26-year-old patient is still complaining about persistent fatigue symptoms and sweating. She denies any significant problem otherwise. Today's visit is to discuss the test results of 10 days ago.

O: No examination today because detailed examination was done at the last visit. Recent blood test shows hemoglobin 13.4, hematocrit 38.6, platelet count 240,000 with a normal differential count, and WBC count of 5.6. The only abnormality in the CBC noticed was macrocytosis with MCV of 102 and MCH of 353. Folic acid level reported normal at 12.3, glucose of 122, which is slightly elevated, but still under the 126, so it is suggestive of impaired glucose function. Vitamin B_{12} reported 429 as normal. Total cholesterol 214, slightly elevated with normal HDL and LDL. Liver function tests are normal, as is the thyroid function test.

1. Impaired glucose function with elevated blood sugar, but not to the point of being classified as diabetes type II

2. Macrocytosis, could be related to smoking or alcohol use because vitamin B_{12}, folic acid, and thyroid function tests are all normal

3. Mild elevation of the total cholesterol, but HDL, LDL, and triglycerides are normal

4. Normal liver function test

P: The above results were explained to the patient in detail. I spent 25 minutes out of a 25-minute visit on counseling. I suggested at this time that I would not recommend anything else. Symptoms may abate and disappear by themselves. I do not have any clear-cut reason for the symptoms of fatigue and sweating after going through all the blood tests and recent physical. I can only suspect the probability of a recent viral infection, especially mononucleosis infection, in light of a positive EBV, IgG titer. This was discussed with the patient. The patient will return in 2 weeks for reevaluation or sooner if new symptoms develop or her condition gets worse.

Answer:

History: _____

Examination: _____

Medical Decision Making: _____

E/M Code: _____

CMS-1500 Excerpt: _____

21. DIAGNOSIS OR NATURE OF ILLNESS OR INJURY Relate A-L to service line below (24E)		ICD Ind.		22. RESUBMISSION CODE		ORIGINAL REF. NO.				
A. |_____ B. |_____ C. |_____ D. |_____										
E. |_____ F. |_____ G. |_____ H. |_____				23. PRIOR AUTHORIZATION NUMBER						
I. |_____ J. |_____ K. |_____ L. |_____										

24. A. DATE(S) OF SERVICE From / To	B. PLACE OF SERVICE	C. EMG	D. PROCEDURES, SERVICES, OR SUPPLIES (Explain Unusual Circumstances) CPT/HCPCS | MODIFIER	E. DIAGNOSIS POINTER	F. $ CHARGES	G. DAYS OR UNITS	H. EPSDT Family Plan	I. ID. QUAL.	J. RENDERING PROVIDER ID. #
1			99215					NPI	
2								NPI	
3								NPI	
4								NPI	
5								NPI	
6								NPI	

Audit Case #4—Visit Note

Requested by L. Kline, MD

CC: Tired

S: I saw this 42-year-old man last year for evaluation of obstructive sleep apnea. His primary physician again requests him to be evaluated. He had a sleep study done in the past that revealed moderate obstructive sleep apnea syndrome. See past patient questionnaire on waking/sleeping and his update done today. His wife called earlier today in preparation for his appointment to tell us that her husband has been falling asleep every night by at least 7 o'clock for the past month. She reports that he seems to have lost his energy and has no drive to pursue anything, and she feels that his sleep apnea is more severe than it was when we saw him last. He doesn't report as much difference as his wife does. He reports that he did not tolerate the CPAP at all. It created some nasal congestion for him. He takes the mask off during the night and cannot tolerate it. He does awake with headaches frequently as well. He lives with his wife. They have no children. He is employed as an accountant and leads a very sedentary lifestyle.

O: His nose reveals a moderate degree of edema in the left side. His right side is clear today. Oral cavity reveals an elongation hypertrophy of the soft palate. Tonsils are still present with 1+ hypertrophy. He has redundant posterior wall mucosa with a Fujita type II appearance. His nasopharynx, hypopharynx, and larynx are normal. His head and face appear normal, and his neck examination was unremarkable. Cranial nerves 2 through 10 are normal. His weight is stable at 230 lb with BP and vitals WNL.

A: Obstructive sleep apnea syndrome

P: The treatment options were discussed with him. These would include CPAP, which we know he does not tolerate well, a tracheotomy of which the pros and cons are usually fairly obvious, or uvulopalatopharyngoplasty. The patient understands that there is no medication that can make a positive impact. The risks of surgery, including those from general anesthesia, bleeding, and pain, were discussed, as was nasopharyngeal regurgitation. I also discussed with him the potential outcome from surgery, which is a 50 to 70 percent success rate on a long-term basis. He is interested in pursuing a surgical alternative as opposed to the CPAP. He will proceed with this and determine whether he can get approval for this from his insurance company. If approved, he will call our office to schedule surgery.

cc: Dr. L. Kline by fax

Answer:

History: _____

Examination: _____

Medical Decision Making: _____

E/M Code: _____

CMS-1500 Excerpt: _____

21. DIAGNOSIS OR NATURE OF ILLNESS OR INJURY Relate A-L to service line below (24E)		ICD Ind.		22. RESUBMISSION CODE		ORIGINAL REF. NO.

A. _____ B. _____ C. _____ D. _____

E. _____ F. _____ G. _____ H. _____

23. PRIOR AUTHORIZATION NUMBER

I. _____ J. _____ K. _____ L. _____

24. A. DATE(S) OF SERVICE From To						B. PLACE OF SERVICE	C. EMG	D. PROCEDURES, SERVICES, OR SUPPLIES (Explain Unusual Circumstances) CPT/HCPCS MODIFIER	E. DIAGNOSIS POINTER	F. $ CHARGES	G. DAYS OR UNITS	H. EPSDT Family Plan	I. ID. QUAL.	J. RENDERING PROVIDER ID. #
MM	DD	YY	MM	DD	YY									
1								99243					NPI	
2													NPI	
3													NPI	
4													NPI	
5													NPI	
6													NPI	

Audit Case #5—Visit Note

CC—Painful urination

S—This patient has noticed significant dysuria in the past 24 to 48 hours. On Sunday, she had a few slight sharp pains in the right pelvis. On Monday, she developed frequency. On Tuesday, she developed dysuria. She also has a headache today and some slight chills, but no back pain or no documented fever. She has no known drug allergies. To her knowledge, she has never had a urinary tract infection.

O—On examination, she is nontoxic and afebrile. Blood pressure 102/70. Temperature 97.8° F. Her bladder is not tender to palpation. She has no costovertebral angle tenderness. Her urine dip in the office today shows 10 to 25 RBCs per high-power field and 3–5 WBCs per high-power microscopic field.

A—Urinary tract infection.

P—We will treat with Bactrim-DS twice a day for 3 days and Pyridium 200 mg 1 twice a day p.r.n. for the next 2 days. Patient was advised that the Pyridium will turn her urine bright red. She is to call if her symptoms do not improve in the next 2 days or so or if she develops severe backache, shaking, chills, or fever.

Answer:

History: _____

Examination: _____

Medical Decision Making: _____

E/M Code: _____

CMS-1500 Excerpt: _____

21. DIAGNOSIS OR NATURE OF ILLNESS OR INJURY Relate A-L to service line below (24E)		ICD Ind.	22. RESUBMISSION CODE	ORIGINAL REF. NO.

A. |_____| B. |_____| C. |_____| D. |_____|

23. PRIOR AUTHORIZATION NUMBER

E. |_____| F. |_____| G. |_____| H. |_____|

I. |_____| J. |_____| K. |_____| L. |_____|

24. A. DATE(S) OF SERVICE From MM DD YY	To MM DD YY	B. PLACE OF SERVICE	C. EMG	D. PROCEDURES, SERVICES, OR SUPPLIES (Explain Unusual Circumstances) CPT/HCPCS / MODIFIER	E. DIAGNOSIS POINTER	F. $ CHARGES	G. DAYS OR UNITS	H. EPSDT Family Plan	I. ID. QUAL.	J. RENDERING PROVIDER ID. #
1				99212					NPI	
2				81000					NPI	
3									NPI	
4									NPI	
5									NPI	
6									NPI	

Appendix C

Acronyms and Abbreviations

Acronym/ Abbreviation	Name of Organization or Entity
AAAHC	Accreditation Association of Ambulatory Health Care
AAPC	American Academy of Professional Coders
ABN	advanced beneficiary notice
ACOG	American Congress of Obstetricians and Gynecologists
ACS	American College of Surgeons
AHIMA	American Health Information Management Association
ALJ	administrative law judge
AMA	American Medical Association
ANSI	American National Standards Institute
A/R	accounts receivable
ASA	American Society of Anesthesiologists
ASC	ambulatory surgery center
ASC X12	Accredited Standards Committee, Electronic Data Interchange
BC/BS	Blue Cross and Blue Shield
CABG	coronary artery bypass grafting
CC	chief complaint
CCA	certified coding associate
CCI	Correct Coding Initiative
CCS	certified coding specialist
CCS–P	certified coding specialist–physician-based
CCU	cardiac care unit
CDC	Centers for Disease Control and Prevention

CF	conversion factor
CFR	Code of Federal Regulations
CLIA	Clinical Laboratory Improvement Amendments
CMS	Centers for Medicare and Medicaid Services
CMT	chiropractic manipulative treatment
CNS	central nervous system
COB	coordination of benefits
COMP	comprehensive
CPC	certified professional coder
CPT	Current Procedural Terminology
CRNA	certified registered nurse anesthetist
CT	computed tomography
CTS	carpal tunnel syndrome
CWF	common working file
D&C	dilation and curettage
DET	detailed
DG	documentation guideline
DME	durable medical equipment
DMEMAC	durable medical equipment Medicare administrative contractor
DMERC	durable medical equipment regional carrier
DX	diagnosis
ECCE	extracapsular cataract extraction
EDI	electronic data interchange
EEG	electroencephalogram
EHR	electronic health record
E/M	evaluation and management
EMG	electromyogram
EMR	electronic medical record
EOB	explanation of benefits
EPF	expanded problem focused
ER	emergency room
ERA	electronic remittance advice
ESRD	end-stage renal disease
FAHIMA	Fellow of the American Health Information Management Association
FCA	False Claims Act
FDA	Food and Drug Administration

FOIA	Freedom of Information Act
GPCI	geographic practice cost index
HCFA	Health Care Financing Administration (now CMS)
HCPCS	Healthcare Common Procedure Coding System
HEDIS	Healthcare Effectiveness Data and Information Set
HHS	Department of Health and Human Services
HIM	health information management
HIPAA	Health Insurance Portability and Accountability Act of 1996
HMO	health maintenance organization
HPI	history of present illness
HPSA	health professional shortage area
ICCE	intracapsular cataract extraction
ICD-9-CM	International Classification of Diseases, Ninth Revision, Clinical Modification
ICD-10-CM	International Classification of Diseases, Tenth Revision, Clinical Modification
ICF	intermediate care facility
ICU	intensive care unit
IOL	intraocular lens
IPA	independent practice association
IPO	integrated provider organization
IPPB	intermittent positive pressure breathing
IV	intravenous
LBW	low birth weight
LCD	local coverage determination
LEEP	loop electrode excision procedure
LMRP	local medical review policy
MAC	Medicare administrative contractor
MAC	monitored anesthesia care
MCO	managed care organization
MDM	medical decision making
MDS	minimum data set
MPFS	Medicare physician fee schedule
MGMA	Medical Group Management Association
MPFSDB	Medicare Provider Fee Schedule Data Base
MPI	master population/patient index

MRI	magnetic resonance imaging
MSO	management service organization
MSP	Medicare secondary payer
MUGA	multiple gated acquisition
NB	newborn
NCCI	National Correct Coding Initiative
NCD	national coverage determination
NCHS	National Center for Health Statistics
NCQA	National Committee for Quality Assurance
NCS	nerve conduction study
NCVHS	National Committee on Vital and Health Statistics
NMJ	neuromuscular junction studies
Non-PAR	nonparticipating provider
NPBD	National Practitioner Data Bank
NPF	national provider file
NPI	national provider identifier
OB	obstetrics
OB/GYN	obstetrics and gynecology
OBRA	Omnibus Budget Reconciliation Act
OCR	optical character recognition
OIG	Office of the Inspector General
OMT	osteopathic manipulative treatment
ORT	Operation Restore Trust
PAR	participating provider
PC	professional component
PCI	percutaneous coronary intervention
PCP	primary care physician
PEG	percutaneous endoscopic gastrostomy tube
PF	Problem focused
PFSH	Past, family, and/or social history
PHO	physician–hospital organization
PHR	personal health record
PI	performance improvement
PICC	peripherally inserted central venous catheter
PICU	pediatric intensive care unit
PIN	provider identification number

PMD	primary medical doctor
PMPM	per member per month
POL	physician office laboratory
POMR	problem-oriented medical record
POS	point of service/place of service
PPO	preferred provider organization
PTCA	percutaneous transluminal coronary angioplasty
QI	quality improvement
RA	remittance advice
RAI	resident assessment instrument
RAP	resident assessment protocol
RBRVS	resource-based relative value scale
RHIA	registered health information administrator
RHIT	registered health information technician
R/O	rule out
ROS	review of systems
RVU	relative value unit
SEPs	Somatosensory evoked potentials
SF	straightforward
SMI	supplemental medical insurance (Medicare Part B)
SNF	skilled nursing facility
SOF	signature on file
SSA	Social Security Administration
SSN	social security number
TC	technical component
TCS	transaction and code sets
TEFRA	Tax Equity and Fiscal Responsibility Act of 1982
UACDS	Uniform Ambulatory Care Data Set
U/C	usual and customary
UCR	usual, customary, and reasonable
UPIN	unique physician identification number
UPP	urethral pressure profile
VBAC	vaginal birth after C-section
VLBW	very low birth weight
V/Q	ventilation-perfusion

Appendix D

Glossary

Accreditation: 1. A voluntary process of institutional or organizational review in which a quasi independent body created for this purpose periodically evaluates the quality of the entity's work against preestablished written criteria. 2. A determination by an accrediting body that an eligible organization, network, program, group, or individual complies with applicable standards

Actinotherapy: The use of ultraviolet light therapy in the treatment of skin diseases

Add-on codes: CPT codes indicated with a "+" symbol that cannot be coded alone. They must be used in addition to the primary procedure code and are exempt from use of the –51 modifier

Administrative data: Coded information contained in secondary records, such as billing records, describing patient identification, diagnoses, procedures, and insurance

Advance beneficiary notice (ABN): A statement signed by the patient when he or she is notified by the provider, prior to a service or procedure being done, that Medicare may not reimburse the provider for the service, wherein the patient indicates that he or she will be responsible for any charges

Allowable charge: Average or maximum amount a third party payer will reimburse providers for a service; *See* **allowable fee**

Allowable fee: *See* **allowable charge**

Analyte: Any material or chemical substance subjected to analysis

Anatomical modifiers: Two-digit HCPCS codes that provide information about the exact body location of procedures, such as –LT, Left side, and –TA, Left great toe

Antegrade: Extending or moving forward

Appeal: A request for reconsideration of a negative claim decision

Assignment of benefits: The transfer of one's interest or policy benefits to another party, typically the payment of medical benefits directly to a provider of care

Attorney–client privilege: An understanding that protects communication between client and attorney

Audit: A review process conducted by healthcare facilities (internally and/or externally) to identify variations from established baselines; *See* **external review**

Balance billing: A reimbursement method that allows providers to bill patients for charges in excess of the amount paid by the patients' health plan or other third-party payer (not allowed under Medicare or Medicaid)

Biofeedback: The process of providing visual or auditory evidence to a person on the status of an autonomic body function (such as the sounding of a tone when blood pressure is at a desirable level) so that he or she learns to exert control over the function

Birthday rule: A method of determining which insurance company is the primary carrier for dependents when both parents carry insurance on them. The rule states that the policyholder with the birthday earliest in the calendar year carries the primary policy for the dependents. If the policyholders are both born on the same day, the policy that has been in force the longest is the primary policy. Birth year has no relevance in this method

Carrier: The insurance company; the insurer that sold the policy and administers the benefits

Case management services: Services in which a physician is responsible for direct care of a patient, as well as for coordinating and controlling access to, or initiating and/or supervising other healthcare services for, the patient

Category II codes: CPT codes that describe services or test results that are agreed upon as contributing to positive health outcomes and high-quality patient care. They are for performance measurement, and use of these codes is optional

Category III codes: CPT codes that describe new and emerging technology. New codes are released semi-annually, rather than on the annual publication cycle, and can be found on the AMA website (www.ama-assn.org/go/cpt) for the most current listing. They are published annually and are located immediately preceding the Alphabetic Index in the CPT codebook

Certificate holder: Member of a group for which an employer or association has purchased group healthcare insurance; *See* **insured, member, policyholder**, and **subscriber**

Charge ticket: The tool used to collect data for the billing process; also known as superbill, fee ticket, encounter form, charge slip, route tag, route slip, fee slip, or billing slip

Chemical destruction: The application of chemicals to destroy tissue

Chief complaint: The principal problem a patient reports to a healthcare provider

Claim: A request for payment for services, benefits, or costs by a hospital, physician or other provider that is submitted for reimbursement to the healthcare insurance plan by either the insured party or by the provider

Clean claim: A claim that has all the billing and coding information correct and can be paid by the payer the first time it is submitted

Clearinghouse: An organization that processes and/or reformats electronic claims to insurers on behalf of multiple healthcare providers

Clinical brachytherapy: The use of radioactive sources placed directly into a tumor area to generate local regions of high-intensity radiation

Clinical data: Data captured during the process of diagnosis and treatment

Clinical Laboratory Improvement Amendments (CLIA): The federal regulation that governs physician office laboratories. A CLIA waiver or certificate is necessary for the performance and billing of laboratory services in the physician office

Clustering: The practice of coding/charging one or two middle levels of service codes exclusively, under the philosophy that some will be higher, some lower, and the charges will average out over an extended period

CMS-1500 form: A Medicare claim form used to bill third-party payers for provider services, for example, physician office visits

Code edit: An accuracy checkpoint in the claim-processing software, such as female procedures done only on female patients

Coding: The process of assigning numeric representations to clinical documentation

Coinsurance: Cost-sharing in which the policy or certificate holder pays a preestablished percentage of eligible expenses after the deductible has been met

Compliance: 1. The process of establishing an organizational culture that promotes the prevention, detection, and resolution of instances of conduct that do not conform to federal, state, or private payer healthcare program requirements or the healthcare organization's ethical and business policies. 2. The act of adhering to official requirements 3. Managing a coding or billing department according to the laws, regulations, and guidelines that govern it

Computerized internal fee schedule: The listing of codes and associated fees maintained in the practice's computer system, along with the additional data fields necessary for completing the CMS-1500 claim form

Conization: The removal of a cone-shaped portion of tissue such as from the cervix

Consultation: The response by one healthcare professional to another healthcare professional's request to provide recommendations or opinions regarding the care of a particular patient/resident

Contralateral: Pertaining to, located on, or occurring in or on the opposite side

Contrast material: An ingested or injected substance that enhances the appearance of anatomic structures when they undergo imaging

Credentialing: The process of reviewing and validating the qualifications (degrees, licenses, and other credentials), of physicians and other licensed independent practitioners, for granting medical staff membership to provide patient care services

Critical care: The care of critically ill patients in a medical emergency requiring the constant attention of the physician

Current Procedural Terminology, Fourth Edition (**CPT®**): A comprehensive, descriptive list of terms and numeric codes used for reporting diagnostic and therapeutic procedures and other medical services performed by physicians; published and updated annually by the American Medical Association

Customary fee: The fee normally charged by physicians of the same specialty, in the same geographic area

Denial: The circumstance when a bill has been accepted, but payment has been denied for any of several reasons (for example, sending the bill to the wrong insurance company, patient not having current coverage, inaccurate coding, lack of medical necessity, and so on)

Destruction: The ablation of benign, premalignant, or malignant tissues, by any method, with or without curettement, including local anesthesia, and not usually requiring closure. "Any method" includes electrocautery, electrodesiccation, cryosurgery, laser, and chemical treatment. Typical lesions include condylomata, papillomata, molluscum contagiosum, herpetic lesions, warts, milia, or other benign, premalignant, or malignant lesions

Diagnosis: A word or phrase used by a physician to identify a disease from which an individual patient suffers or a condition for which the patient needs, seeks, or receives medical care

Diagnostic mammography: Breast imaging, either unilateral or bilateral, done to provide information on a patient with a suspected breast condition

Direct laryngoscopy: The procedure that allows the larynx to be viewed through an endoscope

Documentation: The recording of pertinent healthcare findings, interventions, and responses to treatment as a business record and form of communication among caregivers

Documentation guideline (DG):   A statement that indicates what health information must be recorded to substantiate use of a particular CPT code

Duplex scan: An ultrasonic scanning procedure that displays both two-dimensional structure and motion with time. This process utilizes Doppler ultrasonic signal documentation with spectral analysis and/or color flow velocity mapping or imaging

Electrodesication: The destruction of tissue by way of a small needle heated by passing electricity through it

Emergency department: An organized hospital-based facility providing unscheduled episodic services to patients who present for immediate medical attention

Encounter history database: A transaction file that summarizes all the coded data for each patient seen in the physician office

Established patient: A patient who has received professional services from the physician or another physician of the same specialty in the same practice group within the past three years

Evaluation and management (E/M) services: The history, examination, and medical decision-making services that physicians must perform in evaluating and treating patients in all healthcare settings

Examination: The act of evaluating the body to determine the presence or absence of disease

Examination types: The levels of E/M services define four types of examination:

- *Problem focused* (an examination that is limited to the affected body area or organ system)

- *Expanded problem focused* (an examination of the affected body area or organ system and other symptomatic or related organ systems)

- *Detailed* (an extended examination of the affected body area[s] and other symptomatic or related organ systems)

- *Comprehensive* (a complete single-system specialty examination or a general multisystem examination)

Excisional breast biopsy: A breast biopsy that includes the removal of the entire lesion, whether benign or malignant

Explanation of benefits (EOB): A statement issued to the insured and the healthcare provider by an insurer to explain the services provided, amounts billed, and payments made by a health plan

External fee schedule: The maximum amount an insurance company is willing to pay for the listed services; also known as schedule of benefits or maximum benefits

External review: A performance or quality review conducted by a third-party payer or consultant hired for the purpose; *See* **audit**

Extracapsular lens extraction: The surgical removal of the front portion and nucleus of the lens, leaving the posterior capsule in place. A posterior chamber intraocular lens is generally inserted after this procedure

Fee schedule: A list of healthcare services and procedures (usually CPT/HCPCS codes) and the charges associated with them developed by a third-party payer to represent the approved payment levels for a given insurance plan; also called table of allowances

Fraud: That which is done erroneously to purposely achieve gain from another

Gender rule: A method of determining which insurance company is the primary carrier for dependents when both parents carry insurance on them. The rule states that the insurance for the male of the household is considered primary

Global Package: *See* **Surgical package**

Gonioscopy: The examination of the angle of the anterior chamber of the eye with a lens, or gonioscope

Healthcare Common Procedure Coding System (HCPCS): A classification system that identifies healthcare procedures, equipment, and supplies for claim submission purposes; the three levels are as follows: I, *Current Procedural Terminology* codes, developed by the AMA; II, codes for equipment, supplies, and services not covered by *Current Procedural Terminology* codes as well as modifiers that can be used with all levels of codes, developed by CMS; and III (eliminated December 31, 2003 to comply with HIPAA), local codes developed by regional Medicare Part B carriers and used to report physicians' services and supplies to Medicare for reimbursement

Health Insurance Portability and Accountability Act of 1996 (HIPAA): The federal legislation enacted to provide continuity of health coverage, control fraud and abuse in healthcare, reduce healthcare costs, and guarantee the security and privacy of health information. The act limits exclusion for preexisting medical conditions, prohibits discrimination against employees and dependents based on health status, guarantees availability of health insurance to small employers, and guarantees renewability of insurance to all employees regardless of size

Hemodialysis: The process of removing metabolic waste products, toxins, and excess fluid from the bloodstream, accessed by an indwelling dialysis port

History: The pertinent information about a patient, including chief complaint, past and present illnesses, family history, social history, and review of body systems

History of present illness (HPI): A chronologic description of the development of the patient's present illness from the first sign or symptom or from the previous encounter to the present

History types: The levels of E/M services define four types of history

- *Problem focused* (chief complaint; brief history of present illness or problem)

- *Expanded problem focused* (chief complaint; brief history of present illness; problem-pertinent system review)

- *Detailed* (chief complaint; extended history of present illness; extended system review; pertinent past, family, and/or social history)

- *Comprehensive* (chief complaint; extended history of present illness; complete system review; complete past, family, and social history)

Hospital inpatient: A patient who is provided with room, board, and continuous general nursing services in an area of an acute care facility where patients generally stay at least overnight; *See also* **Inpatient**

Hyperthermia: The use of heat to raise the temperature of a specific area of the body in an attempt to increase cell metabolism

Immunoassay: Detection and evaluation of substances by serological (immunologic) methods

Incisional breast biopsy: A type of breast biopsy done through an incision that does not include removal of the entire lesion

Indirect laryngoscopy: A procedure that enables the larynx to be viewed with a laryngeal mirror

Inpatient: A patient who is provided with room, board, and continuous general nursing services in an area of an acute-care facility where patients generally stay at least overnight; *See also* **hospital inpatient**

Insured: Individual or entity that purchases healthcare insurance coverage; *See* **certificate holder, member, policyholder**, and **subscriber**

International Classification of Diseases, Ninth Revision, Clinical Modification (ICD-9-CM): A classification system used in the United States to report morbidity and mortality information

International Classification of Diseases, Tenth Revision, Clinical Modification (ICD-10-CM): The newest revision of the disease classification system developed and used by the World Health Organization to track morbidity and mortality information worldwide. ICD-10-CM will be adopted for use by physicians in coding diagnostic statements on October 1, 2014

Interventional radiology: Defined as the branch of medicine that diagnoses and treats a wide range of diseases using percutaneous or minimally invasive techniques under imaging guidance

Intracapsular lens extraction: The surgical removal of the entire lens and its capsule. An anterior chamber intraocular lens is generally inserted after this procedure

Ipsilateral: Situated or appearing on the same side, or affecting the same side of the body

Laser: The acronym for "light amplification by stimulated emission of radiation"; may be used to cut or destroy tissue. Types of lasers currently in use are the argon laser and the Nd: YAG laser

Linking: The assignment of diagnosis codes to individual line items (1 through 4) on a CMS-1500 claim form to cross-reference the procedure to the diagnosis code, establishing the medical necessity of the procedure

Local codes: Also known as HCPCS Level III codes, these codes were developed by local Medicare and/or Medicaid carriers and were eliminated December 31, 2003 to comply with HIPAA

Magnetic resonance image (MRI): The generation of a powerful magnetic field that surrounds the patient, creating computer-interpreted radiofrequency imaging

Medical decision making: The process of establishing a diagnosis and management option for a patient

Medical necessity: The concept that procedures are only reimbursed as a covered benefit when they are performed for a specific diagnosis or specified frequency; insurers develop their own payment policies regarding medical necessity

Medicare fee schedule (MFS): A feature of the resource-based relative value system that includes a complete list of the payments Medicare makes to physicians and other providers

Medicare nonparticipation: The status with the Medicare program in which the provider has not signed a participation agreement. The provider does not accept the Medicare allowable fee as payment in full. In this case, the payment goes directly to the patient and the patient must pay the bill up to Medicare's limiting charge of 115 percent of the approved amount. The practice also does not receive an explanation of Medicare benefits about the claim

Medicare participation: The status with the Medicare program in which the provider signs a participation agreement with Medicare and agrees to accept the allowable fee as payment in full. The payment and an explanation of Medicare benefits are sent to the provider, and the patient pays any remaining balance, up to the allowed fee

Member: Individual or entity that purchases healthcare insurance coverage; *See* **certificate holder**, **insured**, **policyholder**, and **subscriber**

Modifier: A two-digit numeric or alphanumeric code listed after a procedure code that indicates that a service was altered in some way from the stated CPT or HCPCS descriptor without changing the definition; also used to enhance a code narrative to describe the circumstances of each procedure or service and how it individually applies to a patient

Mohs' micrographic surgery: A type of surgery performed to remove complex or ill-defined skin cancer. This technique requires that a single physician act in two integrated, but separate and distinct, capacities: surgeon and pathologist. Mohs' micrographic surgery does not routinely require wound repair

National Correct Coding Initiative (NCCI): A national initiative designed to improve the accuracy of Part B claims processed by Medicare carriers

National Permanent Codes: These HCPCS Level II codes provide a standard coding system that is managed by private and public insurers and provide a stable environment for claims submission and processing

New patient: An individual who has not received professional services from the physician, or any other physician of the same specialty in the same practice group before or within a designated time frame; an individual who has not received professional services from any provider of a organization/healthcare facility before or within a designated time frame

No man's land: The zone in the palmar, or volar, surface of the hand between the distal palmar crease (the crease in the palm closest to the fingers) and the middle of the middle phalanx (middle finger)

Noncovered procedures: Services not reimbursable under an insurance plan

Nonselective catheter placement: Catheter placement into the aorta, vena cava, or the vessel punctured

Nuclear medicine: A method of examination in which technologists introduce radioactive substances into the body orally, intravenously, or by ventilated aerosol or gas. A special camera is used to detect the radioactive substances as they circulate through the body and produce an image

Office of the Inspector General (OIG): The office through which the federal government established compliance plans for the healthcare industry

Optimization: The process of thoroughly reviewing the health record to identify all procedures performed and services rendered by the physician; must be accurately and completely coded to ensure optimum reimbursement

Outpatient: A patient who receives ambulatory care services in a hospital-based clinic or department

Panel: A group of tests commonly performed together for a given purpose, usually for one diagnosis

Partial mastectomy: The partial removal of breast tissue, leaving the breast nearly intact and includes specific attention to adequate surgical margins surrounding the breast mass or lesion; sometimes called a lumpectomy

Past, family, and/or social history (PFSH): The patient's past experience with illnesses, hospitalizations, operations, injuries, and treatments; a review of medical events in the patient's family, including diseases that may be hereditary or place the patient at risk; and an age-appropriate review of past and current activities

Payer remittance report: A report generated by the insurance company that states the outcome of the claim and how the insurer's share of the reimbursement was determined; *See* **Explanation of benefits (EOB)**

Peritoneal dialysis: A continuous or intermittent procedure in which dialyzing solution is introduced into and removed from the peritoneal cavity to cleanse the body of metabolic waste products

Phacoemulsification: A cataract extraction technique that uses ultrasonic waves to fragment the lens and aspirate it out of the eye

Phacofragmentation: A technique whereby the lens is broken into fragments by a mechanical means or by ultrasound

Photochemotherapy: The combination of light and chemical therapy in treating skin diseases

Physical status modifier: The two-digit code (P1–P6) attached to a CPT code to describe the patient's condition and therefore the complexity of the anesthesia service

Place of service: A two-digit code used in box 24b of the CMS-1500 claim form to describe the location where the service was performed

Policyholder: An individual or entity that purchases healthcare insurance coverage; *See* **insured, certificate holder, member**, and **subscriber**

Primary insurer: The insurance company responsible for making the first payment on a claim

Procedure: An action of a medical professional for treatment or diagnosis of a medical condition

Qualifying circumstances: Unusual situations that complicate the provision of anesthesia. Special CPT codes are provided for extreme age, total body hypothermia, controlled hypotension, and emergency situations

Questionable covered procedure: A procedure that may or may not be covered, depending on the patient's diagnosis and other factors

Radioactive ribbon: A small plastic tube (ribbon) that has radioactive sources spaced at regular lengths along it. *Ribbon* refers to temporary interstitial placement

Radioactive source: Radioactive elements packaged in a small configuration used for permanent implantation into tumors

Radioimmunoassay: A procedure that combines the use of radioactive chemicals and antibodies to detect hormones and drugs in a patient's blood

Reagent: Any substance added to a solution of another substance to participate in a chemical reaction

Relative value unit (RVU): A number assigned to a procedure that describes its difficulty and expense in relationship to other procedures by assigning weights to such factors as personnel, time, and level of skill

Resubmittal: The process of sending a corrected, or now complete, claim to an insurance company for reconsideration of the original payment or denial; also known as rebilling

Retinal detachment: The separation of two layers of the retina from each other. This usually occurs when the vitreous adheres to the retina (the sensitive layer of the eye) and "pulls," resulting in retinal holes and tears that may lead to retinal detachment. The repair involves the surgical reattachment of minor or major separations of the retina from the choroid (the membranous lining inside the sclera, or white of the eye), which contains many blood vessels that supply the eye with nutrients

Retrograde: Moving backward, against the normal flow

Revenue: The charges generated from providing healthcare services; earned and measurable income

Review of systems (ROS): An inventory of body systems obtained through a series of questions seeking to identify signs or symptoms that the patient may be experiencing or has experienced

Screening mammography: Breast imaging, usually done with two views bilaterally, to detect unsuspected cancer in an asymptomatic woman

Secondary insurer: The insurance carrier that pays benefits after the primary payer has determined and paid its obligation

Selective catheter placement: Catheter placement into any arterial or venous vessel other than the aorta, vena cava, or the original vessel that was punctured

Separate procedure: A procedure that is commonly part of another, more complex procedure, but which may be performed independently or be otherwise unrelated to the other procedure

Shaving: The sharp removal, by transverse incision or horizontal slicing, of epidermal and superficial dermal lesions without a full-thickness dermal excision. This includes local anesthesia and chemical or electrocauterization of the wound. The wound does not require suture closure

Simple complete mastectomy: The removal of all of the breast tissue without removing lymph nodes or muscle

Skin graft: Skin tissue that is completely detached from its blood supply in the donor area and reattached to a blood supply from the base of the wound or the recipient area

Specimen: Tissue submitted for individual and separate attention, requiring individual examination and pathologic diagnosis

Speech-language therapy: A treatment intended to improve or enhance a resident's ability to communicate and/or swallow

Speech recognition technology: Technology that translates speech to text

Spirometry: The measurement of the breathing capacity of the lungs

Subcutaneous mastectomy: The removal of breast tissue, leaving the skin of the breast and nipple intact. This type of mastectomy usually requires that a breast implant be inserted

Subpoena: A command to appear at a certain time and place to give testimony on a certain matter

Subscriber: Individual or entity that purchases healthcare insurance coverage; *See* **certificate holder**, **insured**, **member**, and **policyholder**

Surgical package: A payment policy of bundling payment for the various services associated with a surgery into a single payment, covering professional services for preoperative care, the surgery itself, and postoperative care

Tonometry: The measurement of tension or pressure, especially the indirect estimation of the intraocular pressure, from determination of the resistance of the eyeball to indentation by an applied force

Ultrasound: A diagnostic imaging technique that uses high-frequency, inaudible sound waves that bounce off body tissues. The recorded pattern provides information about the anatomy of an organ

Unbundling: The practice of using multiple codes to bill for the various individual steps in a single procedure rather than using a single code that includes all of the steps of the comprehensive procedure

Unique physician identification number (UPIN): A unique numerical identifier created by the Health Care Financing Administration (now called the Centers for Medicare and Medicaid Services) for use by physicians who bill for services provided to Medicare patients

Unique provider identification number (UPIN): A unique number assigned by the Centers for Medicare and Medicaid Services to identify physicians and suppliers who provide medical services or supplies to Medicare beneficiaries

Unlisted procedure codes: Codes available in each section of CPT to describe procedures that have no specific procedure code assigned because the procedure is new or unusual

Usual fee: The amount a physician normally charges the majority of the patients seen for that service

Utilization: The number of times a service is performed or supply is provided during a given period of time

Vascular family: A group of blood vessels that is fed by a branch, or primary division, of a major blood vessel

Vascular order: The furthest point to which the catheter is placed into the branches of a vessel originating off the aorta, vena cava, or vessel punctured if the aorta is not entered, and is referred to the level of selectivity

VBAC: The acronym for vaginal birth after a previous cesarean delivery

Vitrectomy: An ocular surgical procedure involving removal of the soft jelly-like material (vitreous humor) that fills the area behind the lens of the eye (vitreous chamber) and replacement with a clear solution. This is necessary when blood and scar tissue accumulate in the vitreous humor

Waiver: *See* **Advance beneficiary notice**

Wound repair: Wound repair is classified according to the following definitions

- *Simple repair* refers to the repair of superficial wounds, involving primarily epidermis or dermis or subcutaneous tissues without significant involvement of deeper structures. This repair requires simple one-layer closure/suturing, including local anesthesia and chemical or electrocauterization of wounds not closed.

- *Intermediate repair* involves the repair of wounds that require layered closure of one or more of the deeper layers of subcutaneous tissue and superficial (nonmuscle) fascia, in addition to the skin (epidermal and dermal) closure. These wounds usually involve deeper layers of subcutaneous tissue and fascia with one of the layers requiring separate closure. Single-layer closure of heavily contaminated wounds that require extensive cleaning or removal of particulate matter also constitutes intermediate repair.

- *Complex repair* designates the repair of wounds requiring more than layered closures; namely, scar revision, debridement, extensive undermining, stents, or retention sutures. It also may include creation of the defect and necessary preparation for repairs or the debridement and repair of complicated lacerations or avulsions.

Appendix E

Answers to Odd-Numbered Chapter Review Exercises

Exercise 1.1. Introduction to Coding Basics

1. c
3. d
5. Surgery
7. Evaluation and Management
9. Medicine
11. description . . . revised
13. new . . . revised
15. True
17. 45338
19. c

Exercise 2.1. Evaluation and Management Coding

1. a
3. b
5. d
7. 99204
9. 99479
11. 99255–32
13. 99243
15. 99468
17. 99203
19. 99283

Exercise 3.1. Anesthesia

1. a
3. a
5. 01925–AA–53
7. 00400–QY–QS, 00400–QX–QS
9. 00567–P4, 93503, 36620

Exercise 4.1. Surgery Section

1. d
3. c
5. a
7. b
9. b

Exercise 4.2. Integumentary System

1. b
3. d
5. c
7. d
9. c
11. c
13. 15240, 15004
15. 17340
17. 11100, 11101
19. 12032, 12004–51

Exercise 4.3. Musculoskeletal System

1. c
3. b
5. d
7. 29105
9. 29881

Exercise 4.4. Respiratory System

1. a
3. c
5. c
7. 32666, 32667 ×2
9. 32551

Exercise 4.5. Cardiovascular, Hemic, and Lymphatic Systems

1. b
3. c
5. 33533, 33518
7. 33425
9. 33233, 33207

Exercise 4.6. Digestive System

1. a
3. b
5. 44140
7. 43247
9. 47563

Exercise 4.7. Urinary System

1. a
3. c
5. 50390
7. 51701
9. 52353

Exercise 4.8. Male and Female Genital Systems

1. c
3. a
5. 54150
7. 57460
9. 59612

Exercise 4.9. Nervous System

1. c
3. Drainage of cyst
5. 61619
7. 63090
9. 62311

Exercise 4.10. Eye and Ocular Adnexa, and Auditory Systems

1. c
3. 67228–LT
5. 69645–50
7. 69910-RT
9. 66984–LT

Exercise 5.1. Radiology

1. d
3. c
5. a
7. 74400
9. 71035
11. 73090
13. 73502
15. 76946
17. 73090–26
19. 73050

Exercise 6.1. Pathology and Laboratory

1. d
3. c
5. b
7. 86485
9. 80198
11. 85025
13. 80076, 82043
15. 88304, 88304, 88304
17. 82248, 36416
19. 80081

Exercise 7.1. Medicine

1. c
3. c
5. 95800
7. 92014, 92082
9. 99202, 90375, 96372
11. 90937
13. 93010
15. 97761, 97761, 97761
17. 98940–AT
19. 93452

Exercise 8.1. HCPCS Level II Coding

1. 99395–25, 57170, A4266
3. S9442
5. Q4037
7. 96409, 96413, 96415, 96375–59, 96375–59, J1100 ×20, J2405 ×8, J7050 ×3, J0640 ×8, J9190 ×2, J1642 ×60
9. G0268, 92591

Exercise 9.1. Modifiers

1. c
3. b
5. c
7. False
9. False

Exercise 10.1. Reimbursement Process

1. c
3. c
5. b
7. b
9. a
11. f
13. True
15. False
17. 837
19. –GA

Exercise 11.1. Coding and Reimbursement Reports and Databases

1. a
3. b
5. b
7. c
9. d
11. a
13. b
15. a
17. Claim history
19. False

Exercise 12.1. Evaluation of Coding Quality

1. b

3. a

5. d

7. True

9. True

Index

A

Abdomen, peritoneum, and omentum subsection of surgery, 168–169

Abortion, 192

Accessory sinuses, endoscopies of, 138

Accounts receivable (A/R) management,
338–340

   aged accounts receivable and claims
follow-up for, 339

   appeals process in, 340

   definition of, 338

   denial management as part of, 339

   tracking amounts using days in accounts
receivable for, 338–339

Accreditation Association for Ambulatory
Health Care (AAAHC), 3

   standards for basic elements of health
records set by, 11

Accreditation organizations and standards, 3

Accredited Standards Committee (ASC)
X12 Electronic Data Interchange
(ASC X12) transaction and code set
standards, 333–334

Acellular dermal grafts, 114

Acellular xenogeneic implant, 114

Acupuncture, 280

ADA Dental Claim Form, 295

Add-on codes

   for anesthesia, 87

   for angioscopy during therapeutic
intervention, 151

   for computer-assisted, image-guided
navigation, 139

   for coronary artery blocked vessels, 268

   for critical care services, 63

   for electrode arrays, 198

   for iliac artery angioplasty, 154

   for intravascular ultrasound, 269

   for mammography, 221

   for photodynamic therapy, 279

   for placement of adjustable suture during
strabismus surgery, 211

   plus symbol (+) to designate, 17, 106

   for previous eye surgery, 211

   for qualifying circumstances for
anesthesia, 282

   for surgery, 106

   for veins harvested for bypass grafts, 151

   for vertebral levels in rhizotomy, 201

Additional codes

   for additional tissue block from same
specimen, 248

   for application of stereotactic headframe,
198

   for arthrodesis, 128

   for audiometric tests, 267

   for breast procedures, 118

   for cardiac catheterization, 271

   for cardiovascular myocardial perfusion
and cardiac blood pool imaging
studies, 227

   for injections, 262, 277–278

   for intracardiac echocardiography during
therapeutic/diagnostic intervention, 272

   for multiple vessels in procedure, 26

   for operating microscope for surgical
services, 211

   for physician standby services, 66

   for reconstruction procedures on ear, 211

   for skin grafts in addition to primary
procedures, 114

   for spinal instrumentation, 128

   when to use, 31–33

Additional procedures, separate codes for,
104

Adenoidectomy, 166

Adjacent tissue transfer or rearrangement,
113

Administration of contrast materials, 229–230

Administrative law judge (ALJ) hearing for reimbursement decision, 340

Advance beneficiary notice (ABN), 328
modifiers for, 328, 330
sample, 329

Aged accounts receivable, 339

AHA *Coding Clinic for ICD-10-CM*, 13

ALJ hearing. *See* Administrative law judge (ALJ) hearing

Allergen immunotherapy, 274

Allergy and clinical immunology, 273–274

Allergy testing, 273–274

Allograft (human skin), 114
corneal endothelial, 206
definition of, 114
tissue cultured, 114

Ambulatory coding guidelines for ICD-10-CM, 30–33
accessing and downloading current, 30

Ambulatory surgery, diagnosis for, 33

American Academy of Professional Coders (AAPC), 35

American Dental Association, *Current Dental Terminology* (CDT) of, 166, 295

American Health Information Management Association (AHIMA)
certifications by, 35
ICD–10 resources of, 13

American Medical Association (AMA)
CPT code book first developed by, 13–14
E/M service documentation guidelines by CMS (HCFA) and, 40
revisions of CPT code book by, 14

American Society of Anesthesiologists (ASA)
ranking system of, 88
time units and relative values system of, 93

Amount and/or complexity of data to review for medical decision making, 47

Anastomosis
arteriovenous, 153
of multiple-vein segments, 151
preparation of artery for, 151
in stomach, 166–167

Anatomic pathology
consultations for, 243, 247–248
physician services for, 245

Anesthesia, general, ophthalmological examination performed under, 266

Anesthesia section, 21, 85–96
codes used in reporting qualifying circumstances in, 90–91

format and arrangement of codes in, 86
modifiers for, 87–89

Anesthesia services
anesthesia package for, 86–87
fees for, calculating, 91–92
medical direction of, Medicare and Medicaid coverage of, 92–93
qualifying circumstances for, 90–91, 281–282
regional, as separate from surgical package, 186
steps in coding, 90–91
team approach for providing, 92
time charges for, 91–92

Anesthesia types included and not included in surgical package, 103

Anesthesiologist assistant (AA), 86–87
time charges for, 91

Aneurysm, 156
abdominal aortic, 151

Angiography, 229

Angioplasty
balloon, 268–269
iliac artery, 154
transluminal, 144, 268

Angioscopy, 151

Antepartum and/or postpartum care only, 190–191

Anterior segment of eye, 205–206

Anticoagulant management, 67

Anus, surgery on, 168

Appendectomy, 167–168

Aqueous shunt to extraocular reservoir, 207

Arterial catheterizations, 152

Arteriogram, 156

Arteriovenous fistulas, 153

Arthrodesis codes, 127

Arthroscopies, diagnostic and surgical, 131

Atherectomy, 268–269

Attorney–client privilege, 378–379

Audiologic function tests, 211, 267

Audiometry, 211

Audit
to analyze coding information, 373
attorney–client privilege for completing, 378–379
baseline, physician office, 387
conducting, 41, 379–381
determining size of sample for, 380
factors that trigger, 378
following up, 380–381
identifying need for, 378
preparing for, 378–379
steps in performing, 379–380
steps in performing internal, 379–380
time required to complete, 380

Auditory system subsection of surgery, 209–211
  diagram of, 210
Audit tool to assess quality of coding, 373
  based on 1995 guidelines, 375–376
  based on 1997 guidelines, 377
Autograft (autologous) skin graft
  definition of, 114
  tissue cultured skin in, 114

B
Bad debt write-off, 338
Balanced Budget Act of 1997 (BBA), 330, 385
Bariatric surgery, laparoscopic, 167
Benign lesions, 110
Biliary tract, 160, 168
Biller, teamwork of coder and, 363–364
Billing abuse
  as audit trigger, 378
  avoiding allegations of, 41. See also Fraud and abuse
  inflated medical billing as, 385
Billing, component, 275, 331
Billing database, physician, 348
Biofeedback, 264
Biopsies
  bladder/urethra, 177
  bone, 125
  bone marrow, 125, 244
  breast, 118–119, 155
  digestive system, 161
  excisional versus incisional, 118
  female genital system, 186
  hysteroscopic, 189
  lung and pleura, 140
  lymph node, 155
  male genital system, 183–185
  mediastinum, 155
  miscoding, 382
  prostate, 185, 247
  sentinel node, 155
  ureter, 178
Birthday rule for primary and secondary payers, 335
Birthing room attendance, 71
Bladder, 178–180
Blood draws (venipuncture), 240–241
Blood flow to and from heart, diagram of, 145–147
Blood gases and information data stored in computers, 63
Blood or blood component transfusion, 330
Blood transfusions and provision of blood products, 251

Body size, measuring, 115
Boldface for main terms in CPT code book index, 20
Bone density study, 230
Bone flaps, 195
Bone grafts, 126–127, 200–201
Bone marrow biopsy codes, 125, 244
Bone scans, 227
Bones of foot, diagram of, 129
Brachytherapy
  clinical, 226
  definition of, 224
  for radiation oncology, 224–225
Breast procedures, 118–120
Bronchial valves, 140
Bronchoscopies, 139–140, 279
Bullet (•) in CPT code book to designate new code, 16, 294
Bundling of services, improper, 362
Bunion repairs, 128–129
  errors in coding, 382
Burch procedure, 188
Burns
  debridement of, 110
  local treatment of, 117
Bypass graft, veins and arteries harvested for, 148, 151

C
C codes as inappropriate for billing professional services, 295
Capitation payment arrangement, 321
Cardiac anomalies, complex, 150
Cardiac catheterizations, 144, 155, 271–272
Cardiac procedures, HCPCS codes for, 285
Cardiac scans, 227–228
Cardiac valves, 148
Cardiography and cardiovascular monitoring services, 270
Cardiopulmonary resuscitation, 269
Cardiovascular device monitoring, 270
Cardiovascular, hemic and lymphatic systems of surgery, 144–156
Cardiovascular monitoring services, 270
Cardiovascular subsection of medicine, 267–272
Cardiovascular system subsection of surgery, 144–156
  diagram of, 145–147
  miscellaneous guidelines for, 155–156
Care plan oversight services, 68
Case management services, 67–68
Casts and strapping, 124, 130

Cataract extraction
    common errors in coding, 383
    ECCE and ICCE, 208
    implant procedures in, 208
    procedures included in, 207
    terminology for, 207
Catheters
    arterial, 87
    bronchoscopic placement of, 139
    cardiac, 144, 155, 271–272
    codes for placement of, 152, 270
    epidural, 95–96
    hyperalimentation or hemodialysis, 144
    inserted by physician rather than nurse,
        152
    intra-arterial, 87
    nonselective and selective, in
        interventional radiology, 223
    in pelvic organs and/or genitalia, 185
    removal of, 152
    suprapubic, 187
    ureteral, 178–179
    venous, 152
Cell washings and brushings, 139–140
Centers for Medicare and Medicaid Services
    (CMS)
    ambulatory coding guidelines by NCHS
        and, 30
    claim form for billing. *See* CMS-1500
        claim form
    CPT code book included in Healthcare
        Common Procedure Coding System
        by, 13
    E/M service documentation guidelines by
        AMA and, 40
    National Codes updated by, 294
    National Correct Coding Initiative
        developed by, 331
    payment for consultation codes eliminated
        by, 60
    statistics for comparative graph available
        from, 354–355
    website of, 241, 294, 296, 309, 322, 328,
        331, 333–334, 354
Central line catheter placement, 152
Central nervous system assessments/tests,
    276
Central nervous system, diagram of, 195
Central venous access procedures, 152
Central venous lines (CVPs), 87
Certified Coding Associate (CCA), 35
Certified Coding Specialist (CCS), 35
Certified Coding Specialist–Physician-Based
    (CCS–P), 35
Certified Professional Coder (CPC), 35

Certified Registered Nurse Anesthetist
    (CRNA), 86, 87, 89
    fees for services of, 91
    modifiers for services of, 89
    time charges for, 91
Cervical or vaginal cancer screening; pelvic
    and clinical breast examination,
    330–331
Cervix uteri, 187
Charge summary report, 348, 351
    sample, 350
Charge ticket
    items included on, 24
    sample office services, 26
    submission for payment of, 372
    used in audit, 379
Chemistry, 243
Chemotherapy, 225
    administration of, 278
Chest x-rays, 63, 220
Chief complaint used for coding, 30
    definition of, 44
    in history component of E/M service, 44
Childbirth and parenting classes, 192
Chiropractic manipulative treatment (CMT),
    280–281
Chronic diseases, coding, 32
Circumcision, 184
Claim adjustment reason codes, Washington
    Publishing Company tables of, 363
Claim denial
    C codes on CMS-1500 form resulting in,
        295
    caused by failure to perform steps in
        claims process, 337
    denial management for, 339
    diagnosis codes as cause of, 362
    NCCI edits signaling, 333
    noncoding reasons for, 363
    nonspecific diagnosis code causing, 41
    preventing, 331
    speeding Medicare, 330
Claim history, patient, 348
    sample, 349
Claims process
    appeals process for Medicare in, 340
    steps in, 337–340
    submission of CMS-1500 form in, 333–336
Clean claims
    goal of submitting, 333
    percentage of, as key indicator, 364
Clinic/office setting for charges, 22
Clinical brachytherapy, 226–227
Clinical Laboratory Improvement
    Amendments of 1988 (CLIA), 241

Clustering of service codes, 359
CMS-1500 claim form
    billing professional services on, 295
    claims process for, 337–340
    code edits for missing information on, 362
    completing, 333–335
    date of accident or injury on, 33
    electronic format of, 334–335, 338
    HIPAA transaction and code set for,
        333–334
    internal fee schedule for, 336–337,
        360–361
    linking diagnoses to procedures or
        services on, 264, 335
    reporting allergy tests performed on, 273
    reporting units on, 125
    submission of paper or electronic,
        334–335, 338
    used in audit, 379
Codable diagnostic statements, identifying,
    29–34
Codable physician office documentation
    statements, identifying, 34–35
Codable procedural statements, identifying,
    27–29
Coders. See also Certified Coding Associate
        (CCA); Certified Coding Specialist
        (CCS); Certified Coding Specialist–
        Physician-based (CCS–P); Certified
        Professional Coder (CPC)
    and billers as team, 363–364
    as validating code selection, 41
Coding
    anesthesia, 85–96
    audit of, 373, 375–381, 386
    basics of, introduction to, 1–35
    diagnostic, 13
    evaluation and management, 39–76
    main body of CPT code books used for
        assigning, 21, 27
    medicine, 259–286
    operative report used for, 28–29
    pathology and laboratory, 239–251
    radiology, 219–231
    surgery, 101–211
Coding credentials earned from AHIMA and
        AAPC, 35
Coding errors
    common CPT, 381–383
    identified through reports, 357–360
    payer remittance report revealing, 361–364
Coding fraud. See Fraud and abuse
Coding quality, evaluation of, 371–387
Coexisting conditions, coding, 32
Colon, cross section diagram of, 167

Colonoscopy
    coding, 162–164, 382
    distinguished from protosigmoidoscopy
        and sigmoidoscopy, 163
Colposcopy/vaginoscopy, 187
Combination code, 271
Communication tools
    complex, 373
    simple, 372
Comparative study for service distribution
        report
    creating, 354–355
    purpose of, 352
    sample, 354
Complete blood counts (CBCs), 244
Complex repair of wounds, 112
Compliance, definition of, 383
Compliance programs for physician practices,
        386–387
    OIG work plans for, 387
Compliance regulations, 383–387
Complications, surgical package as not
        including encounters for, 102–103
Component billing, 275, 331
Comprehensive history in E/M service level,
        43
Computed tomography (CT), 220–221
    performed with stereotactic biopsy, 197
    spinal, 201
    ultrafast or cine, 230
Computerized corneal topography (CCT),
        266
Computerized internal fee schedule reports,
        336–337, 360–361
Concurrent care, appropriate ICD-10-CM code
        for each service provided in, 42–44
Confirmatory consultations, 61
Conization of cervix, 187
Conscious sedation, 282
    ⊙ symbol indicating code that includes, 17
    codes including, in appendix G of CPT
        code book, 20
Consultations, 60–62
    anatomic pathology, 243, 247–248
    clinical pathology, 243
    definition of, 60
    documentation of, 23
    inpatient, 61
    for minor diagnoses, audits triggered by,
        378
    modifiers for, 61
    outpatient, 61
Consulting physicians, guidelines for roles
        of, 60
Contact lenses, HCPCS codes for, 285

Contact lens service, 266
Contrast materials
    administration of, 229–230
    for diagnostic radiology, 220, 230
    HCPCS codes for, 230
Contributing components of E/M services, 43
Coordination of care as contributing E/M
    component, 43
Coronary arteries with potential blockages,
    diagram of, 149
Coronary artery bypass grafting (CABG),
    148–149, 151–152
Coronary thrombolysis, 270
Corporate integrity agreement, definition of,
    385
Corpus uteri, 187–189
Corrected claim, 337, 339
Counseling
    as contributing E/M component, 43
    to promote health and prevent illness or
        injury, 70
    CPT Assistant
    allergy tests and treatments in, 273–274
    AMA as publisher, 13–14
    aspiration and trigger point injection codes
        in, 125
    bilateral codes for tonsillectomy and
        adenoidectomy in, 166
    biopsy and excision of lesions in, 118, 163
    breast procedures in, 119
    cholecystectomy in, 168
    circumcision, in newborn, 184
    electrodiagnostic medicine (EDX) testing
        in, 275
    history and physical performed on
        newborn in, 71
    interventional radiology defined in, 222
    multiple gestation vaginal deliveries in,
        191–192
    narcosynthesis in, 263
    orchiopexy with hernia repair in, 170
    Pap smear results in, 245–246
    reporting open and laparoscopic
        procedures in, 162
    separate coding for lysis of adhesions in,
        167
    surgical laparoscopy in, removal of
        adnexal structures during, 189
    surgical margins of lesions in, attention
        to, 118
    uses of urodynamics in, 178
CPT code book
    add-on codes in appendix D of, 17, 20
    alphabetic index of, 240
    appendixes of, 17, 20
    assignment of codes for services from, 13
    clinical examples for E/M coding in
        appendix C of, 19, 44
    code formats in, 16–17
    code organization in, 21
    codes assigned from main body rather
        than index of, 21, 27
    codes exempt from use of –51 modifier in
        appendix E of, 17, 20
    codes exempt from use of –63 modifier in
        appendix F of, 20
    codes including conscious sedation in
        appendix G of, 20
    coding notes and instructions in, 19
    criteria for inclusion of procedures in, 15
    crosswalk to deleted CPT codes in, 20
    HCPCS Level I as, 14
    headings in, 21
    index of, 20–21, 26–28
    main entry in, semicolon (;) to designate
        common portion of indented portions
        of, 17–19
    modifiers list in appendix A of, 19, 302
    modifiers to use with genetic testing codes
        in appendix I of, 20
    new, revised terminology, and deleted
        codes in appendix B of, 19
    non-add-on codes exempt from use of –51
        modifier in appendix E of, 17, 20
    performance measurement codes in
        appendix H of, 20
    professional edition of, 129, 209
    revisions by AMA of, 14, 330
    sections of, 21
    structure and conventions of, 14–21
    subheadings in, 21
    subsections of, 21
    symbols in, 16–17
    used in audit, 379
    vascular families described in appendix L
        of, 223
CPT codes
    add-on, plus sign (+) to designate, 17, 20
    Category I of, 14, 15
    Category II service and/or test, 14–15
    Category III new and emerging
        technology, 14–15
    for catheter insertions by physicians, 152
    code assignment hierarchy for National
        Codes and, 294
    deleted, 19–20
    development of new HCPCS codes to
        replace, 330
    examples of, 14
    format of, 16–17

general instructions for using, 26–27

for internal fee schedule, 336–337

new and revised text in coding notes for, facing triangles (►◄) to indicate, 17

new, filled-in dot (•) in CPT code book to designate, 16

non-add on, exempt from using –51 modifier, null zero (⊘) to designate, 17, 20

out of numerical sequence, 17, 20

revised, triangle (▲) in CPT code book to designate, 16–17, 294–295

for unlisted procedures, 19

CPT Editorial Panel (AMA), 14

Craniectomy, 194

Craniotomy, 20, 194

Critical care services, 63

care settings for, 63

neonatal and pediatric inpatient, 63, 72–74

Crosswalk to deleted CPT codes in Appendix M of CPT code book, 20

Current Dental Terminology (CDT) coding system, 166, 295

Current Procedural Terminology, Fourth Edition, 13. *See also* CPT code book

Custom reports for assessing coding quality, 355–360

Cystectomy, 178

Cystometrogram, simple and complex, 178

Cystoscopy, 177, 179

Cystourethroscopy, 179

Cytogenetic studies, 247

Cytopathology, 245–247

D

D codes of HCPCS comprising *Current Dental Terminology* (CDT), 295

Database

billing, physician, 348

in problem-oriented medical record, 4

reports based on encounter history, 355–360

of services using CPT and HCPCS codes and fee schedule, 336–347, 360

Data collection form for each place of service, 24–26

Data elements of computerized internal fee schedule, 336–337

Data evaluation, qualitative and quantitative, 348–360

Days in accounts receivable, 338–339

Days or units information, 337

Debridement and decontamination of wounds, 113–114, 130

Debridement and removal of granulations or avulsion in skin grafts, 114

Debridement of burns, 110

Debridement of mastoid cavity, 211

Debridement of multiple wounds, 110

Decubitus (pressure) ulcers, 117

Deleted codes in HCPCS, strike-through to indicate, 294

Delivery services, 71, 190–192

Denial management for claims, 339

Dental-related services, billing for, 295

Dentoalveolar structures, 165

Department of Health and Human Services, Medicare program administered by CMS under, 385

Detailed history in E/M service level, 44–45

Developmental screening, 276

Diabetes, HCPCS codes for, 286

Diagnoses

falsifying, 384

not to code under ICD-10-CM, 31

Diagnosis distribution report, 351–352

sample of, showing problem areas, 351

Diagnosis/procedure mismatch, 360

Diagnostic coronary angiography, codes and injection codes, 268

Diagnostic imaging. *See* Diagnostic radiology

Diagnostic nuclear medicine scans, 227–228

Diagnostic procedures, reports of, 11

Diagnostic radiology, 220–221

contrast materials for, 220

HCPCS codes for, 230

Diagnostic services, sequencing, 32

Diagnostic statement

assignment of code number to describe physician's, 13

definition of, 12

identifying codable, 29–34

for laboratory- or radiology-only appointment, 29

in physician's notes, 29

Diagnostic ultrasound

coding guidelines for, 222

HCPCS codes for, 230

types of, 222

Dialysis, 264–265

Diaphragmatic hernia, 170

Dictation matched to handwritten notation, 373

Digestive system subsection of surgery, 160–171

common coding errors for, 382

diagram of, 161

modifiers for, 163, 164

Dilatation and curettage (D&C), 187–188

Discharge services, nursing facility, 64–65

Discounted charges for medical services, 320
Dislocation treatment codes, 126–127
Documentation guidelines
    for E/M services, 40–41, 44, 46
    for physicians, 27
Documentation sources that generate
    physician codes and charges, 22–26
Documentation that supports charges and
    diagnoses of physician, 41, 360
    communication tools to request, 372–373
Domiciliary, rest home, or custodial care
    services, 65
Domiciliary, rest home, or home care
    oversight services, 66
Donor site of skin flaps or skin grafts,
    115–116
Dressing changes, 116
Drug testing, 242
    table of codes for drug names and classes
    in, 243
Duplex scan, 272
Durable medical equipment (DME)
    HCPCS codes used for, 131–133, 296
    for Medicare beneficiaries, 296
    provider number for, 132, 285, 296
Durable medical equipment Medicare
    administrative contractors (DME
    MACs), 296

E
E codes for external causes of injury, 33–34
Echocardiography, 270
Education and training for patient self-
    management, 281
Electrocardiograms (ECGs or EKGs), 270
    screening, 69
Electroencephalography (EEG), 275
    automated monitoring of, 285
Electromyography (EMG), 275
    of muscle activity during voiding, 179
    surface, 285
Electronic claims for CMS-1500
    claim submission using, 334
    signatures for, 334
    submission error management for, 335
    time savings using, 334
Electrophysiologic (EP) procedures, 147, 272
Emergency department services, 62
    modifiers for, 62–63
Emergency department setting for charges,
    23–24
End-stage renal disease (ESRD), 264
Endarterectomy, 151
Endocrinology, 274–275
Endomicroscopy, optical, 163

Endoscopy. See also Laparoscopies
    bladder, 178–179
    diagnostic endoscopy as included in
        surgical procedure, 139
    digestive system, 160–179, 382
    genitourinary, 179
    larynx, 138–139
    posterior segment, 208
    renal, 177
    sinus, 138
    ureteral, 178
Endoscopy/arthroscopy, 130–131
Endovascular repair of abdominal aortic
    aneurysm, 156
Endovascular revascularization, 154
Errors, reports for identifying
    claim history and charge summary
        qualitative analysis, 348, 351
    comparative, 352, 354–355
    computerized internal fee schedule, 360–361
    diagnosis distribution and service
        distribution quantitative analysis,
        351–355
    status, 335
    types of errors revealed by, 357, 359–360
Esophageal motility studies, 265
Esophagogastric fundoplasty, 166
Esophagoscopy, 163, 279
Established patient defined for E/M services,
    41
    for domiciliary, rest home, or custodial
        care services, 65
    for home services, 66
    for office or other outpatient services, 56
Evaluation and management (E/M) section,
    21, 190, 191, 225, 243, 278, 280, 274
    categories and subcategories for, 41,
        54–76
    categories that identify new versus
        established patient for, 42, 265
    coding for, 39–76, 103, 264
    documentation guidelines for, 40–41
    format of service codes for, 40
    modifiers for, 52–54, 61, 67, 71
    1995 guidelines for, 40, 47, 375–376
    1997 guidelines for, 40, 47, 266, 377
Evaluation and management (E/M) services
    case example for selecting level of, 50–51
    code, psychotherapy with, 263
    health and behavior assessment/
        intervention with, 276
    levels of, 43–52, 265, 375, 377
    other, 76
    special, 71
    terms used in reporting, 41–42

Evaluation of coding quality, 371–388

Evocative/suppression testing, 243

Examination
four types of, 46–47
as key E/M component, 42, 46–47, 55, 373

Excision-debridement of skin, 110

Excision inferior turbinate, 138

Excisional biopsies, 118

Expanded problem focused history in E/M service level, 43

Explanation of benefits (EOB), 338, 361, 363
codes and code edits for, 362–363
payer information about, 362

External causes of injury (E codes), 33–34

External fixation of fracture, 126

Extracapsular cataract extraction (ECCE), 208

Extracranial nerves, peripheral nerves, and autonomic nervous system, 201–202

Extraction of lens, extracapsular and intracapsular, 208

Extraspinal regions, 281

Eye and ocular adnexa subsection of surgery, 205–209
common coding errors for, 383
diagram of, 205
modifiers for, 209

Eyeball, 206

F

F wave test, 275

Facing triangles (▶◀) to indicate new and revised text in coding notes, 16

Fallopian tubes (oviducts), 189

False Claims Act (FCA), Federal, criminal penalties for fraud under, 385

Federal Register
listing of global surgical days in, 380
Medicare conversion factors published annually in, 321
National Physician Fee Schedule Relative Value File as electronic, 322

Fee problem log, 325

Fee schedule management, 324–325
computerized reports for, 360–361

Fee schedule management worksheet, 324–325

Fee schedule, negotiated, 321

Fee survey report, national, 325

Female genital system subsection of surgery, 186–192
diagram of, 186

Fertilization services, 192

Fetal repairs, HCPCS codes for, 192

Filled-in dot (•) in CPT code book to designate new code, 16, 294

Fine needle aspiration of prostate, 185

First-listed diagnosis in outpatient setting, 31

Fistulectomy, 168

Fistulization of sclera, 206

Flaps
donor site for, 116
procedures included in reporting use of, 120
types of, 116

Follow-up care
for diagnostic and therapeutic surgical procedures, 104
postoperative, 103

Food and Drug Administration (FDA), *N* symbol for approval of vaccines by, 17, 262

Foot, bones of, diagram of, 129

Foreign bodies, removal of
from external ear, 211
from eye, 206
from wound, 113, 124

Fracture treatment codes, 124, 126–127, 132

Fraud and abuse
changing or manipulating codes as constituting, 364
civil monetary penalty for, 385
HIPAA provisions to address, 384
reducing risk of allegation of, 330
submission of undocumented code as constituting, 41
terminology of, 385
unsubstantiated charges as constituting, 2

Freedom of Information Unit, 326

Full-thickness skin graft, 114

G

Gastrectomy, 166

Gastric and duodenal intubation and aspiration, 166

Gastric bands, bariatric surgery using, 167

Gastric intubation, 63, 265

Gastroenterology, 265

Gastrointestinal subsection endoscopies, 162

Gastrostomy (feeding) tube (PEG), 166

Genetic testing codes, modifiers used with, 20, 312

Genital system. *See* Female genital system subsection of surgery; *See* Male genital system subsection of surgery

Geographic practice cost index (GPCI) for Medicare payments, 322

Gestational diabetes, 191

Glaucoma screening, 266

Glaucoma, surgical treatment of, 206–207
Global surgical days listed in *Federal Register*, 380
Global surgical procedure. *See* Surgical package
Gonioscopy with medical diagnostic evaluation, 266
Goniotomy, 206
GPCI. *See* Geographic practice cost index (GPCI) for Medicare payments
Grafts. *See* Bone grafts; *See* Coronary artery bypass grafting (CABG); *See* Skin grafts
Growth factor preparation, 120

H
Hammertoe, errors in coding, 382
HCPCS codes
  assignment of, 13
  C outpatient, 295
  D Current Dental Terminology, 295
  durable medical equipment, 296
  effect of HIPAA on, 295
  J medication. *See* J codes, HCPCS
  Level I of. *See* CPT code book
  Level II of. *See* National Codes
  new, 330–331
  symbols used with, 294
  temporary, 295–296
  used in audit, 380
  website to obtain, 294
HCPCS coding system. *See Healthcare Common Procedure Coding System* (HCPCS)
Health and behavior assessment/intervention, 276
Health Care Fraud and Abuse Control Program created under HIPAA, 384
Health Insurance Portability and Accountability Act (HIPAA) (Public Law 104–193)
  code sets for use for third-party payers under, final rule for, 384
  effect on HCPCS of, 295
  fraud and abuse provisions of, 384
  Health Care Fraud and Abuse Control Program created under, 384
  major provisions of, 384
  Transaction and Code Sets (TCS) of, 333, 384
Health record
  addendum to, 12
  administrative data in, 6–8
  assignment of benefits form and Medicare signature on file in, 8
  changes to, 12
  clinical data in, 8–11
  content of, 3, 5–11
  documentation elements of accrediting agencies for, 11–12
  formats of, 4–5
  fraud and abuse involving, 41, 363, 384
  integrated, 4
  primary functions of, 2
  purposes of, 2
  registration record within, 6
Healthcare Common Procedure Coding System (HCPCS)
  for contrast material, 220
  CPT codes included in, 14
  for diagnostic radiology, 230
  for diagnostic ultrasound, 230
  for female genital system, 186
  for integumentary system, 119
  master list of services by CPT codes and, 336
  for medicine, 282–283
  modifiers in, 14, 335. *See also* Modifiers, HCPCS
  for musculoskeletal system, 124, 131–133
  for nervous system, 202
  for ophthalmology, 266
  for pathology and laboratory, 249–250
  for radiology services, 230–231
  requests for new codes in, 330–331
  for supplies in internal fee schedule, 336
Heart, veins, and arteries, diagram of, 145, 146–147
Hematology and coagulation, 244
Hemic and lymphatic systems, 155
Hemilaminectomy, 200
Hemodialysis, 264–265
Hemodialysis access, intervascular cannulation for extracorporeal circulation or shunt insertion, 153
Hemorrhoidectomy, 160
Hepatobiliary (HIDA) scans, 228
Hernia repair, 169–171
Hiatal hernia, 166, 170
History
  as key E/M component, 43, 44–46, 373
  psychiatric, 262–264
History of present illness (HPI) in history component of E/M service, 45
Home health agencies, physician supervision of patients for, 68
Home health procedures/services, 283
Home infusion procedures, 283
Home services, 66
Home visit hemodialysis, 265

Home visit setting for charges, 23

Hospital discharge services, 59

Hospital inpatient services, 57–59
    modifiers for, 59

Hospital observation services, 56–57

Hospital outpatient prospective payment
    system (OPPS) reimbursement, 295

H-reflex test, 275

Hybrid format of health record, 5

Hyperthermia, 225

Hysterectomy
    abdominal, 188
    vaginal, 188

Hysteroscopy, 188–189

I

ICD-10-CM. *See International Classification
    of Diseases, Ninth Edition, Clinical
    Modifications* (ICD-10-CM)

ICD-10-CM code book
    annual update of, 13
    Index to External Causes in, 33–34

ICD-10-CM codes
    assigned to highest level of specificity, 32,
        41, 362
    coding reason for encounter using, 31
    linking CPT/HCPCS codes to, 330, 338
    physician office uses for, 12
    role in billing and receiving payment for
        concurrent care services of, 42

ICD-10-CM diagnostic codes, 13

ICD-10-PCS procedure coding system, 13

Immune globulins, serum or recombinant
    products, 260

Immunization administration for vaccines/
    toxoids, 261–262

Immunization against disease, 260–262

Immunization pending FDA approval, *N*
    symbol in CPT code book to note, 17, 262

Immunization services, HCPCS codes for, 284

Immunology, 244

Immunotherapy, allergen, 273–274

Implant, removal of, 126

Implanted material in eye, removal of, 206

"Incident to" services and supplies, billing,
    378

Incisional biopsies, 118

Incision and drainage of skin, simple and
    complicated, 109

Index of CPT code book, avoiding assigning
    codes from, 21, 27

Index to External Causes in ICD-10-CM
    code book, 33–34

Induction dilution studies, 271

Infants, critical care services for, 63, 72–74

Information analysis, 373. *See also* Audit

Information collection, charge ticket for, 372

Information correction, tools for, 372–377

Infusion pumps, 144, 152

Infusions, therapeutic, prophylactic, or
    diagnostic, 276–279

Inhalation bronchial challenge testing, 273

Initial hospital care, 22, 58
    to neonate of 28 or fewer days, 74

Initial observation care, 57

Initial plan in problem-oriented medical
    record, 4

Initial preventive physical examination
    (IPPE) for Medicare patients, 69–70

Injections
    anesthetic agent, 96, 184, 186
    hydration, therapeutic, prophylactic, and
        diagnostic, 276–279
    joint, 201
    of medication into joint or ganglion cyst,
        125
    neurolytic, 201
    nonneurolytic, 201
    spinal, 198, 201
    trigger point, 125–126

Injury, E codes for external causes of, 33–34

Inpatient consultations, 61

Inpatient hospital setting for charges, 22–23

Inpatient neonatal and pediatric critical care,
    72–74

Insurance company appeals process, 340

Insurance company claim processing, 338

Insurance company fact sheet, 326
    sample blank, 327

Integrated health record, 4

Integumentary system subsection of surgery,
    109–119, 138
    HCPCS codes for, 119–120

Intermediate repair of wounds, 112

Internal elective electrical cardioversion of
    arrhythmia, 270

Internal fee schedule
    computerized reports for, 360–61
    data elements of computerized, 336–337

Internal fixation of fracture, 126

*International Classification of Diseases,
    Ninth Edition, Clinical Modifications*
    (ICD-10-CM)
    ambulatory coding guidelines for, 30–33
    benign versus malignant neoplasms in, 111
    code book for, index and tabular sections
        of, physician offices' use of, 13
    understanding which diagnostic statements
        are codable using, 30–33
    used in audit, 379

Intersex surgery, 185
Interventional radiology, 222–224
Intestines, 167–168
    diagram of, 167
Intracapsular cataract extraction
    (ICCE), 207
Intracardiac electrophysiologic procedures/
    studies, 272
Intraocular lens prosthesis (IOL), 208
Intravascular cannulization or shunt, 152
Intravascular ultrasound, 269
Intravenous (IV) infusion, 277–278
Inventory discrepancies on service
    distribution report, 352, 354
Iridotomy/iridectomy by laser
    surgery, 207

J
J codes, HCPCS
    for evocative/suppression testing, 243
    for medications, 125, 273, 276, 296
    for nebulizer treatment, 273
Joint, aspiration or injection of medication
    into, 125
Joint Commission, 3
    medication list required to be included in
        health record by, 8
    problem list required for continuing
        ambulatory services by, 8–9
    standards for basic elements of health
        records set by, 11
Joint scans, 227

K
Keratoplasty (corneal transplant), 206
Key components of E/M services
    for consultation codes, 60
    for domiciliary, rest home, or custodial
        care services, 65
    for home services, 66
    for nursing facility services, 64, 65
    in selecting level of E/M service, 42–52,
        54
Kidney, 177–178
Knee arthroscopy, diagram of, 131

L
Laboratory-only appointments, diagnosis for,
    29
Laboratory reports in health record, 11
Laboratory tests
    evocative/suppression testing in, 243
    kit or transportable instrument for, 308
    medical necessity of, 328
    repetition of, audits triggered by, 378

Laminectomy, laminotomy,
    hemilaminectomy, 200
Laparoscopic surgical approach, 105
Laparoscopies
    diagram of, 188
    digestive system, 160, 166, 167
    female genital system, 186–187
    male genital system, 183
    surgical, diagnostic laparoscopy included
        in, 162, 170, 188–189
    urinary system, 175–180
Laparotomy for abdomen, peritoneum, and
    omentum, 168–169
Laryngoscopies, indirect and direct, 138–139
Larynx, 138–139
LEEP procedures, 187
Lens extraction. See Cataract extraction
Lesions, biopsies of genital, 186
Lesions, breast, 118
Lesions, digestive system, 162, 164
Lesions, eyelid, 208
Lesions, penile, 184
Lesions, renal mass, 177
Lesions, skin
    destruction of, 117, 279, 382
    excision of, 109, 110–111, 382
    malignant versus benign, 382
    measurement of, 110
Lesions, skull base, 195–196
Lesions, surgical margins of, 118
Lesions, tongue, 165
Lesions, vulva, 187
Levels of E/M services, 42–52
    audits triggered by billing unsupported,
        378
    components of, key and contributing,
        43–52, 54, 61
    examples of selecting among, 50–51
    time as factor in selecting, 50–52
Ligation as part of wound repair, 113
Lips, repairs of, 165
Lithotripsy to destroy urinary stones, 177
Local Coverage Determinations (LCDs), 326,
    328, 331
LOOP procedures, 187
Lower gastrointestinal endoscopies, 163–164
Lumpectomy, breast, 118
Lung excision, 140
Lung scans, 228
Lungs and pleura, 140–141
Lymph nodes
    biopsy or excision of, 155
    removal during cystectomy of, 179
    removal during mastectomy of, 118
Lymphadenectomies, 155

M

Magnetic resonance imaging (MRI), 220, 231

Main terms in CPT code book index, 20, 29

Male genital system subsection of surgery, 175, 183–185

    diagram of, 184

Malignant lesions, 111

Mammography, screening and diagnostic, 221, 230

Managed care organizations, capitation used by, 321

Manipulation of fracture, 126

Mastectomies, 118–120

Mastoidectomy cavity, 211

Maternity care and delivery, 190–192

Mechanical thrombectomy, 269

Mediastinoscopy, 155

    diagram of, 155

Mediastinum, 155

Medicaid

    certification number for lab on file for test coverage by, 241

    reduced reimbursement by, 93

Medical and/or surgical complications during pregnancy, 191

Medical decision making as key E/M component, 43, 44, 47–49, 54, 55, 373

    factors in, 48

    four types of, 47

Medical history in health record, 9

Medical imaging report in health record, 11

Medical necessity, 326, 328–230

    in office visits, 378

Medical nutrition therapy, 280

Medical record. *See* Health record

Medicare Appeals Council, 340

Medicare appeals process, 340

Medicare audit, factors triggering, 378

Medicare carriers

    anesthesiology coverage by, 86

    appeals process of, 340

    certification number for lab on file for test coverage by, 241

    CMS-1500 form used for claims to. *See* CMS-1500 claim form

    durable medical equipment supplies reimbursed by, 285

    HCPCS Level II codes required for claims to, 294

    information on coding and payments from, 326

    National Codes used for, 294

    participating provider agreements with, 324

    point scales of, 51

    RBRVS used by, 321

    reduced reimbursement by, 93

    supplies and materials provided by physicians reported to, 282

    time increments recognized by, 91

    venipuncture coverage by, 241

Medicare Claims Processing Manual

    appeals process detailed in, 340

    Medicare surgical package defined in, 102

    NCCI edits concept in, 386

Medicare Integrity Program, 384

Medicare National Correct Coding Initiative (NCCI) edits. *See* National Correct Coding Initiative (NCCI) edits

Medicare Physician's Fee Schedule Database (Relative Value File), code status in, 294

Medicare Prescription Drug, Improvement, and Modernization Act of 2003 (MMA), 69

Medicare signature on file form, 8

Medicare summary notice, 361

Medicare surgical package, 102, 103

Medication administration. *See* J codes, HCPCS

Medication list required by Joint Commission in health record, 8

Medication therapy management services (MTMS), 283

Medicine section, 21, 144, 155, 190, 211, 259–286

    anatomical modifiers for, 284

    content and structure of, 260

    HCPCS codes for, 284–286

    modifiers for, 271, 275, 280, 283

Meninges of brain, diagram of, 197

Meniscectomies, 130

Metric measurement conversions, 110

Microbiology, 244

Minimal service history in E/M service level, 43

Minimum data set (MDS) included in RAI, 64

Missed abortion, 192

Missed charges

    definition of, 359–360

    sample, 344–345

    service distribution report to reveal, 352–355

Moderate (conscious) sedation, 282

    ⊙ symbol indicating code that includes, 17

    codes including, in appendix G of CPT code book, 20

Modifiers, 301–314
    claim form convention for separating
        codes from, 302
    index of, 311–313
    types of, 302–313
Modifiers, anatomical
    assigned to digits, list of, 107, 284
    for breast procedures, 118
    list of, 107
    for medicine, 284
    for radiology, 229
    for surgery (–LT and –RT), 107, 118
Modifiers, CPT, 302–309
    for ABN waiver, 249, 328, 330
    for anesthesia, 87–88, 95
    in CPT code book, appendix A, 19, 302
    to define service further, 337
    for E/M services, 52–53, 56, 59, 62, 71
    for genetic testing codes, 20
    for medicine, 267, 271, 273, 275, 276, 280,
        283
    for pathology and laboratory, 238, 240,
        242, 249–51
    for physician claims, 302–308, 325
    for radiology, 226–27, 228–229, 331
    for surgery, 105, 107, 111–112, 117,
        124, 127, 131, 132, 138, 141, 162,
        166–169, 170, 184, 186, 188–189,
        197, 200
Modifiers, CRNA, 87
Modifiers, HCPCS, 14, 309–310
    for anesthesia, 93
    component billing, 331
    Level II anesthesia, 89
    Level II E/M, 53, 93
    Level II radiologic, 229
    Level II technical component (–TC), 229,
        275, 284, 310, 331
    for medicine services, 280
    for radiology, 226, 228–229, 331
    for surgery, 191, 209
Modifiers list
    –AA, anesthesia services performed
        personally by anesthesiologist, 89, 93,
        309
    –AD, medical supervision by a physician:
        more than four concurrent anesthesia
        procedures, 89, 309
    –AI, principal physician of record, 309
    –AP, determination of refractive state not
        performed in the course of diagnostic
        ophthalmological examination, 283
    –AT, acute treatment, 283
    –E1–E4, eyelids, 107, 209, 311, 332
    –EJ, subsequent claims for defined course
        of treatment, 284

    –F1–F4, left hand digits, 107, 229, 284,
        311, 324
    –F5–F9, right hand digits, 107, 229, 284,
        311, 332
    –FA, left hand thumb, 107, 229, 284, 311,
        332
    –FP, service provided as part of Medicaid
        family planning program, 53
    –G6, ESRD patient, 284
    –G8, monitored anesthesia care (MAC)
        for deep complex, complicated, or
        markedly invasive surgical procedure,
        89, 94, 309
    –G9, monitored anesthesia care (MAC)
        for patient who has history of severe
        cardio-pulmonary condition, 89, 94,
        309
    –GA, waiver of liability statement on file,
        249, 309, 328, 330
    –GC, service performed in part by a
        resident under the direction of a
        teaching physician, 53, 93, 309
    –GE, service performed by a resident
        without the presence of a teaching
        physician under the primary care
        exception, 54, 309
    –GG, performance and payment of a
        screening mammogram and diagnostic
        mammogram on the same patient,
        same day, 309
    –GH, diagnostic mammogram converted
        from screening mammogram same day,
        229, 310
    –GT, via interactive audio and video
        telecommunication systems, 54
    –GX, notice of liability issued, voluntary
        under payer policy, 310, 328
    –GY, item or service statutorily excluded
        or does not meet the definition of any
        Medicare benefit, 310, 330
    –GZ, item or service expected to be
        denied as not reasonable and necessary,
        310, 330
    –LC/LCX, left circumflex artery, 269,
        305
    –LCA/LMCA, left main artery, 269
    –LAD, left anterior descending artery,
        269, 305
    –LT, left side, 107, 118, 229, 284, 310, 332
    –P1, normal healthy patient, 88, 309
    –P2, patient with mild systemic disease,
        88, 309
    –P3, patient with severe systemic disease,
        98, 309
    –P4, patient with severe system disease
        that is a constant threat to life, 88, 309

–P5, moribund patient who is not expected to survive without the operation, 88, 309

–P6, declared brain-dead patient whose organs are being removed for donor purposes, 88, 309

–Q5, service furnished by a substitute physician under a reciprocal billing arrangement, 54, 309

–Q6, service furnished by a locum tenens physician, 54, 309

–QK, medical direction of two, three, or four concurrent anesthesia procedures involving qualified individuals, 89, 93, 309

–QS, monitored anesthesia care service, 84, 94, 310

–QW, CLIA waived test, 241, 249, 309

–QX, CRNA service: with medical direction by a physician, 89, 93, 310

–QY, medical direction of one certified registered nurse anesthetist (CRNA) by an anesthesiologist, 89, 310

–QZ, CRNA service: without medical direction by a physician, 89, 93, 310

–RCA, right coronary artery, 269

–RI, ramus intermedius artery, 269

–RT, right side, 107, 118, 229, 284, 310, 332

–SA, nurse practitioner rendering service in collaboration with a physician, 310

–SB, nurse midwife, 310

–T1–T4, left foot digits, 107, 229, 284, 311, 332

–T5–T9, right foot digits, 107, 229, 284, 311, 332

–TA, left foot, great toe, 107, 229, 284, 311, 332

–TC, technical component, 229, 275, 284, 310, 331

–XE, separate encounter, 112, 163, 228

–XP, separate practitioner, 112, 163, 228

–XS, separate structure (or organ), 112, 163, 229

–XU, unusual non-overlapping service, 112, 163, 229

–1P, exclusion to performance measure, 15

–2P, exclusion to performance measure, 15

–3P, 15

–8P, 15

–22, increased procedural services, 88, 106, 167, 191, 221, 228, 248, 302–03, 335, 336

–23, unusual anesthesia, 89, 106, 303

–24, unrelated evaluation and management service by the same physician during a postoperative period, 52, 56, 59, 303

–25, significant, separately identifiable evaluation and management service by the same physician on the day of a procedure or other service, 52, 54, 56, 59, 61, 62, 69, 71, 185, 276, 280, 303, 332

–26, professional component, 106, 178, 228, 248, 271, 275, 283, 303–304, 331

–27, as being reserved for facility use only, 302

–32, mandated services, 53, 61, 248, 304

–33, preventive services, 304

–47, anesthesia by surgeon, 106, 185, 186, 304

–50, bilateral procedure, 106, 118, 138, 154, 171, 177, 180, 202, 209, 302, 304

–51, multiple procedures, 17, 20, 89, 105, 106, 118, 127, 131, 138, 149, 162, 168, 178, 180, 197, 200, 209, 211, 212, 272, 275, 283, 304

–52, reduced services, 106, 166, 185, 228, 248, 267, 283, 304, 335

–53, discontinued procedure, 89, 106, 164, 228, 248, 283, 305

–54, surgical care only, 106, 302, 305

–55, postoperative management only, 53, 106, 305

–56, preoperative management only, 53, 106, 305

–57, decision for surgery, 53, 56, 59, 61, 106, 305

–58, staged or related procedure or service by the same physician during the postoperative period, 105, 106, 111, 113, 180, 305, 332

–59, distinct procedural service, 87, 89, 95, 105, 106, 112, 154, 162, 228–229, 249, 283, 306, 332

–62, two surgeons, 106, 226, 306

–63, procedure performed on infants less than 4 kg, 20, 106, 306

–66, surgical team, 106, 226, 306

–73, discontinued outpatient hospital/ ambulatory surgery center (ASC) procedure prior to the administration of anesthesia, 228, 302

–74, discontinued outpatient hospital/ ambulatory surgery center (ASC) procedure after administration of anesthesia, 228, 302

–76, repeat procedure or service by same physician or other qualified health care professional, 105–106, 283, 307

–77, repeat procedure by another physician or other qualified health care professional, 105, 106, 283, 307

Modifiers list *(continued)*
  –78, unplanned return to the operating/ procedure room by the same physician or other qualified health care professional following initial procedure for a related procedure during the postoperative period, 106, 307, 332
  –79, unrelated procedure or service by the same physician during the postoperative period, 104, 105, 106, 307, 332
  –80, assistant surgeon, 106, 308
  –81, minimum assistant surgeon, 106, 308
  –82, assistant (when qualified resident surgeon not available), 106, 308
  –90, reference (outside) laboratory, 249, 308
  –91, repeat clinical diagnostic laboratory test, 243, 249, 308, 332
  –92, alternative laboratory platform testing, 249, 308
Modifiers, missing, 360
  example of, 350
Modifiers, physical status, 88, 91, 309
Monitored anesthesia care (MAC), 86, 94–95
Monitoring coding functions and errors, 381–383
Multiple codes, indented information for procedures requiring, 18
Multiple gestation, 191
Multiple surgical procedures, claims-generation guidelines for, 335
Multiple wound repairs, 112
Musculoskeletal system subsection of surgery, 124–133, 138
  common coding errors for, 382
  general codes for, 124
  HCPCS codes for, 131–133
  modifiers for, 127, 130
Myocutaneous flap, 116

N
Narcosynthesis, 263
Nasal polyps, 136. *See also* Polypectomies
National Codes, 293–296
  for intravenous drug and supplies furnished by physician, 295
  as Level II of HCPCS, 14
  process for assigning, 294
  required for Medicare claims, 294
  sections of, 294
  to specify radiopharmaceutical agent, 227
National Committee for Quality Assurance (NCQA), 3

standards for basic elements of health records set by, 3, 11
National Correct Coding Initiative (NCCI) edits
  in claims-processing systems of Medicare contractors, 386
  denial messages for application of, 333
  development of, 331–333
  tables of, 332
National Coverage Determinations (NCDs), 326, 328
National Physician Fee Schedule Relative Value File
  as electronic *Federal Register*, 321
  example of, 323
  status indicators in, 330
National provider identifier (NPI) of physician or provider for covered entities, 333
Nature of presenting problem as contributing E/M component, 43
Nebulizer treatment, 273
Needle core biopsies, 118
Negotiated fee schedule, 321
Neonatal critical care, 63, 72–74
Neonates, neonatal critical care for
  inpatient, 63, 72–74
  outpatient, 63, 72
Neoplasms, benign and malignant, 111
Nephrectomy, 178
  laparoscopic, 177
Nephrolithotomy to remove urinary stones, 177
Nerve conduction studies (NCS), 275
Nerve graft, 202
Nervous system subsection of surgery, 194–202
  modifier for, 197–198
Neurology and neuromuscular procedures, 275
  HCPCS codes for, 285
Neurolytic injections, 198
Neuroplasty, 202
Neurorrhaphy, 202
Neurostimulators, 198, 275
New and emerging technologies, Category III CPT codes for, 15–16
New patient defined for E/M services, 44
  for domiciliary, rest home, or custodial care services, 65
  for home services, 66
  for office or other outpatient services, 54–56
  for preventive medicine services, 68–70
New patient defined for ophthalmology, 265

Newborn care, 71–75

Newborn resuscitation services, 71

Noncovered service, assigning code for, 386

Non-face-to-face nonphysician services, 70–71, 220

Noninvasive vascular diagnostic studies, 272

Nonneurolytic injections, 201

Nonphysician services, billing, 22

Nose, 136–137

Nuclear medicine, 227–28
    applications of coding for, 227–228

Null zero (⊘) to designate non-add-on code exempt from using –51 modifier, 17

Number of diagnoses or management options for medical decision making, 47, 52

Numerical sequence, CPT codes not in, 20
    appendix N of CPT code book listing, 20
    symbol # indicating, 17

Nursing facilities, physician supervision of patients for, 64–65

Nursing facility services
    discharge services as, 64–65
    initial nursing facility care for, 64
    subsequent care using key components in, 64

Nursing facility setting for charges, 23

O

Observation area setting for charges, 23

Observation or inpatient care services (including admission and discharge services), 59–60

Observer to assist with conscious sedation, 282

Ocular adnexa, 208–9
    modifiers for, 208–209

Ocular implant, 208

Ocular prostheses, 267

Office of Inspector General (OIG)
    audit size recommendations by, 380
    audits and investigations by, 385
    compliance program guidance documents of, 386–387
    website of, 387

Office or other outpatient consultations, 61–62

Office or other outpatient services category, 54–56
    for established patient, 55–56
    modifiers for, 56
    for new patient, 55
    preventive medicine services distinguished from, 68–69

Office service report, 355
    sample of, 356

Office visit
    in addition to immunotherapy, 274
    level of, 27, 378

Omentectomy, 190

Online medical evaluation, 71, 281–282

On-site testing for pathological and laboratory section, 240

Oophorectomy (ovariectomy), 190

Open prostatectomy, 175–176

Operating microscope
    for eye and ocular adnexa, and auditory system procedures, 208
    for larynx procedures, 138–139
    in male genital system procedures, 183–184
    in neural repair, 202
    in posterior segment procedures, 208

Operation Restore Trust (ORT), 385

Operative report
    coding from, 28–29
    lesion measurement taken from, 110
    reviewed in assigning endoscopy/arthroscopy codes, 130–131
    reviewed in assigning flap codes, 116
    reviewed in assigning proctectomy codes, 167–168

Ophthalmology, 265–267

Ophthalmoscopy
    extended, with retinal drawing, 266–267
    ophthalmologic services erroneously reported as, 266–267

Optical endomicroscopy, 163

Orbital implant, 208

Orchiectomy, 183

Orchiopexy, 185
    with hernia repair, 170–171

Organ or disease-oriented panels, 242

Organ systems documented in physical examination, 9–10

Organizations and agencies directing health record content, 3

Osteopathic and chiropractic manipulative treatment, 280–281
    modifiers for, 281

Other evaluation and management services, 76

Other procedures for integumentary system, 116

Other services and procedures for medicine, 282–283

Outpatient hospital setting for charges, 23

Outpatient services, basic coding guidelines for, 30–33

Ovary, 190

Oviduct, 189

P

Pacemaker or pacing cardioverter-defibrillator, 144, 147
Pain management services, 96–97
Pap smears, 245–247
Participating provider agreements, 324
Past medical, family, and social history (PFSH) in history component of E/M service, 45
Pathology and laboratory section, 21, 239–251
   alphabetic index main terms for, 240
   guidelines for subsections of, 242–248
   HCPCS codes for, 249–250
   modifiers for, 238, 240, 244–245
   quantitative and qualitative studies for, 242
   structure and content of, 240–241
Patient contact, face-to-face, for prolonged services, 67
Patient record as audit tool, 379
Patient self-management, education and training for, 281
Patient transport, physician attendance during, 72
Payer remittance report, 338, 361–362
   coder and biller as team for, 363–364
   codes and code edits for, 362–363
   sample, 362
Payer-specific guidelines for procedures, supplies, and services, 277, 326, 328–332
Payers, primary and secondary, 335–336
PCI. See Percutaneous coronary interventions (PCI)
Pediatric critical care services
   initial, 73
   for patient transport, 63, 71–72
   subsequent, 73
Pedicle flap, 116, 197
Penis, 184–185
Per member, per month (PMPM) rate, 321
Percutaneous coronary interventions (PCI), 268–269
Percutaneous lysis of epidural adhesions, 198
Percutaneous transluminal coronary angioplasty (PTCA), 144, 267–268
Peritoneal dialysis, 264
Phacoemulsification, 207
Phacofragmentation, 207
Pharmacologic management, 263–264
Pharynx, adenoids, and tonsils, 166
Photochemotherapy, 279
Photodynamic therapy, 279

Physical examination in health record, body areas, organ systems, and diagnosis statement components of, 9–10
Physical medicine and rehabilitation, 279
Physical status modifiers for anesthesia, 88, 309
Physician office documentation
   differences between most health records and, 11
   documentation guidelines by AMA and CMS for, 40–41
   education about deficiencies in, 386
   identifying codable statements in, 34–35
Physician office laboratories (POLs), 241–242
Physician orders in health record, 10
Physician services, billing, 294–295
   modifiers for, 302–308, 332
Physician standby services requested by another physician, 67
Pinch graft, 114
Place of service charges, 22–24, 336
Place of service (POS) codes matched to service, 362
Plus symbol (+) to designate add-on codes, 17, 20, 105–106
Polypectomies, 189, 382. See also Nasal polyps
   performed through colonoscope, 164–165
   simple versus extensive, 136, 138
Polysomnographies, 275
Positron emission tomography (PET) imaging, 230
Posterior segment of eye, 208
Postoperative care included in global service, 103
Postpartum care, 190–191
Prenatal visits, outpatient, 33
Preoperative evaluations, sequencing, 33
Pressure (decubitus) ulcers, 117
Preventive medicine services, 68–70
Principal diagnosis, definition of, 30
Problem focused history in E/M service level, 43
Problem list
   for continuing ambulatory services, 8–9
   in problem-oriented medical record, 4
Problem-oriented medical record (POMR), 4–5
Procedural statements, identifying codable, 27–29
Proctectomy, 168
Proctosigmoidoscopy, 163
Professional services, billing, 295
   modifiers for, 302–308

Progress notes
    content of, 10
    in problem-oriented medical record, 4–5
    reviewed in assigning surgery codes, 102
Prolonged services, 66–67
Prostate, 185
    needle biopsy of, 185, 222
Provider identification numbers for
        physicians and nonphysicians, 24
Provider remittance advice (RA), 361
Psychiatric services, HCPCS codes for, 284
Psychiatry, 262–264
Psychotherapy, 263
    with E/M service codes, 263
Pulmonary services, HCPCS codes for, 286
Pulmonary subsection, 273
Pulse oximetry, 63, 273
Pyramid (▲) in CPT code book to designate
        revised terminology, 16–17

Q
Qualified independent contractor (QIC),
        reconsideration of Medicare appeals
        decision by, 340
Qualifying circumstances for anesthesia,
        90–92, 282
Qualitative analysis, reports for, 348, 351
    custom, 355–360
Quality and validation reviews, 41
Quality of coding, 371–387
    audit to analyze, 373–377
    tools for correcting and verifying,
        372–377
Quantitative analysis
    definition of, 348
    diagnosis distribution report for,
        351–352
    service distribution report for, 352–355
Quantitative and qualitative studies for
        pathology and laboratory, 242
Qui tam (whistleblower) actions for fraud and
        abuse, 385–386

R
Radiation oncology, 220, 224–227
    coding guidelines for, 226–227
    consultations and treatment planning for,
        225
    unlisted procedure codes for, 225
Radiation therapy. See Brachytherapy; See
        Teletherapy
Radiation treatment delivery, 225
    coding guidelines for, 226–227
Radiation treatment management, 225
    coding guidelines for, 226–227

Radiologic supervision and interpretation
        subsection, coding guidelines in, 222
Radiological supervision and interpretation
        for biopsies
    of breast, 118
    of lungs and pleura, 140
Radiology, interventional, 222–224
Radiology-only appointments, diagnosis for,
        29, 33
Radiology reports in health record, 11
Radiology section, 21, 219–231
    format and arrangement of, 220–228
    HCPCS codes for, 230–231
    modifiers for, 226–227, 228–229
    subsections of, 220
Radiopharmaceuticals
    provision of, 227
    used in brachytherapy, descriptions of, 227
Reason for accident or injury, 33
Reason for encounter/visit, 32
Reduction of fracture, 126
Reference lab testing for pathology and
        laboratory section, 240
Registered Health Information
        Administrators (RHIAs), 35
Registered Health Information Technicians
        (RHITs), 35
Registration record of demographic data, 6–7
Reimbursement
    modifiers for component billing and, 331
    optimizing, 2
    reduced Medicare or Medicaid, 93
Reimbursement guidelines, sources of, 318,
        328–332
Reimbursement process, 319–340
    claims in, 333–336, 337–340
    fee schedule management in, 324–325,
        336–337
    master list of services kept for, 336
    mechanisms for, 320–324
    payer-specific guidelines for, 326, 328–332
    sources of guidelines for, 326
Relative value file for physician fee schedule,
        322
    example of, 323
Relative Value Guide (ASA), 91
Relative value unit (RVU) data on service
        distribution reports, 355
Relative value units (RVUs) specific to CPT
        code, 337
Remark codes, Washington Publishing
        Company tables of, 363
Removal of hardware, 126
Removal of sutures, 116
Renal scans, 228

Renal transplantation, 178
Repairs
    of tendons, 127
    of wounds, 112–113
Reports and databases, coding and
    reimbursement, 347–364
Reproductive system procedures, 185
Resident assessment instrument (RAI), 64
Resident assessment protocols (RAPs), 64
Resource-based relative value system
    (RBRVS)
    applying fee for standard charge to, 320
    elements of formula to compute, 322
    as national fee scale for Medicare, 321
Resources to assign diagnostic and procedure
    codes, 12–14
Respiratory syncytial virus monoclonal
    antibodies, 260–261
Respiratory system subsection of surgery,
    136–141
    diagrams of, 137
    modifiers for, 136, 138, 139, 140
Retinal detachment, 207, 208
Retrograde pyelogram (ureteropyelography),
    176, 179
Revascularization code series, procedures
    included in, 154
Revenue production report, 324–325
    sample, 359
Review of systems (ROS) in history
    component of E/M service, 44–45
Rhinoplasties, secondary, 138
Risk of significant complications, morbidity,
    and/or mortality for medical decision
    making, 47
Rotational flap, 113
Rotator cuff repair, 131

S
Sample for audit, 380
Schedule of benefits, insurance, 320
Screening cytopathology, 249–250
Sedation, moderate (conscious), 282
    symbol indicating code that includes, 17
    codes including, in appendix G of CPT
        code book, 20
See cross-reference, use of in CPT code book
    index for other possible terms, 21
Semicolon (;) to designate common portion of
    indented portions for main entry, 17–19
Separate procedures in surgery section,
    104–105
Service distribution report, 352, 355
    comparative report for, 354
    sample of, showing problem areas, 353

Service-mix report, 357
    sample, 358
Service record for variety of physician
    services, sample blank, 26
Sigmoidoscopy, 163
Signatures
    for assignment of benefits form specific
        to Medicare (Medicare signature on
        file), 8
    for services during patient encounter at
        time of service, 12
Signs and symptoms
    chief complaint reflected in, 30
    codes describing, when to use, 31
Simple repair of wounds, 112
Single nerve conduction study, 275
Sinusotomy, 138
Skin and components, diagram of, 109
Skin grafts, 113–115
    extensive, 197
Skin layers, 109
Skin lesions. See Lesions, skin
Skin tags removal, 110
Skin traction, 127
Skull base surgery, 195–197
Skull, meninges, and brain, 195, 197
Sleep-testing codes, 275
SNOCAMP progress notes, 5
SOAP progress notes, 10
    in problem-oriented medical record, 5
Source-oriented health record, 4
Special dermatological procedures, 279
Special evaluation and management services
    category, 71
Special otorhinolaryngologic services, 267
Special services, procedures, and reports, 282
    HCPCS codes for, 285–286
Specimen, blood, 153, 240–241
Specimen slides, 245–247
Spectacles
    lenses for, 285
    prescription for, 266
Spermatic cord, 185
Spinal column, diagram of, 196
Spinal injections/infusions, 201
Spinal punctures and injections,
    documentation for, 198
Spine
    bone graft codes for, 127–128
    modifiers for, 127
Spine and spinal cord, 198–201
Spirometry tests, 273
Split-thickness skin graft, 114
Standard charges for medical services, 320
Standard fee, 336

Statistical summary in audit follow-up, 380–381
Stents
  ductal, 150
  indwelling, 180
  temporary ureteral, 180
Stereotaxis, 197–198
Stomach, 166
Strabismus surgery, 209
Submucous resection inferior turbinate, partial or complete, any method, 138
Subsequent hospital care, 22, 58, 63, 71
Subsequent nursing facility care, 64
Subterms in CPT code book index, 20, 29
Surgery, ambulatory. *See* Ambulatory surgery
Surgery center, same-day, as setting for charges, 23
Surgery section, 21, 101–211
  add-on codes in, 105–106
  common coding errors for, 382–383
  laparoscopic approach in, 105
  modifiers for, 105, 118, 130, 136, 138–139, 140, 162–163, 164–168, 171, 177–180, 202
  reporting more than one procedure or service in, 105
  separate procedures in, 104–105
  subsections of, 102. *See also* specific subsections
Surgical dressings, 119
Surgical package
  anesthesia types included in, 87, 102, 125
  Medicare, 103
  surgical procedures included in, 104
Surgical pathology, 247
Surgical procedures, multiple, 106, 335
Surgical services, documentation of, 22
Surgical tray for procedures of integumentary system, 119–120
Susceptibility testing, 244
Sutures, removal of, 116
  cerclage, 190
Swan-Ganz (pulmonary artery) catheters, 87
Symbols in CPT code book, 16–17, 294–295
Sympathectomy, 158

T
Table of drugs and associated testing codes for pathology and laboratory section, 244
TAVI codes. *See* Transcatheter aortic valve implantation (TAVI) codes
TAVR codes. *See* Transcatheter aortic valve replacement (TAVR) codes
Team conferences, 68

Technical component of service, –TC HCPCS modifier for, 229, 283–284
Telephone services by physician, 71, 281–282
Teletherapy for radiation oncology, 224–225
Temporary codes of HCPCS (G, H, K, Q, S, and T), 295–296
Temporary transcutaneous pacing, 63
Tendon repair, revision, and/or reconstruction, 127
Testis, 185
Therapeutic procedures, follow-up care for, 104
Therapeutic, prophylactic, or diagnostic injections and infusions, 276
Therapeutic services
  for cardiovascular subsection of medicine, 267–269
  sequencing, 32
Third-party payer policies, 61, 277
Thoracoscopy, diagnostic and surgical, 140
Thrombolysis, coronary, 270
Thyroid scans, 228
Time
  for anesthesia services, 91–92
  for cardiovascular monitoring, 270
  for care plan oversight services, 68
  as contributing E/M component, 43, 50–52
  for critical care services, 63
  for hydration services, 276
  for injections and infusions, 277–278
  for medical nutrition therapy, 280
  for patient transport, 63, 72
  for prolonged services, 66–67
  for psychiatric care provider, 263
Tongue and floor of mouth, 165
Tonsillectomy, 166
Trabeculectomy ab externo, 207
Trabeculoplasty using laser, 207
Trabeculotomy ab externo, 206
Tracer claim, 364
Trachea and bronchi, 139–140
Tracheostomy, 139
Traction, skeletal and skin, 126–127
Transaction and Code Sets (TCS), HIPAA, 333
Transcatheter aortic valve implantation (TAVI) codes, 148
Transcatheter aortic valve replacement (TAVR) codes, 148
Transluminal dilation of aqueous outflow canal, 207
Transport, coding time physician spends in attendance during patient, 63, 72
Transurethral cystoscopy with bladder/urethra biopsy, 177

Transurethral destruction of prostatic tissue by microwave and radiofrequency thermotherapy, 180
Triangle (▲) in CPT code book to designate revised terminology, 16–17, 294
Trigger point injections, 125–126
Trigger, release of, 382
Tubal ligation, 189
Tumor removal
    benign, 110
    soft tissue and bone, 124
Tympanostomy, 211
Type of service categorization, 337

U
Ultrasound
    B-scan, for abdominal aortic aneurysm scanning, 231
    diagnostic, 221–222, 230
    intravascular, 269
    obstetrical or pregnancy (abdominal), 222
    paranasal sinus, 230
Unbundling of code packages, 105, 220, 359, 384
Uniform Hospital Discharge Data Set (UHDDS), principal diagnosis defined in, 30
Unique physician identifier number (UPIN)
    lack of, as noncoding reason for denied claim, 363
    NPI as replacing, 333
Unique service identifier, 336
Unlisted procedure codes, 19
Upcoding, 378
Upper gastrointestinal endoscopies, 163
Ureter, 178
Ureteral stent
    insertion of, 179
    removal of, 180
Urethra, 180
Urethral pressure profile (UPP), 179
Urethral stricture or stenosis, 179
Urethroplasty, 180
Urethroscopy, 179
Urgent care visits setting for charges, 24
Urinary stones
    lithotripsy to destroy, 177
    nephrolithotomy in kidney to remove, 177
    surgical removal of, 178
Urinary stress incontinence, 177, 187
Urinary system subsection of surgery, 175–180
    common coding errors for, 383
    diagram of, 176
    laparoscopic codes for, 177

miscellaneous guidelines for, 176–177
    modifiers for, 178
Urodynamics subgrouping of urinary system, 176, 178–179
Uroflowmetry, 179
US Government Printing Office, National Codes available from, 294
Usual and customary (U/C) fee profile, 320–321
Uterine monitor, home, 192
Utilization guidelines included in RAIs, 64

V
V codes
    for circumstances other than disease or injury, 31
    for histories, 32
    for prenatal visits, 33
    for preoperative evaluations, 33
    for reason for encounter, 31
    for vision services, 285
Vaccines/toxoids
    assignment of codes during approval process for, 262
    immunization administration for, 261, 284
    products used in, 262
Vagina, 187
Vaginal birth after cesarean (VBAC) delivery, 191
Vas deferens, 185
Vascular access procedures, 63
Vascular family defined for interventional radiology, 223
Vascular injection procedures, 152, 156
Vascular order, 223
Venipuncture. See Blood draws (venipuncture)
Venous catheterizations, 152
Ventilation-perfusion (V/Q) scans, 228
Ventilator management, 63
Vertebral column (spine), 127–128
Vertebral corpectomy, arthrodesis, 201
Vertebral segment, single, diagram of, 199
Vertebra with spinal cord, diagram of, 199
Vestibular tests, 211
Vision services, HCPCS codes for, 285
Vitrectomy, 208
Voiding pressure studies, 179
Vulva, perineum, and introitus, 187
Vulvectomy, 187
V-Y plasty, 113

W
Waiver, ABN, 328
    modifiers for, 249, 328, 330
    sample, 329

Waiver, CLIA, 241
Washington Publishing Company
    publications, 334, 363
Websites
    AHA, 13
    AHIMA, 13
    AMA, 14
    CMS, 230, 242, 294, 296, 322, 328, 331,
        333–334, 354
    FDA, 241
    ICD-10, 13
    NCHS, 30
    OIG, 387
    Washington Publishing
        Company, 363
Weed, Lawrence L., POMR developed
    by, 4
Wire localization biopsies, 118

Workman's compensation payers,
    requirements of, 86
Work plan, OIG, 387
Wound exploration codes, 113
Wound repairs, 112–113, 382
W-plasty, 113

X
X-ray (radiology) reports in health record, 11
X-rays, 220–221
    included in critical care codes, 62
    transportation and setup of equipment for,
        230
Xenograft, 116

Y–Z
Zipped files, unzipping, 322
Z-plasty, 113